THE HYPERTROPHIED HEART

PROGRESS IN EXPERIMENTAL CARDIOLOGY

Edited by Naranjan S. Dhalla, Ph.D., M.D. (Hon.), D. Sc. (Hon.)

1. S. Mochizuki, N. Takeda, M. Nagano, N.S. Dhalla (eds.): *The Ischemic Heart*. 1998
   ISBN 0-7923-8105-X

2. N.S. Dhalla, P. Zahradka, I. Dixon, R. Beamish (eds.): *Angiotensin II Receptor Blockade: Physiological and Clinical Implications*. 1998.
   ISBN 0-7923-8147-5

3. N. Takeda, M. Nagano, N.S. Dhalla (eds.): *The Hypertrophied Heart*. 2000.
   ISBN 0-7923-7741-9

THE HYPERTROPHIED HEART

Edited by
NOBUAKIRA TAKEDA, M.D., Ph.D.
Associate Professor
Department of Internal Medicine
Aoto Hospital
Jikei University School of Medicine
Tokyo, Japan

MAKOTO NAGANO, M.D., Ph.D.
Professor Emeritus
Jikei University School of Medicine
Tokyo, Japan

NARANJAN S. DHALLA, Ph.D., M.D. (Hon.), D.Sc. (Hon.)
Distinguished Professor and Director
Institute of Cardiovascular Sciences
St. Boniface General Hospital Research Centre
Faculty of Medicine, University of Manitoba
Winnipeg, Canada

KLUWER ACADEMIC PUBLISHERS
BOSTON

Distributors for North, Central and South America:
Kluwer Academic Publishers
101 Philip Drive
Assinippi Park
Norwell, Massachusetts 02061 USA

Distributors for all other countries:
Kluwer Academic Publishers Group
Distribution Centre
Post Office Box 322
3300 AH Dordrecht, THE NETHERLANDS

Library of Congress Cataloging-in-Publication Data

The hypertrophied heart / editors, Nobuakira Takeda, Makoto Nagano, Naranjan S. Dhalla.
    p. ; cm.— (Progress in experimental cardiology ; 3)
    Selected papers from the International Conference on Cardiac Hypertrophy, held in
Tokyo, Japan. Oct. 8–10, 1998.
    Includes Index.
    ISBN 0-7923-7741-9 (alk. paper)
    1. Heart—Hypertrophy—Congresses. I. Takeda, Nobuakira. II. Nagano, Makoto, 1928–
III. Dhalla, Naranjan S. IV. International Conference on Cardiac Hypertrophy (1998 : Tokyo,
Japan) V. Series.
    [DNLM: 1. Heart Hypertrophy—physiopathology—Congresses. 2.
Heart—physiopathology—Congresses. WG 210 H998 2000]
    RC685.H9 H959 2000
    616.1′207—dc21
                                                  00-024807

Printed on acid-free paper.

Printer in the United States of America

CONTENTS

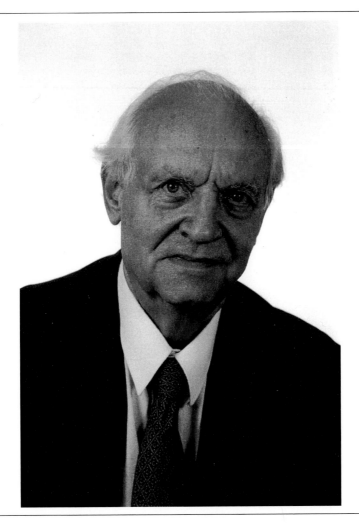

Ruthard Jacob, M.D.

This book is dedicated to Dr. Ruthard Jacob for his outstanding leadership in the field of cardiac physiology and biochemistry, with particular emphasis on cardiac hypertrophy. He promoted cardiovascular science as the Chief Editor of *Basic Research in Cardiology* and as Professor and Director of the Second Department of Physiology at Tübingen University, Tübingen, Germany. He is known for his kindness, compassion, and inspiration to numerous young investigators in the field of heart research.

Whenever the heart is challenged with an increased work load for a prolonged period, it responds by increasing its muscle mass—a phenomenon known as *cardiac hypertrophy*. Although cardiac hypertrophy is commonly seen under physiological conditions such as development and exercise, a wide variety of pathological situations such as hypertension (pressure overload), valvular defects (volume overload), myocardial infarction (muscle loss), and cardiomyopathy (muscle disease) are also known to result in cardiac hypertrophy. Various hormones such as catecholamines, thyroid hormones, angiotensin II, endothelin, and growth factors have also been shown to induce cardiac hypertrophy. Although the exact mechanisms underlying the physiological or pathological forms of cardiac hypertrophy are poorly understood, an increase in the intraventricular pressure is believed to represent the major stimulus for the development of cardiac hypertrophy. In this regard, stretching of the cardiac muscle has been shown to induce the hypertrophic response, but the role of metabolic influences in this process cannot be ruled out. Furthermore, different hormones and other interventions in the absence of stretch have been observed to stimulate protein synthesis in both isolated cardiomyocyte and vascular myocyte preparations. Nonetheless, it is becoming clear that receptor as well as phospholipid-linked signal transduction pathways are activated in some specific manner depending upon the initial hypertrophic stimulus, and these then result in an increase in the size and mass of cardiomyocytes.

Since the size and shape of the heart are altered in cardiac hypertrophy, the cardiomyocytes are considered to be remodeled. This remodeling of cardiomyocytes is not only due to changes in the extracellular matrix (particularly in the collagen content) but also has been shown to be associated with subcellular remodeling, whereas the molecular structure and composition of organelles such as sarcolemma, sarcoplasmic reticulum, myofibrils, and mitochondria are altered in the hypertrophied heart. Although cardiac hypertrophy at initial stages is compensatory in nature, the hypertrophied heart becomes the failing heart over a period of time if the hypertrophic stimulus is not removed. It has been suggested that oxidative stress and/or Ca^{2+}-handling abnormalities may play a crucial role in the transition of cardiac hypertrophy to heart failure; however, exact mechanisms in this process are not fully understood. Furthermore, the changes in different signal transduction pathways in the failing heart remain to be investigated in greater detail. Extensive studies at the level of gene transcription and gene translation need to be carried out in the failing heart for understanding the pathophysiology of heart dysfunction as well as for improving the therapy of heart failure. In particular, the relationship among changes in subcellular remodeling, myocardial metabolism, and molecular events in the hypertrophied nonfailing and failing hearts remains to be carefully defined.

In order to understand the molecular and cellular mechanisms for the genesis of cardiac hypertrophy as well as for the transition of cardiac hypertrophy to heart failure, the International Conference on Cardiac Hypertrophy was organized in Tokyo, Japan, from October 8–10, 1998. Those who attended the conference witnessed an extraordinary exchange of multidisciplinary information among basic scientists and clinical investigators in the field of cardiovascular medicine. The state-of-the-art presentations in the area of molecular biology, cellular physiology, and signal transduction in cardiac hypertrophy and heart failure helped the formulation of new concepts and new approaches for stimulating research. In this book, we have presented some selected papers to highlight the major issues and problems in the hypertrophied and failing hearts. These 37 chapters were organized in two sections, namely, (1) Mechanisms of Cardiac Hypertrophy and (2) Cardiac Failure in the Hypertrophied Heart. It is hoped that both students and scientists, as well as clinical and experimental cardiologists, will find this book useful in understanding the molecular and cellular events underlying the development of cardiac hypertrophy, as well as the transition of cardiac hypertrophy to heart failure.

Nobuakira Takeda, Tokyo, Japan
Makoto Nagano, Tokyo, Japan
Naranjan S. Dhalla, Winnipeg, Canada

ACKNOWLEDGMENTS

This book contains invited chapters that are based on the selected symposia program for the International Conference on Cardiac Hypertrophy held in Tokyo, Japan, from October 8–10, 1998. We are indebted to Ms. Susan Zettler for her help in the preparation of this book. We are also grateful to Mr. Zachary Rolnik, Ms. Melissa Ramondetta, Ms. Laura Walsh, and the editorial staff at Kluwer Academic Publishers for their interest in assembling this volume. In addition, we wish to extend special thanks to the following institutions for their sponsorship and corporations for their generous contributions in support of the International Conference on Cardiac Hypertrophy:

A. INSTITUTIONS
Japan Heart Foundation
Japanese Circulation Society
International Academy of Cardiovascular Sciences
International Society for Heart Research
World Heart Federation

B. CORPORATIONS
Uehara Memorial Foundation
Astra Japan Co. Ltd.
Banyu Pharmaceutical Co. Ltd.
Bayer Pharmaceutical Co. Ltd.
Chugai Pharmaceutical Co. Ltd.
Daiichi Pharmaceutical Co. Ltd.
Dainippon Pharmaceutical Co. Ltd.
Eisai Co. Ltd.
Fujisawa Pharmaceutical Co. Ltd.
Hoechst Marion Roussel Co. Ltd.
Kowa Co. Ltd.
Kyowa Hakkou Kogyo Co. Ltd.
Mitsubishi Tokyo Pharmaceutical Co. Ltd.
Nippon Boehringer Ingelheim Co. Ltd.
Nippon Shinyaku Co. Ltd.
Novartis Pharma Co. Ltd.
One Pharmaceutical Co. Ltd.

Otsuka Pharmaceutical Co. Ltd.
Sankyo Co. Ltd.
Shionogi Co. Ltd.
Sumitomo Pharmaceutical Co. Ltd.
Takeda Chemical Industries Co. Ltd.
Tanabe Pharmaceutical Co. Ltd.
Toa Eiyo Co. Ltd.
Yamanouchi Pharmaceutical Co. Ltd.
Yoshitomi Pharmaceutical Co. Ltd.

A. MECHANISMS OF CARDIAC HYPERTROPHY

N. Takeda, M. Nagano and N.S. Dhalla
(eds). The Hypertrophied Heart. Copyright
© 2000. pp. 3–16. Kluwer Academic
Publishers. Boston. All rights reserved.

SIGNAL TRANSDUCTION IN THE ADAPTED HEART: IMPLICATION OF PROTEIN KINASE C-DEPENDENT AND -INDEPENDENT PATHWAYS

JOHN DEBARROS and **DIPAK K. DAS**

Department of Surgery, University of Connecticut School of Medicine, Farmington, Connecticut 06032, USA

Summary. Cardioprotection as a result of myocardial adaptation to cellular stress is a product of evolution. Myocardial adaptation potentiates intracellular signaling involving diverse signal transduction pathways. Ischemic preconditioning, a specific form of myocardial adaptive response, occurs through both G proteins and receptor tyrosine kinase. Such preconditioning, mediated by cyclic episodes of brief reversible ischemia each followed by another brief period of reperfusion, leads to improvement in infarct size and ventricular recovery. Adaptation can also be achieved through other environmental stresses, including oxidative stress. Several triggers for signal transduction have been identified, including catecholamines, bradykinin, and adenosine. The processing of stress signals from signal initiation to propagation to eventual termination is the focus of this chapter. Signal initiation occurs through G-protein as well as receptor tyrosine kinase activation. Complex signaling processes involving MAP kinases, MAPKAP kinase 2, and protein kinase C have become central to our understanding of signal propagation. Signal termination resulting in biological expression of signal propagation by means of gene expression and transcription regulation is the ultimate outcome of cellular stress response. This chapter especially examines these complex signal transduction processes that lead to the stress response and eventual adaptation, focusing primarily upon protein kinase C-dependent and -independent pathways.

INTRODUCTION

Clinicians and basic scientists since the modern understanding of cardiac physiology have been concerned with the problems associated with myocardial preservation. With the advent of coronary artery angioplasty and recent developments in cardiac surgery such as coronary artery bypass grafting, fantastic leaps in myocardial preservation have been accomplished. However, myocardial ischemia and subsequent reperfusion injury remain an unsolved problem, despite a great deal of research to understand the mechanisms of reperfusion injury. Conventional techniques for myocardial protection have focused on extracellular interventions or invasive procedures. The recent decade has witnessed increasing interest and breakthroughs in the understanding of the cardiomyocyte's own inherent ability for self-preservation. To this end, in the past decade several researchers have been studying the concept of myocardial preservation based on myocytes' endogenous cellular defense mechanism, which allows the cell to manufacture proteins to aid in its ongoing struggle for self-preservation. Several investigators have demonstrated that cyclic episodes of short durations of ischemia and reperfusion can delay the onset of further irreversible injury and even improve postischemic ventricular dysfunction and arrhythmias [1–22]. Since the findings that repeated episodes of short-term reversible ischemia could improve myocardial function and reduce the incidence of ventricular arrhythmias, the concept of myocardial adaptation has become a focal point of efforts to understand endogenous cellular protection. This chapter will examine the evolution of the signal transduction pathway triggered by ischemic preconditioning.

ISCHEMIC PRECONDITIONING

In the early 1980's, several researchers noted that brief periods of reversible ischemia led to an improvement in expected infarct size and ventricular function [1–10]. These small periods of ischemia protected the myocyte by making it resistant to further damage when later subjected to longer periods of ischemia. This adaptive mechanism came to be known as ischemic preconditioning (IP). Although the exact mechanism remains controversial, a number of hypotheses have been investigated as to the etiology of this stress adaptation. Most believe that the protection afforded by IP lies in the complex mechanisms of cell signaling and subsequent induction of gene expression. The possibility of interorgan protection was recently addressed by McClanahan et al., who demonstrated in rabbits that brief renal artery occlusion followed by reperfusion preceding a 45 minute coronary artery occlusion reduced infarct size [23]. This finding adds another layer to the mechanism of IP: not only is intracellular signaling important but also we must consider the vast array of events related to the intercellular signaling cascade.

TRIGGERS FOR SIGNAL TRANSDUCTION

Some of the initial hypotheses implicated adenosine as a likely suspect in initiating preconditioning. Adenosine is formed from the breakdown of adenosine triphosphate (ATP). Under normal aerobic conditions, ATP is hydrolyzed to adenosine diphosphate (ADP) and then, utilizing the cell's capacity for aerobic metabolism, ADP is converted rapidly to ATP again. Under ischemic conditions, however, ADP is hydrolyzed to adenosine monophosphate (IMP) and adenosine [24]. Adenosine in turn is rapidly metabolized into inosine. Both inosine and IMP are then further metabolized to hypoxanthine, which is then metabolized further to xanthine and uric acid. It is during the hypoxic conditions that adenosine accumulates in the interstitial space. In 1991, Liu et al. observed that through the use of adenosine agonists and antagonists, myocardial infarct size could be modulated [13]. Although there is general agreement that adenosine does have cardioprotective effects, the question of whether adenosine functions as the trigger for ischemic preconditioning remains controversial because of adenosine's extremely short life. Nevertheless, a small amount of adenosine may trigger the activation of G proteins located within the plasma membrane of the cell, which in turn could open ATP-sensitive potassium channels (K-ATP) [13,25,26]. In 1993, Lawson et al., however, called the G-protein theory into question when their study failed to demonstrate that pertussis toxin could influence the proarrhythmic effects by preconditioning [27].

Subsequently, many other triggers for ischemic preconditioning became apparent. For example, the angiotensin II receptor antagonist EXP 3174 was found to reduce the infarct size to an extant comparable with enalaprilat and to augment preconditioning in the pig heart [28]. In another study, activation of AT_1 receptors by angiotensin II produced locally in the heart contributed to the limitation of infarct size by preconditioning [29,30]. Angiotensin-converting enzyme inhibitors was shown to augment ischemic preconditioning through bradykinin B_2-receptor activation [31]. Consistent with these results, selective blockade of AT_1 angiotensin II receptors was found to abolish ischemic preconditioning in isolated rabbit hearts [30]. A direct effect of bradykinin has also been implicated in the pathophysiology of ischemic preconditioning. In a recent study, bradykinin was found to play an essential role in classical preconditioning [32]. In another study, bradykinin could mediate ischemic preconditioning against free-radical injury in guinea pig isolated heart [33]. In another related study, preconditioning protected the endothelial function in coronary resistance arteries of the rat by activating bradykinin B1 receptors.

PROCESSING OF SIGNALS

Once a physiological signal is generated, it must be processed using a cascade of signaling elements before it can exert its biological effects. Generally, extracellular signals are transmitted into the cells through a receptor-mediated process.

SIGNAL INITIATION

G Proteins

Guanine nucleotide-binding regulatory proteins (G proteins) play a major role in the regulation of a variety of physiological processes, including modulation of adenylate cyclase activity and gating of ion channels [34,35]. Myocardial ischemia and reperfusion induce the changes in receptor G-protein signal transduction system in the heart [36]. Among the three types of G proteins, Gi and Gs proteins readily loses their functional activity during ischemia [37]. Based on the findings that pertussis toxin, a Gi-protein blocker, greatly attenuated the cardioprotective effects of preconditioning, Gi protein is believed to play a role in ischemic preconditioning [38]. Consistent with this report, Niroomand et al. demonstrated that although during the first 5 minutes of ischemia the function of Gi protein was significantly reduced, during a following 15 minute period of reperfusion, this decreased responsiveness was completely reversed, exceeding control activities [39]. This finding suggests that the underlying mechanism of ischemic preconditioning is the increased responsiveness of Gi proteins after a brief period of ischemia and reperfusion. In contrast, Fu et al. could not find any changes in Gs proteins and the activity of adenylate cyclase in the preconditioned myocardium [40]. Another study from Lawson et al. also did not find any role of G proteins in ischemic preconditioning [27].

Receptor tyrosine kinase

Protein phosphorylation plays a crucial role in a wide variety of cellular processes that control signal transduction. Protein phosphorylation is a rapidly reversible process that regulates the intracellular signaling in response to a specific stress, e.g., environmental changes. Protein phosphorylation is mediated by a number of protein kinases that can be grouped into two major classes: (1) those that phosphorylate serine/threonine residues, e.g., protein kinase A, protein kinase C (PKC), and casein kinases; and (2) those that phosphorylate proteins on their tyrosine residues, e.g., tyrosine kinases. Tyrosine kinases can activate a number of different intracellular signaling pathways, including tyrosine phosphorylation in the case of phospholipase C (PLC) and phospholipase D (PLD). Conformational changes are induced by binding of the SH2 domain to phosphotyrosine for P13 kinases as well as by translocation to the plasma membrane for stimulation of Ras guanine nucleotide exchange by Sos [41,42]. Protein tyrosine kinase is triggered when a ligand produced from a stimulus binds the tyrosine kinase receptor on the cell surface. Such interaction induces a conformational change in the tyrosine kinase receptor–ligand complex. The dimerization leads to intermolecular autophosphorylation followed by transphosphorylation. This step, which seems to be crucial, then leads to cytosolic substrate phosphorylation. Through complex interactions, the autophosphorylated substrate recruits other substrates having affinity for the receptor. Signaling by activated tyrosine kinase receptor protein is initiated by the phosphorylation of cytoplasmic proteins, which in turn potentiate the intracellular signaling cascade. In a sense, tyrosine kinase signal production is dependent on tyrosine kinase activity.

In a recent study, a link between tyrosine and PLD was established as a potential pathway for ischemic preconditioning [43–45]. PLD plays an important role in the intracellular signaling process. In 1996, Cohen et al. demonstrated that PLD is critical in ischemic preconditioning [46]. Other investigators documented activation of PLD in preconditioned hearts. PLD was also documented in ischemic reperfused hearts [47] through the use of analogues that potentiated PLD activity and was also shown to be beneficial to the effects of preconditioning antagonists that blocked this effect. PLD catalyzes the terminal diester bond of phosphatidylcholine, which results in the formation of choline and phosphatidic acid [48]. Phosphatidic acid then serves as the substrate for diacylglycerol synthesis by the action of phosphatidic acid on phosphohydrolase. Diacyl glycerol may itself serve as a second messenger by activating PKC [49]. Work done by Eskildsen-Helmond et al. suggests a link between preconditioning and activation of PLD, eventually resulting in the potentiation of PKC isoenzymes [50]. In a more recent study, Fryer et al. demonstrated that pretreatment with tyrosine kinase inhibitors partially attenuated ischemic preconditioning in the rat heart [51].

SIGNAL TRANSMISSION

Protein kinase C

As mentioned earlier, it has been demonstrated that cellular PKC activation is an important step in the mechanism of adaptive protection of the heart [6,52]. The PKC hypothesis received further support from observations that any agent that can activate PKC can also precondition the heart. For example, phenylephrine, an α_1-agonist; angiotensin AT_1; and bradykinin B_2-receptors can activate PKC [8,53] and can also precondition the hearts when infused prior to ischemia [11,13,14,54,55].

A variety of stress signals have been found to translocate and activate PKC. For example, mechanical stress induced by stretching can activate PKC in cultured myocytes [56]. Immediately after stretching, activation of phosphatidyl inositol turnover was observed, suggesting a role of PLC in PKC activation. Even a short-term ischemia or ischemia followed by a reperfusion was previously shown to translocate and activate PKC [3]. Furthermore, both α_1-receptor stimulation and Ca^{2+} ion can translocate and activate PKC [4,5]. Given the fact that both α_1-receptor activation and intracellular Ca^{2+} overloading are the manifestations of ischemia reperfusion injury, it was not surprising when ischemic preconditioning consisting of repeated ischemia and reperfusion was also found to translocate and activate PKC.

MITOGEN-ACTIVATED PROTEIN KINASES

The mitogen-activated protein kinases (MAPKs), a serine/threonine protein kinase family, play an essential role in mediating intracellular signal transduction events [41,57]. In response to extracellular stimulation, MAPKs are rapidly activated and in turn regulate cellular functions by inducing the phosphorylation of proteins, such as an oncogene product c-jun, S6 ribosomal protein kinase, and MAPK-activated protein kinase [17,58]. MAPKAP kinase 2 has been implicated in a novel mammalian stress-activated signal transduction pathway initiated by a variety of mitogens, proinflammatory cytokines, or environmental stresses, where it regulates its substrate molecules by serine/threonine phosphorylation [42,59]. Stimulation of cultured cardiomyocytes with α_1-selective adrenergic analogues, endothelin-1, fibroblast growth factors, and mechanical stress activates MAPK signaling cascade [60]. In the case of the rat heart, a mitogen-activated protein kinase cascade has already been identified by Lazov et al. [61]. These authors have demonstrated that the MAPK isoforms p42MAPK and p44MAPK and two peaks of MEK were activated by more than 10-fold in perfused hearts or in ventricular myocytes exposed to PMA for 5 minutes. In our study, we identified the participation of MAPK cascades in the ischemic preconditioning of rat hearts [62]. The results of our study demonstrated that a kinase cascade involving tyrosine kinase–PLD–MAPKs–MAPKAP kinase 2 is triggered after ischemic stress.

In a recent study, MAPK activation was found to be essential during the bombesin-induced, PKC-mediated sustained contraction in smooth muscle cells, and the redistribution of MAPKs were colocalized with the redistribution of HSP-27 in smooth muscle cells [63]. In view of the evidence that the HSP-27 gene is induced after ischemic preconditioning [1,64,65], it seems likely that MAPKs are involved in signal transduction leading to this gene expression. Indeed, in another related study, activation of cardiac gene expression during phenylephrine-induced hypertrophy seemed to require ERK activation [66].

Recently, a new member of the MAPK family, namely, p38MAPK, has been identified [67]. This MAPK seems to possess a dual phosophorylation motif: Thr-Gly-Tyr in place of the Thr-Pro-Tyr motif present in Jnk and in place of the Thr-Glu-Tyr modtif present in Erk. A recent study from our laboratory has demonstrated that p38MAPK is translocated and activated after ischemic preconditioning. Additionally, a inhibitor of p38MAPK blocked the effects of ischemic preconditioning.

The MAPK signal transduction pathway is likely to involve activation of Ras and Raf-1, which in turn induces mitogen-activated protein kinase kinase (MKK) and MAPKs. It is also known that Raf-1 kinases possess MAPKKK activity and lie upstream from MAPKK and MAPKs in various cell types [68,69]. Hypoxia and hypoxia/reoxygenation activated raf-1, MKK, and MAPKs in cultured rat cardiomyocytes [70]. Raf-1 operates downstream from cell surface-associated tyrosine kinases and upstream from MAPKs. Raf is not strictly a member of the MEKK family, but it is functionally analogous. Ras is part of the signal transduction chain extending from extracellular signals to transcriptional regulation in the nucleus. Upon activation, tyrosine kinase recruits a number of proteins, including RAS-specific guanine nucleotide-releasing proteins, which then regulate the binding of Ras with GTP, thereby potentiating the Ras signal. Ras proteins then interact with Raf kinases to induce downstream signals that activate MAPKs and other protein kinases. Once Raf is activated, then Ras is no longer required. The precise mechanism by which Ras controls Raf-1 is poorly understood. The binding of Raf-1 to Ras is largely GTP dependent and requires the effector region of Ras and the regulatory region of Raf-1.

MAPKAP kinase 2

Evidence suggests that MAPKAP kinase 2 is a crucial step leading to gene expression and myocyte adaptation, resulting in adaptive cardioprotection. This unique protein kinase is highly expressed in heart muscle, suggesting that it also may be expressed and functioning in the myocardium in response to stress. MAPKAP kinase 2 also has been shown to have increased activity when subjected to oxidative stress as well as heat shock [62,71]. This increased activity of MAPKAP kinase 2 in association with heat shock protein gives rise to the hypothesis that this kinase may be one of the critical factors involved with ultimate transcription of proteins, leading to adaptive protection of the heart. In cultured myocytes, the activity of MAPKAP kinase 2 was found to increase when the myocytes were subjected to oxidative stress as well as heat shock [64,78]. Heat shock proteins (HSPs) are early targets of phosphorylation by a variety of stress conditions [72–74]. HSP-27, HSP-32, and HSP-70 can be induced by oxidative stress and ischemic preconditioning [35,75,76]. Not only have heat shock proteins been found to be cardioprotective through reduction

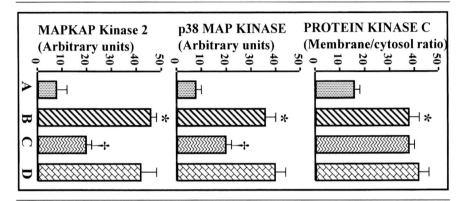

Figure 1. Effects of ischemic preconditioning, DMTU, a hydroxyl radical scavenger, and SN50 peptide, a NFkB blocker, on the activities of PKC, p38MAPK, and MAPKAP kinase 2 in heart. Results are expressed as means ± SEM of six animals per group. Each experiment was run in duplicate. $*p < 0.05$ compared to preconditioned group (**A**) control; (**B**) preconditioned; (**C**) DMTU; (**D**) SN50. Data reproduced with permission from Mol Cell Biochem 1999.

of infarct size but also evidence suggests that they important in delayed protection against infarction—the so-called "second window" of protection.

The precise physiological role of MAPKAP kinase 2 remains unknown; however, this kinase has been implicated as a downstream protein of the stress-activated protein kinase cascade. And as previously mentioned, MAPKAP kinase 2 has been shown to activate HSP directly in response to stress, suggesting its important role in myocardial adaptation and ultimate preservation.

In a recent study, we detected enzymatic activity in in vitro kinase assay by using MBP as a substrate resulted from the activation of the tissue Erk and/or p38MAPKs. In in vitro studies, both Erk and p38MAPK can phosphorylate and activate MAPKAP kinase 2 [74,77]. Another study demonstrated that p38MAPKs not ERK MAPK, lead to the activation of MAPKAP kinase 2 in vivo [78].

SIGNAL TRANSDUCTION BY PKC-DEPENDENT AND PKC-INDEPENDENT PATHWAYS

A recent study from our laboratory demonstrated the inhibition of enhanced tyrosine kinase phosphorylation during ischemic adaptation by DMTU [79]. DMTU also inhibited preconditioning-mediated increased phosphorylation of p38MAPK and MAPKAP kinase 2 activity. However, DMTU had no effect on the translation and activation of protein kinase C (PKC) resulting from preconditioning (figure 1). Preconditioning reduced myocardial infarct size as expected. This cardioprotective effect of preconditioning was abolished by both DMTU and SN50. Preconditioning resulted in the nuclear translocation and activation of NFkB. Increased NFkB binding was blocked by both DMTU and SN50. The results of this study demonstrate that reactive oxygen species play a crucial role in signal transduction medi-

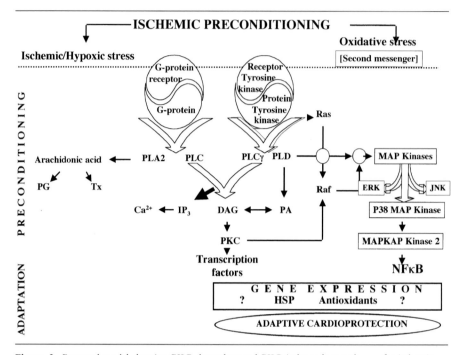

Figure 2. Proposed model showing PKC-dependent and PKC-independent pathways for ischemic preconditioning of heart.

ated by preconditioning. This signaling process appears to be potentiated by tyrosine kinase phosphorylation, resulting in the activation of p38MAPK and MAPKAP kinase 2, which in turn leads to the activation of NFκB. This process suggests a role of oxygen free radicals as second messenger. Free-radical signaling seems to be independent of PKC, although PKC is activated during the preconditioning process, which suggests a role for two separate signaling pathways in ischemic preconditioning (figure 2).

TERMINATION OF SIGNALS: GENE EXPRESSION AND TRANSCRIPTION REGULATION

The signal transduction potentiated by G-protein or tyrosine kinase receptor and propagated by multiple kinases is terminated by the induction of the expression of genes. Activation by diacylglycerol PKC and MAPKAP kinase 2 is likely to induce expression of a variety of genes, presumably at the transcription level. The synthesis of stress proteins such as oxidative stress and heat shock proteins, as well as those genes that are related to growth factors, appears to be regulated at the same transcriptional level [80]. Some proto-oncogenes, such as c-fos and c-myc, are also potential targets of PKC action. Constitutively expressed Ras or Raf-1 can not only mimic the action of α-receptor signaling but also regulate the action of multiple

kinases [81]. The current hypothesis is that genes such as ras, raf, src, and mos trans-
form cells by prolonging the activated stage of MAPKs and of components downstream in the signaling pathway [82].

Alteration in the expression patterns of many "early response" genes have been
reported to be expressed in mammalian systems in response to environmental stress.
These genes include c-fos, egr-1, c-jun, and c-myc, which encode transcription
factors and thus have the power to further modulate gene expression [83,84]. Most
proto-oncogenes are involved in the transcription regulation of a variety of genes,
including the stress-inducible genes. The proto-oncogene c-fos is known to be
expressed under any kind of stress that leads to the alteration of the redox state
within the system [85]. It has also been shown that a transient accumulation of c-
fos and c-myc mRNAs occurs in response to hemodynamic overload [86]. We and
others have shown that a number of proto-oncogenes, including c-fos and c-myc,
are rapidly induced in the preconditioned myocardium [21]. Such induction
increases with the number of preconditioning cycle, i.e., the induction of c-fos and
c-myc in the heart is greatly enhanced after four cycles of ischemia and reperfusion compared to the induction found after only one cycle of ischemia and reperfusion [73]. A recent study from our laboratory documented an induction of bcl-2
in the ischemically adapted rat myocardium [87]. Interestingly, bcl-2 was found to
be downregulated after ischemia and reperfusion [34,87].

Both ischemia/reperfusion and ischemic adaptation result in the induction of the
expression of several HSPs, including HSP-27, HSP-32, HSP-70, and HSP-89, as
well as oxidative stress-inducible genes such as genes for SOD and catalase
[21,62,73]. After heat shock, HSP is rapidly phosphorylated, and its synthesis is then
enhanced. Such enhancement not only makes the cells resistant to subsequent heat
stress but also makes them more resistant to oxidative stress. Using subtractive
hybridization and differential display techniques, our laboratory has also documented
the expression of several mitochondrial genes after ischemia and reperfusion, indicating a sequential upregulation of energy metabolism genes induced by ischemia
[1,64].

The nuclear transcription factor, NFκB, was found to play a role in the signaling process. We recently demonstrated nuclear translocation and activation of NFκB
in response to preconditioning [34,87]. Increased binding of NFκB was found to
be dependent on both tyrosine knase and p38MAPK. NFκB is a member of the
Rel transcription factory family, which is involved in the regulation of stress-defense
mechanisms. Since ischemic adaptation was also found to reduce apoptosis, we speculated a direct role of NFkB in apoptosis. AP-1 is another redox-sensitive signaling
molecule that also plays an important regulatory role in cellular responses to stress
induced by external factors, including UV radiation, phorbol esters, and TNFα [88].
The binding site of AP-1 is recognized by Jun family-member homodimers and
Jun/Fox family-member heterodimers. The balance between Jun and Fos is very
critical for gene expression. Induction of apoptosis by elevated level of c-Jun is a
crucial event in growth factor-deprived nerve cells. Stress induced by
ischemia/reperfusion was previously shown to induce the activation of c-Jun [10].

A recent study from our laboratory revealed significant upregulation of AP-1 in the ischemic reperfused myocardium. Ischemic preconditioning decreased such upregulation almost to the baseline level [87].

CONCLUSIONS

Throughout evolution, adaptation has been the result of genotypic heredity, mutation, and natural selection. This essential scientific dogma has come to be the mainstay of medicine. As a result of environmental stresses, selective expression of genes has resulted in the adaptation and survival of a particular organism. The heart is no exception. Environmental stresses can result in adaptation of cell death, depending on the severity of the stress. Long-term myocardial hypoxia may lead to various changes in myocardial subcellular organelles as an adaptation to ischemic conditions. Takeda et al. studied adaptive changes in two myosin isoenzymes and found small but definite adaptive changes, possibly due to long-term ischemia [89]. *Short-term* can be subdivided into *immediate* and *delayed*. Hypoxic bursts of 5 to 10 minutes duration followed by reperfusion "ischemic preconditioning" can lead to both an immediate and delayed response. The immediate response, discussed previously, leads to the production of intracellular second messengers that can help the myocyte to adapt to stress.

Ischemic preconditioning is the manifestation of the earlier stress response that occurs during repeated episodes of brief ischemia and reperfusion, and it can render the myocardium more tolerant to a subsequent potential lethal ischemic injury. This transient adaptive response has been demonstrated to be associated with decreased reperfusion-induced arrhythmias, increased recovery of postischemic contractile functions, and reduction of infarct size. The adaptive protection is believed to be mediated by gene expression and transcriptional regulation. Recent findings indicate that multiple kinases, including MAPKs and MAPKAP kinase 2, are likely to be involved in the adaptive signaling process. The acutely developing adaptive effect is short-lived, lasting for only up to 2 to 3 hours. Hearts can subsequently undergo a secondary and delayed adaptation to stress, presumably through the induction of the expression of new genes and their subsequent translation into proteins. A number of genes and proteins have been identified as possibly involved in the development of delayed preconditioning, including heat shock proteins (HSPs), superoxide dismutase (SOD), catalase nitric oxide synthase, and ATPase 6 and cytochrome b subunits [90]. Such an adaptive response becomes evident only after approximately 24 hours of stress treatment and may include stress induced by heat shock, oxidants, and other stress-inducible agents. MAPKAP kinase 2 and PKC appear to link the early preconditioning effect to the delayed adaptive response [41].

The results of our study indicate that preconditioning can be achieved by PKC-dependent as well as PKC-independent pathways [91]. It appears that preconditioning reduces cellular injury in two ways: (1) by decreasing ischemic/reperfusion injury; and (2) by decreasing oxidative injury. Based on our recent results, we speculate that preconditioning ameliorates the ischemic component of injury via a PKC-dependent mechanism, while the free-radical component of injury is reduced via a

PKC-independent mechanism. Both signal transduction pathways appear to involve MAPKs. As mentioned previously, the MAPK cascade plays an essential role in intracellular signal transduction. MAPKs and tyrosine kinase appear to function as integral messengers in cardiomyocyte adaptation by triggering gene expression, resulting in adaptive cardioprotection.

REFERENCES

1. Das DK, Moraru II, Maulik N, Engelman, RM. 1994. Gene expression during myocardial adaptation to ischemia and reperfusion injury. Ann NY Acad Sci 723:292–307.
2. Das, DK. 1993. Ischemic preconditioning and myocardial adaptation to ischemia. Cardiovasc Res 27:2077–2079.
3. Prasad MR, Jones RM. 1992. Enhanced membrane protein kinase C activity in myocardial ischemia. Basic Res Cardiol 87:19–26.
4. Henrich CJ, Simpson PC. 1988. Differential acute and chronic response to protein kinase C in cultured neonatal rat heart myocytes to alphal-adrenergic and phorbol ester stimulation. J Mol Cell Cardiol 20:1081–1085.
5. Fearon CW, Tashjian AH. 1985. Thyrotropin-releasing hormone induces redistribution of protein kinase C in GH4C1 rat pituitary cells. J Biol Chem 260:8366–8371.
6. Ytrehus K, Liu Y, Downey JM. 1994. Preconditioning protects ischemic rabbit heart by protein kinase C activation. Am J Physiol 266:H1145–H1152.
7. Mitchell MB, Meng X, Brown J, Harken AH, Banerjee A. 1995. Preconditioning of isolated rat heart is mediated by protein kinase C. Circ Res 76:73–81.
8. Nishizuka Y. 1986. Studies and perspectives of protein Kinase C. Science 233:305–312.
9. Maulik N, Sharma HS, Das DM. 1996. Induction of the haem oxygenase gene expression during the reperfusion of ischemic rat myocardium. J Mol Cell Cardiol 28:1261–1270.
10. Das DK, Maulik N, Moraru II. 1995. Gene expression in acute myocardial stress. Induction by hypoxia, ischemia, reperfusion, hyperthermia, oxidative stress. J Mol Cell Cardiol 27:181–193.
11. Heads RJ, Latchman DS, Yellon DM. 1995. Differential stress protein mRNA expression during early ischemic preconditioning in the rabbit heart and its relationship to adenosine receptor function. J Mol Cell Cardiol 27:2133–2148.
12. Liu X, Engelman RM, Moraru II, Rousou JA, Flack JE, Deaton DW, Maulik N, Das DK. 1992. Heat shock: a new approach for myocardial preservation in cardiac surgery. Circulation 86(Suppl II):358–363.
13. Liu GS, Thornton J, Van Winkle DM, Stanley AWH, Olsson RA, Downey JM. 1991. Protection against infarction afforded by preconditioning is mediated by A1 adenosine receptors in rabbit heart. Circulation 84:350–356.
14. Vegh A, Komori S, Szekeres L, Parratt JR. 1992. Antiarrhythmic effects of preconditioning in anaesthetized dogs and rats. Cardiovasc Res 26:487–495.
15 Schott RJ, Rohman S, Brown ER, Schaper W. 1990. Ischemic preconditioning reduces infarct size in swine myocardium. Circ Res 66:1133–1142.
16 Yellon DM, Baxter GF. 1995. "Second window of protection" or delayed preconditioning phenomenon: future horizons for myocardial protection? J Mol Cell Cardiol 27:1023–1034.
17 Anderson NG, Maller JI, Tonks NK, Sturgill TW. 1990. Requirement for integration of signals from two distinct phosphorylation pathways for activation of Mapkinase. Nature (Lond) 343:651–653.
18. Asimakis GK, Inners-McBride K, Medellin G, Conti VR. 1992. Ischemic preconditioning attenuates acidosis and postischemic dysfunction in isolated rat heart. Am J Physiol 263:H887–H894.
19. Banerjee A, Locke-Winter C, Rogers KB, Mitchess MB, Brew EC, Cairns CB, Bensard DD, Hartken AH. 1993. Preconditioning against myocardial dysfunction after ischemia and reperfusion by an alpha-1, -adrenergic mechanism. Circ Res 73:656–670.
20. Billah MM. 1993. Phospholipase D and cell signaling. Curr Opin Immunol 5:114–123.
21. Das, DK, Engelman RM, Kimura Y. 1993. Molecular adaptation of cellular defenses following preconditioning of the heart by repeated ischemia. Cardiovasc Res 27:578–584.
22. Tosaki A, Cordis GA, Szerdahelyi P, Engelman RM, Das DK. 1994. Effects of preconditioning on reperfusion arrhythmias, myocardial functions, formation of free radicals, and ion shifts in isolated ischemic/reperfused rat hearts. J Cardiovasc Pharmacol 23:365–373.

23. McClanahan TB, Nao LJ, Wolke BJ, Martin TE, Metz KP, Gallagher KP. Brief renal occlusion and reperfusion reduces myocardial infarct size in rabbits. FASEB J 7:A118, 682.
24. Gross GJ, Mizumura T, Nithipatikom K, Mei DA. Myocardial preconditioning via ATP sensitive potassium channels, interactions with adenosine. Adv Organ Biol 6:81–100.
25. Gross GJ, Auchampach JA. 1992. Blockade of ATP-sensitive potassium channels prevents myocardial preconditioning in dogs. Circ Res 73:656–670.
26. Kirsch GE, Condina J, Birnbaumer L, Brown AM. 1990. Coupling of ATP sensitive K+ channels to A-1 receptors by G proteins in rat ventricular myocytes. Am J Physiol 259:H820–H826.
27. Lawson CS, Coltart DJ, Hearse DJ. 1993. The antiarrhythmic action of ischemic preconditioning in rat hearts does not involve functional Gi proteins. Cardiovasc Res 27:681–687.
28. Schwarz ER, Montino H, Fleischhauer J, Klues HG, vom Dahl J, Hanrath P. 1997. Angiotensin II receptor antagonist EXP 3174 reduces infarct size comparable with enalaprilat and augments pre-conditioning in the pig heart. Cardiovasc Drugs Ther 11:687–695.
29. Nakano A, Miura T, Ura N, Suzuki K, Shimamoto K. 1997. Role of angiotensin II type 1 receptor in preconditioning against infarction. Coronary Artery Dis 8:343–350.
30. Diaz RJ, Wilson GJ. 1997. Selective blockade of AT-1 angiotensin II receptors abolishes ischemic preconditioning in isolated rabbit hearts. J Mol Cell Cardiol 29:129–139.
31. Morris SD, Yellon DM. 1997. Angiotensin-converting enzyme inhibitors potentiate preconditioning through bradykinin B2 receptor activation in human heart. J Am Coll Cardiol 29(7):1599–1606.
32. Schulz R, Post H, Vahlhaus C, Heusch G. 1998. Ischemic preconditioning in pigs: a graded phe-nomenon: its relation to adenosine and bradykinin. Circulation 98:1022–1029.
33. Jin AQ, Chen X. 1998. Bradykinin mediates myocardial ischemic preconditioning against free radical injury in guinea-pig isolated heart. Clin Exp Pharmacol Physiol 25(11):932–935.
34. Li C, Browder W, Kao RL. 1999. Early activation of transcription factor NF-kappaB during ischemia in perfused rat heart. Am J Physiol 276(2, Pt 2):H543–H552.
35. Scholich K, Mullenix JB, Wittpoth C, Poppleton HM, Pierre SC, Lindorfer MA, Garrison JC, Patel TB. 1999. Facilitation of signal onset and termination of adenylyl cyclase. Science 283(5406): 1328–1331.
36. Ohyanagi M, Iwasaki T. 1996. The guanine nucleotide-binding regulatory proteins (G proteins) in myocardium with ischemia. Mol Cell Biochem 160/161:153–158.
37. Strasser RH, Marquetant R. 1990. Supersensitivity of adenylyl cyclase system in acute myocardial ischemia: evaluation of three independent mechanisms. Basic Res Cardiol 85:67–78.
38. Thornton JD, Liu GS, Downey JM. 1993. Pretreatment with pertussis toxin blocked the protective effects of preconditioning: evidence of a G-protein mechanism. J Mol Cell Cardiol 25:311–320.
39. Niroomand F, Weinbrenner C, Weis A, Bangert M, Schwencke C, Marquetant R, Beyer T, Strasser RH, Kubler W, Rauch B. 1995. Impaired function of inhibitory G proteins during acute myocar-dial ischemia of canine heart and its reversal during reperfusion and a second period of ischemia. Possible implications for the protective mechanism of ischemic preconditioning. Circ Res 76:861–870.
40. Fu L-X, Kirkeboen KA, Liang Q-M, Sjogren K-G, Jhalmarson A, llebekk A. 1993. Free radical scav-enging enzymes and G protein mediated receptor signaling systems in ischemically preconditioned porcine myocardium. Cardiovasc Res 27:612–616.
41. Blumer KJ, Johnson GL. 1994. Diversity in function and regulation of MAP kinase pathway. Trends Biochem Sci 19:236–240.
42. Bogoyevitch MA, Glennon PE, Andersson MB, Clerk A, Lazou A, Marshall CJ, Packer PJ, Sugden PH. 1994. Endothelin-1 and fibroblast growth factors stimulate the mitogen-activated protein kinase signaling cascade in cardiac myocytes. J Biol Chem 269:1110–1119.
43. Bourgoin S, Grinstein S. 1992. Peroxides of vanadate induce activation of phospholipase D in HL-60 cells. Role of tyrosine phosphorylation. J Biol Chem 267:11908–11916.
44. Rivard N, Rydzewska G, Lods JS, Martinex LJ, Morisset J. 1994. Pancreas growth, tyrosine kinase, Ptdlns 3-kinase, and PLD involve high-affinity CCK-receptor occupation. Am J Physiol 266: G62–G70.
45. Schmidt M, Huwe SM, Fasselt B, Homann D, Rumenapp U, Sandmann J, Jakobs KH. 1994. Mechanisms of phospholipase D stimulation by M3 muscarinic acetylcholine receptors. Evidence for involvement of tyrosine phosphorylation. Eur J Biochem 225:667–675.
46. Cohen MV, Liu Y, Liu GS, Wang P, Cordis GA, Das DK, Downey JM. 1996. Phospholipase D plays a major role in ischemic preconditioning in rabbit heart. Circulation 94:1713–1718.
47. Moraru II, Popescu LM, Liu X, Engelman RM, Das DK. 1993. Role of phospholipase A2, C, and D activities during myocardial item and reperfusion. Ann NY Acad Sci 723:328–332.

48. Kanfer JN. 1980. The base exchange enzymes and phospholipase D of mammalian tissue. Can J Biochem 58:1370–1380.
49. Ha KS, Exton JH. 1993. Differential translocation of protein kinase C isozymes thrombin and platelet derived growth factor. A possible function for phosphatidylcholine-derived diacylglycerol. J Biol Chem 268:10534–10539.
50. Eskildensen-Helmond YEG, Gho BCG, Bezstarosti K, Dekkers DHW, Loek S, VanHeusten HAA, Vierdouw PD, Lamers JMJ. Exploration of the possible roles of phospholipase D and protein kinase C in the mechanism of ischemic preconditioning in the myocardium. Ann NY Acad Sci 793:210–225.
51. Fryer RM, Schultz JE, Hsu AK, Gross GJ. 1998. Pretreatment with tyrosine kinase inhibitors partially attenuates ischemic preconditioning in rat hearts. Am J Physiol 275(6, Pt 2):H2009–H2015.
52. Bugge E, Ytrehus K. 1995. Ischemic preconditioning is protein kinase C dependent but not through stimulation of alpha adrenergic or adenosine receptors in the isolated rat heart. Cardiovasc Res 29:401–406.
53. Dixon BS, Sharma RV, Dickerson T, Fortune J. 1994. Bradykinin and angiotensin II: activation of protein kinase C in arterial muscle. Am J Physiol 266:C1406–C1420.
54. Goto M, Liu Y, Yang X-M, Ardell JL, Cohen MV, Downey JM. 1995. Role of bradykinin in protection of ischemic preconditioning in rabbit hearts. Circ Res 77:611–621.
55. Tosaki A, Maulik N, Engelman DT, Engelman RM, Das DK. 1996. The role of protein kinase C in ischemic/reperfused preconditioning isolated rat hearts. J Cardiovasc Pharmacol 28:723–731.
56. Yazaki Y, Komuro I, Yamazaki T, Tobe K, Maemura K, Kadowaki T, Nagai R. 1993. Role of protein kinase system in the signal transduction of stretch-mediated protooncogene expression and hypertrophy of cardiac myocytes. Mol Cell Biochem 119:11–16.
57. Segar R, Krebs EG. 1995. The MAPK signaling cascade. FASEB J 9:726–735.
58. Novak-Hofer I, Thomas G. 1984. An activated S6 kinase in extracts from serum- and epidermal growth factor-stimulated Swiss 3T3 cells. J Biol Chem 259:5995–6000.
59. Cobb MH, Goldsmith EJ. 1995. How MAP kinases are regulated? J Biol Chem 270:14843–14846.
60. Yamazaki T, Komuro I, Kudoh S, Zou Y, Shiojima I, Hiroi Y, Mizuno T, Maemura K, Kurihara H, Aikawa R, Takano H, Yazaki Y. 1996. Endothelin-1 is involved in mechanical stress-induced cardiomyocyte hypertrophy. J Biol Chem 271:3221–3228.
61. Lazou A, Bogoyevitch MA, Clerk A, Fuller SJ, Marshall CJ, Sugden PH. 1994. Regulation of mitogen-activated protein kinase cascade in adult rat heart preparations in vitro. Cite Res 932–941.
62. Das DK, Engelman RM, Rousou JA, Breyer RH, Otani H, Lemeshow S. 1986. Role of membrane phospholipids in myocardial injury induced by ischemia and reperfusion. Am J Physiol 251:H71–H79.
63. Yamada H, Strahler J, Welsh MJ, Bitar KN. 1995. Activation of MAP kinase and translocation with HSP 27 in bombesin-induced contraction of rectosigmoid smooth muscle. Am J Physiol 269:G683–G691.
64. Das DK, Maulik N, Moraru II. 1995. Gene expression in acute myocardial stress. J Mol Cell Cardiol 27:181–193.
65. Das DK, Maulik N. 1997. Reprogramming of gene expression during myocardial adaptation to stress. In Adaptation Biology and Medicine. Ed. BK Sharma, N Takeda, PK Ganguly, PK and Singal, ••. Narosa Publishing House.
66. Thorburn J, Carlson M, Mansour SJ, Chien KR, Ahn NG, Thorburn A. 1995. Inhibition of a signaling pathway in cardiac muscle cells by active mitogen-activated protein kinase. Mol Biol Cell 6:1479–1490.
67. Han J, Lee J-D, Bibbs L, Velvitch RJ. 1994. A new map kinase targeted by endotoxin and hyperosmolarity in mammalian cells, Science 265:808–811.
68. Force T, Bonventrem JV, Heidecker G, Rapp U, Avruch J, Kyriakis LM. 1994. Enzymatic characteristics of the Raf-1 protein kinase. Proc Nat Acad Sci U S A 91:1270–1274.
69. Galchva-Gorgova, Z, Deriard B, Wu I-H, Davis RJ. 1994. An osmosensing signal transduction pathway in mammalian cells. Science 265:806–808.
70. Seko Y, Tobe K, Ueki K, Kadowaki T, Yazaki Y. 1996 Hypoxia and hypoxia/reoxygenation activate raf-1, mitogen-activated protein kinase kinase, mitogen-activated protein kinases, and S6 kinase in cultured rat cardiac myocytes. Circ Res 78:82–90.
71. Maulik N, Watanabe M, Zu Y-L, Huang C-K, Cordis GA, Schley JA, Das DK. 1996. Ischemic preconditioning triggers the activation of MAP kinases and MAPKAP kinase 2 in rat hearts. FEBS Lett 396:233–237.

72. Ciocca DR, Oesterreich S, Charoness GC, McGuire WL, Fuqua SAW. 1993. Biological and clinical implications of heat shock protein 27,000 (HSP 27): a review. J Nat Cancer Inst 85:1558–1570.
73. Das DK, Maulik N. 1995. Cross talk between heat shock and oxidative stress inducible genes during myocardial adaptation of ischemia. In Cell Biology of Trauma. Ed. JJ Lemasters and C Oliver, 193–211. Boca Raton, FL: CRC Press.
74. Stokoe D, Engel K, Campbell DG, Cohen P, Gaeste M. 1992. Identification of MAPKAP kinase 2 as a major enzyme responsible for the phosphorylation of the small mammalian heat shock proteins. FEBS 313:307–313.
75. Maulik N, Das DK. 1996. Hunting for differentially expressed MRNA species in preconditioned myocardium. Ann NY Acad Sci 793:240–258.
76. Benjamin IJ, McMillan R, 1998. Stenn (Heat Shock) Proteins Molecular Chaperones.
77. Zu Y-L, Ai Y, Gilchrist A, Labadia ME, Sha'afi RI, Huang CK. 1996. Activation of MAPkinase-activated protein kinase 2 in human neutrophils after phorbol ester or fMLP peptide stimulation. Blood 87:5287–5296.
78. Maulik N, Yoshida T, Zu YL, Sato M, Banerjee A, Das DK. 1998. Ischemic preconditioning triggers tyrosine kinase signaling: a potential role for MAPKAP kinase 2. Am J Physiol 275(5, Pt 2): H1857–H1864.
79. Das DK, Engelman RM, Maulik N. 1990. Oxygen free radical signaling in ischemic preconditioning. N Y Acad Sci 874:1–18.
80. Lee YJ, Corry PM. 1998. Metabolic oxidative stress-Induced HSP70 gene expression is mediated through SAPK pathway. Role of Bcl-2 and c-Jun Nh2-terminal kinase. J Biol Chem 273(45): 29857–29863.
81. Cook SJ, Aziz N, McMahon M. 1999. The repertoire of fos and jun proteins expressed during the G1 phase of the cell cycle is determined by the duration of mitogen-activated protein kinase activation. Mol Cell Biol 19(1):330–341.
82. Das DK. 1998. Ischemic preconditioning: role of multiple kinases in signal amplication and modulation. In Advanced Organ Biology: Myocardial Preservation and Cellular Adaptation, 101–124. Stamford: Jai Press.
83. Slinker BK, Stephens RL, Fisher SA, Yang Q. 1996. Immediate-early gene responses to different cardiac loads in the ejecting rabbit left ventricle. J Mol Cell Cardiol 28(7):1565–1574.
84. Larsen TH, Skar R, Frotjold EK, Haukanes K, Greve G, Saetersdal T. 1998. Regional activation of immediate-early response gene c-fos in infarcted rat hearts. Int J Exp Pathol 79 (3):163–172.
85. Wechsler AS, Entwistle JC 3rd, Yeh T Jr, Ding M, Jakoi ER. 1994. Early gene changes in myocardial ischemia. Ann Thorac Surg 58(4):1282–1284.
86. Komuro I, Kurabayashi M, Shibazaki Y, Katoh Y, Hoh E, Kadia T, Leki K, Takaku F, Yazaki Y. 1990. Molecular mechanism of cardiac hypertrophy. Jpn Circ J 54(5):526–534.
87. Maulik N, Goswami S, Galang N, Das DK. 1999. Differential regulation of Bcl-2, Ap-1 and NF-kappaB on cardiomyocyte apoptosis during myocardial ischemic stress adaptation. FEBS Lett 443(3):331–336.
88. Pinkus R. 1996. Role of oxidants and antioxidants in the induction of AP-1, NFkB and glutathione S-transferase gene expression. J Biol Chem 271:13422–13429.
89. Takeda N, Ota Y, Tanaka Y, Shikata C, Hayashi Y, Nemoto S, Tanamura A, Iwai T, Nakamura I. 1996. Myocardial adaptive changes and damages in ischemic heart disease. Ann NY Acad Sci 793:282–288.
90. Moraru II, Engelman DT, Engelman RM, Rousou JA, Flack JE, Deaton DW, Das DK. 1994. Myocardial ischemia triggers rapid expression of mitochondrial genes. Surg Forum 45:315–317.
91. Das DK, Maulik N, Sato M, Ray P. 1999. Reactive oxygen species function as second messenger during ischemic preconditioning of heart. Mol Cell Biochem, in press.

N. Takeda, M. Nagano and N.S. Dhalla
(eds). The Hypertrophied Heart. Copyright
© 2000. pp. 17–30. Kluwer Academic
Publishers. Boston. All rights reserved.

GLUCOSE-6-PHOSPHATE DEHYDROGENASE: A MARKER OF CARDIAC HYPERTROPHY

HEINZ-GERD ZIMMER

Carl-Ludwig-Institute of Physiology, University of Leipzig, Liebigstrasse 27, D-04103 Leipzig, Germany

Summary. The pentose phosphate pathway is the link between carbohydrate and fatty acid metabolism as well as purine and pyrimidine nucleotide metabolism. The oxidative branch of this pathway is poorly expressed in the heart. The occurrence, function, and regulation of this pathway and the intervention into it are described. It is then examined whether glucose-6-phosphate dehydrogenase (G-6-PD), the first and regulating enzyme, may be a marker of cardiac hypertrophy. Three rat models of cardiac hypertrophy were studied.

1. Left ventricular (LV) hypertrophy was induced by continuous i.v. infusion of norepinephrine (NE, 0.2 mg/kg i.v.) for 3 days. NE stimulated the activity and mRNA level of cardiac G-6-PD. Carvedilol, an α- and β-adrenergic blocker, prevented the NE-induced increase in cardiac G-6-PD mRNA and activity, in functional parameters, and in the heart weight/body weight ratio. Also, the combination of the β-adrenergic blocker metoprolol and the α-adrenergic blocker prazosin prevented both the development of NE-induced cardiac hypertrophy and the increase in myocardial G-6-PD-activity.
2. Treatment of spontaneously hypertensive rats (SHR) with triiodothyronine (T_3) for 14 days induced additional cardiac hypertrophy as well as an increase in cardiac function and G-6-PD activity. Discontinuation of T_3 treatment for another 14 days normalized all parameters.
3. Right ventricular (RV) hypertrophy was induced by exposure of rats to intermittent hypoxia for 4 weeks. G-6-PD activity was enhanced exclusively in the right ventricle in which systolic pressure was elevated and which developed hypertrophy. The hypoxia-induced increase in RV pressure, RV weight, and RV G-6-PD activity, which all occurred exclusively in the RV, were attenuated by the AT_1 receptor blocker losartan. Thus, there was a good correlation between G-6-PD activity, heart function, and heart weight in these experimental models. It is concluded that G-6-PD may be a marker of cardiac hypertrophy.

THE OXIDATIVE PENTOSE PHOSPHATE PATHWAY

The pentose phosphate pathway (PPP) is important for cardiac metabolism in several respects. The oxidative branch of this pathway is the link between carbohydrate and

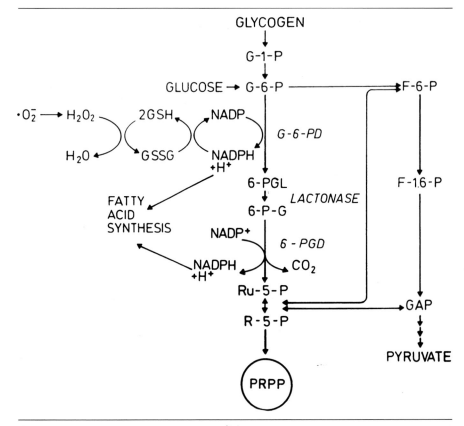

Figure 1. Schematic representation of the oxidative PPP (center) and its connections to glycolysis (right-hand side) via the transaldolase and transketolase reactions (arrows) and to purine and pyrimidine nucleotide synthesis via 5-phosphoribosyl-1-pyrophosphate (PRPP).
Abbreviations: G-1-P: glucose-1-phospate; G-6-P: glucose-6-phosphate; F-6-P: fructose-6-phosphate; F-1,6-phosphate: fructose-1,6-biphosphate; GAP: glyceraldehyde-3-phosphate; 6-PGL: 6-phosphogluconolactone; 6-PG: 6-phosphogluconate; Ru-5-P: ribulose-5-phosphate; R-5-P: ribose-5-phosphate; NADP⁺: nicotinamide adenine dinucleotide phosphate; GSH: reduced glutathione; GSSG: oxidized glutathione; G-6-PD: glucose-6-phosphate dehydrogenase; 6-PGD: 6-phosphogluconate dehydrogenase.

fatty acid metabolism as well as purine and pyrimidine nucleotide metabolism (figure 1). Glucose-6-phosphate originating from glycogenolysis or from glucose taken up by the myocardial cell is metabolized predominantly via glycolysis. A small portion of glucose-6-phosphate, however, enters the oxidative branch of the pentose phosphate pathway. Glucose-6-phosphate dehydrogenase (G-6-PD) is the first and rate-limiting enzyme. It was discovered in 1931 by Warburg and Christian [1], is widely distributed, and catalyzes the dehydrogenation of glucose-6-phosphate, a reaction that is essentially irreversible. This enzyme is highly specific for $NADP^+$. The product is 6-phosphoglucono-δ-lactone. The next step is the hydrolysis of 6-phosphoglucono-δ-lactone by a specific lactonase to produce 6-phosphogluconate, which is then oxidatively decarboxylated by 6-phosphogluconate dehydrogenase to yield ribulose-5-phosphate. $NADP^+$ is again the electron acceptor. The final step is the isomerization of ribulose-5-phosphate by phosphopentose isomerase to produce ribose-5-phosphate, which can be transformed into 5-phosphoribosyl-1-pyrophosphate (PRPP) by ribophosphate pyrophosphokinase (figure 1).

The oxidative branch of the PPP serves mainly two functions:

1. It provides reducing equivalents in the form of NADPH, which can be used for the synthesis of free fatty acids and for the conversion of oxidized (GSSG) to reduced glutathione (GSH). This is important for the detoxification of reactive oxygen species via glutathione peroxidase (figure 1). The regeneration of reduced glutathione is catalyzed by glutathione reductase, which is a dimer of 50 kDa subunits.
2. Ribose-5-phosphate is generated, which is transformed into PRPP. This substance is an essential precursor for the de novo synthesis of purine nucleotides, for the utilization of orotic acid for UTP synthesis, and for the salvage of the purine bases adenine and hypoxanthine.

The capacity of the oxidative PPP was assessed in several rat organs. The activity of G-6-PD and the available pool of PRPP were measured. There was a parallel behavior of these parameters: They were highest in the kidney, followed by the liver, heart, and skeletal muscle (figure 2). Thus, the capacity of the oxidative PPP is very low in muscular organs [2,3]. In the heart, this finding becomes of critical importance when there is a need for restoration of the ATP pool, as during the reperfusion following severe ischemia [4,5]. The oxidative PPP plays an important role quantitatively in the metabolism of the liver, adipose tissue, adrenal cortex, thyroid gland, lactating mammary gland, testes, and erythrocytes.

The low capacity of the oxidative PPP is not confined to the rat heart. Studies on a variety of animal species, including guinea pig, rat, rabbit, dog, calf, monkey, and man, have shown that the activity of cardiac G-6-PD is on the same order of magnitude and always lower than the activity of 6-phosphogluconate dehydrogenase. Thus, the cardiac oxidative PPP is poorly developed in all animal species examined [6]. Therefore, a characteristic metabolic feature of the heart is that this organ restores its adenine nucleotide pool only very slowly once that pool has been depleted by a brief period of ischemia. Upon reperfusion, it takes several days both in the dog and rat heart until normal ATP levels are reestablished [4,5], because the degradation products of ATP such as adenosine, inosine, and hypoxanthine that are produced during ischemia can permeate the cell membrane. These products are washed out and lost from the heart and thus are not available for reutilization via the salvage pathways. The repletion of the ATP pool can therefore be attained only via the de novo synthesis (biosynthesis) of adenine nucleotides. This process,

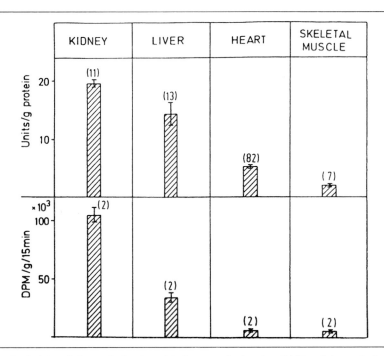

Figure 2. Activity of glucose-6-phosphate dehydrogenase (top) and availability of the pool of 5-phosphoribosyl-1-pyrophosphate (bottom) in several rat organs. Data are mean values ± SEM; the number of experiments is in parentheses.

however, is very slow [7], since the available pool of PRPP is limited in the heart due to the low capacity of the oxidative PPP.

In erythrocytes, the oxidative PPP is important for the production of reduced glutathione (GSH in figure 1), which is essential for maintaining the normal structure of red cells and for keeping hemoglobin in the ferrous state. Cells with a lower level of reduced glutathione are more susceptible to hemolysis. A deficiency of G-6-PD activity was discovered in red cells of persons sensitive to the hemolytic effect of the antimalarial compound primaquine. This deficiency was also found to be one of the causes of infection-induced hemolysis, hereditary nonspherocytic hemolytic anemia, fava bean–induced hemolytic anemia, and, in some populations, severe neonatal jaundice leading to kernicterus [8]. The most likely mechanism is that free radicals and hydrogen peroxide damage hemoglobin and red cell components. The PPP is the only source of NADPH in red cells, since these cells lack mitochondria, so the production of NADPH is markedly diminished by this deficiency. The major role of NADPH in these cells is to reduce the disulfide form of glutathione (GSSG in figure 1) to the sulfhydryl form (GSH). The reduced form of glutathione, a tripeptide with a free sulfhydryl group, serves as a sulfhydryl buffer that maintains the cystein residues of hemoglobin and other red cell protein in the reduced state. The ratio of GSH/GSSG is normally about 500.

REGULATION OF THE PATHWAY

In rat liver, G-6-PD is always inhibited by NADPH. This inhibition is competitive with $NADP^+$ [9,10]. Since the enzyme is almost completely inhibited at physiological concentrations of free $NADP^+$ and free NADPH, the regulation of G-6-PD is a matter of deinhibition. It turned out that among over 100 cell constituents tested, only two counteracted the inhibition by NADPH—namely, AMP and oxidized glutathione (GSSG)—and only GSSG was highly effective at concentrations that may occur physiologically. In isolated perfused rat hearts, a 40-fold elevation of the GSSG concentration was induced by perfusion with the oxidizing agent tert-butyl hydroperoxide. In addition, the $NADP^+$/NADPH ratio was increased twofold. Under these conditions, the incorporation of ^{14}C-adenine into myocardial adenine nucleotides, a relative measure of the PRPP pool, was increased threefold within the first 15 minutes after tert-butyl hydroperoxide administration. Since the increase in both the GSSG and the $NADP^+$ concentration is known to overcome the NADPH-mediated inhibition of G-6-PD, it was difficult to decide which of these two factors may be more relevant. Since GSSG was elevated more markedly than the $NADP^+$/NADPH ratio and since the latter may still be inhibitory, it was concluded that it is the GSSG that is more important for the regulation of G-6-PD. This appears to be a rapid control mechanism that becomes effective within minutes [11]. Such a mechanism may be activated when oxygen free radicals are produced. In the neutrophils, the activation of the oxidative PPP has been shown to be associated with the respiratory burst and with the process of phagocytosis [12].

Apart from this "fine" control mechanism exerted by NADPH that is involved in the short-term regulation of G-6-PD, there is a long-term mechanism. This is also directed at G-6-PD and involves the increase in the new synthesis of enzyme protein. This mechanism can be activated in skeletal muscle and in the rat heart during the development of cardiac hypertrophy and under the influence of catecholamines [13].

ALTERATIONS OF THE PATHWAY IN PATHOPHYSIOLOGICAL STATES

After constriction of the abdominal aorta in rats, the first increase in cardiac G-6-PD activity occurred after 48 hours and reached the maximum after 3 and 4 days. This stimulation correlated with the elevation of adenine nucleotide and protein synthesis that occurred prior to the development of cardiac hypertrophy [14]. A similar picture was seen in the nonischemic part of the heart after ligation of the descending branch of the left coronary. The rates of adenine nucleotide and protein synthesis were elevated after 48 hours.

Stimulation of cardiac β-adrenergic receptors with isoproterenol also resulted in the development of cardiac hypertrophy in rats. This hypertrophy was characterized by an elevation of G-6-PD activity, adenine nucleotide, and protein synthesis. However, the sequential increase was different. Cardiac adenine nucleotide de novo synthesis was maximally stimulated already after 5 hours, at a time when there was no change in G-6-PD activity. Protein synthesis reached its peak after 12 hours, at a time when G-6-PD activity had just started to be elevated [3]. This finding can be explained by two phases that became activated sequentially. The first phase was characterized by an immediate increase in the cAMP and glucose-6-phosphate contents. Parallel to these metabolic changes, heart rate and contractility were also elevated. After 12 and 24 hours, these parameters had returned to the respective control levels. However, myocardial adenine nucleotide biosynthesis, which was also enhanced very early, remained elevated, though at a somewhat lower level. In the second phase, which started at about 12 hours subsequent to isoproterenol injection, protein synthesis began to increase, and when this had achieved the maximum, G-6-PD activity became stimulated. From this time course, it can be concluded that cAMP may be the trigger for the stimulation of cardiac G-6-PD activity and that G-6-PD activation is dependent on protein synthesis and thus may reflect an increased new synthesis of enzyme protein. When the isoproterenol-induced increase in cAMP was prevented with the β-receptor blocker atenolol, the stimulation of enzyme activity was completely prevented. Inhibition of protein synthesis with cycloheximide, which inhibits translation, and with actinomycin D, which interferes with transcription, blunted the isoproterenol effect. Thus, cardiac β-adrenergic receptors and enzyme protein synthesis appear to be involved in the isoproterenol-mediated increase in G-6-PD activity [3].

Likewise, continuous infusion of norepinephrine in rats for 3 days induced cardiac hypertrophy [15] and increased both the mRNA and activity of cardiac G-6-PD. This increase was antagonized by simultaneous administration of carvedilol, a β-adrenergic blocker and vasodilator with α_1-blocking activity. Thus, both α- and β-adrenergic agonists promote specifically gene expression of cardiac G-6-PD [13]. Triiodothyronine (T_3) also induces cardiac hypertrophy. However, daily injections of T_3 for 5 days have no effect on the activity of cardiac G-6-PD [14], although there is a substantial stimulation of both adenine nucleotide and protein synthesis [16].

After administration of catecholamines, there is an immediate stimulation of glycogenolysis and glycolysis and a positive chronotropic and inotropic effect as well as a concomitant elevation in the PRPP pool and in adenine nucleotide biosynthesis. There was no change in G-6-PD activity in this first phase. It was only in the subsequent second phase that cardiac G-6-PD activity was enhanced. A mechanism other than an enhanced flow through the oxidative PPP must therefore be responsible for the elevation of the PRPP pool and for the stimulation of adenine nucleotide biosynthesis in the first phase. One possibility is that PRPP becomes elevated via the nonoxidative branch of the PPP through the transaldolase and transketolase reactions. This may also be true for thyroid hormone action [17] and represents a very likely mechanism, since the activities of the enzymes of the nonoxidative PPP are much higher than those of the oxidative branch in muscle [18]. Furthermore, the large amounts of NAD^+ present in the heart [19] may favor glycolysis, whereas the small quantity of NADP$^+$ may be limiting rather than stimulating the oxidative PPP.

INTERVENTION INTO THE PATHWAY

Apart from affecting the mRNA and activity of cardiac G-6-PD, there is another intervention into the oxidative PPP that ultimately results in an elevation of the myocardial PRPP pool and consequently of adenine nucleotide de novo synthesis. This is the administration of ribose. Ribose bypasses the critical and rate-limiting step in the pathway and leads via ribose-5-phosphate to the formation of PRPP.

This metabolic approach has been utilized in many experimental models, e.g., in isolated cardiac myocytes [20], after catecholamine stimulation of the intact rat heart [3,13,21], during development of cardiac hypertrophy [22], during recovery from temporary oxygen deficieny in the isolated rat [23,24] and guinea pig heart [25], in the vivo rat [5] and dog heart [26–29], after permanent coronary artery ligation [30], in chronic alcoholic cardiomyopathy as assessed in the isolated working rat heart [31], and in primary rat muscle cultures [32]. In all these studies, ribose proved to be an intervention that either attenuated or prevented entirely the decline of the myocardial ATP pool. For instance, after 15 minutes of reversible regional ischemia, the ATP fell by about 40%. During the reperfusion period, the ATP pool recovered to some extent, most probably due to the rephosphorylation of ADP and AMP. However, even after 3 days, ATP was still lower than the respective control value of sham-operated rats [5]. This finding corresponded well with the results obtained in dogs [4]. However, when ribose was administered as continuous i.v. infusion, ATP was already normalized after 12 hours. So the metabolic recovery period was shortened by at least 60 hours [5].

In some pathophysiological situations in the intact rat, there was a good correlation between the restoration of the cardiac ATP pool and heart function. Two experimental models were examined to determine whether a depressed heart function may be improved when the cardiac ATP pool is normalized with ribose. In the first model, depression of all hemodynamic parameters was induced in rats by severe constriction of the abdominal aorta in combination with a single s.c. dose of isoproterenol. Twenty-four hours after this combined intervention, both the ATP level and heart function had deteriorated in animals that had received continuous i.v. infusion of 0.9% NaCl. When ribose had been administered for 24 hours, the biosynthesis of cardiac adenine nucleotides was stimulated to such an extent that the depression of ATP and of the total adenine nucleotide pool was prevented. This metabolic normalization was accompanied by an elevation of the depressed left ventricular pressure and LV dp/dt_{max}. Also, the pressure–rate product had returned to a near normal value [33]. Thus, ribose was able to normalize an impaired global heart function concomitantly with the restoration of the cardiac adenine nucleotide pool.

A marked impairment of heart function was also induced by experimental myocardial infarction by ligation of the descending branch of the left coronary artery in rats. There was a progressive decline in left ventricular systolic pressure, in LV dp/dt_{max}, and in the pressure–rate product [30]. Left ventricular end-diastolic pressure was elevated. Cardiac output and stroke volume were depressed. The ATP content in the nonischemic region was lower than in the control after 24 hours and recovered spontaneously toward the control within the following 3 days. Continuous i.v. infusion of ribose attenuated the fall and promoted the restoration of the ATP level in the nonischemic myocardium within 4 days after coronary artery ligation. The elevation of left ventricular end-diastolic pressure was attenuated with ribose after 2 and 4 days [30].

The great advantage of ribose is that it has purely metabolic effects and is entirely neutral in functional terms as far as the heart and circulatory system are concerned, in contrast to purine nucleosides such as adenosine [34] and inosine [35]. Another characteristic feature of ribose is that it can be combined with drugs that are used in the conventional therapy of heart diseases. It was found that ribose did not alter the hemodynamic effects of the calcium antagonist verapamil and of the β-adrenergic receptor blocker metoprolol in the intact rat. The negative chronotropic and inotropic effects of metoprolol and verapamil were fully expressed, and neither the verapamil-induced decrease in total peripheral resistance nor the metoprolol-induced reduction of cardiac output was changed in the presence of ribose. On the other hand, ribose retained its typical metabolic effect, i.e., the stimulation of cardiac adenine nucleotide biosynthesis, despite the pronounced hemodynamic changes brought about by these drugs [36]. Thus, ribose appears to be a suitable and appropriate adjunct in the medical therapy of certain heart diseases.

GLUCOSE-6-PHOSPHATE DEHYDROGENASE AND EXPERIMENTAL CARDIAC HYPERTROPHY

To examine whether G-6-PD may be a marker of experimentally induced cardiac hypertrophy, several in vivo rat models of left ventricular (LV) and right ventricular (RV) hypertrophy were studied. Essentially, two approaches were used. In the first, an effective and appropriate stimulus was applied to induce cardiac hypertrophy, which was then characterized hemodynamically and morphologically; then G-6-PD activity was examined to determine whether it was elevated in the respective heart chamber. In the second approach, cardiac hypertrophy was prevented or reversed, and G-6-PD activity was then measured.

Left ventricular hypertrophy induced by norepinephrine

LV hypertrophy was induced by continuous i.v. infusion of NE (0.2 mg/kg/h) for 3 days. NE stimulated the activity and mRNA level of cardiac G-6-PD in a time-dependent manner [13]. Furthermore, it induced LV hypertrophy that was due solely to the stimulation of α- and β-adrenergic receptors. The elevation of total peripheral resistance did not contribute to the development of LV hypertrophy, since normalization of peripheral resistance with verapamil did not influence cardiac

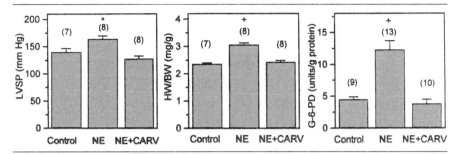

Figure 3. Changes in left ventricular systolic pressure (LVSP), heart-weight/body-weight (HW/BW) ratio, and glucose-6-phosphate dehydrogenase (G-6-PD) activity in rats under control conditions, after i.v. infusion of norepinephrine (NE, 0.2 mg/kg/h) without and with carvediolol (CARV, 0.5 mg/kg/h) for 3 days. Data are means ± SEM; the number of experiments is in parentheses. $\star$, $p < 0.01$; +, $p < 0.0005$.

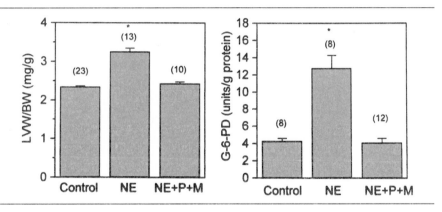

Figure 4. Changes in left ventricular-weight/body-weight (HW/BW) ratio and glucose-6-phosphate dehydrogenase (G-6-PD) activity in rats under control conditions, after i.v. infusion of norepinephrine (NE, 0.2 mg/kg/h) without and with simultaneous administration of prazosin (P, 0.1 mg/kg/h) and metoprolol (M, 1 mg/kg/h) for 3 days. Data are means ± SEM; the number of experiments is in parentheses. $\star$, $p < 0.05$.

hypertrophy appreciably [15]. Carvedilol, an α- and β-adrenergic blocker, prevented the NE-induced increase in cardiac G-6-PD mRNA and activity [13], in functional parameters, and in the heart-weight/body-weight ratio [15]. Figure 3 shows the increase in LVSP, heart-weight/body-weight ratio, and G-6-PD activity 3 days after continuous NE infusion without and with simultaneous treatment with carvedilol, a combined α- and β-adrenergic receptor blocker. The NE-induced changes were all prevented to the same extent. The combined administration of the α-adrenergic blocker prazosin together with the β-blocker metoprolol had the same effect as carvedilol. Both the NE-induced increase in heart-weight/body-weight ratio and in G-6-PD activity were prevented with this combined receptor blockade (figure 4).

Thus, there was a parallel behavior of heart weight and G-6-PD activity in this model of experimentally induced cardiac hypertrophy.

Triiodothyronine treatment and withdrawal in spontaneously hypertensive rats

In the second experimental model of LV hypertrophy, in which there was a good correlation between G-6-PD activity and heart weight, spontaneously hypertensive rats (SHR) were treated with triiodothyronine (T_3) for 14 days. Application of T_3 for 5 days did not induce an increase in G-6-PD activity in control rat hearts [14]. The time of the treatment period may have been too short for G-6-PD activity to become enhanced. However, a 14-day treatment period with T_3 of SHR that had already developed a marked degree of cardiac hypertrophy induced additional myocardial cell growth as well as an increase in cardiac function and G-6-PD activity [37]. Discontinuation of T_3 treatment for another 14 days normalized all parameters (figure 5). It is surprising, however, that there was no elevation in G-6-PD activity in the hearts of SHR that were already hypertrophied (figure 5). It may be that mechanisms other than activation of the oxidative PPP and, in particular, an increase in G-6-PD activity prevail in genetically induced cardiac hypertrophy.

Right ventricular hypertrophy induced by intermittent hypoxia

The notion that G-6-PD is a marker of established cardiac hypertrophy applies not only to LV hypertrophy but also to RV hypertrophy. RV hypertrophy was induced by exposure of rats to intermittent hypoxia. Hypoxia has been shown to induce an immediate elevation of pulmonary arterial pressure in cats [38]. This hypoxic vaso-constriction is a unique feature of the pulmonary circulation and is in striking contrast to the systemic circulation, which responds to hypoxia with vasodilation. It is therefore not surprising that long-term exposure to high altitude in humans leads to an increase in pulmonary artery pressure [39]. Such increased pulmonary artery pressure has an effect on the right heart to such a degree that the normal difference between the wall thickness of the left and right heart is eliminated, as autopsies of children living at high altitude have revealed [40]. Also, there is a pronounced muscularization of the terminal arterial lung vessels at high altitudes [41].

When rats were exposed to intermittent hypoxia (10% O_2, 8 hours/day, 5 days/week, 20 days exposure), G-6-PD activity was enhanced exclusively in the right ventricle in which systolic pressure was elevated and which had developed hypertrophy, in contrast to the LV, which did not respond to chronic intermittent hypoxia. Figure 6 shows the effects of hypoxia that led to an elevation in RV weight and RV G-6-PD. When the AT_1 receptor blocker losartan was simultaneously administered during the entire hypoxic exposure period, this increase was attenuated to about the same extent [42]. These experimental studies again showed a good parallel behavior of G-6-PD activity and heart weight.

From the studies of these three cardiac hypertrophy models, it appears that there was a good correlation between G-6-PD activity, heart function, and heart weight.

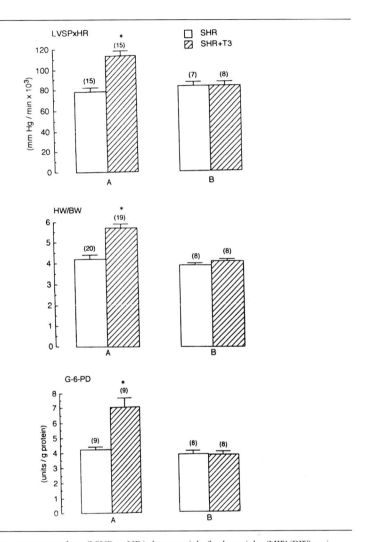

Figure 5. Heart rate–pressure product (LSVP × HR), heart-weight/body-weight (HW/BW) ratio, and glucose-6-phosphate dehydrogenase (G-6-PD) activity in SHR with daily injections of 0.9% NaCl (blank bars) and with daily injection of T_3 (hatched bars) at the end of the treatment period of 14 days duration (**A**) and at the end of 14 days after discontinuation of T_3 treatment (**B**). Data are mean values ± SEM; the number of experiments is in parentheses. ★, $p < 0.01$.

The importance of G-6-PD for cell growth was also demonstrated in studies on several cell lines, in which inhibition of G-6-PD activity abrogated cell growth and overexpression of G-6-PD stimulated cell growth. Moreover, it was shown that when G-6-PD activity was inhibited by dehydroepiandrosterone (DHEA), the NADPH/NAD ratio was also lowered. This decrease seemed to be detrimental to cell growth. It was therefore concluded that the intracellular redox potential that is

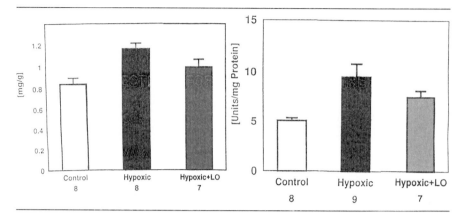

Figure 6. Heart-weight/body-weight ratio (left-hand panel) and activity of cardiac glucose-6-phosphate dehydrogenase (right-hand panel) in control rats, after 4 weeks of intermittent hypoxia without and with losartan treatment (LO, 12 mg/kg/d). Data are mean values ± SEM; the number of experiments is below the respective experimental groups. The hypoxic values are statistically significant ($p < 0.05$ vs. controls).

determined by NADPH, the principal intracellular reductant, may play an important role in the regulation of cell growth [43]. When these findings are taken together, it appears that G-6-PD activity and the intracellular redox potential are related to cell growth and that, in the rat heart, G-6-PD seems to be a marker of experimentally induced cardiac hypertrophy.

REFERENCES

1. Warburg O, Christian W. 1931. Über Aktivierung der Robinsonschen Hexose-Mono-Phosphorsäure in roten Blutzellen und die Gewinnung aktivierender Fermentlösungen. Biochem Z 242:206–227.
2. Meijer AE. 1991. The pentose phosphate pathway in skeletal muscle under pathophysiological conditions. A combined histochemical and biochemical study. Progr Histochem Cytochem 22:1–118.
3. Zimmer H-G, Ibel H, Suchner U. 1990. β-Adrenergic agonists stimulate the oxidative pentose phosphate pathway in the rat heart. Circ Res 67:1525–1534.
4. Reimer KA, Hill ML, Jennings RB. 1981. Prolonged depletion of ATP and of the adenine nucleotide pool due to delayed resynthesis of adenine nucleotides following reversible myocardial ischemic injury in dogs. J Mol Cell Cardiol 13:229–239.
5. Zimmer H-G, Ibel H. 1984. Ribose accelerates the repletion of the ATP pool during recovery from reversible ischemia of the rat myocardium. J Mol Cell Cardiol 16:863–866.
6. Zimmer H-G, Ibel H, Suchner U, Schad H. 1984. Ribose intervention in the cardiac pentose phosphate pathway is not species-specific. Science 223:712–714.
7. Zimmer H-G, Trendelenburg C, Kammermeier H, Gerlach E. 1973. De novo synthesis of myocardial adenine nucleotides in the rat. Acceleration during recovery from oxygen deficiency. Circ Res 32:635–642.
8. Yoshida A, Beutler E (eds). 1986. Glucose-6-Phosphate Dehydrogenase. New York: Academic Press.
9. Negelein E, Haas E. 1936. Über die Wirkungsweise des Zwischenferments. Biochem Z 282:206–220.
10. Eggleston LV, Krebs HA. 1974. Regulation of the pentose phosphate cycle. Biochem J 138:425–435.
11. Zimmer H-G, Bünger R, Koschine H, Steinkopff G. 1981. Rapid stimulation of the hexose monophosphate shunt in the isolated perfused rat heart: possible involvement of oxidized glutathione. J Mol Cell Cardiol 13:531–535.

12. Borregaard N, Schwartz JH, Tauber AI. 1984. Proton secretion by stimulated neutrophils. Significance of hexose monophosphate shunt activity as source of electrons and protons for the respiratory burst. J Clin Invest 74:455–459.

13. Zimmer H-G, Lankat-Buttgereit B, Kolbeck-Rühmkorff C, Nagano T, Zierhut W. 1992. Effects of norepinephrine on the oxidative pentose phosphate pathway in the rat heart. Circ Res 71:451–459.

14. Zimmer H-G, Ibel H, Gerlach E. 1980. Significance of the hexose monophosphate shunt in experimentally induced cardiac hypertrophy. Basic Res Cardiol 75:207–213.

15. Zierhut W, Zimmer H-G. 1989. Significance of myocardial α- and β-adrenoceptors in catecholamine-induced cardiac hypertrophy. Circ Res 65:1417–1425.

16. Zimmer H-G. 1996. Regulation of and intervention into the oxidative pentose phosphate pathway and adenine nucleotide metabolism in the heart. Mol Cell Biochem 160/161:101–109.

17. Seymour A-ML, Eldar H, Radda GK. 1990. Hyperthyroidism results in increased glycolytic capacity in the rat heart. A ^{31}P-NMR study. Biochim Biophys Acta 1055:107–116.

18. Wagner KR, Kauffman FC, Max SR. 1978. The pentose phosphate pathway in regenerating skeletal muscle. Biochem J 170:17–22.

19. Glock GE, McLean P. 1955. Levels of oxidized and reduced diphosphopyridine nucleotide and triphosphopyridine nucleotide in animals tissues. Biochem J 61:388–390.

20. Dow JW, Nigdikar S, Bowditch J. 1985. Adenine nucleotide synthesis de novo in mature rat cardiac myocytes. Biochim Biophys Acta 847:223–227.

21. Zimmer H-G, Ibel H, Steinkopff G, Korb G. 1980. Reduction of the isoproterenol-induced alterations in cardiac adenine nucleotides and morphology by ribose. Science 207:319–321.

22. Zimmer H-G, Peffer H. 1986. Metabolic aspects of the development of experimental cardiac hypertrophy. Basic Res Cardiol 81(Suppl 1):127–137.

23. Chatham JC, Challiss RAJ, Radda GK. 1985. Seymour A-ML: studies on the protective effect of ribose in myocardial ischaemia by using ^{31}P-nuclear-magnetic-resonance spectroscopy. Biochem Soc Trans 13:885–886.

24. Pasque MK, Spray TL, Pellom GL, van Trigt P, Peyton RB, Currie W, Wechsler AS. 1982. Ribose-enhanced myocardial recovery following ischemia in the isolated working rat heart. J Thorac Cardiovasc Surg 83:390–398.

25. Seifart HI, Delabar U, Siess M. 1980. The influence of various precursors on the concentration of energy-rich phosphates and pyridine nucleotides in cardiac tissue and its possible meaning for anoxic survival. Basic Res Cardiol 75:57–61.

26. Haas GS, DeBoer LWV, O'Keefe DD, Bodenhamer RM, Geffin GA, Drop LJ, Teplick RS, Daggett WM. 1984. Reduction of postischemic myocardial dysfunction by substrate repletion during reperfusion. Circulation 70(Suppl I):I-65–I-74.

27. Mauser M, Hoffmeister HM, Nienaber C, Schaper W. 1985. Influence of ribose, adenosine, and "AICAR" on the rate of myocardial adenosine triphosphate synthesis during reperfusion after coronary artery occlusion in the dog. Circ Res 56:220–230.

28. Ward HB, St Cyr JA, Cogordan JA, Alyono D, Bioanco RW, Kriett JM, Foker JE. 1984. Recovery of adenine nucleotide levels after global ischemia in dogs. Surgery 96:248–253.

29. Wyatt DA, Ely SW, Lasley RD, Walsh R, Mainwaring R, Berne RM, Mentzer RM. 1989. Purine-enriched asanguineous cardioplegia retards adenosine triphosphate degradation during ischemia and improves postischemic ventricular function. J Thorac Cardiovasc Surg 97:771–778.

30. Zimmer H-G, Martius PA, Marschner G. 1989. Myocardial infarction in rats: effects of metabolic and pharmacologic interventions. Basic Res Cardiol 84:332–343.

31. Clay MA, Stewart-Richardson P, Tasset DM, Williams JF. 1988. Chronic alcoholic cardiomyopathy. Protection of the isolated ischaemic working heart by ribose. Biochem Internat 17:791–800.

32. Zoref-Shani E, Shainberg A, Sperling O. 1982. Characterization of purine nucleotide metabolism in primary rat muscle cultures. Biochim Biophys Acta 716:324–330.

33. Zimmer H-G. 1983. Normalization of depressed heart function in rats by ribose. Science 220:81–82.

34. Isselhard W, Hamaji M, Mäurer W, Erkens H, Welter H. 1985. Adenosine-induced increase in myocardial adenine nucleotides without adenosine-induced systemic hypotension. Basic Res Cardiol 80:47–61.

35. Seesko RC, Zimmer H-G. 1990. Hemodynamic effects of inosine in combination with positive and negative inotropic drugs: studies on rats in vivo. J Cardiovasc Pharmacol 16:249–256.

36. Zimmer H-G, Zierhut W, Marschner G. 1987. Combination of ribose with calcium antagonist and β-blocker treatment in closed-chest rats. J Mol Cell Cardiol 19:635–639.

37. Heckmann M, Zimmer H-G. 1992. Effects of triiodothyronine in spontaneously hypertensive rats. Studies on cardiac metabolism, function, and heart weight. Basic Res Cardiol 87:333–343.
38. von Euler US, Liljestrand G. 1946. Observations on the pulmonary arterial pressure in the cat. Acta Physiol Scand 12:301–320.
39. Rotta A, Canepa A, Hurtado A, Velasquez T, Chavez R. 1956. Pulmonary circulation at sea level and at high altidues. J Appl Physiol 9:328–336.
40. Arias-Stella J, Recavarren S. 1962. Right ventricular hypertrophy in native children living at high altitude. Am J Pathol 41:55–64.
41. Arias-Stella J, Saldana M. 1963. The terminal portion of the pulmonary arterial tree in people native to high altitudes. Circulation 28:915–925.
42. Irlbeck M, Iwai T, Lerner T, Zimmer H-G. 1997. Effects of angiotensin II receptor blockade on hypoxia-induced right ventricular hypertrophy in rats. J Mol Cell Cardiol 29:2931–2939.
43. Tian W-N, Braunstein LD, Pang J, Stuhlmeier KM, Xi Q-C, Tian X, Stanton RC. 1998. Importance of glucose-6-phosphate dehydrogenase for cell growth. J Biol Chem 273:10609–10617.

N. Takeda, M. Nagano and N.S. Dhalla
(eds). The Hypertrophied Heart. Copyright
© 2000. pp. 31–40. Kluwer Academic
Publishers. Boston. All rights reserved.

REGULATION OF RIBOSOMAL DNA TRANSCRIPTION DURING CARDIOMYOCYTE HYPERTROPHY

TORU ARINO,[1] ROSS D. HANNAN,[2] KIYOFUMI SUZUKI,[3]
and LAWRENCE I. ROTHBLUM[3]

[1] Department of Internal Medicine 4, Aoto Hospital, Jikei University, School of Medicine, Katsushika-ku,

Tokyo, Japan; [2] Molecular and Physiology Laboratory, Baker Medical Research Institute, Melbourne,

Victoria, Australia; [3] Henry Hood Research Program, Weis Center for Research, Geisinger Clinic,

Danville, Pennsylvania, USA

Summary. Cardiomyocyte hypertrophy, induced by norepinephrine, endothelin-I, and contraction, is associated with increased rates of protein synthesis and reexpression of genes associated with the fetal gene program. The signal transduction pathways that link these stimuli to alterations in phenotype and protein accumulation are poorly understood. The increased rate of protein synthesis associated with cardiac hypertrophy is facilitated by an increase in the rate of transcription of the ribosomal genes (rDNA). We have demonstrated that norepinephrine or contraction-induced changes in the expression of an rDNA transcription factor, UBF, can account for the increased rates of rDNA transcription. Endothelin-1 stimulated the phosphorylation of UBF but not the cellular content of UBF. These results suggest that norepinephrine or contraction and endothelin-1 modulate both ribosome biogenesis and cardiomyocyte hypertrophy via different signal transduction pathways.

RIBOSOME BIOGENESIS DURING CARDIAC GROWTH

There is significant evidence, from experiments with intact hearts and from studies on neonatal cardiomyocytes in culture, that hypertrophic cardiac growth is the result of increased protein accumulation. Accelerated cellular protein synthesis can be regulated at the level of efficiency of protein elongation and/or by the capacity to produce new protein by elevating functional ribosome content. Available evidence indicates that the latter mechanism is the most likely to account for increased protein synthesis during cardiac hypertrophy. This conclusion has been draw from two major observations. First, at least 80–90% of existing ribosomes in nongrowing adult hearts are in the form of polysomes (i.e., they are already engaged in protein synthesis) [1,2]. Thus, the availability of components of the translation pathway and the rate of peptide chain initiation do not appear to be limiting to growth. Second, hypertrophy associated with the administration of either thyroid or adrenergic hormones that observed in response to pressure overload is associated not only with increased cardiac ribosomal RNA content and RNA synthesis [2–4] but also with accelerated ribosome formation [3,5].

Clearly, the increase in ribosome content is a significant event that occurs during the hypertrophic growth of the heart. These findings have led to the examination of the control of ribosome biogenesis as an initial step in the elucidation of the mechanisms that regulate cardiac hypertrophic growth.

rDNA TRANSCRIPTION AND THE CONTROL OF CARDIOMYOCYTE GROWTH

Ribosome biogenesis is a complex process. Potentially, the process could be regulated at one or more steps. Possible sites for regulation would include transcription of the ribosomal precursor genes (45S and 5S), preribosomal RNA processing, assembly of the preribosomal subunits, and transport from the nucleus to the cytoplasm. The relative contributions of each and every step to the accumulation of ribosomes during cardiac hypertrophy has not been investigated. However, studies on ribosome biogenesis in cardiomyocytes as well as in other systems, such as cultured skeletal muscle cells, have demonstrated that the initiation of transcription of the rDNA (45S pre-rRNA genes) is a key step in the regulation of ribosome biogenesis [4,6–8].

Evidence that the accelerated rates of rDNA transcription observed during hypertrophy are sufficient for increased ribosome accumulation has been obtained using primary cultures of neonatal cardiomyocytes [4,6–8]. Under the appropriate culture conditions, the neonatal cardiomyocytes maintain their phenotype for up to 10 days and exhibit hypertrophic growth in response to the appropriate stimuli [9]. This growth process is accompanied by many of the phenotypic changes observed during certain forms of hypertrophy of adult cardiomyocytes in vivo [10–12].

Both humoral and mechanical agents promote hypertrophy in this system (figure 1). When neonatal cardiomyocytes are plated at a relatively high density and are allowed to spontaneously contract, the cells accumulate more protein than cells that are contraction arrested [13]. Vasoactive agents, such as norepinephrine [14] and endothelin-1 [16], and activators of protein kinases, such as the active phorbol ester phorbol 12-myristate 13-acetate (PMA) [7,16], also induce hypertrophic growth to various degrees. It is important to note that the hypertrophic effects of norepinephrine and endothelin-1 are independent of their effects on cardiomyocyte contractility, since hypertrophic growth is observed in contraction-arrested cardiomyocytes.

As with in vivo studies, experiments in vitro have clearly substantiated the role of rDNA transcription in the hypertrophic growth of neonatal cardiomyocytes induced by diverse stimuli, including adrenergic agents [14], phorbol esters [7,16], and endothelin-1 [16] (figure 2). In each case, the increased rDNA transcription correlates temporally and quantitatively with the observed increases in protein synthesis. The weight of current evidence supports the hypothesis that increased rDNA

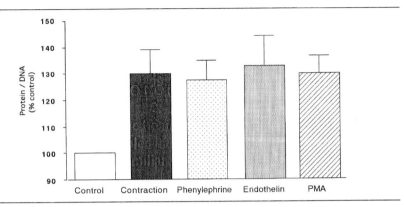

Figure 1. Protein accumulation in cultured neonatal cardiomyocytes in response to contraction, treatment with norepinephrine, PMA, or endothelin-1. Contraction-arrested neonatal cardiomyocytes cultured at 4×10^6 cells/60 mm plate were treated and allowed to contract or treated with either norepinephrine (1 μM), PMA (0.1 μM), or endothelin-I (0.1 μM), and after 48 hours total cellular protein was determined by standard methods and normalized for the DNA content per plate. Results are expressed as the percentage increase in protein-to-DNA ratio of norepinephrine-treated cells over time as compared to control cells. Vertical lines represent standard deviation from the mean for five or more independent experiments.

transcription is an important regulatory step in protein accumulation during cardiomyocyte hypertrophy [1].

rDNA TRANSCRIPTION FACTORS AND CARDIOMYOCYTE HYPERTROPHY

Increased rates of rDNA transcription can be due to alterations in the chromatin structure or changes in the amounts and/or activities of RNA polymerase I and/or of the associated rDNA transcription factors. To fully characterize the mechanisms of rDNA transcription during hypertrophy of the heart will require a detailed examination of each of these potential control points. However, studies (summarized below) demonstrate that RNA polymerase I itself does not appear to be a target of the regulation during cardiomyocyte hypertrophy. Rather, there is a strong correlation between the expression/phosphorylation of upstream binding factor (UBF) and the growth status of cardiomyocytes in culture [17–19]. Such studies indicate that this gene product may contribute to the regulation of ribosome biogenesis during cardiomyocyte hypertrophy.

REGULATION OF RNA POLYMERASE I DURING HYPERTROPHY

The increased level of transcription by RNA polymerase I that was demonstrated in the nuclear run on assay (figure 2) could result from (1) an increased amount of RNA polymerase I, (2) an increase in the specific activity of the enzyme, or (3) an increase in the fraction of the enzyme that was engaged in actively transcribing the ribosomal chromatin. Measurement of total enzyme activity present in solubilized

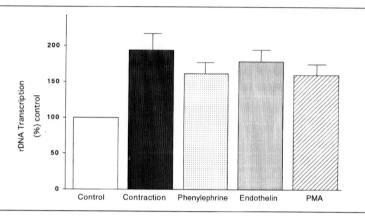

Figure 2. rDNA transcription in cultured neonatal cardiomyocytes that were allowed to spontaneously contract, or in arrested cardiomyocytes following exposure to norepinephrine, PMA, or endothelin-1. Neonatal cardiomyocytes, cultured at 4×10^6 cell/60 mm plate and stimulated for 24 hours with norepinephrine ($1 \mu M$), PMA ($0.1 \mu M$), or endothelin-1 ($0.1 \mu M$), were allowed to spontaneously contract (beating) for 24 hours, and nuclei were isolated from 16×10^6 cells per time point. RNA polymerase I transcription was measured by nuclear run-on assays, hybridization of the radiolabeled transcripts to 45 S rDNA (clone pU5.1E/X), and visualization of the hybrids by autoradiography. Control cells were contraction arrested by the addition of 50 mM KCl and were treated with vehicle for 24 hours before rDNA transcription was measured.

cell extracts of hypertrophic (either contracting or contraction-arrested cells stimulated with norepinephrine) cardiomyocytes demonstrated that the hypertrophic myocytes contained essentially the same amount (106%) of enzyme activity as the control (contraction-arrested) cardiomyocytes [13]. Moreover, Western analysis of whole-cell extracts using a monospecific antibody to the 194 kDa subunit of RNA polymerase I confirmed that the number of RNA polymerase-1 molecules was unaltered during hypertrophy [13]. Thus, it is likely that the increased rate of rDNA transcription demonstrated in the nuclear run on assays reflects an increase in the fraction of RNA polymerase I engaged in transcription. This in turn suggests that the hypertrophic stimuli must be linked to a mechanism(s) that results in the more efficient recruitment of RNA polymerase I to the ribosomal chromatin. It is formally possible that this event is mediated by one or more of the known rDNA transcription factors or is even due to the activity of a novel factor. However, there was sufficient evidence from studies on the mechanism of rDNA transcription to examine the hypothesis that the various hypertrophic stimuli were in fact altering the cellular activity of the rDNA transcription factor referred to as UBF, which in turn would alter the efficiency of rDNA transcription.

EVIDENCE FOR THE REGULATION OF UBF DURING THE HYPERTROPHIC GROWTH OF CULTURED NEONATAL CARDIOMYOCYTES

Experiments utilizing the cultured neonatal cardiomyocyte model described above demonstrated an association between UBF expression and ribosome biogenesis

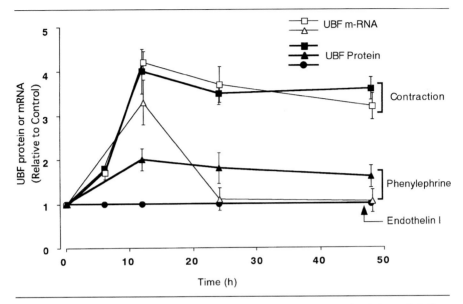

Figure 3. UBF protein levels in neonatal cardiomyocytes in response to norepinephrine, endothelin-1, or contraction. Total cellular protein was extracted from arrested neonatal cardiomyocytes cultured at 4×10^6 cells/60 mm plate at the times indicated after treatment with vehicle, norepinephrine, or endothelin-1. Alternatively, total cellular protein was extracted at the times indicated from spontaneously contracting neonatal cardiomyocytes cultured at 4×10^6 cells/60 mm plate. After SDS-PAGE and Western transfer, UBF1 and UBF2 protein was detected with a rabbit anti-UBF antibody and visualized by ECL (Amersham). UBF mRNA levels in neonatal cardiomyocytes were measured following treatment with norepinephrine, with endothelin-1, or after spontaneously contraction. Total RNA was extracted from the contraction-arrested (50 mM KCl), percoll-purified neonatal cardiomyocytes after 12 hours of treatment with vehicle, norepinephrine, or endothelin-1, or from spontaneously contracting cardiomyocytes. After electrophoresis and Northern blotting, the RNA was hybridized to [^{32}P]-labeled UBF cDNA, and UBF mRNA transcripts were detected by autoradiography.

[14,20]. For example, when the rDNA transcription rate is elevated in neonatal cardiomyocytes in response to norepinephrine or contraction, the levels of UBF increased (2–2.5- and 3–4-fold, respectively) compared to time-matched contraction-arrested cells [13,14] (figure 3). The increased UBF protein content in the cardiomyocytes was first observable 6–12 hours following initiation of the stimuli, and the UBF content remained elevated for up to 4 days [14]. Elevations in UBF content in response to contraction or norepinephrine correlated both temporally and quantitatively with the accelerated rates of rDNA transcription observed in response to the two stimuli. For example, the increase in UBF content in response to norepinephrine was maximal after 12 hours; thus, accumulation of UBF preceded the time of maximal rates of rDNA transcription (24 hours). Second, the increase in UBF protein following norepinephrine stimulation was less than that observed in response to contraction, paralleling the relative rates of rDNA transcription

observed in response to the two stimuli [14]. These experiments provided correlative evidence for the hypothesis that alterations in the level of UBF protein were responsible for the elevated rates of rDNA transcription observed during the hypertrophy that resulted from contraction and norepinephrine stimulation. Additional evidence for this hypothesis has been provided by experiments in which we have been able to demonstrate that the overexpression of UBF in contraction-arrested cardiomyocytes can drive rDNA transcription [15].

POSTTRANSLATIONAL MODIFICATION OF UBF

UBF is a phosphoprotein [17], and studies with cell-free extracts have shown that hypophosphorylated UBF is less efficient at stimulating rDNA transcription than phosphorylated forms of the protein [21,22]. It is interesting to note that the relative degree of phosphorylation of UBF per molecule was no greater in spontaneously contracting, hypertrophying cells than that observed in contractile-arrested, nongrowing neonatal cardiomyocytes [13]. Thus, increases in the overall cellular content, rather than alterations in the degree of phosphorylation, appear to contribute to changes in the transcriptional activity of this rDNA transcription factor during contraction and norepinephrine-induced cardiomyocyte hypertrophy. These results do not eliminate possible qualitative differences in the sites of UBF phosphorylated during periods of cardiomyocyte growth and quiescence.

In fact, studies on the regulation of UBF activity in response to treatment with PMA and endothelin-1 suggest the importance of the regulation of phosphorylation of UBF during hypertrophy. Treatment of cells with endothelin-1 and PMA, agents that can induce hypertrophy [14,23–26] and rDNA transcription, did not increase UBF mRNA [14] or protein levels (figure 3). Instead, similar to what was observed when the response of CHO cells to serum starvation and refeeding was examined [17], the protein was hyperphosphorylated [16]. In fact, the kinetics of UBF phosphorylation paralleled the rate of increase in rDNA transcription observed in response to these agents, and the hyperphosphorylation was maintained for at least 24 hours [16]. Since the ability of UBF to activate transcription is proportional to its phosphorylation state, it would seem that treatment with PMA and endothelin-1 affect rDNA transcription at the same regulatory step as do norepinephrine and contraction, but through a different pathway(s).

These findings also suggest that an increase in the level of cellular UBF is not necessary for the induction of neonatal cardiomyocyte hypertrophy in response to all stimuli. Thus, UBF may contribute to accelerated rDNA transcription through two mechanisms: (1) an increase in the amount of active UBF and (2) an increase in the activity of preexisting UBF.

TRANSCRIPTIONAL CONTROL OF UBF EXPRESSION

Possible mechanisms by which increased amounts of UBF protein are effected by hypertrophic stimuli include pre- and posttranslational regulation. Northern blot analysis reveals that increased UBF mRNA levels contribute, at least in part, to the accumulation of UBF protein in response to norepinephrine [14] and contraction. Moreover, similar results were obtained from neonatal cardiomyocytes that had been purified by centrifugation through Percoll density gradients [27]. Cardiomyocyte cultures prepared in such a manner contain less than 1% nonmyocardial cells (NMCs) as determined immunohistochemically. Therefore, these studies indicate that NMCs are not required for the induction of UBF mRNA during norepinephrine-induced hypertrophy. We have carried out similar experiments with cardiomyocytes plated at densities as low as 0.5×10^6 cells/60 mm plate and have found that the quantitative induction of UBF by adrenergic agents is not affected by cell-plating density [14].

The rate of increase in UBF mRNA is rapid. Elevated levels of UBF mRNA are detectable within 3–6 hours following either norepinephrine or contraction stimulus. Nuclear run-on experiments demonstrate that an increased rate of transcription of the UBF gene could account for the elevation in UBF mRNA. Interestingly, UBF mRNA levels are sustained in response to contraction; the increases in UBF transcripts following norepinephrine treatment are transient, returning to the levels found in untreated cells within 24–36 hours [14]. Since UBF protein content remains elevated during norepinephrine stimulation, posttranslational mechanisms of control, such as protein stabilization, may also contribute to the regulation of this transcription factor [14].

Nuclear run-on assays demonstrated that increased transcription of the UBF gene was at least partly responsible for the accrued cellular content of UBF mRNA observed in response to contraction [13] or norepinephrine stimulation. Thus, the UBF gene must contain cis-acting elements capable of responding to these stimuli. While adrenergic agents can effect altered levels of gene expression through several different combinations of cis-acting elements and trans-acting factors, there are no studies to suggest the mechanism through which a mechanical stimulus, such as contraction, might affect cardiomyocyte transcription. Moreover, attempts to unravel the signal transduction pathways that link contraction to hypertrophy have failed, since the traditional protein kinase and phosphatase inhibitors used to study these pathways also inhibit contraction. Therefore, it is of considerable interest to determine the cis-acting elements that link contraction to UBF transcription, since this will facilitate the elucidation of the signal transduction pathways that couple these two events. As a first step in this process, we examined the hypothesis that the UBF gene contains such cis-acting elements.

To test the hypothesis that the UBF gene contains cis-acting elements that respond to contraction, we transfected arrested and contracting cultured neonatal cardiomyocytes with various UBF/CAT constructs and compared the levels of CAT activity expressed (figure 4). As demonstrated in figure 4, phenylephrine-stimulated or -contracting [13] cardiomyocytes transfected with a fragment of the UBF gene extending from −3124 to +93 (+1 being the transcription initiation site) demonstrated a threefold increase in CAT activity as compared to noncontracting cardiomyocytes. On the other hand, a construct that extended from −665 to +93 did not respond to either stimulus. These results suggested that the UBF gene contains

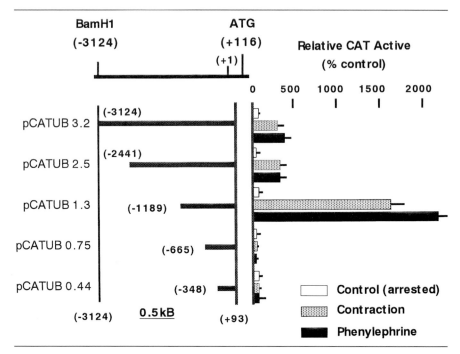

Figure 4. Analysis of UBF promoter activity by transient expression in arrested and contracting cardiomyocytes. Neonatal cardiomyocytes were transfected with either pCAT0.44, pCATUB0.75, pCATUB1.3, pCATUB2.5, or pCATUB3.2 and were either arrested by the addition of 50 mM KCl to the serum-free defined media, arrested and treated with norepinephrine (0.1 μM), or allowed to contract. Twenty-four hours later, extracts were made from the cardiomyocytes and assayed for CAT activity. Neonatal cardiomyocytes were cotransfected with the indicated constructs of the UBF prompter linked to the bacterial chloramphenicol acetyltransferase gene and the pCMV-β-gal construct, and treated as described above. Twenty-four hours after transfection, cells were harvested, and extracts were prepared and assayed for CAT and β-galactosidase activity. The CAT activity in each extract was normalized for the recovery of β-galactosidase activity to correct for differences in transfection efficiency. The normalized activity of pCATUB3.2 in arrested cardiomyocytes is indicated as 100%. The normalized activities of the remainder of the constructs are shown as a percentage of pCATUB3.2.

cis-acting elements capable of responding to both phenylephrine and contraction and that these elements lie between −3124 and −665. Subsequent experiments with a more complete set of 5′ deletion mutants demonstrated that this element lies between −1189 and −665 of the UBF gene. In addition, these experiments suggest that the region between −2441 and −1189 is capable of repressing the induction of transcription from the UBF gene, since deleting this segment resulted in an amplification of the response to both contraction and phenylephrine.

REFERENCES

1. Morgan HE, Chua BHL, Russo L. 1992. Protein synthesis and degradation. In: The Heart and Cardiovascular System. Ed. G. Fozzard et al., 1505–1524. New York: Raven Press.

2. Siehl D, Chua BH, Lautensack-Belser N, Morgan HE. 1985. Faster protein and ribosome synthesis in thyroxine-induced hypertrophy of rat heart. Am J Physiol 248:C309–C319.

3. Morgan HE, Gordon EE, Kira Y, Chua HL, Russo LA, Peterson CJ, McDermott PJ, Watson PA. 1987. Biochemical mechanisms of cardiac hypertrophy. Annu Rev Physiol 49:533–543.

4. Cutilletta AF, Rudnik M, Zak R. 1978. Muscle and non-muscle cell RNA polymerase activity during the development of myocardial hypertrophy. J Mol Cell Cardiol 10:677–687.

5. Watson PA, Haneda T, Morgan HE. 1989. Effect of higher aortic pressure on ribosome formation and cAMP content in rat heart. Am J Physiol 256:C1257–C1261.

6. McDermott PJ, Rothblum LI, Smith SD, Morgan HE. 1989. Accelerated rates of ribosomal RNA synthesis during growth of contracting heart cells in culture. J Biol Chem 264:18220–18227.

7. Allo SN, McDermott PJ, Carl LL, Morgan HE. 1991. Phorbol ester stimulation of protein kinase C activity and ribosomal DNA transcription. Role in hypertrophic growth of cultured cardiomyocytes. J Biol Chem 266:22003–22009.

8. McDermott PJ, Morgan HE. 1989. Contraction modulates the capacity for protein synthesis during growth of neonatal heart cells in culture. Circ Res 64:542–553.

9. Simpson P, McGrath A, Savion S. 1982. Myocyte hypertrophy in neonatal rat heart cultures and its regulation by serum and by catecholamines. Circ Res 51:787–801.

10. Parker TG, Schneider MD. 1991. Growth factors, proto-oncogenes, and plasticity of the cardiac phenotype. Annu Rev Physiol 53:179–200.

11. Bilsen M, Chien KR. 1993. Growth and hypertrophy of the heart. J Cardiovasc Res 27:P1140–P1149.

12. Chien KR, Knowlton KU, Zhu H, Chien S. 1991. Regulation of cardiac gene expression during myocardial growth and hypertrophy: molecular studies of an adaptive physiologic response. FASEB J 5:3037–3046.

13. Hannan RD, Luyken J, Rothblum LI. 1996. Regulation of ribosomal DNA transcription during contraction-induced hypertrophy of neonatal cardiomyocytes. J Biol Chem 271:3213–3220.

14. Hannan RD, Luyken J, Rothblum LI. 1995. Regulation of rDNA transcription factors during cardiomyocyte hypertrophy induced by adrenergic agents. J Biol Chem 270:8290–8297.

15. Hannan RD, Stefanovsky V, Taylor L, Moss T, Rothblum LI. 1996. Overexpression of the transcription factor UBF1 is sufficient to increase ribosomal DNA transcription in neonatal cardiomyocytes: implications for cardiac hypertrophy. Proc Natl Acad Sci USA 93:8750–8755.

16. Luyken J, Hannan RD, Cheung JY, Rothblum LI. 1996. Regulation of rDNA transcription during endothelin-1-induced hypertrophy of neonatal cardiomyoctes. Hyperphosphorylation of upstream binding factor, an rDNA transcription factor. Circ Res 78:354–361.

17. O'Mahony DJ, Xie WQ, Smith SD, Singer HA, Rothblum LI. 1992. Differential phosphorylation and localization of the transcription factor UBF in vivo in response to serum deprivation. In vitro dephosphorylation of UBF reduces its transactivation properties. J Biol Chem 267:35–38.

18. Larson DE, Xie W, Glibetic M, O'Mahony D, Sells BH, Rothblum LI. 1993. Coordinated decreases in rRNA gene transcription factors and rRNA snythesis during muscle cell differentiation. Proc Natl Acad Sci USA 90:7933–7936.

19. Glibetic M, Taylor L, Larson D, Hannan R, Sells B, Rothblum L. 1995. The RNA polymerase I transcription factor UBF is the product of a primary response gene. J Biol Chem 270:4209–4212.

20. Xie WQ, Rothblum LI. 1993. rDNA transcription and cardiac hypertrophy. Trends Cardiovasc Med 3:7–11.

21. O'Mahony DJ, Smith SD, Xie W, Rothblum LI. 1992. Analysis of the phosphorylation, DNA-binding and dimerization properties of the RNA polymerase I transcription factors UBF1 and UBF2. Nucleic Acids Res 20:1301–1308.

22. Voit R, Schnapp A, Kuhn A, Rosenbauer H, Hirschmann P, Stunnenberg HG, Grummt I. 1992. The nucleolar transcription factor mUBF is phosphorylated by casein kinase II in the C-terminal hyperacidic tail which is essential for transactivation. EMBO J 11:2211–2218.

23. Simpson PC, Kariya K, Karns LR, Long CS, Karliner JS. 1991. Adrenergic hormones and control of cardiac myocyte growth. Mol Cell Biochem 104:35–43.

24. Henrich CJ, Simpson PC. 1988. Differential acute and chronic response of protein kinase C in cultured neonatal rat heart myocytes to alpha 1-adrenergic and phorbol ester stimulation. J Mol Cell Cardiol 20:1081–1085.

25. Puceat M, Hilal-Dandan R, Strulovici B, Brunton LL, Brown JH. 1994. Differential regulation of protein kinase C isoforms in isolated neonatal and adult rat cardiomyocytes. J Biol Chem 269:16938–16944.

26. Bogoyevitch MA, Parker PJ, Sugden PH. 1993. Characterization of protein kinase C isotype expression in adult rat heart. Protein kinase C-epsilon is a major isotype present, and it is activated by phorbol esters, epinephrine, and endothelin. Circ Res 72:757–767.
27. Iwaki K, Sukhatme VP, Shubeita HE, Chien KR. 1990. Alpha- and beta-adrenergic stimulation induces distinct patterns of immediate early gene expression in neonatal rat myocardial cells. fos/jun expression is associated with sarcomere assembly; Egr-1 induction is primarily an alpha 1-mediated response. J Biol Chem 265:13809–13817.

N. Takeda, M. Nagano and N.S. Dhalla
(eds). The Hypertrophied Heart. Copyright
© 2000. pp. 41–49. Kluwer Academic
Publishers. Boston. All rights reserved.

MITOCHONDRIAL GENE EXPRESSION IN HYPERTROPHIC CARDIAC MUSCLES IN RATS

TARO MURAKAMI,[1] YOSHIHARU SHIMOMURA,[1] LI ZHIHAO,[1]
KAZUYUKI SHIMIZU,[2] and SATORU SUGIYAMA[3]

[1] Department of Bioscience, Nagoya Institute of Technology, Gokiso-cho, Showa-ku, Nagoya 466-8555, Japan;
[2] Department of Medicine, Nagoya City Higashi General Hospital, Nagoya 464-8547, Japan; and [3] Institute of
Applied Biochemistry, Gifu 505-01, Japan

Summary. Mitochondrial gene expression and enzyme activities were analyzed in exercise-induced hypertrophic rat heart and SHR heart muscles. Exercise-induced hypertrophic hearts (7% increase in weight relative to body weight compared to that of sedentary rats) were prepared by endurance training of rats for 12 weeks (90 min/day, 5 days/week). Although the activity of cytochrome oxidase and concentrations of cytochrome *b* mRNA and mitochondrial DNA (mtDNA) in gastrocnemius muscle were increased approximately 1.5-fold by training, those in the heart were not altered, suggesting that adaptation in the heart to endurance training is attained by increasing the muscle mass, not by mitochondrial gene expression. The concentration of mtDNA in the SHR heart, which increased in relative weight by 62% compared to that of normal rats, was not altered by hypertrophy, but the concentration of cytochrome *b* mRNA and activities of citrate synthase and cytochrome oxidase in the heart tended to be decreased by hypertrophy. These results suggest that the adaptive response of mitochondrial gene expression to cardiac hypertrophy is different in exercise- and hypertension-induced hypertrophy.

INTRODUCTION

The energy demand for the contraction of muscle cells may be an exclusive factor in determining the oxidative capacity of these cells, which is reflected by the expression of genes that encode enzymes involved in oxidative metabolism. Mitochondria in skeletal muscle adapt to a change of cellular energy status with a coordinated expression of both nuclear and mitochondrial genomes [1–3]. It is well known that endurance training increases the biogenesis of mitochondria in skeletal muscle [4,5]. In contrast, genetic information about the adaptation of mitochondria in cardiac muscle to exercise training is wanting, although the muscle is an exclusively aerobic tissue containing a greater mass of mitochondria in comparison to skeletal muscle [6].

Regular strenuous exercise induces cardiac hypertrophy, although this phenomenon does not occur in skeletal muscle [7–10]. In this case, mitochondrial oxidative capacity is proportional to cardiac hypertrophy [7–10]. These results suggest that gene expression of mitochondrial proteins encoded by nuclear DNA and mitochondrial DNA (mtDNA) are coordinately increased with the gene expression of other cellular proteins during cardiac hypertrophy. Like exercise training, chronic hypertension also induces cardiac hypertrophy [11–13]. In hypertension-induced hypertrophic cardiac muscle, it has been reported that mitochondrial oxidative activity is not proportional to cardiac hypertrophy [11–13]. Therefore, it becomes necessary to characterize the differences between exercise-induced and hypertension-induced cardiac hypertrophy.

The first purpose of the present study was to determine the difference between skeletal and cardiac muscles in the adaptive responses of their mitochondrial gene expression to endurance exercise. The second purpose was to examine the differences in mitochondrial oxidative activity and gene expression between exercise-induced and hypertension-induced hypertrophy in cardiac muscles. We report here that the oxidative activity and content of mtDNA, and its message level relative to those of the other components in cardiac muscle cells, were not altered in exercise-induced cardiac hypertrophy, although some of these measures decreased in hypertension-induced cardiac hypertrophy. These results suggest that the adaptive response of mitochondrial gene expression to cardiac hypertrophy is different in exercise-induced and hypertension-induced hypertrophy.

MATERIALS AND METHODS

Animal care and experimental design

All procedures involving animals were approved by the experimental animal care committee of Nagoya Institute of Technology.

Experiment 1: Effects of exercise-induced cardiac
hypertrophy on mitochondrial gene expression [10]

Sixteen female Sprague-Dawley rats (7 weeks old) were obtained from CLEA Japan, Tokyo. The rats were housed in an animal room at 22°C with light from 12:00 noon to 12:00 midnight and with free access to water and food (commercial rat chow). The animals (at 8 weeks old) were randomly divided into two groups; exercise training ($n = 8$) and sedentary ($n = 8$) groups. The former group of rats was trained for 12 weeks by treadmill running according to our previous study [4] at a speed of 25 m/min at a 6° incline for 90 min/day in the morning, 5 days/week. Twenty-four hours after the final bout of running, rats were anesthetized with ether and sacrificed by exsanguination. Heart and gastrocnemius muscle were immediately removed, freeze-clamped at liquid nitrogen temperature, and stored at −80°C until use.

Experiment 2: Effect of hypertension-induced cardiac
hypertrophy on mitochondrial gene expression

Eight male Wistar rats and spontaneous hypertensive rats (SHR) (7 weeks old) were obtained from SLC, Hamamatsu, and HOS, Yashio, respectively. The rats were housed in an animal room at 22°C with light from 5:00 a.m. to 5:00 p.m. and with free access to water and food (commercial rat chow). After 17 weeks (age of rats: 24 weeks old), heart rate and blood pressure were determined by the tail-cuff method [14] using BP-98A, Softron, Tokyo. On the next day, the rats were anesthetized with ether and sacrificed by exsanguination. The heart was immediately removed, freeze-clamped at liquid nitrogen temperature, and stored at −80°C until use.

Analyses

Extraction of cytochrome oxidase and citrate synthase from tissues was carried out as described previously [4], and the enzyme activities were measured at 25°C by the methods of Smith [15] and Srere [16], respectively. Total cellular DNA was fluorometrically [17] determined using a calf thymus DNA as a standard. Cytochrome *b* mRNA and mtDNA concentrations in gastrocnemius and cardiac muscles were determined by the standard Northern and Southern blot analyses, respectively, using human cytochrome *b* cDNA probe as described previously [4].

Statistics

To evaluate differences between the sedentary and the training groups, data were analyzed by two-tailed Student's *t*-test [18], and $p < 0.05$ was defined as statistically significant.

RESULTS

Experiment 1 [10]

Body weight, heart, and gastrocnemius muscle weights

After 12 weeks of treadmill training, heart weight was significantly greater in trained rats than in sedentary rats (table 1). Also, the ratio of heart weight to body weight showed the same trend (table 1). These results indicate that exercise-induced cardiac hypertrophy occurred after 12 weeks of endurance training. However, the body weight and gastrocnemius muscle weight were not different between sedentary and trained rats (table 1).

Cytochrome oxidase activities in cardiac and gastrocnemius muscles

Cytochrome oxidase is one of the key enzymes in the mitochondrial electron transport chain, and the activity is used as a marker of the mitochondrial oxidative

Table 1. Body weight and cardiac and gastrocnemius muscle weights

	Sedentary	Trained
Body weight (g)	285 ± 7	286 ± 6
Heart (g)	0.73 ± 0.01	0.79 ± 0.02[a]
Heart/Body weight ($\times 10^{-3}$)	2.54 ± 0.07	2.72 ± 0.03[a]
Gastrocnemius muscle (g)	3.55 ± 0.06	3.66 ± 0.09

[a] $p < 0.05$.
Note: Values are means ± SE for eight rats.

capacity. In our previous study [4], we reported that cytochrome oxidase activity in the soleus muscle was increased about 1.5-fold after varying periods (3, 6, and 12 weeks) of treadmill training in rats and that 12 weeks of training were sufficient to increase the oxidative capacity in the skeletal muscle. In the present study, the activity of cytochrome oxidase in gastrocnemius muscle was significantly higher (1.5-fold) in trained rats than in sedentary rats, whereas the enzyme activity in the cardiac muscle was not different between trained and sedentary rats (figure 1A). The enzyme activity in cardiac muscle was approximately eightfold higher than that in gastrocnemius muscle of sedentary rats (figure 1A).

Cytochrome b *mRNA and mitochondrial DNA in heart and gastrocnemius muscle*

In skeletal muscle, endurance training increases the expression of mRNA for mitochondrial enzymes, which are encoded by both nuclear and mitochondrial genomes [4,19], and also increases replication of mitochondrial DNA [4]. It is of interest whether endurance training increases mitochondrial gene expression and replication in cardiac muscle. Northern blot analyses showed that the concentration of mitochondrially encoded cytochrome *b* mRNA in the gastrocnemius muscle was greater (1.5-fold) in trained rats than in sedentary rats; however, the concentration in the cardiac muscle was not different between these groups (figure 1B). Also, Southern blot analyses showed that the mtDNA concentration in gastrocnemius muscle was greater (1.5-fold) in trained rats than in sedentary rats; however, the concentration in the cardiac muscle was not different between these groups (figure 1C). Although concentrations of cytochrome *b* mRNA and mtDNA in the cardiac muscle were not affected by training, these values of sedentary rats were 3.3-fold and 1.7-fold higher, respectively, than those in gastrocnemius muscle of sedentary rats (figures 1B and 1C).

Experiment 2

Body and heart weights

Heart weight was not different between SHR and control rats at the age of 24 weeks (table 2). However, the body weight of SHR was significantly smaller than that of normotensive control rats (table 2). Therefore, the ratio of heart weight to body weight of SHR was significantly greater (1.6-fold) than that of control rats (table 2).

Table 2. Body weight and cardiac muscle weight

	Control	SHR
Body weight (g)	508 ± 9	343 ± 10
Heart (g)	1.18 ± 0.02	1.26 ± 0.04
Heart/body weight ($\times 10^{-3}$)	2.32 ± 0.06	3.67 ± 0.06[a]

[a] $p < 0.001$.
Note: Values are means ± SE for eight rats.

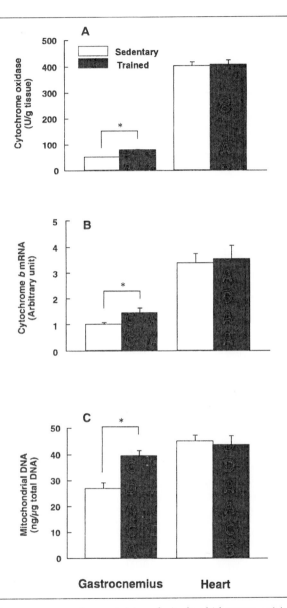

Figure 1. Adaptive responses to endurance training of mitochondrial enzyme activity and mitochondrial gene expression and replication in skeletal and cardiac muscles [10]. (**A**) Cytochrome oxidase activity in gastrocnemius and cardiac muscles of sedentary and trained rats. One unit (U) of cytochrome oxidase catalyzed the oxidation of 1 μmol of reduced cytochrome c/min. (**B**) Relative cytochrome b mRNA expression in gastrocnemius and cardiac muscles of sedentary and trained rats. Northern blots of total RNA (10 μg) from gastrocnemius and cardiac muscles were prepared by capillary blotting after electrophoresis in 1.0% agarose-formaldehyde gels. Cytochrome b mRNA was shown relative to the level of expression of β-actin mRNA. (**C**) Mitochondrial DNA concentration in gastrocnemius and cardiac muscles of sedentary and trained rats. Total DNA (1 μg) extracted from gastrocnemius and cardiac muscles of trained and sedentary rats and purified mitochondrial DNA (10, 20, 50, and 100 ng for standard) were treated with Bgl II restriction endonuclease, followed by Southern blot analysis. Values are means ± SE for eight rats. $\star$, $p < 0.05$.

Table 3. Hemodynamic measurements

	Control	SHR
Heart rate (bpm)	474 ± 23	373 ± 28[a]
Blood pressure (mmHg)		
Mean	103 ± 6	194 ± 5[a]
Systolic	121 ± 8	215 ± 7[a]
Diastolic	96 ± 6	184 ± 4[a]

[a] $p < 0.001$.
Note: Values are means ± SE for eight rats.

Hemodynamic measurements

At the end of the experiment, the heart rate of SHR was significantly lower than that of control rats (table 3). On the other hand, mean systolic and diastolic blood pressures were approximately twofold higher in SHR than in control rats (table 3).

Activities of citrate synthase and cytochrome oxidase in cardiac muscle

Citrate synthase is one of the key enzymes in the tricarboxylic acid (TCA) cycle, and the activity is used as a marker of the mitochondrial oxidative capacity. The activity of citrate synthase was significantly lower in SHR cardiac muscle (0.79-fold) than in control rats (figure 2A). Also, the activity of cytochrome oxidase was significantly lower in SHR hearts (0.75-fold) than in hearts of control rats (figure 2B).

Cytochrome b mRNA and mitochondrial DNA in cardiac and gastrocnemius muscles

Northern blot analyses showed that the concentration of mitochondrially encoded cytochrome *b* mRNA in SHR cardiac muscle was trend to be lower (0.87-fold, $p = 0.09$) than that in control rats (figure 3A). However, Southern blot analyses showed that the mtDNA concentrations in cardiac muscles were not different between SHR and control rats (figure 3B).

DISCUSSION

In the present study, it was found that both endurance exercise training and chronic hypertension induce cardiac hypertrophy. However, the adaptive response of mito-chondrail enzyme activity and gene expression were different between exercise-induced and hypertension-induced cardiac hypertrophy.

Cardiac muscle does not undergo an adaptive increase in the activity of cytochrome oxidase or in the concentrations of cytochrome *b* mRNA and mtDNA by endurance training, although heart weight was significantly increased by training [10]. These responses to training of gene expression and replication of mtDNA in cardiac muscle are different from those in skeletal muscle. Our results are supported by the findings of Oscai et al. [7–9], who have reported that strenuous programs of

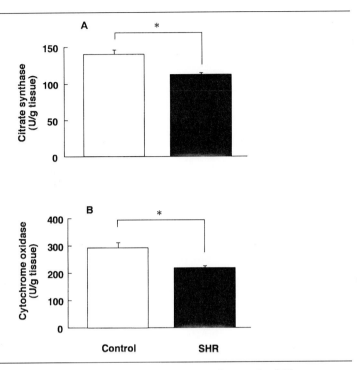

Figure 2. Activities of citrate synthase and cytochrome oxidase in cardiac muscle of Wistar rat and SHR. Values are mean ± SE for eight rats. *, $p < 0.05$. One unit (U) of enzymes catalyzed the formation of 1 μmol of free CoA/min for citrate synthase and oxidation of 1 μmol of reduced cytochrome c/min for cytochrome oxidase.

treadmill running or daily swimming training for rats did not alter the activities of citrate synthase and cytochrome oxidase or the concentrations of cytochrome c or total mitochondrial protein. These findings suggest that gene expression and replication of mtDNA in cardiac muscle is coordinated with gene expression of nuclear DNA for other cell components in exercise-induced cardiac hypertrophy.

In contrast to the mitochondrial adaptation of exercise-induced cardiac hypertrophy, the activities of citrate synthase and cytochrome oxidase in the muscle were decreased by hypertension-induced cardiac hypertrophy. Furthermore, the expression of cytochrome b mRNA tended to be lower in the hypertrophic cardiac muscle. It has been reported that there is a dissociation between mitochondrial and myofibrillar masses in cardiac muscle responding to pressure-induced hypertrophy [6,11–13] or thyroid hormone administration [6]. Tokoro et al. [11,12] reported that activities of isocitrate dehydrogenase, superoxide dismutase, and cytochrome oxidase were lower in cardiac muscle of SHR. They also found two deletions of mtDNA in SHR cardiac muscle and speculated that the lower scavenging activity against oxidative stress in mitochondria might induce alteration of the membrane system

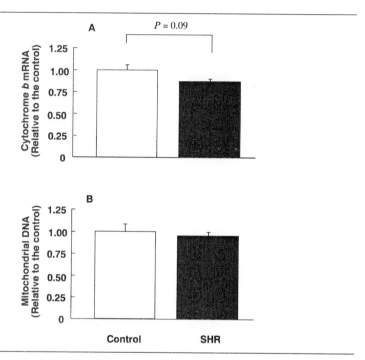

Figure 3. Cytochrome *b* mRNA and mitochondrial DNA concentrations in cardiac muscle of Wistar rat and SHR. Values are means ± SE for eight rats.

of mitochondria and deletions of mtDNA [11,12]. One possible mechanism of lower oxidative activity in SHR cardiac muscle observed in their experiments and ours might be a decrease in accurate mitochondrial gene expression because of the deletions of mtDNA. These findings suggest that mechanisms for mitochondrial adaptation are different in cardiac hypertrophy under normal conditions (such as exercise) and under abnormal conditions. More intensive study is required to clarify the genetic regulation of cardiac hypertrophy.

It should be noted that the activity of cytochrome oxidase and the concentrations of cytochrome *b* mRNA and mtDNA in the cardiac muscle of sedentary rats were 9.4-, 2.3-, and 1.2-fold greater compared to even those in gastrocnemius muscle of trained rats, although the increase in oxidative capacity in the cardiac muscle was not observed via the training. The results obtained in the present study using rats are consistent with those reported for the rabbit and mouse [20,21]. These findings suggest that mitochondrial gene expression in cardiac muscle is regulated at both transcriptional and translational steps. Furthermore, these findings suggest that mitochondrial oxidative capacity in cardiac muscle may have attained a maximal level; therefore, the increase in muscle mass of the heart may be required to meet the increased demands for ATP imposed by endurance training.

REFERENCES

1. Anderson SA, Bankier T, Barrell BG, de Bruijn MHL, Coulson AR, Drouin J, Eperon IC, Nierlich DP, Roe BA, Sanger F, Schreier PH, Smith AJH, Staden R, Young IG. 1981. Sequence and organization of the human mitochondrial genome. Nature 290:457–465.
2. Tzagoloff A, Myers AM. 1986. Genetics of mitochondrial biogenesis. Annu Rev Biochem 55:249–285.
3. Clayton DA. 1991. Replication and transcription of vertebrate mitochondrial DNA. Annu Rev Cell Biol 7:453–479.
4. Murakami T, Shimomura Y, Fujitsuka N, Nakai N, Sugiyama S, Ozawa T, Sokabe M, Horai S, Toduyama K, Suzuki M. 1994. Enzymatic and genetic adaptation of soleus muscle mitochondria to physical training in rats. Am J Physiol 267:E388–E395.
5. Holloszy JO, Booth FW. 1976. Biochemical adaptations to endurance exercise in muscle. Annu Rev Physiol 38:273–291.
6. Rabinowits M, Zak R. 1975. Mitochondria and cardiac hypertrophy. Circ Res 36:367–376.
7. Oscai LB, Molé PA, Brei B, Holloszy JO. 1971. Cardiac growth and respiratory enzyme levels in male rats subjected to a running program. Am J Physiol 220:1238–1241.
8. Oscai LB, Molé PA, Holloszy JO. 1971. Effects of exercise on cardiac weight and mitochondria in male and female rats. Am J Physiol 220:1944–1948.
9. Hickson RC, Hammons GT, Holoszy JO. 1979. Development and regression of exercise-induced cardiac hypertrophy in rats. Am J Physiol 236:H268–H272.
10. Murakami T, Shimomura Y, Fujitsuka N, Sugiyama S. 1995. Different adaptation to endurance training between heart and gastrocnemius muscle mitochondria in rats. Biochem Mol Biol Int 36:285–290.
11. Tokoro T, Ito H, Maenishi O, Suzuki T. 1995. Mitochondrial abnormalities in hypertrophied myocardium of stroke-prone spontaneously hypertensive rats. Clin Exp Pharmacol Physiol Suppl 1:S268–S269.
12. Tokoro T, Ito H, Suzuki T. 1996. Alterations in mitochondrial DNA and enzyme activities in hypertrophied myocardium of stroke-prone SHRs. Clin Exp Hypertens 18:595–606.
13. Chen L, Tian X, Song L. 1995. Biochemical and biophysical characteristics of mitochondria in the hypertrophic hearts from hypertensive rats. Clin Med J (Engl) 108:361–366.
14. Bunag RD. 1973. Validation in awake rats of tail-cuff method for measuring systolic pressure. J Appl Physiol 34:279–282.
15. Smith L. 1955. Spectrophotometric assay of cytochrome c oxidase. Methods Biochem Anal 2:427–434.
16. Srere PA. 1969. Citrate synthase. Methods Enzymol 13:3–5.
17. Labarca C, Paigen K. 1980. A simple, rapid, and sensitive DNA assay procedure. Anal Biochem 102:344–352.
18. Ott RL. 1993. An Introduction to Statistical Methods and Data Analysis (4th ed.). Belmont, CA: Wadsworth.
19. Morrison PR, Biggs RB, Booth FW. 1989. Daily running for 2 wk and mRNAs for cytochrome c and α-actin in rat skeletal muscle. Am J Physiol 257:C936–C939.
20. Annex BH, Kraus WE, Dohm GL, Williams RS. 1991. Mitochondrial biogenesis in striated muscles: rapid induction of citrate synthase mRNA by nerve stimulation. Am J Physiol 260:C266–C270.
21. Williams RS. 1986. Mitochondrial gene expression in mammalian striated muscle. Evidence that variation in gene dosage is the major regulatory event. J Biol Chem 261:12390–12394.

N. Takeda, M. Nagano and N.S. Dhalla
(eds). The Hypertrophied Heart. Copyright
© 2000. pp. 51–66. Kluwer Academic
Publishers. Boston. All rights reserved.

SERCA2 AND ANF PROMOTER-ACTIVITY STUDIES IN HYPERTROPHIC CARDIOMYOCYTES USING LIPOSOME-, GENE GUN-, AND ADENOVIRUS-MEDIATED GENE TRANSFER

KARIN EIZEMA,[1] HAN A.A. VAN HEUGTEN,[1] KAREL BEZSTAROSTI,[1] MARGA C. VAN SETTEN,[1] SONJA SCHNEIDER-RASP,[2] WOLFGANG C. POLLER,[2] and JOS M.J. LAMERS[1]

[1] Department of Biochemistry, Cardiovascular Research Institute COEUR, Erasmus University Rotterdam, P.O. Box 1738, 3000 DR Rotterdam, The Netherlands; [2] Department of Cardiology and Pneumology, University Hospital Benjamin Franklin, Free University, Hindenburgdamm 30, D-122200 Berlin, Germany

Summary. Myocardial hypertrophy is known as the process of enlargement of ventricular cells, which is also accompanied by changes in the phenotype. The latter changes include, e.g., downregulation of the expression of sarcoplasmatic reticulum Ca^{2+} ATPase (SERCA2), phospholamban (PL), and β-adrenergic receptor and upregulation of the expression of atrial natriuretic factor (ANF) and β-myosin heavy chain (β-MHC). Analysis of the transcriptional regulation of a promoter fragment of the SERCA2 gene using liposome-mediated transfection revealed that the SERCA2 gene may not respond to the general increase in transcription upon stimulation of neonatal rat cardiomyocytes by 10^{-8} M endothelin-1. Liposome-mediated transfection used in these promoter activity studies yields no more than 1% transfection efficiency (the percentage of cells expressing the transgene). To obtain higher efficiency, we set out to develop the gene-gun biolistics method for transfection of cardiomyocytes. An efficiency up to approximately 10% can be achieved by the gene gun as tested using a RSV-β-Gal construct. Here, we demonstrate the efficacy of the method by use of an endothelin-1 inducible ANF promoter fragment coupled to a CAT reporter. Therefore, gene-gun biolistics is ideally suited as a quick and reliable method to test DNA constructs on their activity. The ANF promoter is normally only active to a very low extent in ventricular adult cells; it is upregulated by hypertrophic stimuli. We used the latter property for generating DNA constructs encompassing the antisense PL gene under the control of the endothelin-1 inducible ANF promoter fragment. Adenovirus infection with almost 100% efficiency is required to measure the functional consequences of the overexpressed antisense PL. Here, we present the first results with the ANF-promoter–PL-antisense adenovirus infection of rat neonatal cardiomyocytes.

INTRODUCTION

In response to chronically increased workload, compensatory mechanisms in the heart are activated that result in increase of the mass and changes of phenotype of the ventricular myocytes [1]. This apparent salutory response to excess load is accompanied by reversion to a fetal program of cardiac gene expression [1–4]. The autocrine and paracrine formation of hormones such as angiotensin II, noradrenaline, endothelin-1 (ET-1), and atrial natriuretic factor (ANF) are partially involved in mediating the hypertrophic and gene expression responses (see, e.g., [5–7]). The underlying cause of heart failure, which ultimately develops, is thought to partially reside in the reprogramming of gene expression [3,8–11]. This hypothesis is consistent with the observed relative downregulation of key proteins involved in (β-adrenergic regulation of) the uptake and release of Ca^{2+} from the cardiac sarcoplasmic reticulum: the β-adrenergic receptor, Ca^{2+} ATPase (SERCA2), and phospholamban (PL) [2,3,9–14]. On the other hand, the genes encoding, e.g., ANF, β-myosin heavy chain, and α-skeletal actin are found to be upregulated during hypertrophy [1,3,4,8]. the nuclear mechanisms involved in coordinately regulating these cardiac genes during hypertrophy are fully unknown, although binding sites for several transcription factors, including serum response factor (SRF), transcription enhancer factor (TEF1), AP-1 (a heterodimer of jun/fos), and transcription factor Sp1 were shown to be important for activation of fetal cardiac genes in response to hypertrophy [15–18].

Most of the previous studies on nuclear factors concern upregulation of cardiac genes during hypertrophy (see, e.g., [4,15–19]). To initiate studies on the nuclear factors involved in transcriptional downregulation of the SERCA2 gene during hypertrophy, we employed the model of cultured neonatal rat ventricular myocytes as used successfully for promoter studies by many other groups [2,4,16–21]. In the latter model, we were previously able to show that ET-1 is a strong inducer of hypertrophy by its increasing effect on the rate of amino acid incorporation in total protein after 24 and 48 hours [2,21,22]. The increased amino acid incorporation is due to an increase in protein synthesis and not solely due to an augmented protein turnover rate, since the protein content per cell (measured as protein/DNA ratio) was increased as well, as in the in vivo situation. The development of hypertrophy in the cultured cardiomyocytes was associated with several phenotypic changes, including upregulation of ANF and downregulation of SERCA2 and PL [2,21,22]. We have isolated, characterized, and tested the activity (by liposome-mediated transfection) of an isolated SERCA2 promoter fragment in order to make a first step in the search for the *cis*-acting elements and *trans*-acting factors responsible for downregulation of this gene during cardiomyocyte hypertrophy. The results of our study [22] confirmed the findings of many other groups [15–19] that the use of traditional methods, such as liposome-mediated transfection of cardiomyocytes, can be of value for studying promoter regulation. However, the efficiency (percentage of cells expressing the transgene) and level of expression (total amount of protein expressed) obtained by these traditional methods are extremely low, generally no more than 1%, and therefore only suitable when the sensitivity of the assay employed to detect reporter gene expression is sufficiently high. Expression may then also be detectable in a high percentage of the cell population even if the intrinsic efficiency of gene transfer is low. For certain, liposome-mediated transfection does not work in functional testing of the effects of overexpression of cardiac proteins, although the use of strong promoters (CMV or RSV) can be of help when a reasonable transfection efficiency is reached. Other transfection methods, including cationic lipid/plasmid DNA complexes, incubations with "naked" plasmid DNA, and calcium phosphate precipitation, do usually not achieve higher efficiencies in cardiac cells [23]. A recently reported new transfection method that combines the convenience of plasmid DNA with the unique targeting properties of adenovirus vectors [24] did not, however, in our hands give the expected results.

Recombinant adenoviral vectors offer several significant advantages. These viruses can be prepared at high titer, infect nonreplicatory cells, and allow the incorporation of relatively large or even multiple cDNAs. The recombinant replication-defective human adenovirus can transfect primary cardiac cultures with near to 100% efficiency [25]. Other studies could demonstrate that the overexpression of SERCA2 and/or PL leads to the expected functional changes in cardiomyocytes Ca^{2+} handling [26,27]. Since recombinant adenoviruses overexpressing cardiac Ca^{2+}-handling proteins are time consuming to prepare, there remains a need for methods with high-efficiency transfection of cardiomyocytes with so-called "naked" DNA that can be tested for its functionality. Recently, a new product for transfection, Fugene6 (Boehringer), and a gold-particle-mediated transfer technology, the Helios Gene Gun (Biorad) [28,29], have become available. The Helios Gene Gun uses helium pressure to propel DNA-coated gold particles into cells (biolistics [30]), a process originally developed for in vivo gene transfer into the somatic tissues of live animals. Generally, elemental gold has been chosen for mammalian gene transfer, because pure gold is chemically inert and does not produce cytotoxicity. The high density of gold also permits grater momentum, allowing deeper penetration into target cells. In recent reports, we presented the first results with the Helios Gene Gun system in cardiomyocytes; we used a reported plasmid harboring the β-Galactosidase (β-Gal) gene under the control of the Rous sarcoma virus (RSV) promoter [31,32]. We could demonstrate that the Gene Gun method is applicable for the transfection of beating rat cardiomyocytes and gives superior results when compared to other traditional and new transfection reagents such as DOTAP and Fugene6, respectively.

The purpose of the present work is to briefly describe our previous results concerning the use of liposome-mediated transfer of SERCA2-CAT promoter plasmid to primary cultures of rat neonatal cardiomyocytes in order to study downregulation of the SERCA2 promoter, and the use of the Helios Gene Gun to increase transfection efficiency for testing the ET-1 inducibility of an ANF-promoter/CAT-reporter plasmid. Next, we show that cardiomyocytes infected with an adenoviral vector expressing antisense PL mRNA under control of the ET-1-inducible ANF promoter fragment contain less PL.

METHODS

DNA constructs

The SERCA2 5′ upstream regulatory region (1.9 kb, including 0.4 kb of the 5′ UTR of the mRNA) was subcloned in a chloramphenicol acetyltransferase (CAT) reporter vector (pCAT-Basic, Promega) (CatSpro$_{1.9}$) [22,31]. The RSV-β-Gal construct was a kind gift from the department of Endocrinology and Reproduction (Erasmus University Rotterdam). The ANF promoter (680 bp KpnI-BamHI)—a kind gift from K.R. Chien (University of California, San Diego)—was cloned in pCAT3 (Promega) (ANFCAT) to test its ET-1 inducibility (see also [33]). The DNAs were isolated and purified with the Wizard midiprep kit (Promega) in the study aimed at SERCA2 promoter regulation and CsCl purified for the gene gun experiments.

Trans(in)fection and induction of hypertrophy by ET-1

Rat neonatal ventricular cardiomyocytes were isolated as described in detail previously [20], preplated, and cultured in 20 cm^2 (7.5 × 10^4 cells/cm^2 for the SERCA2 promoter regulation studies) or 1.8 cm^2 dishes (1.5 × 10^5 cells/cm^2 for the Gene Gun-mediated gene transfer with the RSV-β-Gal construct, 7.5 × 10^4 cells/cm^2 for the ANF promoter studies and adenoviral infection studies), up to 24 hours in DMEM/M199 (4:1) supplemented with 5% fetal calf serum and 5% horse serum (HS). Hereafter, the medium was changed to DMEM/M199 (4:1) with only 5% HS. After 64 hours, the medium was changed to serum-free DMEM/M199. Infection with the viruses (see below) was subsequently done in serum-free medium in 200 μl (1.8 cm^2 dishes) for 3 hours followed by the addition of serum-free medium (600 μl). The amounts of virus used are indicated. Transfection was performed in serum-free medium by standard calcium phosphate (0.5–3 μg DNA per well, 25 mM Hepes buffer (pH 70.5), and overnight incubation), Fugene6 and DOTAP methodologies according to instructions provided by Boehringer Mannheim Germany (Fugene6/DNA ratio: 1.5 μl/0.5 μg DNA or 3.6 μl/1.44 μg DNA; DOTAP/DNA ratio: 15 μg/5 μg DNA, 18 hours), or by Gene Gun biolistics (see below). Subsequently, cells were washed with serum-free DMEM/M199 (4:1) and fresh medium was added. After 3 hours, ET-1 (10^{-8} M) was added for 48 or 72 hours to induce hypertrophy [9,21,22].

Gene Gun-mediated biolistics transfection

The most recent hand-held version of the pulse gene gun (Biorad), using helium gas-driven force to propel the gold particles into cultured cells, was used. DNA capsules were 1.2 cm pieces of Tefzel® tubing inner-coated with gold particles loaded by CsCl-purified DNA. These capsules were then inserted into the Gene Gun cartridges, which hold 12 capsules, allowing 12 transfections per single loading. The cartridges were prepared according to the manufacturer's protocol, with slight but essential modifications [29,31]. Per shot, 0.5 μg DNA was delivered, which was coated on 0.1 mg gold particles (DLR: 0.5, MLQ: 0.1). A special delivery device on top of the Gene Gun was developed at our laboratory to specifically enable high-efficiency bombardment of cardiomyocytes in a 1.8 cm^2 well. The medium was first aspirated from the cells, followed by immediate bombardment with the Helios Gene Gun system (Biorad) at 100-psi helium pressure; then new serum-free medium was carefully layered back on the cells. ET-1 was added 3 hours after bombardment.

Adenoviruses CMVβ-Gal and ANFPLAS

The CMVβ-Gal adenovirus encoding the β-Gal reporter gene under the control of the Cowpea Mosaic virus (CMV) promoter was developed in the laboratory of Dr. W.C. Poller (Free University Berlin). The details of the construction of the ANFPLAS virus will be described elsewhere [32]. Briefly, a part of the isolated PL cDNA covering the ATG start codon (EcoRI-TaqI [230 bp]) was used for the generation of the antisense construct, and this fragment of the PL cDNA was cloned in the antisense direction in the ANFCAT constructs, thereby eliminating the CAT reporter and introducing a chimeric intron between the ANF promoter and the PL fragment. The EcoRI-BamHI fragments of the constructs were subsequently cloned in the EcoRI-BglII sites of the shuttle vector pΔElspl (Microbix, UK). All constructs were purified using the Endo-free plasmid maxi kit (Qiagen, Westburg, The Netherlands). The shuttle constructs were cotransfected with an adenovirus-derived plasmid, pJM17, into 293 cells. The homologous recombination between the two vectors in 293 cells led to the generation of recombinant adenovirus containing the gene of interest. The adenoviruses were verified by PCR and subsequently propagated, purified by CsCl gradient centrifugation, and plaque titered according to standard procedures. The titers of the virus preparation were CMVβ-Gal-4.6 × 10^8 particles/μl ANFPLAS-1.3 × 10^9 particles/μl.

Northern blotting

Total RNA was isolated by the guanidinium isothiocyanate method, quantified by spectrophotometry, separated on 1% denaturing formaldehyde-agarose gels, and blotted onto Hybond (Amersham). Probes described below were labeled by random priming using [α-^{32}P]dCTP (Amersham). The CAT probe was excised from the CAT reporter plasmid [22]. The glyceraldehyde-3-phosphate dehydrogenase (GAPDH), and ANF probes were developed by RT-PCR on rat heart RNA based on published sequences. A SERCA2 cDNA (RHCa-117) was a kind gift from A-M Lompre (Universite Paris-Sud, Paris, France) [34]. Hybridization was performed as described [22]. The hybridization signal was quantified by the Molecular Imager (Biorad).

Analysis of reporter gene expression

Quantificantion of the β-Gal and CAT protein was performed by ELISA according to the manufacturer's protocol (Boehringer, Mannheim).

Western blotting

After the indicated infection time (72 hours), cells were homogenized using a mikro-dismembrator U (Braun, Biotech, International, Germany), and protein content was determined by the Lowry method. Ten μg of protein in SDS-loading dye (not boiled, to keep the PL pentamers intact) was separated using an SDS-PAGE gradient gel 7.5–15% and blotted onto PVDF (Amersham). Blots were incubated with monoclonal anti-PL (1 : 2500; ABR) as primary antibody followed by GAMIgG [125]I (1 : 1000) (ICN) as secondary antibody. After washing, the blots were exposed in the molecular imager (Biorad) and quantified. The primary band detected represented the pentameric form of PL. The monomer was detected at only very low intensities and, therefore, was not quantified.

Statistical analysis

Significance was set at $p < 0.05$, using the Student–Newman–Keuls test, for at least four independent experiments.

RESULTS

Analysis of SERCA2-promoter activity using liposome-based transfection

The observed changes in cardiac gene expression in hypertrophic conditions are mimicked by stimulating cultured rat neonatal cardiomyocytes with 10^{-8} M ET-1. We determined the changes in gene expression that are characteristic of cardiac hypertrophy and failure in vivo by measuring the changes in the mRNA levels of ANF and SERCA2 after 24 hours of ET-1 stimulation (figure 1). A general increase in transcriptional activity occurs, as proven by an increase in GAPDH messenger. To correct for this general increase in RNA, mRNA levels of the ANF and SERCA2 genes were calculated relative to those of the GAPDH gene (figure 1, table 1). Our observation that the ANF gene was upregulated and the SERCA2

Table 1. Transcriptional regulation of the SERCA2 gene by ET-1 in neonatal rat cardiomyocytes

	Untransfected cells	Transfected cells
GAPDH mRNA		
mRNA level (% of unstimulated control)	138% ± 10%[a]	210% ± 42%
SERCA/GAPDH		
mRNA ratio (% of unstimulated control)	81% ± 9%[a]	74% ± 7%[a]
CAT/GAPDH		
mRNA ratio (% of unstimulated control)		56% ± 19%[a]

[a] $p < 0.05$.

The CATspro$_{1.9}$ DNA construct was transfected into neonatal rat cardiomyocytes using DOTAP, and hypertrophy was induced by stimulation of the cells with 10^{-8} M ET-1 for 48 hours. Subsequently, mRNA levels were quantified as described under Materials and Methods. Hybridization signals are represented as a percentage of unstimulated (without ET-1) control cells for GAPDH mRNA, while the (endogenous) SERCA2 and CAT mRNA signals were first corrected for the increase in total RNA by dividing them through the signal of GAPDH mRNA. Date represent mean ± SEM for 4–8 independent experiments.

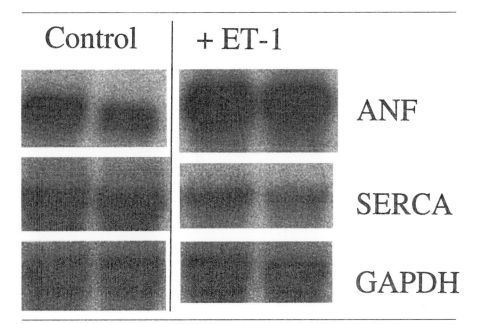

Figure 1. Effect of ET-1 stimulation on the mRNA levels of ANF and SERCA2 in neonatal rat cardiomyocytes. Twenty-four hours after stimulation with ET-1 (10^{-8} M), total RNA was isolated and analyzed, as described under Materials and Methods. The same blot was hybridized with the different specific probes. Representative blots are shown in duplicate to demonstrate the strong upregulation of the ANF messenger paralleled by the downregulation of the SERCA2 messenger.

gene was downregulated in hypertrophied cardiomyocytes is consistent with the findings of numerous other reports (e.g., [35–37]). We have isolated a genomic fragment of the SERCA2 gene containing 1.5 kb of the promoter region and 0.4 kb of the 5'UTR, which was subcloned into the CAT reporter plasmid (nucleotide sequences were published in [22]). The SERCA2 promoter activity was studied by liposome-mediated transfection in cardiomyocytes that were stimulated for 48 hours with ET-1 (10^{-8} M) to become hypertrophied. Since the CAT protein was found to have a very low turnover in these cells, it was not possible to measure reduction in activity of the SERCA2 promoter by measuring CAT protein. Therefore, mRNA was isolated, and CAT mRNA levels were measured by Northern blotting. Table 1 shows that downregulation of CAT relative to GAPDH mRNA is present, which indicates that this promoter fragment contains all the necessary elements for the cellular response to hypertrophic stimuli. As a control, the genomic SERCA2 promoter activity was determined too, in order to demonstrate that the observed downregulation of the SERCA2 promoter–CAT construct was not due to quenching of promoter elements. Of note is that absolute CAT mRNA (without correction for the GAPDH increase) remained unchanged upon ET-1 stimulation (results not shown).

Gene Gun-mediated biolistic versus other vehicle-mediated gene transfer

The data in table 1 demonstrate that it is possible to investigate SERCA2 promoter regulation in rat neonatal cardiomyocytes using "traditional" transfection methods. However, these methods (liposome- as well as calcium phosphate-based methods) are known to give rise to very low transfection efficiencies (see below). The study of other promoters with very low activities may be difficult using these transfection methods. Moreover, much higher transfection efficiencies are required to analyze the functional consequences of, e.g., SERCA2 gene overexpression or PL synthesis disabled by antisense oligonucleotides, in both cases by exogenously introduced DNA constructs in these cardiomyocytes. Therefore, we set out to develop a technology that made use of biolistics, which recently became commercially available: the Gene Gun for in situ bombardment of tissue [28,29]. We have optimized the biolistics transfection for its use with primary cultures of cardiomyocytes and have analyzed its efficacy by using a plasmid containing the β-Gal reporter under control of the RSV promoter [31]. Forty-eight hours after bombardment, cells were stained for β-Gal and the cellular morphology examined [31]. Next, we determined quantitatively the β-Gal expression in bombarded cells by ELISA and compared these results with other traditional transfection reagents. In this respect, it is important to note that, with both traditional methods and the Gene Gun, only $0.5\,\mu g$ DNA was transfected. Figure 2 depicts the results of the comparison of transfection methods using the RSV-β-Gal DNA construct, as measured by ELISA. Transfection efficiencies were based on comparing the obtained results to the amount of β-Gal measured by ELISA after 100% infection of cardiomyocytes with an adenovirus encoding β-Gal under the control of a CMV promoter. Transfection efficiencies of up to 10% of the bombarded cells were obtained. Thus, it is clear that the biolistics method of transfection gives superior results compared to the traditional methods. The use of more DNA for the transfections with Fugene6 and calcium phosphate raises the efficiencies obtained with these methods only for the calcium phosphate method, although the amount of β-Gal measured after calcium phosphate transfection is still considerably lower compared to the biolistics results (figure 2). The new Fugene6 transfection reagent does not give any measurable transfection in our test conditions (figure 2). As expected based upon previous studies [25–27,38–40], infection with an adenovirus encoding β-Gal under the control of the CMV promoter still gave superior results in comparison with the Gene Gun transfection method. Therefore, when transfection efficiencies of near 100% are desired, adenoviral infection should be the method of choice.

Analysis of transcriptional regulation of the ANF gene using Gene Gun biolistics

The ANF gene is strongly upregulated upon hypertrophic stimulation of cultured neonatal cardiomyocytes (figure 1; [36–38]), as well as in hypertrophied and/or failing hearts in vivo [1,41,42]. The ANF promoter fragment used in the present study was previously used by others to demonstrate upregulation upon induction

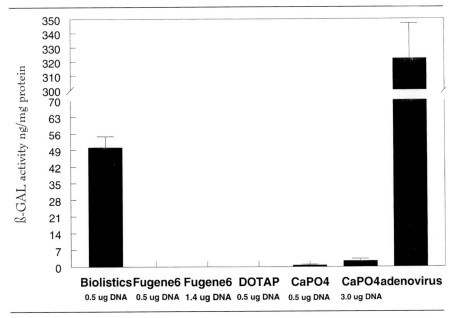

Figure 2. Gene Gun-mediated compared to other-vehicle-mediated gene transfer. In all experiments, the same plasmid (RSV-β-Gal) was used. Forty-eight hours after transfection, cells were homogenized and protein expression measured by ELISA. Data are represented as ng β-Gal per mg protein (±SEM). Cells were subjected to biolistic bombardment using 0.1 mg of gold particles coated with 0.5 μg of DNA (biolistics), or transfected using Fugene6, DOTAP, or calcium phosphate. The amount of DNA used per 1.8 cm² well in the transfection experiments is indicated. For the adenovirus infection, 6.9×10^9 particles per well were used.

Table 2. Upregulation of CAT reporter controlled by an ANF promoter fragment after ET-1 stimulation of cardiomyocytes transfected with the Gene Gun

	CAT activity
Control	100%
ET-1 $(10^{-8}\,M)$	256 ± 40%★

Cells were bombarded with DNA encoding the ANF-CAT construct and were stimulated with ET-1 to induce hypertrophic responses. Forty-eight hours after Gene Gun-mediated transfection, cells were homogenized and CAT activity was measured (absolute activity in control cells was 5.15 ± 1.67 ng CAT/mg protein). Data represent mean ± SEM for six independent experiments. ★, $p < 0.05$.

of hypertrophy (see, e.g., [33]). We used this ANF promoter fragment to demonstrate the feasibility of analyzing transcriptional regulation by the use of biolistics transfection techniques. The activity of this promoter fragment was tested (after 48 hours) in the presence or absence of ET-1 $(10^{-8}\,M)$. Table 2 depicts the results of Gene Gun transfection of the ANF-CAT reporter construct. The ANF promoter is upregulated approximately 2.5-fold by ET-1 stimulation. This is the first report on Gene Gun-mediated transfection used for analysis of promoter activity in cardiomyocytes.

Infection with an adenovirus encoding antisense phospholamban under the control of the ANF promoter fragment

To improve the contractile properties of failing hearts in vivo, infection of a large proportion of the ventricular myoctes with DNA constructs that display specific activity in the heart, and preferably in those myocytes that are failing, will be required. As stated before, the ANF promoter is known to be upregulated during the initially hypertrophying and ultimately failing state of the myocardium observed in vivo as well as in vitro [1,35–37,41,42]. Similarly, in the currently used in vitro model of cardiomyocytes, a hypertrophic stimulus such as ET-1 upregulated ANF expression (figure 1, table 2). We designed DNA constructs aimed at a further downregulation of PL (endogenous inhibitor of the SR-Ca^{2+} pump) by using an antisense strategy. A part of the PL cDNA was cloned in the antisense direction in a suitable vector under control of an ET-1 inducible ANF promoter fragment (see Materials and Methods above). To show whether the adenovectors containing ANF promoter fragments are still inducible by a hypertrophic stimulus, we stimulated infected cardiomyocytes with ET-1. Figure 3 depicts the results on PL protein expression obtained after infection for 72 hours with ANFPLAS with or without ET-1 stimulation. In unstimulated cells, ANF mRNA appears to be present in low amounts in ventricular tissue, thus representing a low basal activity of this promoter (compare also figure 1). Therefore, it was not surprising to see that, in the absence of ET-1, a decrease in PL protein is detectable (figure 3; 82% ± 7% relative to the unstimulated control cells). However, infection with ANFPLAS and ET-1 stimulation resulted in a further reduction of PL protein (67% ± 13% compared to the control cells with only ET-1 treatment). The latter results demonstrate that the PL antisense cDNA under control of the ANF promoter fragment results in a significant and ET-1-dependent reduction of PL protein in cardiomyocytes.

DISCUSSION

Previously, we isolated and determined the sequence of the rat SERCA2 gene 5′-regulatory region (1.8 kb) and analyzed its function in rat neonatal cardiomyocytes in the presence or absence of a hypertrophy-inducing stimulus (ET-1). Liposome-mediated transfection of the SERCA2 promoter fragment in these cells did not change the genomic downregulation of the SERCA2 mRNA level during hypertrophy, showing that transcription factors did not become limited by the exogenous SERCA2 promoter fragment. A 1.5 kb 5′ regulatory region together with a 360 bp 5′ UTR dictates the downregulation of a reporter gene similar to that observed for the genomic SERCA2 downregulation (table 1 [22,31]). It indicates that (most) cis-acting elements responsible for hypertrophy-associated downregula-

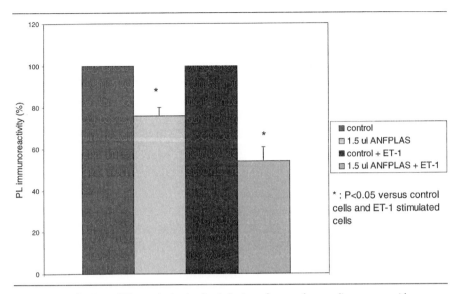

Figure 3. Reduction of PL protein levels after infection of neonatal rat cardiomyocytes with ANFPLAS virus. Cells were infected with the ANFPLAS virus; 72 hours after the start of infection, the cells were homogenized and levels of PL protein were analyzed as described. Data are represented as percentage of the control PL immunoreactivity ± SEM for five independent experiments. PL protein is reduced as a consequence of the antisense virus infection. The ANF promoter is slightly active when the cells are cultured without ET-1. Upon addition of ET-1 (10^{-8} M), the ANF promoter is upregulated, a finding that can be derived from the further reduction of the PL protein. *, $p < 0.05$ versus control cells (without virus infection).

tion of SERCA2 expression are confined to this regulatory region. During hypertrophy, SERCA2 mRNA level was only reduced when expressed relative to the GAPDH mRNA, but in fact the absolute SERCA2 mRNA levels remained unchanged. Therefore, the observed downregulation of the SERCA2 promoter may be interpreted as not responding to the general increase in transcription that accompanies hypertrophic growth. At present, there are two other studies showing SERCA2 downregulation in cultured neonatal cardiomyocytes, but in response to another hypertrophic stimulus, namely, phorbol 12-myristate 13-acetate (PMA) [43,44]. As we and others have demonstrated, ET-1 and phorbolester are both potent activators of protein kinase C isotypes in these cells [45–47]. Qi et al. [43] reported that a reduction in the stability of the SERCA2 message may be causally related to the PMA-induced downregulation of SERCA2 expression. PMA is a potent activator of PKC-α, -ε, and -δ isotypes, whereas ET-1 only translocates/activates PKC-ε [45]. Interestingly, a recent study of Cadre et al. [48] shows that cyclic stretch induces a decrease of SERCA2 mRNA level as well, in parallel with an increase of total protein synthesis. Unpublished results obtained in our laboratory demonstrated, however, that no activation of PKC isotypes occurs early after exposure of the cells to cyclic stretch.

Recently, we presented the first results with the Helios Gene Gun system in cardiomyocytes using a reporter plasmid harboring the β-Gal gene under the control of the RSV promoter [31,32]. The use of helium pressure to propel DNA-coated gold beads into the cardiomyocytes could also be suitable for directly testing promoter/reporter-gene DNA constructs, since the transfection efficiency appears to be appreciably higher as compared with more traditional transfection methods (figure 2 [31,32]). A transfection efficiency of approximately 10% of the cells in the bombarded area can be achieved. Presently, we tested the activity of an ANF promoter fragment (680 bp) via biolistic-mediated transfection on cardiomyocytes and stimulated with ET-1 to induce hypertrophy (figure 1; table 2). A marked increase of transcriptional activity of this ANF promoter fragment is observed after ET-1 (10^{-8} M) stimulation. The results of these experiments indicate that biolistic transfection has no negative influence on the viability of the cardiomyocytes and that the cells remain capable of responding to hypertrophic stimuli in the characteristic manner. If these results are taken together, we could demonstrate that the hand-held gene gun is a quick and reliable method to achieve high transfection efficiencies with primary rat neonatal cardiomyocytes as target cells, and could, therefore, be used as well for promoter analysis. Additional experiments on the 5'-flanking regions of SERCA2 and PL genes using the Gene Gun transfection methodology are currently in progress. The methodology may even be useful for testing the functional changes by over- or underexpression of a specific gene, since approximately 10% of the cells in the bombarded area are usually transfected.

The cardiac hypertrophic phenotype in vivo as well as in vitro is characterized by an increase in muscle cell size, an increase in contractile protein content, and the transcriptional activation of distinct genes, including the ANF gene [1,35–37,41,42,49–51]. Therefore, the ANF promoter could potentially be used to direct gene expression specifically in the hypertrophied and/or failing myocardium. For instance, the downregulation of SERCA2 in hypertrophied and/or failing myocardium is generally believed to be part of the underlying mechanism of diastolic dysfunction. Drug-induced activation of the sarcoplasmic reticulum Ca^{2+} pump might improve the contractile function of the chronically overloaded myocardium. For this reason, we chose the endogenous inhibitor phospholamban as a target for gene manipulation [52,53]. The functional importance of PL in the regulation was indeed substantiated in studies on PL heterozygous mice, which contain only one targeted PL allele [54]. The reduced PL expression is associated with increases in the affinity of the cardiac sarcoplasmatic reticulum Ca^{2+} pump for Ca^{2+} and the expected increase in contractile parameters in the intact myocardium [54]. In the present study, the effect of infection of the cardiomyocyte with an adenoviral vector was tested. The vector, designed by us, expresses antisense PL mRNA under the control of the Gene Gun-tested ANF promoter fragment. After 72 hours of infection, a decrease in PL immunoreactivity was detectable already without ET-1 stimulation. These results with the ANF-CAT reporter construct, transfected in the cells by the Gene Gun and described in table 2 (see legends), are in agreement with the findings on the adenoviral ANFPL antisense vector. However, in vivo, the expression of ANF in the ventricular compartment is downregulated in the adult myocardium, leading to atrial-specific expression of the ANF gene [55]. It is not completely clear why considerable expression of ANF mRNA was found in unstimulated cardiomyocytes, but this outcome may be partially due to the presence of atrium-derived myocytes. Under hypertrophic conditions (stimulation with ET-1) the ANF promoter is upregulated (table 2), resulting in a further reduction of the PL protein in the cardiomyocytes infected with the ANFPLAS (figure 3). This is the first demonstration of the feasibility of using a heart-specific promoter that is only active in hypertrophied and failing ventricles for gene therapy. The obvious advantage of using this particular promoter in in vivo experiments is the expected low activity in the nonmyocyte cells in the myocardium and the likely ability of this promoter to shut itself off when contractile function improves, thereby reducing the workload of the myocardium. In vivo experiments can be performed using the method first reported by Hajjar and coworkers [56] to obtain high infection rate specifically in the ventricle. The first experiments using a control adenovirus expressing green fluorescent protein in our laboratory are promising.

ACKNOWLEDGMENTS

This work was supported by Grant No 95.109 from the Netherlands Heart Foundation and by the Deutsche Forschungsgemeinschaft through a Heiseberg fellowship to W.P. Grant No. 378/2-1,2.

REFERENCES

1. Schwartz K, Carrier L, Mercadier J-J, Lompre A-M, Boheler KR. 1993. Molecular phenotype of the hypertrophied and failing myocardium. Circulation 87:VII5–VII10.
2. Van Heugten HAA, De Jonge HW, Goedbloed MA, Bezstarosti K, Sharma HS, Verdouw PD, Lamers JMJ. 1995. Intracellular signaling and genetic reprogramming during development of hypertrophy in cultured cardiomyocytes. In Heart Hypertrophy and Failure Ed. NS Dhalla, GN Pierce, VN Panagia, and L Beamish, 79–92. Boston: Kluwer Academic Publishers.
3. Van Heugten HAA, Lamers JMJ. 1997. Changes in cardiac phenotype in hypertrophy and failure: from receptor to gene. Heart Failure Rev 2:95–106.
4. Komuro I, Yazaki Y. 1993. Control of cardiac gene expression by mechanical stress. Annu Rev Physiol 55:55–75.
5. Love MP, McMurray JJV. 1996. Endothelin in chronic heart failure: current position and future prospects. Cardiovasc Res 31:665–774.
6. Baker KM, Booz GW, Dostal DE. 1992. Cardiac actions of angiotensin II: role of an intracardiac renin–angiotensin system. Annu Rev Physiol 54:227–241.
7. Simpson P. 1983. Norepinephrine-stimulated hypertrophy of cultured neonatal rat cardiomyocytes. J Clin Invest 72:732–738.
8. Swynghedauw B. 1986. Developmental and functional adaptation of contractile proteins in cardiac and skeletal muscles. Physiol Rev 66:710–771.
9. Morgan JP, Erny RE, Allen PD, Grossman W, Gwathmey JK. 1990. Abnormal intracellular Ca^{2+} handling. A major cause of systolic and diastolic dysfunction in ventricular myocardium from patients with heart failure. Circulation 81(Suppl III):21–32.
10. Arai M, Matsui H, Periasamy M. 1994. Sarcoplasmic reticulum gene expression in cardiac hypertrophy and heart failure. Circ Res 74:555–564.
11. Hasenfuss G, Meyer M, Schillinger W, Preuss M, Priske B, Just H. 1997. Calcium handling proteins in the failing human heart. Basic Res Cardiol 92(Suppl 1):87–93.

12. Flesch M, Schwinger RHG, Schnabel P, Schiffer F, Van Gelder I, Bavendiek U, Südkamp M, Kuhn-Regnier F, Böhm M. 1996. Sarcoplasmic reticulum Ca^{2+}-ATPase and phospholamban mRNA and protein levels in end-stage heart failure due to ischemic or dilated cardiomyopathy. J Mol Med 74:321–332.

13. Zarain-Herzberg A, Afzal N, Elimban V, Dhalla NS. 1996. Decreased expression of sarcoplasmic reticulum Ca^{2+} pump ATPase in congestive heart failure due to myocardial infarction. Mol Cell Biochem 163/164:285–290.

14. Linck B, Boknik P, Eschenhagen T, Müller FU, Neumann J, Nose M, Jones LR, Schmitz W, Scholz H. 1996. Messenger RNA expression and immunological quantification of phospholamban and SR-Ca^{2+}-ATPase in failing and nonfailing human hearts. Cardiovasc Res 31:625–632.

15. Kovacic-Milivojevic B, Wong VSH, Gardner DG. 1996. Selective regulation of the atrial natriuretic peptide gene by individual components of the activatorprotein-1 complex. Endocrinology 137:1108–1117.

16. Karns LR, Kariya K, Simpson PC. 1995. M-CAT, CarG, and Sp1 elements are required for α-adrenergic induction of the skeletal α-actin promoter during cardiac myocyte hypertrophy. J Biol Chem 270:410–417.

17. Sadoshima J, Izumo S. 1993. Signal transduction pathways of angiotensin II-induced c-fos gene expression in cardiac myocytes in vitro. Circ Res 73:424–438.

18. Kariya K, Karns LR, Simpson PC. 1994. An enhancer core element mediates stimulation of the rat α-myosin heavy chain promoter by an α$_1$-adrenergic agonist and activated protein kinase C in hypertrophy of cardiac myocytes. J Biol Chem 269:3775–3782.

19. Molkentin JD, Lu J-R, Antos CL, Markham B, Richardson J, Robbins J, Grant SR, Olson EN. 1998. A calcineurin-dependent transcriptional pathway for cardiac hypertrophy. Cell 93:215–228.

20. Van Heugten HAA, Bezstarosti K, Dekkers DHW, Lamers JMJ. 1994. Homologous desensitization of the endothelin-1 receptor evoked phosphoinositide response in cultured neonatal rat cardiomyocytes. J Mol Cell Cardiol 25:41–52.

21. Van Heugten HAA, De Jonge HW, Bezstarosti K, Sharma HS, Verdouw PD, Lamers JMJ. 1995. Intracellular signalling and genetic reprogramming during agonist-induced hypertrophy of cardiomyocytes. Ann NY Acad Sci 752:343–352.

22. Van Heugten HAA, Van Setten MC, Eizema K, Verdouw P, Lamers JMJ. 1998. Sarcoplasmic reticulum Ca^{2+} ATPase promoter activity during endothelin-1 induced hypertrophy of cultured rat cardiomyocytes. Cardiovasc Res 37:503–514.

23. Antin PB, Mar JH, Ordahl CP. 1988. Single cell analysis of transfected gene expression in primary heart cell cultures containing multiple cell types,. Biotechnology 6:630–648.

24. Kohout TA, O'Brian JJ, Gaa ST, Lederer WJ, Rogers TB. 1996. Novel adenovirus component system that transfects cultured cardiac cells with high efficiency. Circ Res 78:971–977.

25. Hajjar RJ, Schmidt U, Kang JX, Matsui T, Rosenzweig A. 1997. Adenovirus gene transfer of phospholamban in isolated rat cardiomyocytes. Rescue effects by concomitant gene transfer of sarcoplasmic reticulum Ca^{2+}ATPase. Circ Res 81:145–153.

26. Meyer M, Dillmann WH. 1998. Sarcoplasmic Ca^{2+}ATPase overexpressing by adenovirus mediated gene transfer and in transgenic mice. Cardiovasc Res 37:360–366.

27. Hajjar RJ, Kang JX, Gwathmey JK, Rosenzweig A. 1997. Physiological effects of adenoviral gene transfer of sarcoplasmic reticulum Ca^{2+}ATPase in isolated rat myocytes. Circulation 95:423–429.

28. Yang N-S, Sun WH, McCabe D. 1996. Developing particle-mediated gene-transfer technology for research into gene therapy of cancer. Mol Med Today (Nov):476–481.

29. Yoshida Y, Kobayashi E, Endo H, Hamamoto T, Yamanaka T, Fujimura A, Kagawa Y. 1997. Introduction of DNA into rat liver with a hand-held Gene gun: Distribution of the expressed enzyme, [^{32}P] DNA, and Ca^{2+} flux. Biochem Biophys Res Commun 234:695–700.

30. Sanford JC. 1988. The biolistic process. Trends Biotechnol 6:299–302.

31. Eizema K, van Heugten HAA, Bezstarosti K, van Setten MC, Lamers JMJ. 1999. In vitro analysis of SERCA2 gene regulation in hypertrophic cardiomyocytes and increasing transfection efficiency by Gene-Gun biolistics. Ann NY Acad Sci 874:111–124.

32. Eizema K, van Heugten HAA, Bezstarosti K, van Setten MC, Lamers JMJ. 2000. Endothelin-1 responsiveness of a 1.4 kb phospholamban promoter fragment in rat cardiomyocytes transfected by the gene gun. J Mol Cell Cardiol 32:311–321.

33. Decock JB, Gillespie-Brown J, Parker PJ, Sugden PH, Fuller SJ. 1994. Classical, novel and atypical isoforms of PKC stimulate ANF and TRE/AP-1 regulated promoter activity in ventricular cardiomyocytes. FEBS Lett 356:275–278.

34. Lompre A-M, De La Bastie D, Boheler KR, Schwartz K. 1989. Characterization and expression of the rat sarcoplasmic reticulum $Ca^{2+}ATPase$ mRNA. FEBS Lett 249:35–41.

35. Shubeita HE, McDonough PM, Harris AN, Knowlton KU, Glembotski CC, Heller Brown J, Chien KR. 1990. Endothelin induction of inositol phospholipid hydrolysis, sarcomere assembly, and cardiac gene expression in ventricular myocytes. A paracrine mechanism for cell hypertrophy. J Biol Chem 265:20555–20562.

36. Kovacic-Milivojevic B, Gardner DG. 1993. Regulation of the human atrial natriuretic peptide gene in atrial cardiocytes by the transcription factor AP-1. Am J Hypertens 6:258–263.

37. Kovacic-Milivojevic B, Gardner DG. 1995. Fra-1, a fos gene family member that activates atrial natriuretic peptide gene transcription. Hypertension 25:679–682.

38. Kass-Eisler A, Falck Pedersen E, Alvira M, Revera J, Buttrick PM, Wittenberg BA, Cipriani L, Leinwand LA. 1993. Quantitative determination of adenovirus mediated gene-delivery to rat cardiac myocytes in vitro and in vivo. Proc Natl Acad Sci USA 90:11498–11502.

39. Kirshenbaum LA, Maclellan WR, Mazur W, French BA, Schneider MD. 1993. Highly efficient gene transfer into adult ventricular myocytes by recombinant adenovirus. J Clin Invest 92:381–387.

40. Kirshenbaum LA. 1997. Adenovirus mediated-gene transfer into cardiomyocytes. Mol Cell Biochem 172:13–21.

41. Hasenfuss G, Just H. 1994. Myocardial phenotype changes in heart failure: cellular and subcellular changes and their functional significance. Br Heart J 72:510–517.

42. Chien KR, Ibu H, Knowlton KR, Miller-Honce W, van Bilsen M, Obrein TX, Evans SM. 1993. Transcriptional regulation during cardiac growth and development. Annu Rev Physiol 55:77–95.

43. Qi M, Bassani JW, Bers DM, Samarel AM. 1996. Phorbol 12-myristate 13-acetate alters SR Ca(2+)-ATPase gene expression in cultured neonatal rat heart cells. Am J Physiol 271(3, Pt 2):H1031–1039.

44. Hartong R, Villarreal FJ, Giordano F, Hilal-Dandan R, McDonough PM, Dillmann WH. 1996. Phorbol myristate acetate-induced hypertrophy of neonatal rat cardiac myocytes is associated with decreased sarcoplasmic reticulum Ca^{2+} ATPase (SERCA2) gene expression and calcium reuptake. J Mol Cell Cardiol 28:2467–2477.

45. Eskildsen, YEG, Bezstarosti K, Dekkers DHW, Van Heugten HAA, Lamers JMJ. 1997. Cross-talk between receptor-mediated phospholipase C-β and D via protein kinase C as intracellular signal possibly leading to hypertrophy in serum-free cultured cardiomyocytes. J Mol Cell Cardiol 29:2545–2559.

46. Clerk A, Bogoyevitch MA, Anersson MB, Sugden P. 1994. Differential activation of protein kinase C isoforms by endothelin-1 and phenylephrin and subsequent stimulation of p42 and p44 mitogen-activated protein kinases in ventricular myocytes cultured from neonatal rat heart. J Biol Chem 269:32848–32857.

47. Puceat M, Hilal-Dandan R, Stulovia B, Brunton LL, Heller Brown J. 1994. Differential regulation of protein kinase C isoforms in isolated neonatal and adult cardiomyocytes. J Biol Chem 269:16938–16944.

48. Cadre BM, Qi M, Eble DM, Shannon TR, Bers DM, Samarel AM. 1998. Cyclic stretch down-regulates calcium transporter gene expression in neonatal rat ventricular myocytes J Mol Cell Cardiol 30:2247–2259.

49. Argentin S, Ardiati A, Tremblay S, Lihrmann I, Robitaille L, Drouin J, Nemer M. 1994. Developmental stage-specific regulation of atrial natriuretic factor gene transcription in cardiac cells. Mol Cell Biol 14:777–790.

50. Knowlton KU, Baraccini E, Ross RR, Harris AN, Henderson SA, Evans SM, Glembotski CC, Chien KR. 1991. Coregulation of the atrial natriuretic factor and cardiac myosin-light chain-2 genes during alpha-adrenergic stimulation of neonatal rat ventricular cells. J Biol Chem 266:7759–7768.

51. Rockman HA, Ross R, Harris AN, Knowlton KU, Steinhelper ME, Field LJ, Ross J, Chien KR. 1991. Segregation of atrial-specific and inducible expression of natriuretic factor transgene in an in vivo murine model of cardiac hypertrophy. Proc Natl Acad Sci USA 88:8277–8281.

52. Koss KL, Kranias EG. 1996. Phospholamban: a prominent regulator of myocardial contractility. Circ Res 79:1059–1063.

53. Simmerman HKB, Jones LR. 1998. Phospholamban: protein structure, mechanism of action and role in cardiac function. Physiol Rev 78:921–947.

54. Luo W, Wolska BM, Grupp H, Harrier JM, Haghighi K, Ferguson DG, Slack JP, Grupp G, Doetschman T, Solaro RJ, Kranias EG. 1996. Phospholamban gene dosage effects in the mammalian heart. Circ Res 78:839–847.

55. Wu J, Kovacic-Milivojevic B, La Pointe MC, Nakamura K, Gardner DB. 1991. Cisspreactive determinants of cardiac-specific expression in the human atrial natriuretic peptide gene. Mol Endocrinol 5:1311–1322.
56. Hajjar RJ, Schmidt U, Matsui T, Guerrero JL, Lee K-H, Gwathmey JK, Dec GW, Semigran MJ, Rosenzweig A. 1998. Modulation of ventricular function through gene transfer in vivo. Proc Natl Acad Sci USA 95:5251–5256.

N. Takeda, M. Nagano and N.S. Dhalla
(eds). The Hypertrophied Heart. Copyright
© 2000. pp. 67–81. Kluwer Academic
Publishers. Boston. All rights reserved.

Ca^{2+} TRANSIENTS, CONTRACTILITY, AND INOTROPIC RESPONSES IN RABBIT VOLUME-OVERLOADED CARDIOMYOCYTES

KIYOHARU SAKURAI,[1] HIROMI SUGAWARA,[1] TOMOO WATANABE,[1] SHIGEKAZU NAKADA,[2] HIROYUKI ATSUMI,[2] HITONOBU TOMOIKE,[2] and MASAO ENDOH[1]

[1] Department of Pharmacology and [2] The 1st Department of Internal Medicine, Yamagata University School of Medicine, 2-2-2 Iida-nishi, Yamagata, 990-9585, Japan

Summary. Left ventricular hypertrophy occurs as an adaptation prior to chronic congestive heart failure caused by pressure or volume overload. We examined the modulation of the effects of Ca^{2+} sensitizers, namely, Org 30029 [N-hydroxy-5,6-dimethoxy-benzo[b]thiophene-2-carboximidamide hydrochloride] and JTV-704 (EGIS-9377) [2-(1-methylthio)-5-(2-morpholinoethylamino)-8,9-dihydro-7H-thiopyrano[3,2-d][1,2,4]triazolo[1,5-a]pyrimidine dihydrochloride], in comparison with those of β-adrenoceptor agonists in cardiomyocytes isolated from volume-overloaded rabbits. We isolated ventricular cardiomyocytes by means of collagenase perfusion 12 weeks after the shunt formation, when ventricular weight, aortic flow, left ventricular pressure, and diastolic pressure had been increased significantly. Cell shortening and Ca^{2+} transients were measured in cardiomyocytes loaded with indo-1. In cardiomyocytes isolated from the volume-overloaded heart, cell length and width were increased proportionally. The duration of Ca^{2+} transients and cell shortening was significantly prolonged in volume-overloaded cardiomyocytes compared with that in normal (isolated from sham-operated rabbit) cardiomyocytes. The response of Ca^{2+} transients and cell shortening to the Ca^{2+} sensitizers, namely, Org 30029 and JTV-704, was unaltered in volume-overloaded cardiomyocytes. By contrast, the response to dobutamine and isoproterenol was significantly attenuated in volume-overloaded cardiomyocytes compared with the response in normal cardiomyocytes. These results indicate that in volume-overloaded rabbit cardiomyocytes, the response to the Ca^{2+} sensitizers was maintained when the responsiveness to β-adrenoceptor stimulation had been reduced, an indication that the Ca^{2+} sensitizer may be beneficial for improvement of contractile dysfunction even when β-agonists lose their effectiveness in volume-overloaded cardiomyocytes with hypertrophy.

INTRODUCTION

The myocardium responds to hemodynamic overload with development of myocyte enlargement in association with enhanced and/or suppressed expression of genes of regulatory proteins, including ion channels, ion exchangers, and contractile proteins, as compensatory mechanisms. Hemodynamic overload leading to cardiac hypertrophy is twofold in nature, namely, pressure overload and volume overload, which induce concentric and eccentric hypertrophy, respectively, with distinct and different cellular and molecular events [1,2].

Pressure overload in animal models has been shown to result in impairments of intracellular Ca^{2+} handling and β-adrenoceptor-mediated cardiac regulation [3,4]. In cardiac hypertrophy induced by severe pressure overload in rats, analysis of Ca^{2+} handling by the sarcoplasmic reticulum (SR) has shown that Ca^{2+} uptake and Ca^{2+}–ATPase activity are significantly diminished, while the steady state level of SR Ca^{2+}–ATPase mRNA has been revealed to be significantly decreased [5,6]. In addition, it has been shown that the density of ryanodine receptor (RyR) protein is likewise decreased [7] in association with a decrease in the expression of RyR mRNA in pressure-overloaded hypertrophy [8].

Volume overload, such as aortic regurgitation, mitral regurgitation, and arteriovenous shunt, also induces cardiac hypertrophy, with an increase in the length and width of cardiomyocytes [9]. Relatively little is known about the change in Ca^{2+} handling and contractility that occurs in volume-overloaded cardiomyocytes compared with those in pressure-overloaded cardiomyocytes because of technical difficulties associated with the preparation of volume-overloaded animal models. Volume overload produces alterations that resemble human heart failure in that volume overload is tolerated better than pressure overload and the development of hypertrophy and heart failure occurs more gradually [10]. In the present study, we examined alterations of Ca^{2+} handling and contractility in response to the Ca^{2+} sensitizers Org 30029 and JTV-704, in comparison with the alterations of β-adrenoceptor-mediated regulation in volume-overloaded rabbit ventricular cardiomyocytes loaded with the Ca^{2+}-sensitive fluorescent dye indo-1.

METHODS

Arteriovenous shunt formation

Male Japanese White rabbits (2.5–3.0 kg) were anesthetized with pentobarbital sodium (20 mg/kg, i.v.). Under sponstaneous ventilation with O_2 (2 L/min), the left common carotid artery and jugular vein were excised longitudinally 7 mm in length and anastomosed side by side continuously with single 8-0 nylon thread (Kono Seisakusyo, Tokyo, Japan) using sterile surgical technique. Measurements of carotid artery flow were undertaken just after the shunt operation by electromagnetic flow meter (MFV-3200, Nihon Kohden, Tokyo, Japan). The carotid artery flow in the shunt side was about fourfold of the flow in the contralateral carotid artery.

Isolation of rabbit ventricular cardiomyocytes

Isolation of rabbit ventricular cardiomyocytes was carried out as decribed previously [11]. Briefly, normal rabbits and rabbits at 12 weeks after the shunt operation were anesthetized with pentobarbital sodium (40 mg/kg, i.v.) and given heparin (600 units/kg, i.v.). The heart was rapidly excised, mounted on a Langendorff apparatus, and retrogradely perfused for approximately 1 minute at a perfusion pressure of 80 cmH_2O with HEPES-Tyrode solution containing (in mM): NaCl 136.5, KCl 5.4, $MgCl_2$ 0.53, $CaCl_2$ 1.2, NaH_2PO_4 0.33, glucose 5.0, HEPES 5.0; pH was 7.4 (adjusted with NaOH). The heart was then perfused with nominally Ca^{2+}-free HEPES-Tyrode solution for 5 minutes, followed by perfusion with recirculation of Ca^{2+}-free HEPES-Tyrode solution to which collagenase (0.6 mg/mL) and protease (0.1 mg/mL) had been added. After approximately 20 minutes, when the heart became homogeneously soft, the enzymes were washed out for 1 minute by perfusion with HEPES-Tyrode solution containing 0.2 mM $CaCl_2$. The ventricles were then removed, minced in HEPES-Tyrode solution containing 0.2 mM $CaCl_2$ and filtered through a nylon mesh (200 μm). The myocytes were resuspended in a stepwise manner in HEPES-Tyrode solution containing 0.2, 0.4, and 0.8 mM $CaCl_2$. The myocytes were finally resuspended in HEPES-Tyrode containing 1.2 or 1.8 mM $CaCl_2$ and kept for 1 hour or longer at room temperature (24 to 26°C) before being loading with the acetoxymethyl ester form of the Ca^{2+}-sensitive fluorescent probe indo-1 (indo-1/AM).

Simultaneous measurements of cell length and Ca^{2+} transients

Myocytes were loaded with indo-1/AM, and subsequent experimental procedures were carried out at room temperature (24 to 26°C). The loading solution consisted of 10 μL of 1 mM indo-1/AM, 40 μL pure DMSO, 90 μL fetal bovine serum, 10 μL of 20% pluronic F-127 (wt/wt in DMSO), and 1 mL HEPES-Tyrode solution. The loading solution described above (1.15 mL) was sonicated for 3 minutes, and 1 mL of cell suspension was added to it. The myocytes were allowed to load with indo-1/AM for 1–4 minutes and then centrifuged at 150 rpm for 1 minute. The supernatant was discarded and the pellet was resuspended in HEPES-Tyrode solution. The myocytes were placed in a perfusion chamber on the stage of an inverted microscope (Diaphot TMD 300, Nikon, Tokyo, Japan) equipped for simultaneous recordings of cell length and indo-1 fluorescence. After 10 minutes, the myocytes were perfused at a rate of about 2 mL/min with bicarbonate buffer containing (in mM) NaCl 116.4, KCl 5.4, $MgSO_4$ 0.81, $CaCl_2$ 1.2, NaH_2PO_4 1.02, glucose 5.0, and $NaHCO_3$ 23.8. The buffer was continuously gassed with 95% O_2–5% CO_2 (pH 7.4). Bipolar platinum electrodes placed in the perfusion chamber were used to stimulate the myocyte with square-wave pulses of 5 ms duration and a voltage of 0.5 to 0.7 V at 0.5 Hz.

Indo-1 fluorescence was excited with the light from a xenon lamp with wavelength of 355 nm, reflected by a 380 nm long-pass dichroic mirror, and detected by means of a fluorescence spectrophotometer (CAM-230, Japan Spectroscopic, Tokyo, Japan). Excitation light was applied to the myocyte through a neutral density filter to minimize the photobleaching of indo-1. The emitted fluorescence was collected by an objective lens (CF Fluor DL40, Nikon) after passing through the 380 nm long-pass dichroic mirror; it was first separated by a 580 nm long-pass dichroic mirror (Omega Optical, Brattleboro, VT, USA). The fluorescence light was subsequently split by a 425 nm dichroic mirror to permit simultaneous measurements of both 405 nm and 500 nm wavelength through band-pass filters, respectively, by use of two separate photomultiplier tubes. The fluorescence ratio (405/500 nm) was then used as an index of $[Ca^{2+}]_i$.

The cell length was monitored simultaneously with indo-1 fluorescence using red light (>620 nm) through the normal bright-field illumination optics of the microscope. The bright-field image of the cell was collected by an objective lens and first separated by a 580 nm long-pass dichroic mirror (Omega Optical). This image was projected onto a photodiode array (C6294-01, Hamamatsu Photonics, Hamamatsu, Japan) scanned every 5 ms.

Cell length and indo-1 fluorescence signals were inputted to a computer (Power Macintosh 8100/100AV, Apple Computer, Cupertino, CA, USA) through an A/D converter (MP-100A, BIOPACS Systems, Santa Barbara, CA, USA) at a sampling rate of 5 ms and analyzed after low-pass filtering (cutoff frequency of 25 Hz) and averaging 5 successive signals.

Experimental protocol

Indo-1-loaded myocytes with rod shape and good condition of cell shortening (extent of shortening before the interventions: 6–10%) were selected in normal and volume-overloaded myocytes, and used for these experiments. The myocytes were equilibrated in the bicarbonate buffer at room temperature. To avoid quenching, the indo-1 signal was recorded intermittently. The cell length was monitored continuously throughout the experiment. When the cell shortening reached a steady level at each concentration of the cardiotonic agents or elevation of $[Ca^{2+}]_o$, the indo-1 fluorescence was measured, and then the buffer containing the next higher concentration of the agents was added stepwise.

Drugs and chemicals

The following drugs were used: (−)-isoproterenol hydrochloride, (±)-dobutamine hydrochloride, fetal bovine serum, pluronic F-127 and protease (type XIV) (Sigma Chemical Co, St. Louis, MO, USA); collagenase (class II, Worthington Biochemical, Freehold, NJ, USA); Org 30029 (Organon Laboratories, Lanarkshire, UK); JTV-704, (EGIS-9377: Nihon Tobacco Co, Osaka, Japan); and indo-1/AM (Dojindo Laboratories, Kumamoto, Japan).

Statistical analysis

Experimental values are presented as means ± SEM. Statistical significance of the effects of the agents was evaluated by one-way ANOVA followed by Bonferroni's test. Comparisons between two mean values were carried out by Student's t-test for unpaired values. The difference is considered to be significant when $p < 0.05$.

RESULTS

Hemodynamic changes in volume-overloaded rabbit hearts

In rabbits with shunt at 12 weeks after the operation ($n = 14$), left ventricular end-diastolic pressure (12.0 ± 1.0 mmHg vs. 4.1 ± 0.8 mmHg) and right ventricular systolic pressure (31 ± 2 mmHg vs. 22 ± 3 mmHg) were elevated significantly compared with those in normal (sham-operated) rabbits at 12 weeks after the operation ($n = 11$). No other hemodynamic parameters in rabbits with shunt were significantly different from those in normal rabbits (heart rate: 271 ± 8 vs. 262 ± 9 beats/min; left ventricular systolic pressure: 138 ± 5 vs. 136 ± 4 mmHg; left ventricular + dP/dt_{max}: 7689 ± 424 vs. 6650 ± 419 mmHg/s; left ventricular $-dP/dt_{max}$: -6402 ± 418 vs. -7383 ± 456 mmHg/s; right ventricular $+dP/dt_{max}$: 1452 ± 149 vs. 1137 ± 222 mmHg/s; right ventricular $-dP/dt_{max}$: -1216 ± 99 vs. -1105 ± 154 mmHg/s; $n = 14, 11$, respectively).

Morphological changes in volume-overloaded rabbit hearts

At 12 weeks after the shunt operation, the left and right ventricular chamber sizes of the rabbits with shunt were macroscopically larger than those of normal rabbits. Left and right ventricular weight in shunt rabbits ($n = 6$) was significantly heavier than that in normal rabbits ($n = 5$) (LV: 8.61 ± 0.15 g in shunt vs. 5.48 ± 0.25 g in normal; RV: 2.58 ± 0.11 g in shunt vs. 1.44 ± 0.03 g in normal, respectively). The left and right ventricular-weight/body-weight ratios in rabbits with shunt were also significantly higher (LV: 2.50 ± 0.07 g/kg in shunt vs. 1.65 ± 0.12 g/kg in normal; RV: 0.75 ± 0.03 g/kg in shunt vs. 0.43 ± 0.02 g/kg in normal, respectively).

Morphological and functional changes in volume-overloaded rabbit myocytes

Figure 1 shows a photograph of normal and volume-overloaded myocytes. The diastolic cell length (152.86 ± 4.54 vs. 131.29 ± 3.03 µm) and width (45.21 ± 1.59 vs. 36.80 ± 1.41 µm) in volume-overloaded myocytes ($n = 20$) were significantly larger than those in myocytes of normal rabbits ($n = 19$). The length/width ratio was not significantly altered in rabbits with shunt (3.46 ± 0.16 vs. 3.65 ± 0.15 µm).

When the duration of cell shortening and Ca^{2+} transients in volume-overloaded myocytes ($n = 23$) was compared with that of normal myocytes ($n = 28$) at the level of 90% relaxation of both signals, the duration of cell shortening (553.3 ± 12.4 vs. 472.1 ± 19.1 ms) and Ca^{2+} transients (1152.2 ± 32.9 vs. 1046.3 ± 29.4 ms) was significantly prolonged in volume-overloaded myocytes. The time to peak shortening was also significantly prolonged in volume-overloaded myocytes (374.0 ± 8.5 vs.

Table 1. Baseline cell length and width of normal and volume-overloaded rabbit ventricular myocytes, showing the appropriate cell shortening to be used for the experiment

	Normal ($n = 19$)	Shunt ($n = 20$)
Length	131.3 ± 3.0	152.9 ± 4.5^a
Width	36.8 ± 1.4	45.2 ± 1.6^a
Length/width	3.65 ± 0.1	3.46 ± 0.2

[a] $p < 0.05$ vs. the corresponding control values in myocytes isolated from sham-operated rabbits (normal).

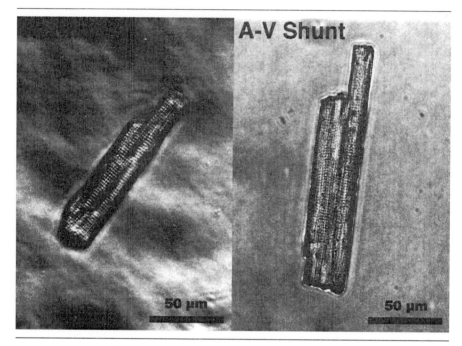

Figure 1. Ventricular cardiomyocytes isolated from normal and volume-overloaded rabbit hearts. In the volume-overloaded myocyte, both cell length and width were proportionally increased.

292.5 ± 12.6 ms). The time required for Ca^{2+} transients to decay to 10% of the peak level was also prolonged significantly in volume-overloaded myocytes (971.9 ± 29.3 vs. 877.5 ± 27.8 ms).

Changes in the effects of cardiotonic agents in volume-overloaded rabbit myocytes

Elevation of $[Ca^{2+}]_0$ increased the cell shortening in a concentration-dependent manner in association with increases in the amplitude of Ca^{2+} transients in sham-operated and volume-overloaded myocytes. There were no significant differences in the response to elevation of $[Ca^{2+}]_0$ between normal ($n = 7$) and volume-overloaded myocytes ($n = 5$).

Isoproterenol, a β-adrenoceptor full agonist (0.3 nM to 30 nM), and dobutamine, a β-adrenoceptor partial agonist (10 nM to 10 μM), exerted a concentration-dependent positive inotropic effect, accompanied by a pronounced increase in the amplitude of Ca^{2+} transients in normal ($n = 7$) and volume-overloaded myocytes ($n = 6$). The response to both isoproterenol and dobutamine in volume-overloaded myocytes was significantly impaired compared with that in normal myocytes.

In myocytes isolated from normal rabbit heart, the Ca^{2+} sensitizers—Org 30029 at 10 to 300 μM and JTV-704 at 1 to 100 μM—induced an increase in cell shortening in a concentration-dependent manner without detectable elevation of the amplitude of Ca^{2+} transients. Actual tracings of the effects of Org 30029 and JTV-704 are presented in figure 2, and the summarized data are shown in figure 3. The diastolic cell length became shorter when the concentration of Ca^{2+} sensitizers was increased, as shown in figures 2 and 4. Total duration, time to peak, and relaxation time of cell shortening were significantly prolonged with no detectable changes in these parameters of Ca^{2+} transients, as shown in figure 5. In contrast to the β-adrenoceptor-mediated response, the increase in systolic cell shortening induced by Org 30029 and JTV-704 in volume-overloaded myocytes was not significantly altered compared with that in normal myocytes.

Relationship between systolic cell shortening and peak Ca^{2+} transients (evaluation of Ca^{2+} sensitivity)

The relationship between the systolic level of Ca^{2+} transients and cell shortening was not modified by volume overload: the relationships during exposure to inotropic interventions, such as elevated $[Ca^{2+}]_o$, isoproterenol, dobutamine, Org 30029, and JTV-704, were similar in normal and volume-overloaded myocytes. The decrease in Ca^{2+} sensitivity induced by isoproterenol and dobutamine in normal myocytes remained unchanged in volume-overloaded myocytes. The increase in Ca^{2+} sensitivity induced by Org 30029 and JTV-704 in normal myocytes was likewise unaltered in volume-overloaded myocytes.

DISCUSSION

Morphological and functional characteristics of volume-overloaded rabbit myocytes

Twelve weeks after the shunt operation, the length and width of myocytes increased proportionally: while the length of myocytes became greater, the ratio of length to width was not significantly changed compared with that in control myocytes isolated from sham-operated rabbits. These findings are consistent with those of Liu and coworkers in rat myocytes with aortocaval fistula [9]. By contrast, in myocytes with pressure overload, cardiac hypertrophy occurs in quite a different manner: primarily the cross-sectional area of myocytes increases, with little or no changes in cell length, and therefore the length/width ratio is decreased in pressure-overloaded myocytes. These changes in the size of volume-overloaded myocytes may be responsible for the macroscopic enlargement (dilatation) of the left and right chambers, which is prominently different compared with pressure-overloaded concentric hypertrophy (wall thickening).

The time for Ca^{2+} transients to decline was prolonged in volume-overloaded myocytes, suggesting that the Ca^{2+} uptake into SR was suppressed in volume-overloaded myocytes. The activity of Ca^{2+} uptake into SR, the energy-consuming process by means of Ca^{2+}–ATPase, may be readily impaired in the failing myocardium [12,13]. This functional derangement may be due to the decrease in mRNA of Ca^{2+}–ATPase in the failing heart [13,14], which provides a potentially reduced

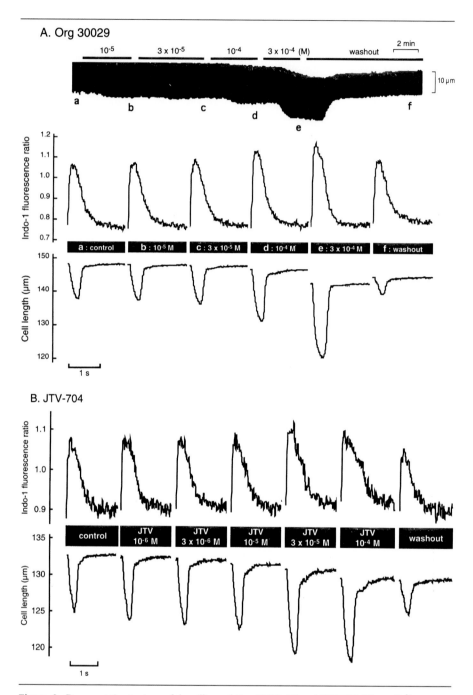

Figure 2. Representative tracings of the effects of Org 30029 (**A**) and JTV-704 (**B**) on Ca^{2+} transients and cell shortening in indo-1-loaded normal rabbit ventricular myocytes. (**A**) The myocyte was exposed to increasing concentrations of Org 30029 that were indicated by horizontal bars. a, control prior to administration of Org 30029; b–e, increasing concentrations of Org 30029; f, after washout of Org 30029. a–f in the lower panels were recorded at the times corresponding to a–f in upper panels. (**B**) The myocyte was exposed to increasing concentrations of JTV-704.

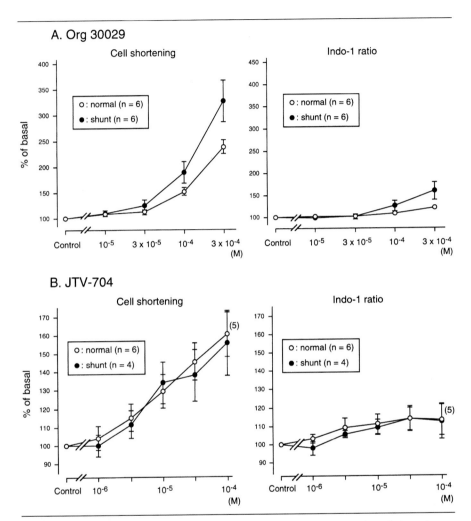

Figure 3. Effects of Org 30029 (**A**) and JTV-704 (**B**) on the amplitude of systolic cell shortening (left panels) and Ca^{2+} transients (right panels) in indo-1-loaded rabbit normal and volume-overloaded myocytes. There were no significant differences in the effects of these Ca^{2+} sensitizers between normal and volume-overloaded rabbit ventricular myocytes. The basal cell lengths of normal and volume-overloaded myocytes were 124.6 ± 8.8 vs. 153.5 ± 7.7 μm in (**A**)($n = 6$ in both normal and volume-overloaded myocytes) and 131.6 ± 5.0 vs. 144.8 ± 16.2 μm in (**B**) ($n = 6$ in normal myocytes, $n = 4$ in volume-overloaded myocytes), respectively. The basal values of the indo-1 ratio in normal and volume-overloaded myocytes were 0.98 ± 0.02 vs. 0.69 ± 0.02 in (**A**) ($n = 6$ in both normal and volume-overloaded myocytes) and 0.93 ± 0.08 vs. 0.79 ± 0.05 in (**B**) ($n = 6$ in normal myocytes, $n = 4$ in volume-overloaded myocytes), respectively.

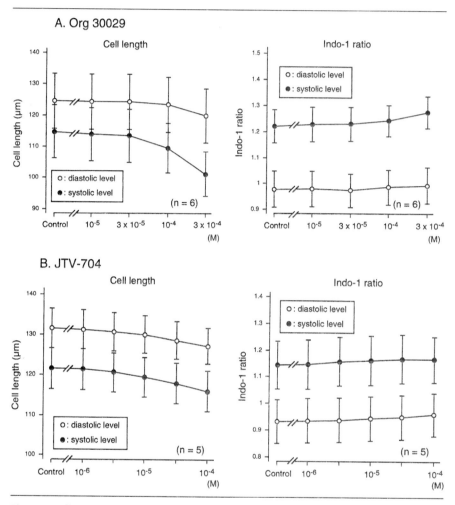

Figure 4. Effects of Org 30029 (**A**) and JTV-704 (**B**) on systolic and diastolic cell length (left panels) and Ca^{2+} transients (right panels) in indo-1–loaded rabbit normal ventricular myocytes.

number of Ca^{2+}–ATPase protein molecules. In adaptive (nonfailing) rat volume-overloaded hypertrophy, Hisamatsu and coworkers have shown that Ca^{2+} uptake into and release from the SR isolated from volume-overloaded heart are both decreased compared with those from the normal heart [15]. In rabbit volume-overloaded myocytes, however, the time to peak Ca^{2+} transients was not significantly longer than that in control myocytes, an indication that the Ca^{2+} release from SR may not be affected, in contrast to a prominent decrease in Ca^{2+} uptake activity in SR in volume-overloaded myocytes.

The time to peak of cell shortening in volume-overloaded myocytes was markedly prolonged compared with that in normal myocytes. It has been reported in the rat

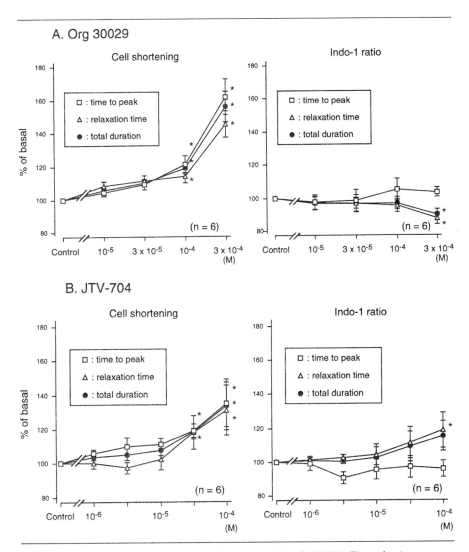

Figure 5. Concentration-dependent effects of Org 30029 (**A**) and JTV-704 (**B**) on the time course of cell shortening (left panels) and Ca^{2+} transients (right panels) in indo-1-loaded rabbit normal ventricular myocytes. *, $p < 0.05$ vs. the corresponding control values. The basal values of time to peak, relaxation time and total duration of cell shortening were 276.3 ± 17.0, 148.3 ± 6.4, and 424.6 ± 23.2 ms in **A** ($n = 6$) and 303.0 ± 34.6, 190.4 ± 19.1, and 493.3 ± 52.9 ms in **B** ($n = 6$), respectively. The basal values of time to peak, relaxation time, and total duration of the indo-1 ratio were 154.6 ± 9.0, 826.3 ± 26.6, and 980.8 ± 27.3 ms in **A** ($n = 6$) and 164.2 ± 4.0, 900.4 ± 66.4, and 1064.6 ± 67.4 ms in **B** ($n = 6$), respectively.

with cardiac hypertrophy that α-myosin is replaced with β-myosin, which has lower ATPase activity and is slower in inducing myocardial contraction but energetically more efficient than α-myosin [16]. Recently, it has been demonstrated that a marked downregulation of α-myosin heavy chain gene expression occurred, being coupled with an upregulation of the β-myosin heavy chain in human heart failure [17]. Therefore, it is likely that the prolongation of the time to peak cell shortening observed in volume-overloaded myocytes might result from the remodeling myosin from α- to β-isoform, while the change in time-to-peak Ca^{2+} transients might contribute to a lesser extent.

Since the time for Ca^{2+} transients to decline was prolonged in volume-overloaded myocytes, it is reasonable to postulate that this prolongation would be reflected in the relaxation time of cell shortening in volume-overloaded myocytes. On the contrary, however, the relaxation time of cell shortening was not prolonged in rabbit volume-overloaded myocytes. This discrepancy could be explained by potential dissociation of both signals under volume overload: since the time to peak shortening was prolonged so prominently by the shift of myosin from α- to β-isoform, cell shortening might have lasted beyond the peak of Ca^{2+} transients, which might have masked the potential prolongation of relaxation time of cell shortening. In addition, it has to be taken into consideration that the procedure for measurements of contractility in single cardiomyocytes is far from ideal: the myocyte is contracting in an auxotonic manner from its slack length in the absence of appropriate stretch to the length close to L_{max}. This disadvantage could disturb the accuracy of the measurements of alterations of contractility that occur during development of volume-overloaded hypertrophy.

The Ca^{2+} influx via L-type Ca^{2+} channels plays a crucial role in cardiac excitation–contraction coupling, which has been reported to be modulated during pressure overload in different manners: L-type Ca^{2+} current density was unchanged [18–21], reduced [22,23], or increased [24] depending on the models used with cardiac hypertrophy and heart failure. In volume-overloaded hypertrophied rabbit myocytes, the baseline L-type Ca^{2+} current amplitude was unchanged or only slightly reduced (unpublished data), a finding that excludes the contribution of L-type Ca^{2+} channels to changes in excitation–contraction coupling induced by volume overload.

Decreased β-adrenoceptor-mediated inotropic response of volume-overloaded rabbit myocytes

The positive inotropic response to the β-adrenoceptor agonists isoproterenol and dobutamine was attenuated significantly in volume-overloaded myocytes compared with that in normal myocytes, in association with the decreased response of amplitude of Ca^{2+} transients to β-stimulation. Atsumi and coworkers have found a persistent elevation of plasma norepinephrine levels after the shunt operation and a decrease in the positive inotropic and chronotropic response to dobutamine, whereas β-adrenoceptors were rather upregulated at 12 weeks after the shunt operation (unpublished data). These results imply that the β-adrenergic pathway may be impaired in the process subsequent to receptor activation, including Gs protein coupling to adenylyl cyclase, protein kinase A, and phosphorylation of functional proteins, which may occur in the course of remodeling to the embryonic phenotype in response to hemodynamic overload of myocardial cells [25].

The enhanced inhibitory pathway via Gi proteins, which has been shown to play a role in attenuation of β-mediated response in heart failure [26–29], might also contribute to the alteration of effects of β-stimulation in the volume-overloaded rabbit model.

Unaltered cardiotonic effects of Ca^{2+} sensitizers on volume-overloaded rabbit myocytes

Org 30029 possesses a pronounced Ca^{2+} sensitizing action and a weak PDE III inhibitory action in intact canine right ventricular trabeculae [30], and Org 30029 could reverse the contractile depression induced by acidosis or BDM [31]. Org 30029 and JTV-704 elicited a positive inotropic effect with little change in Ca^{2+} transients, indicating that these agents act on rabbit myocytes predominantly as Ca^{2+} sensitizers. Important findings in the present study are that the inotropic response to Org 30029 and JTV-704 remained unchanged in the volume-overloaded rabbit myocytes. These results are consistent with previous observations by Hajjar and coworkers [32] in human cardiac muscle that the positive inotropic effect of the Ca^{2+} sensitizers EMD 57033 and Org 30029 in failing myocardium did not differ from that in nonfailing human myocardium. Taken together, these findings indicate that Ca^{2+} sensitizers may be effective in improving the cardiac pump function in myocardial failure induced by both pressure and volume overload, in which the β-adrenoceptor-mediated signal transduction pathway had been impaired.

The potential disadvantage of Ca^{2+} sensitizers in clinical application could be an impairment of ventricular diastolic function due to the Ca^{2+} sensitizing action of the compound over diastolic levels of $[Ca^{2+}]_i$, which might cause the exacerbation of diastolic dysfunction. Hajjar and coworkers have reported that the Ca^{2+} sensitizers EMD 57033 and Org 30029 increased the diastolic force and the duration of cell shortening more readily in failing than in nonfailing human myocardium [32]. Since the diastolic function might have been impaired by abnormal handling of $[Ca^{2+}]_i$ (see, e.g., [33]), further increase in Ca^{2+} sensitivity to diastolic levels of $[Ca^{2+}]_i$ would readily lead to exacerbation of hemodynamics in heart failure patients. Further study will be required, therefore, to elucidate the effect of Ca^{2+} sensitizers on diastolic function in clinical application. In volume-overloaded rabbit myocytes, the extent of diastolic dysfunction induced by Org 30029 and JTV-704 was not different from that in normal myocytes, even in the presence of modified $[Ca^{2+}]_i$ handling, which was evident from the alteration of Ca^{2+} transients in volume-overloaded myocytes.

In conclusion, the present findings indicate that cardiomyocytes isolated from rabbits that have undergone volume overload with arteriovenous shunt for 12 weeks were enlarged proportionally in both longitudinal and transverse directions. The duration of cell shortening and Ca^{2+} transients of volume-overloaded myocytes was prolonged. Although the positive inotropic effect of β-adrenoceptor agonists was markedly impaired, the inotropic effect of the Ca^{2+} sensitizers Org 30029 and JTV-704 remained unaltered in volume-overloaded rabbit ventricular myocytes.

ACKNOWLEDGMENTS

We are grateful to Organon Laboratories (Lanardshire, U.K.) for providing Org 30029 and Nihon Tobacco Co. (Osaka, Japan) for JTV-704. This work was supported in part by a Grant-in-Aid for Scientific Research (B) 11557203 from the Ministry of Education, Science, Sports, and Culture, Japan.

REFERENCES

1. Chien KR, Knowlton KU, Zhu H, Chien S. 1991. Regulation of cardiac gene expression during myocardial growth and hypertrophy: molecular studies of an adaptive physiologic response. FASEB J 5:3037–3046.
2. Calderone A, Takahashi N, Izzo NJ Jr, Thaik CM, Colucci WS. 1995. Pressure- and volume-induced left ventricular hypertrophies are associated with distinct myocyte phenotypes and differential induction of peptide growth factor mRNAs. Circulation 92:2385–2390.
3. Karliner JS, Barnes P, Brown M, Dollery C. 1980. Chronic heart failure in the pig increases cardiac α_1- and β-adrenoceptors. Eur J Pharmacol 67:115–118.
4. Vatner DE, Homcy CJ, Sit SP, Mandders WT, Vatner SF. 1984. Effects of pressure overload, left ventricular hypertrophy on β-adrenergic receptors, and responsiveness to catecholamines. J Clin Invest 73:1473–1482.
5. Komuro I, Kurabayashi M, Shibazaki Y, Takaku F, Yazaki Y. 1989. Molecular cloning and characterization of a Ca^{2+} Mg^{2+}-dependent adenosine triphosphatase from rat cardiac sarcoplasmic reticulum. Regulation of its expression by pressure overload and development stage. J Clin Invest 83:1102–1108.
6. de la Bastie D, Levitsky D, Rappaport L, Mercadier JJ, Marotte J, Wisnewsky C, Brovkovich V, Schwartz K, Lompre AM. 1990. Function of the sarcoplasmic reticulum and expression of its Ca^{2+}-ATPase gene in pressure overload-induced cardiac hypertrophy in the rat. Circ Res 66:554–564.
7. Nandin VN, Rannou OF, Beuve CS, Charlemagne D. 1991. The density of ryanodine receptors decreased with pressure overload-induced rat cardiac hypertrophy. FEBS Lett 285:135–138.
8. Matsui H, Maclennan DH, Alpert NR, Periasamy M. 1995. Sarcoplasmic reticulum gene expression in pressure overload-induced cardiac hypertrophy in rabbit. Am J Physiol 268:C252–C258.
9. Liu Z, Hilbelink DR, Crockett WB, Gerdes AM. 1991. Regional changes in hemodynamics and cardiac myocyte size in rat with aortocaval fistulas. l. Developing and established hypertrophy. Circ Res 69:52–58.
10. Carabero BA, Nakano K, Corin W, Biederman R, Spann JF. 1989. Left ventricular function in experimental volume overload hypertrophy. Am J Physiol 256:H974–H981.
11. Sugawara H, Endoh M. 1998. A novel cardiotonic agent SCH00013 acts as a Ca^{++} sensitizer with no chronotropic activity in mammalian cardiac muscles. J Pharmacol Exp Ther 287:214–222.
12. Cory CR, McCutcheon LJ, O'Grady M, Pang AW, Geiger JD, O'Brien PJ. 1993. Compensatory downregulation of myocardial Ca^{2+} channel in SR from dogs with heart failure. Am J Physiol 264:H926–H937.
13. Gupta RC, Shimoyama H, Tanimura M, Nair R, Lesch M, Sabbah HN. 1997. SR Ca^{2+}-ATPase activity and expression in ventricular myocardium of dogs with heart failure. Am J Physiol 273:H12–H18.
14. Arai M, Matsui H, Periasamy M. 1994. Sarcoplasmic reticulum gene expression in cardiac hypertrophy and heart failure. Circ Res 74:555–564.
15. Hisamatsu Y, Ohkusa T, Kihara Y, Inoko M, Ueyama T, Yano M, Sasayama S, Matsuzaki M. 1997. Early changes in the functions of cardiac sarcoplasmic reticulum in volume-overloaded cardiac hypertrophy in rats. J Mol Cell Cardiol 29:1097–1109.
16. Mercadier JJ, Lompre AM, Wisnewsky C, Samuel JL, Bercovici J, Swynghedauw B, Schwartz K. 1981. Myosin isoenzymic changes in several models of rat cardiac hypertrophy. Circ Res 49:525–532.
17. Lowes BD, Minobe W, Abraham WT, Rizeq MN, Bohlmeyer TJ, Quaife RA, Roden RL, Dutcher DL, Robertson AD, Voelkel NF, Badesch DB, Groves BM, Gilbert EM, Bristow MR. 1997. Changes in gene expression in the intact human heart. Downregulation of α-myosin heavy chain in hypertrophied, failing ventricular myocardium. J Clin Invest 100:2315–2324.
18. Ryder KO, Bryant SM, Hart G. 1993. Membrane current changes in left ventricular myocytes isolated from guinea pigs after abdominal aortic coarctation. Cardiovasc Res 27:1278–1287.

19. Furukawa T, Myerburg RJ, Furukawa N, Kimura S, Bassett AL. 1994. Metabolic inhibition of $I_{Ca,L}$ and I_K differs in feline left ventricular hypertrophy. Am J Physiol 266:H1121–H1131.
20. Scamps F, Mayoux E, Charlimagne D, Vassort G. 1990. Calcium current in single cells isolated from normal and hypertrophied rat heart: effects of β-adrenergic stimulation. Circ Res 67:199–208.
21. Brooksby P, Levi AJ, Jones JV. 1993. The electrophysiological characteristics of hypertrophied ventricular myocytes from the spontaneously hypertensive rat. J Hypertens 11:611–622.
22. Ming Z, Nordin C, Siri F, Aronson RS. 1994. Reduced calcium current density in single myocytes isolated from hypertrophied failing guinea pig hearts. J Mol Cell Cardiol 26:1133–1143.
23. Nuss HB, Houser SR. 1993. T-type Ca^{2+} current is expressed in hypertrophied adult feline left ventricular myocytes. Circ Res 73:777–782.
24. Xiao Y-F, McArkle JJ. 1994. Elevated density and altered pharmacologic properties of myocardial calcium current of the spontaneously hypertensive rat. J Hypertens 12:783–790.
25. Maltsev VA, Ji GJ, Wobus AM, Fleischmann BK, Hescheler J. 1999. Establishment of β-adrenergic modulation of L-type Ca^{2+} current in the early stages of cardiomyocyte development. Circ Res 84: 136–145.
26. Bristow MR, Ginsburg R, Minobe W, Cubicciotti RS, Sageman WS, Lurie K, Billingham ME, Harrison DC, Stinson EB. 1982. Decreased catecholamine sensitivity and beta-adrenergic-receptor density in failing human hearts. N Engl J Med 307:205–211.
27. Fan T-H, Liang C-S, Kawashima S, Banerjee SP. 1987. Alterations in cardiac β-adrenoceptor responsiveness and adenylate cyclase system by congestive heart failure in dogs. Eur J Pharmacol 140: 123–132.
28. Feldman AM, Cates AE, Veazey WB, Hershberger RE, Bristow MR, Baughman KL, Baumgartner WA, Van Dop C. 1988. Increase of the 40,000-mol wt pertussis toxin substrate (G protein) in the failing human heart. J Clin Invest 82:189–197.
29. Bristow MR, Hershberger RE, Port JD, Rasmussen R. 1989. $β_1$ and $β_2$ adrenergic receptor mediated adenylate cyclase stimulation in non-failing and failing human ventricular myocardium. Mol Pharmacol 35:295–303.
30. Kawabata Y, Endoh M. 1993. Effects of the positive inotropic agent Org-30029 on developed force and aequorin light transients in intact canine ventricular myocardium. Circ Res 72:597–606.
31. Watanabe A, Tomoike H, Endoh M. 1996. Ca^{2+} sensitizer Org-30029 reverses acidosis- and BDM-induced contractile depression in canine myocardium. Am J Physiol 271:H1829–H1839.
32. Hajjar RJ, Schmidt U, Helm P, Gwathmey JK. 1996. Ca^{++} sensitizers impair cardiac relaxation in failing human myocardium. J Pharmacol Exp Ther 280:247–254.
33. Hajjar RJ, Gwathmey JK. 1991. Calcium-sensitizing inotropic agents in the treatment of heart failure: critical view. Cardiovasc Drugs Ther 5:961–966.

N. Takeda, M. Nagano and N.S. Dhalla
(eds). The Hypertrophied Heart. Copyright
© 2000. pp. 83–90. Kluwer Academic
Publishers. Boston. All rights reserved.

RESPONSIVENESS OF CONTRACTILE ELEMENTS TO MUSCLE LENGTH CHANGE IN HYPERTHYROID FERRET MYOCARDIUM

TETSUYA ISHIKAWA,[2] HIDETOSHI KAJIWARA,[2] SEIBU MOCHIZUKI,[2] and SATOSHI KURIHARA[1]

Department of Physiology, [1] Department of Cardiology [2] The Jikei University School of Medicine, 3-25-8 Nishishinbashi, Minato-ku, Tokyo 105-8461, Japan

Summary. Hyperthyroidism induces cardiac hypertrophy, which alters the properties of contractile elements. However, the responsiveness of hyperthyroid myocardium to changes in muscle length (the cellular basis of Frank–Starling's law of the heart) is poorly understood. In the present study, we measured the changes in tension and the Ca^{2+} transients monitored with aequorin in the papillary muscles excised from thyroxine-treated hyperthyroid ferrets (Hy) when muscle length was quickly changed during twitch contraction. We also measured the pCa–tension relationship at different muscle lengths in trabeculae treated with Triton X-100. The ratio of heart weight to body weight in Hy was significantly higher than that in age-matched euthyroid ferrets (Eu) ($p < 0.001$). Extra-Ca^{2+} (a transient increase in the intracellular Ca^{2+} concentration in response to quick length change) did not significantly differ in Hy and Eu. The values of pCa_{50}, reflecting the responsiveness of the myofilament to Ca^{2+}, measured at sarcomere lengths of 2.3 and 1.9 μm, were identical at each sarcomere length in Hy and Eu. These results indicate that in the hypertrophied mycoardium induced by hyperthyroidism the responsiveness of the contractile elements to muscle length change is similar to that in euthyroid myocardium.

INTRODUCTION

Thyroid hormone produces various effects on the cardiovascular system [1]. The hyperthyroid state secondarily induces cardiac hypertrophy through the direct effects (a promotion of the synthesis of proteins, etc.) and indirect effects (an increase in the peripheral circulation, etc.) of thyroid hormone on myocardium [1]. Although the properties of the contractile elements in hyperthyroid myocardium have been investigated, the responsiveness of the contractile elements to muscle length change, which is the underlying mechanism of Frank–Starling's law of the heart, has not been fully understood.

   In the present study, we treated ferrets with thyroxine to produce the hyperthyroid state, and investigated how the contractile elements in hyperthyroid myocardium respond to muscle length change in twitch contraction using the aequorin method.

In addition, pCa-tension relations at different muscle length were measured using Triton X-100-treated skinned trabeculae.

METHODS

The methods for the induction of hyperthyroid in ferrets and for the analysis of myosin isoforms have been previously described [2].

Thin papillary muscles or trabeculae were dissected from the right ventricle of ferrets for intact preparations. Both ends of the preparation were tied with silk threads. One end of the preparation was connected to the lever of a motor that was used to alter muscle length, and the other end was connected to the arm of a tension transducer. The preparation was mounted horizontally in an experimental chamber with a pair of platinum black electrodes placed parallel to the preparation for electrical stimulation. The preparation was stimulated with a rectangular pulse at a 1.2-fold threshold with a 5 ms duration. The stimulation frequency was 0.2 Hz unless otherwise mentioned. Before the experiment began, the preparation was slowly stretched to L_{max}, the length at which developed tension reached its maximum.

Measurement of the intracellular Ca^{2+} transients with aequorin has been described by Allen and Kurihara [3]. In order to improve the signal-to-noise ratio, 64 signals were averaged. The constants used in the present experiment were as follows: n, 3.14; K_R, 4,025,000; K_{TR}, 114.6 [4].

In most experiments, Tyrode's solution buffered with HEPES was used, with the following composition (mM): Na^+, 1.28; K^+, 5; Ca^{2+}, 2; Mg^{2+}, 1; Cl^-, 117; SO_4^{2-}, 1; acetate, 20; glucose, 10; and insulin, 5 units/L; pH was adjusted to 7.40, with NaOH at 30°C. The solution was equilibrated with 100% O_2. The temperature of the solution was continuously monitored with a thermocouple and was maintained at 30 ± 0.5°C.

During twitch contraction, muscle length was quickly shortened from L_{max} to 92% L_{max} within 4 ms using an electromagnetic motor. In response to muscle length change, a transient change in the intracellular Ca^{2+} concentration ($[Ca^{2+}]_i$) was observed (extra-Ca^{2+}) [2,3,5–7]. We altered the magnitude of the extra-Ca^{2+} by changing the magnitude of tension reduction in the solution with 2 mM $[Ca^{2+}]_o$.

The method for skinned preparation has also been previously described [2]. The preparations were immersed in the relaxing solution containing 1% Triton X-100 for 60 minutes. After treatment of the preparation with Triton X-100, the preparation was washed with the relaxing solution without Triton X-100. The preparation was cut into a small bundle (length: 1–1.5 mm) in the relaxing solution and used for the experiments. Both ends of the preparation were tied with silk monofilaments, and then the preparation was transferred carefully to a muscle chamber of the same design as that reported by Horiuti [8]. The sarcomere length of the preparations was adjusted to 2.3 μm by measuring the first order of laser diffraction lines.

The composition of the relaxing solution was as follows (mM): K methanesulfonate, 88.6; ATP, 4.5; magnesium methanesulfonate, 5.2; EGTA, 10; PIPES [piperazine-1,4-bis (2-ethanesulfonic acid)], 20; creatine phosphokinase, 10 IU/mL;

dithiothreitol, 0.5. The pH was adjusted to 7.1, with KOH at 20°C. Free Ca^{2+} concentration of the solution was calculated using the binding constant of each ion for each ligand [9]. The calculated apparent dissociation constant of EGTA for Ca^{2+} was 407 nM. The concentrations of free Mg^{2+} and Mg-ATP were kept at 1.0 and 3.5 mM, respectively. The ionic strength was maintained at 0.2 M. The solutions of various pCa ($= -\log[Ca^{2+}]$) were made by mixing the relaxing solution and the solution at a pCa of 4.0. The temperature of the solution was kept at $20 \pm 0.5°C$ throughout the experiment.

We induced contraction of skinned preparations with an activating solution at each pCa by quickly moving the muscle chamber; the solution was changed within 1 second. The measured tension induced by the solution at each pCa was normalized to that of the maximal tension at pCa 5.05, and the relation between the relative tension and pCa was determined. The relationship between pCa and tension in each preparation was fitted by nonlinear least-squares regression to a Hill equation expressed as follows: $T = [Ca^{2+}]^N/(K^N + [Ca^{2+}]^N)$, where T is the tension normalized to the maximal tension, N is the Hill coefficient, and K is the $[Ca^{2+}]_i$ producing 50% of the maximum tension. pCa_{50} is defined as $-\log[K]$.

Statistics

The measured values were expressed as mean ± standard error of the mean (s.e.m.). Unpaired Student's t-test was used, and statistical significance was verified at $p < 0.05$.

RESULTS

Effects of thyroxine on various parameters related to the treatment

In order to confirm that our thyroxine treatment was effective, we compared the following parameters in both groups. The ratios of wet heart weight to body weight (HW/BW) in euthyroid (Eu) and hyperthyroid (Hy) ferrets were 0.0046 ± 0.002 ($n = 7$) and 0.0067 ± 0.002 ($n = 23$), respectively (significant change, $p < 0.001$). Serum free T_3 (pg/mL) and free T_4 (ng/mL) concentrations in Hy were 18.1 ± 6.9 and 7.4 ± 0.6 ($n = 5$), respectively, which were significantly higher than those in Eu (free T_3, 3.7 ± 2.6, $n = 3$; free T_4, 0.92 ± 0.07, $n = 3$) ($p < 0.05$ for T_3 and $p < 0.001$ for T_4). The relative ratio of myosin isoforms was significantly converted from V_3 to V_1 in Hy (100% V_3) compared to that in Eu (27% V_1 and 73% V_3) ($p < 0.001$).

Changes in the Ca^{2+} transients and tension in Hy

We simultaneously measured the Ca^{2+} transients and tension by applying the aequorin method to the papillary muscles dissected from Eu and Hy ferret hearts (figure 1). The time courses of tension and CaT in Hy were significantly faster than those in Eu (figures 1C and 1D), although the magnitude of developed tension and the peak intracellular Ca^{2+} concentration were not significantly different (figure 1A and 1B; table 1).

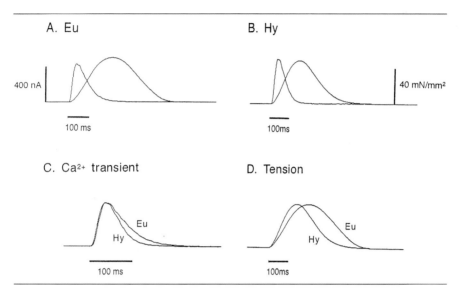

Figure 1. The Ca^{2+} transients and tension in euthyroid (Eu) and hyperthyroid (Hy) myocardium. Representative records of Ca^{2+} transients (aequorin light, faster signals) and tension (slower signals) measured at $2\,mM$ $[Ca^{2+}]_o$ and at L_{max} are shown. (**A**) Eu; (**B**) Hy. The peaks of $[Ca^{2+}]_i$ and developed tension did not significantly differ in both groups (see table 1). In order to observe the differences in the time courses of Ca^{2+} transients and tension, the peaks of Ca^{2+} transients and tension were normalized to match their peaks and superimposed (**C**, **D**, respectively). The decay time was significantly shortened in Hy (see table 1). The time to peak tension and the relaxation time were significantly shortened in Hy (see table 1). From reference 2.

Table 1. Comparison of the measured parameters of the Ca^{2+} transients and tension in euthyroid and hyperthyroid myocardium

	Peak $[Ca^{2+}]_i$ (μM)	TPL (ms)	Decay time (ms)	Tension (mN/mm²)	TPT (ms)	Relaxation time (ms)
Euthyroid (n = 21)	1.8 ± 0.1	38.7 ± 1.5	43.4 ± 1.4	51.0 ± 4.1	194 ± 5	137 ± 6
Hyperthyroid (n = 22)	2.0 ± 0.1	36.4 ± 1.0	33.4 ± 1.0[a]	44.5 ± 6.3	144 ± 3[a]	94 ± 5[a]

[a] Values in hyperthyroid preparations are significantly different from those in euthyroid preparations ($p < 0.001$). Peak $[Ca^{2+}]_i$, the magnitude of CaT that was converted to $[Ca^{2+}]_i$; TPL, time to peak light, the time for aequorin light to reach the peak from the onset of stimulus; decay time, the time for aequorin light to decay from 75% to 25% of the peak; TPT, time to peak tension, the time measured from the onset of stimulus to the peak; relaxation time, the time for tension to decrease from the peak to 50%. From reference 2.

Effects of a quick muscle length change in aequorin–injected papillary muscles in Eu and Hy

Figure 2A shows experimental data of the effects of a quick muscle length change on the Ca^{2+} transients and tension measured in the aequorin-injected papillary muscle in Hy. When the muscle length was quickly shortened from L_{max} to 92%

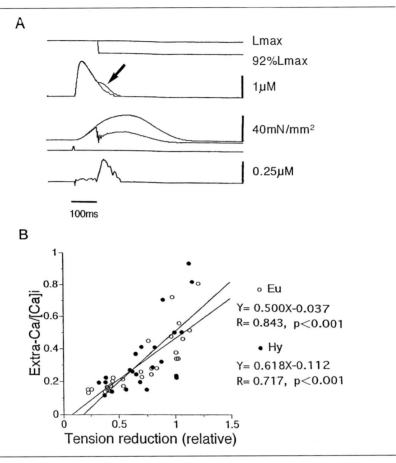

Figure 2. (A) Experimental data of the effects of a quick muscle length change on the Ca^{2+} transient and tension in Hy preparation. Top trace: muscle length. Second trace: $[Ca^{2+}]_i$. Arrow indicates the extra-Ca^{2+}. Third trace: tension. Fourth trace: stimulus. Bottom trace: difference of $[Ca^{2+}]_i$ between two signals (extra-Ca^{2+}). (B) The relation between the amount of extra-Ca^{2+} and tension reduction in Eu (○) and Hy (●) myocardium. The magnitude of the extra-Ca^{2+} normalized to the $[Ca^{2+}]_i$ immediately before length change [Extra-$Ca^{2+}/[Ca^{2+}]_i$] (ordinate) was plotted against the magnitude of tension reduction. These experiments were carried out in the solution with $2\,mM\ [Ca^{2+}]_o$. In order to minimize the disparity of developed tension among all preparations, the magnitude of tension reduction was normalized to the developed tension at L_{max} [Tension reduction (relative)] (abscissa). Equations, correlation coefficients, and the levels of significance are shown in the graphs. Two regression lines in Eu and Hy are not statistically different, although the normalized extra-Ca^{2+} showed a dependence on tension reduction in each preparation. This figure shows pooled data from six experiments for Eu and seven experiments for Hy. From reference 2.

L_{max} during a twitch contraction, developed tension was decreased, and the intracellular Ca^{2+} concentration transiently increased (extra-Ca^{2+}). Extra-Ca^{2+} is considered to reflect Ca^{2+} dissociated from the Tn–Ca^{2+} complex, which is an intermediate between Ca^{2+} signal and tension development. The affinity of Tn–C for Ca^{2+} is influenced by active cross-bridge formation [2,3,5–7]. Therefore, we measured the extra-Ca^{2+} to compare the responsiveness of the contractile elements to the change in active tension in both groups.

Figure 2B shows the relation between the amount of the extra-Ca^{2+} and the magnitude of tension reduction. The extra-Ca^{2+} was a function of the magnitude of tension reduction and the intracellular Ca^{2+} concentration immediately before muscle length change [6]. Therefore, the magnitude of the extra-Ca^{2+} normalized to the intracellular Ca^{2+} concentration immediately before muscle length change was plotted against the magnitude of tension reduction, which was also normalized to the developed tension measured at 2 mM extracellular Ca^{2+} concentration and at L_{max}. Both peaks of the Ca^{2+} transients and tension under control condition (at 2 mM Ca^{2+} and L_{max}) were identical in Eu and Hy (table 1).

Similar regression lines in Eu and Hy indicate that the amount of Ca^{2+} dissociated from the Tn–Ca^{2+} complex through the change in the affinity of Tn–C for Ca^{2+} due to tension reduction was essentially identical in both groups and suggest that the tension-dependent feedback mechanism in Hy works similarly as in Eu.

pCa–tension relation in skinned preparations in Eu and Hy

In order to investigate the responsiveness of the contractile elements to Ca^{2+} at steady state, the pCa–tension relation was measured using thin skinned trabeculae treated with Triton X-100. In addition, the length-dependent change in the Ca^{2+} sensitivity of the contractile elements was also tested in both groups.

In figure 3, pCa–tension relations measured at the sarcomere length of 2.3 μm and at 1.9 μm are shown. Curves were normalized and fitted with the Hill equation. pCa_{50} was not significantly different in both groups, and the length-dependent shift of pCa_{50} was identical in both groups.

Therefore, at steady state, the responsiveness of the contractile elements to muscle length change in Hy was not significantly different from that in Eu.

DISCUSSION

Relevance of thyroxine treatment

The thyroxine treatment in the present study is considered to be effective, because the measured parameters, such as body weight, heart-weight-to-body-weight ratio, serum free T_3 and free T_4 levels, and myosin isoform were all changed as expected from previous reports [10–12]. The cross-bridge cycling rate in Hy is significantly faster compared to that in Eu, because the cross-bridge cycling rate increases depending upon the increase in the relative ratio of the myosin isoform V_1 [13]. In addition, thyroxine is known to increase the amount of Ca^{2+} ATPase mRNA and/or Ca^{2+} ATPase protein and is reported to decrease phospholamban mRNA and/or phospholamban protein in the sarcoplasmic reticulum (SR) [12]. Therefore, in accordance with the increase in the cross-bridge cycling rate and in the Ca^{2+} uptake rate by SR, the time courses of tension and CaT in Hy were significantly shortened compared to those in Eu (table 1) [10,11].

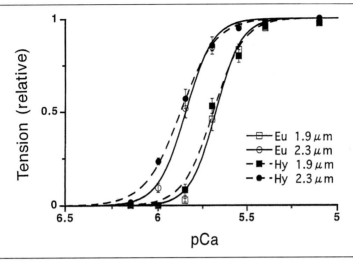

Figure 3. pCa–tension relation in skinned preparations in Eu (solid line) and Hy (dashed line) myocardium at long (2.3 μm) and short (1.9 μm) sarcomere lengths. Curves are normalized and fitted with the Hill equation. Tension at each pCa is expressed as relative values to the maximum tension obtained at pCa 5.05. pCa_{50} values at longer (●) and shorter (■) sarcomere lengths in Hy were similar to those at longer (○) and shorter (□) sarcomere lengths in Eu. The Hill coefficients in Hy were slightly but significantly lower than those in Eu at each length ($p < 0.02$ at longer length, $p < 0.05$ at shorter length). From reference 2.

Properties of the contractile elements of Hy in intact and skinned preparations

When muscle length is quickly shortened during contraction, active cross-bridges detach from thin filaments. The cross-bridge detachment decreases the affinity of Tn–C for Ca^{2+} through the tension-dependent feedback mechanism, and this decrease leads to a transient increase in the myoplasmic Ca^{2+} concentration (extra-Ca^{2+}) [2,3,5–7]. Therefore, the extra-Ca^{2+} is considered to be a function of the amount of Ca^{2+} bound to Tn–C and the magnitude of tension reduction (i.e., the number of detached active cross-bridges). A similar normalized extra-Ca^{2+} in Hy and Eu shows that sufficient Ca^{2+} is on the binding sites of Tn–C in Hy and Eu, and also suggests that the tension-dependent change in the Ca^{2+} affinity of Tn–C works similarly in Hy and Eu (figure 2).

The pCa–tension relation in Hy, which represents the Ca^{2+} responsiveness of the contractile elements, did not differ considerably from that in Eu, and the shift of the pCa–tension relation at the shorter length was similar in both groups. The decrease in the Ca^{2+} sensitivity of the myofilaments induced by shortening the sarcomere length is considered to be mainly due to the increase in interfilament lattice space, which substantially influences the interaction of the cross-bridges with thin filaments [14]. A slight decrease in the Hill coefficient was observed in Hy at both sarcomere lengths. However, the physiological significance of the small change in the Hill coefficient is not clear, because the extra-Ca^{2+} produced by a tension reduction that partly reflects cooperation of the contractile elements did not significantly differ in both groups. Therefore, the contractile elements in Hy at different muscle lengths (relatively within the physiological length) can sufficiently respond to Ca^{2+} as in the case of Eu.

In conclusion, the responsiveness of the contractile elements to muscle length change in hyperthyroid myocardium was essentially similar to that in euthyroid myocardium.

REFERENCES

1. Klein I. 1990. Thyroid hormone and the cardiovascular system. Am J Med 88:631–637.
2. Ishikawa T, Kajiwara H, Kurihara S. In press. Modulation of the Ca^{2+} transient decay by tension and Ca^{2+} removal in hyperthyroid myocardium. Am J Physiol 276:H289–H299.
3. Allen DG, Kurihara S. 1982. The effects of muscle length on intracellular calcium transients in mammalian cardiac muscle. J Physiol (Lond) 327:79–94.
4. Okazaki O, Suda N, Hongo K, Konishi M, Kurihara S. 1990. Modulation of Ca^{2+} transients and contractile properties by β-adrenoceptor stimulation in ferret ventricular muscles. J Physiol (Lond) 423:221–240.
5. Komukai K, Ishikawa T, Kurihara S. 1998. Effects of acidosis on Ca^{2+} sensitivity of contractile elements in intact ferret myocardium. Am J Physiol 274:H147–H154.
6. Kurihara S, Komukai K. 1995. Tension-dependent changes of the intracellular Ca^{2+} transients in ferret ventricular muscles. J Physiol (Lond) 489:617–625.
7. Kurihara S, Saeki Y, Hongo K, Tanaka E, Suda N. 1990. Effects of length change on intracellular Ca^{2+} transients in ferret ventricular muscle treated with 2,3-butanedione monoxine (BDM). Jpn J Physiol 40:915–920.
8. Horiuti K. 1986. Bioassay of calcium in skinned smooth muscle by contraction of skinned skeletal muscle placed nearby. Jikeikai Med J 33:149–156.
9. Martell AE, Smith RM. 1994. Critical Stability Constants. Vol. 1. Amino Acids. New York: Plenum.
10. MacKinnon R, Gwathmey JK, Allen PD, Briggs GM, Morgan JP. 1988. Modulation by the thyroid state of intracellular calcium and contractility in ferret ventricular muscle. Circ Res 63:1080–1089.
11. Fitzsimons DP, Patel JR, Moss RL. 1998. Role of myosin heavy chain composition in kinetics of force development and relaxation in rat myocardium. J Physiol 513:171–183.
12. Kiss E, Jakab G, Kranias EG, Edes I. 1994. Thyroid hormone-induced alterations in phospholamban protein expression. Circ Res 75:245–251.
13. Rossmanith GH, Hoh JFY, Kirman A, Kwan J. 1986. Influence of V_1 and V_3 isomyosins on the mechanical behaviour of rat papillary muscle as studied by pseudo-random binary noise modulated length perturbations. J Muscle Res Cell Motil 7:307–319.
14. Fuchs F, Wang YP. 1996. Sarcomere length versus interfilament lattice spacing as determinants of cardiac myofilament Ca^{2+} sensitivity and Ca^{2+} binding. J Mol Cell Cardiol 28:1375–1383.

N. Takeda, M. Nagano and N.S. Dhalla
(eds). The Hypertrophied Heart. Copyright
© 2000. pp. 91–107. Kluwer Academic
Publishers. Boston. All rights reserved.

CONTRACTION-DEPENDENT HYPERTROPHY OF NEONATAL RAT VENTRICULAR MYOCYTES: POTENTIAL ROLE FOR FOCAL ADHESION KINASE

DIANE M. EBLE,[1,2] MING QI,[1] JAMES STRAIT,[1] and ALLEN M. SAMAREL[1,2]

The Cardiovascular Institute and the Departments of [1] Physiology and [2] Medicine, Loyola University Chicago Stritch School of Medicine, 2160 South First Avenue, Maywood, Illinois 60153 USA

Summary. Focal adhesion kinase (FAK) and other protein tyrosine kinases (PTKs) found in focal adhesions regulate proliferation and cytoskeletal assembly of nonmuscle cells, but their role in hypertrophic growth of cardiac myocytes has not been investigated. Serum-free, primary cultures of spontaneously contracting and contractile-arrested neonatal rat ventricular myocytes (NRVMs) were used to determine the role of FAK and other PTKs in regulating cardiac gene expression and protein turnover associated with the hypertrophic phenotype. FAK was readily detected in focal adhesions and costameres of spontaneously contracting, hypertrophied myocytes, but was reduced in contractile-arrested cells. Chronic treatment of NRVMs with genistein ($50\,\mu M$), a relatively specific PTK inhibitor, prevented NRVM growth, as demonstrated by significant reductions (by 10–35%) in total protein, total protein/DNA ratio, and myofibrillar protein content. Genistein also significantly reduced myosin heavy chain (MHC) and actin synthesis, and increased MHC and actin degradation. Daidzein ($50\,\mu M$), a weakly active analogue, had much less of an effect. Genistein also markedly reduced β-myosin heavy chain (β-MHC) and to a lesser extent atrial natriuretic factor (ANF) gene expression, thus reproducing many of the phenotypic features of cardiac myocyte atrophy produced by contractile arrest. Transient transfection of NRVMs with an expression vector containing the full-length coding sequence of chick FAK along with rat β-MHC and ANF promoter-luciferase constructs resulted in a 2–4-fold increase in luciferase activity, indicating that FAK stimulated transcription of fetal genes associated with the hypertrophic phenotype. Thus, FAK and/or other PTKs found in focal adhesions may play a role in both the transcriptional and posttranslational regulation of cardiac myocyte hypertrophy.

INTRODUCTION

Although there are substantial data demonstrating that hemodynamic overload in vivo causes myocardial growth and cardiac myocyte hypertrophy, it is still unclear exactly how mechanical stimuli are converted to biochemical signals that lead to changes in gene expression and protein turnover characteristic of the hypertrophic phenotype. An important structural site for the transmission of mechanical signals to the cytoskeleton of cardiac muscle cells involves the integrin–extracellular matrix (ECM)–cytoskeletal protein complex. Integrins are transmembrane, cell-surface receptors that bind to and connect specific ECM components to cytoskeletal proteins within the cytoplasm of individual myocytes. This multimeric protein complex forms elements of the costamere, a band-like structure that links the Z-disc to the sarcolemmal membrane [1]. Costamere-like structures are also found in cultured neonatal and adult cardiac myocytes [2]. In addition, focal adhesions (similar to focal adhesions assembled by adherent nonmuscle cells in culture) serve as cell attachment sites to the ECM substratum, which is required for myocyte adhesion and spreading during long-term culture. Focal adhesions and costameres appear to be critical structures involved in the assembly and maintenance of sarcomeres (reviewed in [3]). Both neonatal and adult cardiac myocytes in culture develop focal adhesions and costameres containing β_1-integrins and vinculin, and their organization appears to be highly regulated by externally applied or intrinsically generated mechanical load [4,5].

In addition to their structural role, myocyte focal adhesions and costameres may also be sites of mechanochemical signal transduction during myocyte hypertrophy. Integrin clustering provides binding sites for several protein kinases that rapidly localize to focal adhesions in response to integrin engagement. These cytoplasmic signaling kinases include the protein tyrosine kinases (PTKs) pp125^{FAK} (FAK), pp60^{Src} (Src), and Csk, and the serine/threonine protein kinase PKC (reviewed in [6] and [7]). FAK is one member of a family of nonreceptor PTKs [8] that also includes PYK2 [9]. FAK binds to the cytoplasmic tail of β_1-integrin through specific sequences located in its N-terminus. The C-terminal region of FAK (the so-called *focal adhesion targeting sequence*) also binds directly to paxillin, a cytoskeletal protein that localizes to sites of integrin clustering. Once localized, FAK can phosphorylate paxillin and other cytoskeletal proteins within focal adhesions. These phosphorylation events may be important in regulating cytoskeletal assembly [10]. FAK also phosphorylates itself at a single tyrosine residue (Y-397) during integrin engagement [11] and thus creates a binding site for other nonreceptor PTKs to associate with FAK and other focal adhesion proteins via their SH2 domains [12]. Conceivably, FAK and other PTKs bound to FAK during integrin clustering activate a growth-promoting, signal transduction pathway such as occurs in response to tyrosine autophosphorylation of a peptide growth factor receptor upon binding to its ligand.

Very little is known about the role of FAK in signaling the hypertrophic phenotype of cardiac myocytes. In this report, we provide the first direct evidence for a role for FAK-dependent signaling in both the transcriptional and posttranslational regulation of cardiac myocyte hypertrophy. Using high-density, spontaneously contracting neonatal rat ventricular myocytes (NRVMs) in primary culture, we demonstrate that FAK content, immunolocalization, and phosphorylation are reduced in cells undergoing atrophy in response to contractile arrest. Furthermore, genistein, a relatively specific PTK inhibitor, reproduces many of the atrophic changes associated with contractile arrest. Finally, overexpression of FAK stimulates the transcription of fetal genes associated with the hypertrophic phenotype.

METHODS

Reagents

Dulbecco's Modified Eagle Medium:Nutrient Mixture F12 (Ham) (1:1; DMEM/F12), Joklik's minimal essential medium (MEM), Ca^{2+}-free, Mg^{2+}-free Hanks Balanced Salts (modified) (HBSS), acid-soluble calf skin collagen, and antibiotic/antimycotic solution were obtained from Sigma Chemical Co., St. Louis, MO, USA. PC-1 tissue culture medium was obtained from BioWhittaker, Walkersville, MD, USA. According to the manufacturer, PC-1 medium is formulated in a specially modified DMEM/F12 base and contains a complete HEPES buffering system with insulin ($15\,\mu g/mL$), T_3 ($0.5\,nM$), fatty acids, and proprietary proteins (at a concentration of less than $530\,\mu g/mL$). Collagenase (type CLS II) was obtained from Worthington Biochemical Corp., Freehold, NJ, USA. Tissue culture plates were obtained from Costar, Cambridge, MA, USA. [^{3}H]leucine, [^{35}S]methionine, [γ-^{32}P]ATP and [α-^{32}P]dCTP were purchased from Amersham, Arlington Heights, IL, USA. All other reagents were of the highest grade commercially available and were obtained from Sigma and Baxter S/P, McGaw Park, IL, USA.

Ventricular dissociation and cardiac myocyte isolation

Ventricular myocytes were isolated from the hearts of two-day-old Sprague–Dawley rats by collagenase digestion, as previously described [13]. Released cells were collected by centrifugation, resuspended in PC-1 medium, and plated at a density of 1600 cells per mm^2 onto collagen-coated plastic 35 mm or 100 mm dishes, or Permanox chamberslides, and left undisturbed in a 5% CO_2 incubator (37°C) for 14–18 hours. During this plating period, approximately two thirds of the cells attached [13]. Unattached cells were then removed by aspiration, and cells were maintained in a 2:1 mixture of DMEM/F12:PC-1 (myocyte growth medium). Media were changed daily.

Immunolocalization

Ventricular myocytes grown on collagen-coated chamberslides were fixed (10 minutes, room temperature) with 2% (w/v) paraformaldehyde in sodium phosphate-buffered saline (PBS), washed (15 minutes) in 1% (w/v) glycine in PBS, and permeabilized (15 minutes) with 0.5% (v/v) Triton X-100 in PBS. Cells were then stained with a polyclonal rabbit antibody directed against the C-terminus of chick FAK, followed by FITC-labeled donkey anti-rabbit IgG. To detect focal adhesions and costameres, myocytes were fixed as above and stained with a mouse monoclonal antibody to paxillin, a cytoskeletal protein localized to focal adhesions in nonmuscle cells. Primary antibody binding was detected with rhodamine-labeled goat anti-mouse IgG. Myocytes were also stained with FITC-conjugated phalloidin to visualize F-actin filaments and myofibrillar structure [14]. Fluorescently labeled cells were then viewed with a Zeiss Model 410 laser scanning confocal microscope. Multiple optical sections approximately 1 μm thick were taken of each sample to eliminate out-of-focus fluorescence of the intensely stained myocytes.

Immunoprecipitation and Western blotting

Cell extracts were prepared in modified RIPA lysis buffer (50 mM Tris, pH 7.5 containing 150 mM NaCl, 1 mM EGTA, 1 mM Na vanadate, 30 mM Na pyrophosphate, 1 mM NaF, 0.25% Na deoxycholate, 0.1% Nonidet P-40, 5 mM β-glycerophosphate, 10 μg leupeptin/mL, 10 μg aprotinin/mL, and 1 mM AEBSF [Pefabloc]). Equal amounts of total cell protein were immunoadsorbed with monoclonal anti-FAK antibody bound to agarose (UBI). The immunoadsorbed proteins were then washed twice with RIPA buffer, extracted with SDS sample buffer, heated to 100°C, and separated by SDS-polyacrylamide gel electrophoresis. Separated proteins were then transferred to PVDF membrane, and the blots were probed with anti-FAK monoclonal antibody. Primary antibody binding was detected with horseradish peroxidase-conjugated, goat anti-mouse IgG and was visualized using enhanced chemiluminescence (Amersham). The blots were then stripped and reprobed with a horseradish peroxidase-conjugated phosphotyrosine monoclonal antibody (RC20H, Transduction Labs).

Video-edge detection system

Myocytes plated onto chamberslides were maintained for 24 hours in standard growth medium. The slide was then cut and inserted into a Plexiglas perfusion chamber (Model RC-25; Warner Instrument Corp., Hamden, CT, USA), and the chamber was then placed on the stage of an inverted microscope (Nikon Diaphot). Cells were superfused with modified Kreb's solution (37°C), containing (in mM) NaCl, 135; KCl, 5.9; CaCl$_2$, 1.5; MgCl$_2$, 1.2; HEPES, 11.6; and D-glucose. Cell shortening was measured using a video-edge detection system (Crescent Electronics, Sandy, UT, USA). The analogue signal was digitized using a DI-200 PGH/PGL I/O Board (DATAQ Instruments, Akron, OH, USA) connected to a personal computer, and was stored in a file for off-line analysis using Windaq/200 Data Acquisition software (Ver. 1.30).

Cellular composition

Total cellular protein content was analyzed by the Lowry method using crystalline human serum albumin as standard. DNA content was measured using 33258 Hoecht dye and salmon sperm DNA as standard, as previously described [13]. Data are the means of duplicate or triplicate wells from each treatment group for each cell isolation, and are expressed as μg per well. Total MHC and actin contents were measured by SDS-polyacrylamide gel electrophoresis, Coomassie brilliant blue staining, and laser densitometry [14,15]. Results are the means of duplicate wells from each treatment group for each cell isolation and are expressed as μg of total MHC or actin per well. The fraction of the total MHC that was the β-MHC isoenzyme in

the same cellular protein extracts was assessed by SDS-polyacrylamide gel electrophoresis, silver staining, and laser densitometry, as previously described [13].

[^{3}H]leucine biosynthetic labeling experiments

Pulse biosynthetic labeling experiments were performed to assess MHC and actin
fractional synthetic rates in control, genistein-treated, and daidzein-treated myocytes,
as previously described [14,15]. MHC and actin fractional synthetic rates (K_s, %/h)
were estimated from the following formula:

$$K_s = 100 \cdot [P\star/(F\star \cdot t)],$$

where $P\star$ and $F\star$ are the leucine-specific radioactivities in proteins and medium,
respectively, and t is the labeling time in hours.

Pulse-chase biosynthetic labeling experiments

MHC and actin degradation in control, genistein-treated, and daidzein-treated
NRVMs were assessed in pulse-chase biosynthetic labeling experiments, as previously described [14,15]. In some cultures, protein tyrosine kinases were inhibited
during the chase by the addition of genistein (50 μM) or daidzein (50 μM) to the
chase medium. Cell samples were separated by SDS-polyacrylamide gel electrophoresis on 180 mm-long, 0.7 mm-thick, 7–17% vertical-gradient SDS-polyacrylamide gels. In each experiment, a constant fraction of the total protein of each
culture dish was applied to individual gel lanes. This procedure ensured that, for all
pulse-chase experiments, the amount of radioactivity in MHC and actin declined
by decay rather than by simple dilution. After electrophoresis, gels were autoradi-
ographed with fluorographic enhancement. Dried gels were exposed to unflashed
Kodak XAR-5 film for varying time periods (2–4 days) at −80°C. Individual MHC
and actin bands on the autoradiographs were scanned three times, and the average
area beneath the MHC peak was computed by autointegration. The fractional rate
of MHC and actin degradation (K_d, %/hour) for each condition was estimated by
the following formula:

$$K_d = 100 \cdot [\ln(AU)_0 - \ln(AU)_{24}]/24,$$

where $\ln(AU)_0$ and $\ln(AU)_{24}$ are the natural logarithms of the average absorbance
(in arbitrary absorbance units) of the MHC or actin bands at times 0 and 24 hours
of the chase. Previous studies [14,15] have indicated that MHC and actin degradation in serum-free cultures of NRVMs conforms to a one-compartment model of
protein turnover (i.e., single-event, random decay). MHC and actin K_d values were
converted to apparent half-lives (in hours) according to the following formula:

$$t_{1/2} = 100 \cdot [\ln(2)/K_d]$$

mRNA analysis

Total cellular RNA was isolated by the method of Chomszynski and Sacchi [16].
RNA was quantified by absorbance at 260 nm, and its integrity was determined by

examining the 28S and 18S rRNA bands in ethidium bromide-stained agarose gels. Total RNA ($10\,\mu g$ per lane) was separated by denaturing agarose gel electrophoresis, subjected to alkali pretreatment, transferred to nylon membranes by capillary action, and cross-linked by ultraviolet irradiation. β-MHC mRNA levels were detected by hybridization to a ^{32}P-labeled, 40-base oligo-deoxyribonucleotide probe (Oncogene Science, Inc., Uniondale, NY, USA) complementary to a unique 3' untranslated region of the rat MHC mRNA, as previously described [17]. ANF mRNA levels were detected by hybridization to a ^{32}P-labeled, 786-bp cDNA probe complementary to the rat ANF gene [18]. The Northern blots were also hybridized to a ^{32}P-labeled, 24-base oligodeoxynucleotide probe specific for rat 18S rRNA [19]. The amounts of β-MHC and ANF mRNA species relative to the amount of 18S rRNA were then quantified by autoradiography at $-80°C$ and by laser densitometry.

FAK overexpression studies

An expression vector containing the full-length coding sequence of chick FAK (kindly provided by Dr. J.T. Parsons, University of Virginia) was cotransfected either with an expression plasmid consisting of 3003 bp of upstream regulatory sequences of the rat ANF gene linked to the reporter gene encoding firefly luciferase [20] or with a β-MHC promoter–luciferase reporter construct consisting of $-354/+34\,bp$ of 5' upstream regulatory sequences ligated into the luciferase expression plasmid pLUC [21]. Transient transfections were performed using the calcium phosphate method. The myocytes (grown on 35 mm dishes) were incubated with the DNA/calcium phosphate solution in medium at $37°C$ in 5% CO_2 for 6 hours. At this time the cells were washed and maintained in cell culture media. In some cultures, spontaneous contractile activity was prevented by the addition of verapamil ($10\,\mu M$) to the culture medium. After 48 hours of culture, the cells were lysed and luciferase was measured as relative light units using an Enhanced Luciferase Assay Kit (Analytical Luminescence Laboratory) using a Berthold Luminometer.

Data analysis

Results were expressed as means $\pm$ SEM. Normality was assessed using the Wilk–Shapiro test, and homogeneity of variance was established with Levine's test. One-way, repeated-measures ANOVA followed by the Student–Neuman–Keuls test was used for the statistical comparison of multiple groups. Paired data were compared by the paired t-test. Data were analyzed using SigmaStat Statistical Software Package (Jandel Corp., Ver. 1.0).

RESULTS

Inhibition of spontaneous contractile activity reduces FAK and FAK tyrosine phosphorylation in NRVMs

Previous studies from our laboratory have demonstrated that high-density NRVMs undergo hypertrophy (in the absence of exogenous stimuli) if allowed to beat spon-

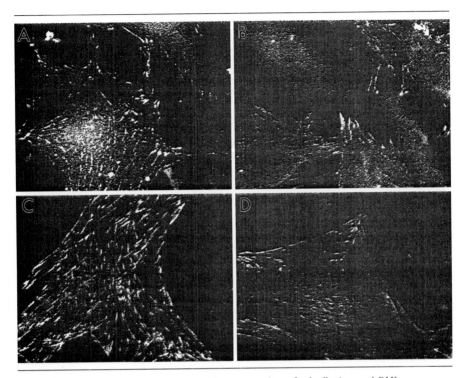

Figure 1. Inhibition of spontaneous contractile activity reduces focal adhesions and FAK immunolocalization in NRVMs. Spontaneously contracting neonatal myocytes grown on collagen-coated chamberslides were maintained (48 hours) in standard growth medium (**A, C**) or medium supplemented with the L-type calcium channel blocker verapamil (10 μM; **B, D**). The myocytes were then fixed, washed, and permeabilized prior to staining for FAK (**A, B**) or paxillin (**C, D**). A polyclonal antibody directed against the C-terminus of chick FAK was detected by FITC-labeled donkey anti-rabbit IgG, and a monoclonal antibody to paxillin was detected by rhodamine-labeled goat anti-mouse IgG. A marked reduction in the central staining of both FAK and paxillin was observed in the verapamil-arrested myocytes as compared to contracting myocytes.

taneously in culture. In contrast, inhibition of spontaneous contractile activity (by L-type Ca^{2+} channel blockade, membrane depolarization, or inhibition of actin–myosin crossbridge formation) prevents contraction-dependent hypertrophy and produces cardiac myocyte atrophy [13,15,22]. We therefore compared the distribution of FAK within focal adhesions of contracting and contractile-arrested NRVMs by immunofluorescence microscopy. As seen in figure 1A, FAK was readily identified within discreet, basilar structures of contracting NRVMs. These sites were identified as focal adhesions by interference reflectance microscopy (not shown) and by localization of paxillin (figure 1C). As previously described [5], the number of focal adhesion sites and costameres and the distribution of paxillin were markedly reduced in noncontracting cells (produced in these experiments by blockade of voltage-sensitive L-type Ca^{2+} channels with the Ca^{2+} channel blocking agent

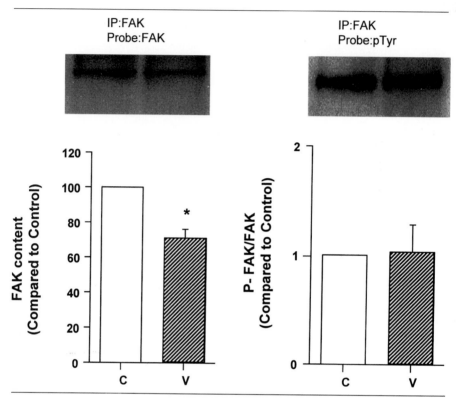

Figure 2. FAK levels and FAK phosphorylation in contracting and arrested NRVMs. Cell lysates from spontaneously contracting neonatal myocytes (Control, C) and myocytes treated with the L-type calcium channel blocker verapamil (V, 10 mM, 48 hours) were prepared using a modified RIPA buffer. Equal amounts of protein were immunoprecipitated (IP) with an anti-focal adhesion kinase (FAK) antibody bound to agarose beads. The immunoadsorbed proteins bound to the beads were washed extensively, extracted with SDS sample buffer, boiled, separated by SDS-polyacrylamide gel electrophoresis, and then transferred to PVDF membrane. The blots were probed with an anti-FAK monoclonal antibody that was detected with horseradish peroxidase-conjugated goat anti-mouse IgG and visualized using enhanced chemiluminescence. The blots were stripped (50°C, 30 minutes) and reprobed with a horseradish peroxidase-conjugated anti-phosphotyrosine (pTyr) monoclonal antibody. The amounts of FAK and phosphorylated FAK (P-FAK) were quantified by laser densitometry. Verapamil-arrested myocytes contained significantly less FAK compared to the control myocytes. However, the ratio of P-FAK to total FAK protein was the same in both control and verapamil-arrested myocytes. Data are the means ± SEM for five cell isolations. Data were compared by paired t-test.

verapamil; figure 1D). The loss of focal adhesions from quiescent NRVMs coincided with a reduction in the amount of immunoreactive FAK detected by confocal microscopy (figure 1B), as well as the time-dependent loss of intact sarcomeres in noncontracting cells ([13,14]; figure 3B). These imaging experiments were confirmed by Western blotting, as depicted in figure 2. Cell extracts were prepared from contracting and contractile-arrested NRVMs, and equal amounts of extracted cellular protein were immunoprecipitated with anti-FAK mAb bound to agarose. The immunoprecipitated FAK was then separated by SDS-PAGE and Western blotting. As seen in figure 2, FAK levels were reduced in noncontracting myocytes, in which contractile activity in these experiments was inhibited by blockade of L-type Ca^{2+} channels with verapamil ($10\,\mu M$). However, the FAK that remained in arrested myocytes showed similar levels of tyrosine phosphorylation as compared to spontaneously contracting cells.

Inhibition of protein tyrosine kinases produces myofibrillar atrophy in spontaneously contracting NRVMs

In order to further investigate the role of FAK and other PTKs in contraction-dependent NRVM hypertrophy, we treated spontaneously contracting NRVMs with the PTK inhibitor genistein ($25\,\mu M$) or the weakly active analogue daidzein ($25\,\mu M$). Genistein treatment reproduced many of the atrophic changes associated with contractile arrest. The PTK inhibitor produced a reduction in the density of myofibrils within each cell, as assessed by laser confocal microscopy of FITC-phalloidin stained cultures (figure 3C). In contrast, NRVMs treated with daidzein ($25\,\mu M$; figure 3D), were indistinguishable from control cultures (figure 3A), which displayed dense arrays of myofibrils throughout the entire thickness of the hypertrophied myocytes. The reduction in myofibrillar density in genistein-treated NRVMs was similar to that observed in cultures treated with the L-type Ca^{2+} channel blocking agent verapamil ($10\,\mu M$, figure 3B), which blocked spontaneous $[Ca^{2+}]_i$ transients and contractile activity [22] and produced sarcomeric disassembly [13,14]. Unlike verapamil, however, genistein had no acute effect on either the amplitude or frequency of spontaneous contractions (table 1). Despite the reduced numbers of myofibrils, NRVMs treated for up to 48 hours with $50\,\mu M$ genistein continued to contract at a rate of 1–2 Hz, as assessed by visual inspection.

Table 1. Genistein has no acute effects on the spontaneous contractile activity of cultured neonatal rat ventricular myocytes

	Control	Genistein	Washout
Contraction amplitude (% of control)	100	90.2 ± 4.2	94.0 ± 8.4
Frequency (bpm)	82 ± 7	93 ± 11	87 ± 14

Spontaneously contracting neonatal myocytes grown on collagen-coated glass coverslips were maintained (24 hours) in standard growth medium. Coverslip cultures were then placed on the stage of an inverted microscope and superfused with modified Kreb's solution during which time the amplitude and frequency of cellular contractions were measured using a video-edge detection system. The superfusion solution was then rapidly switched to Kreb's solution containing genistein ($50\,\mu M$) for 5 minutes, and cell shortening was again measured. Superfusion solution was then switched back to Kreb's solution, and contractile frequency and amplitude were remeasured. Data are the means $\pm$ SEM of four experiments. Data were compared by one-way blocked ANOVA followed by the Student–Newman–Keuls test.

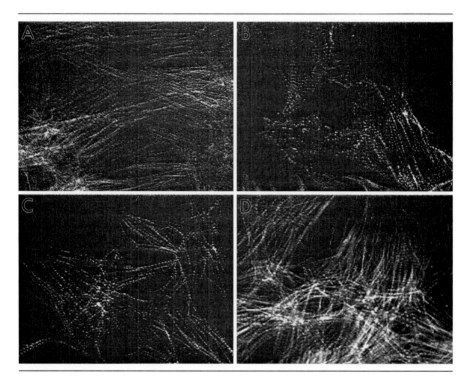

Figure 3. Inhibition of protein tyrosine kinases produces myofibrillar atrophy. Spontaneously contracting neonatal myocytes grown on collagen-coated chamberslides were maintained (48 hours) in standard growth medium (**A**) or medium supplemented with verapamil (10 μM; **B**), genistein (25 μM; **C**), or daidzein (25 μM; **D**). The myocytes were fixed and washed prior to staining with FITC-conjugated phalloidin to visualize F-actin filaments and myofibrillar structure. The control myocytes contained dense arrays of myofibrils throughout the entire thickness of the cell. Protein tryosine kinase inhibition with genistein markedly reduced the density of myofibrils and was comparable to contractile-arrested myocytes such as those treated with verapamil (**B**). The daidzein-treated myocytes were indistinguishable from control myocytes.

In concurrence with the morphological results, we found that treatment of NRVMs with genistein (50 μM) resulted in a reduction in myofibrillar protein content. As seen in table 2, the protein tyrosine kinase inhibitor reduced total protein content and the total protein/DNA ratio, whereas the weakly active analogue daidzein was without effect. Genistein also disproportionately reduced actin and MHC content. In addition, the relative proportion of the β-MHC isoenzyme was selectively reduced in genistein but not in daidzein-treated NRVMs. This isoenzyme switch is similar to that observed by contractile arrest produced with Ca^{2+} channel blocking agents, membrane depolarization, or interference with actin–myosin cross-bridge formation [13,17,23].

The reduced myofibrillar protein content of genistein-treated myocytes resulted from the combined effects of reduced myofibrillar protein synthesis and enhanced

Table 2. Inhibition of protein
tyrosine kinases produces myofibrillar atrophy

	Control	Genistein	Daidzein
Total protein (μg/well)	390 ± 19	230 ± 25[a]	371 ± 23
Total protein/DNA (μg/μg)	67 ± 4	61 ± 3[a]	78 ± 4
Actin (μg/well)	21 ± 2	10 ± 1[a]	21 ± 1
Total MHC (μg/well)	12 ± 1	4 ± 1[a]	10 ± 1[a]
% β-MHC	37 ± 1	24 ± 3[a]	39 ± 1

[a] $p < 0.05$ vs. control.
Spontaneously contracting, neonatal rat ventricular myocytes in 35 mm culture
wells were maintained (72 hours) in control medium or in medium containing
genistein (10–50 μM) or daidzein (10–50 μM). Cells were then harvested for
analysis of total protein, DNA, MHC and actin contents, and the relative concentration of β-MHC. Data are means ± SEM for 3–7 cell isolations. Data were
compared by one-way blocked ANOVA followed by the Student–Newman–Keuls
test.

Table 3. MHC and actin synthesis and degradation
in genistein-treated neonatal rat ventricular myocytes

	Control	Genistein	Daidzein
MHC K_s (%/h)	2.5 ± 0.3	2.1 ± 0.2[a]	2.5 ± 0.3
Actin K_s (%/h)	2.1 ± 0.1	1.7 ± 0.1[a]	2.0 ± 0.1
MHC K_d (%/h)	3.1 ± 0.5	5.9 ± 0.3[a]	3.5 ± 0.2
Actin K_d (%/h)	1.9 ± 0.1	3.6 ± 0.3[a]	2.3 ± 0.3
MHC $t_{1/2}$ (hours)	24 ± 4	12 ± 1	20 ± 1
Actin $t_{1/2}$ (hours)	37 ± 3	20 ± 2	31 ± 5

[a] $p < 0.05$ vs. control.
Spontaneously contracting, neonatal rat ventricular myocytes were maintained (24
hours) in control medium or in medium containing genistein (50 μM) or daidzein
(50 μM). Cells were then pulse-labeled with [³H]leucine (4 hours) for measurement of MHC and actin fractional synthetic rates (K_s). For protein degradation
experiments, contracting myoctyes were biosynthetically labeled with [³⁵S]methio-
nine during the first 24 hours of maintenance culture, followed by chase medium
containing 2 mM unlabeled methionine, or added methionine plus genistein
(50 μM) or daidzein (50 μM). Cells were harvested by SDS lysis for determination of MHC fractional degradative rate (K_d). MHC and actin apparent half-lives
($t_{1/2}$) were derived from the K_d values according to the following formula:
$t_{1/2} = 100 \cdot [\ln(2)/K_d]$. Data are means ± SEM for three cell isolations. Data were
compared by one-way blocked ANOVA followed by the Student–Newman–
Keuls test.

myofibrillar protein degradation. As seen in table 3, both MHC and actin fractional
synthetic rates were inhibited by genistein but not by daidzein. In addition, inhibition of PTKs accelerated the degradation of prelabeled MHC and actin and shortened the intracellular half-lives of these proteins. These results are also similar to
those observed in response to contractile arrest produced by inhibition of phasic

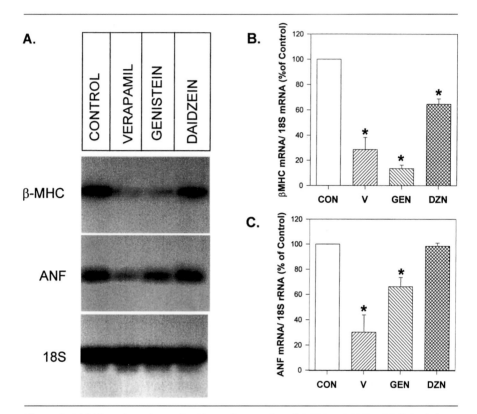

Figure 4. Inhibition of protein tyrosine kinases downregulates β-MHC and ANF mRNA levels in NRVMs. Spontaneously contracting neonatal myocytes were maintained (48 hours) in standard growth medium (CON) or medium supplemented with verapamil (V, 10 μM), genistein (GEN, 25 μM), or daidzein (DZN, 25 μM). Total cellular RNA was isolated and then separated by denaturing agarose gel electrophoresis, subjected to alkali pretreatment, transferred to nylon membranes by capillary action, and cross-linked by ultraviolet irradiation. β-MHC and ANF mRNA levels relative to the amount of 18S rRNA were then quantified by autoradiography at −80°C and by laser densitometry. Representative Northern blots from five individual experiments are shown (**A**) with quantitative analysis for β-MHC (**B**) and ANF (**C**) mRNAs. The high expression of both β-MHC and ANF mRNA levels in spontaneously contracting, CON myocytes was significantly reduced in myocytes treated with genistein but was not greatly affected in myocytes treated with daidzein. The downregulation of both genes with genistein was similar to that seen in verapamil-arrested cultures. Data are expressed as means ± SEM from three different Northern blotting experiments.

$[Ca^{2+}]_i$ transients and contractile activity by membrane depolarization, or blockade of L-type Ca^{2+} channels [13–15].

Furthermore, we found that genistein treatment reduced the expression of secondary response genes characteristic of the hypertrophic phenotype. As seen in figure 4, mRNA transcripts encoding β-MHC and ANF were expressed at high levels in spontaneously contracting, control NRVMs. Genistein reduced both β-MHC and

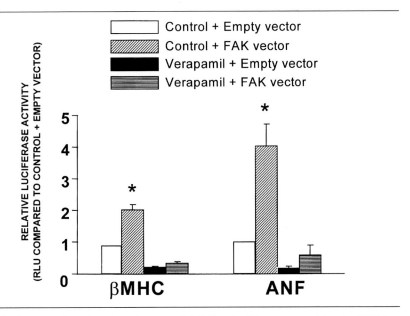

Figure 5. Overexpression of chick FAK activates β-MHC and ANF promoter activities in NRVMs. A constitutively active expression vector containing FAK was transiently transfected into NRVMs using the calcium phosphate method. In addition, an expression plasmid containing 354 bp of the rat β-MHC promoter linked to the gene encoding firefly luciferase or an expression plasmid consisting of 3003 bp of upstream regulatory sequences of the rat ANF gene linked to the gene encoding firefly luciferase were cotransfected with the FAK expression vector or with the empty, parent vector. After 48 hours of culture in either standard growth medium or medium supplemented with verapamil (10 μM), the cells were lysed and luciferase activities were determined. Data are presented as relative light units (RLUs) as a percent of control myocytes transiently transfected with the empty vector. FAK overexpression increased β-MHC promoter activity approximately twofold and ANF promoter activity approximately fourfold in contracting NRVMs but did not significantly increase either ANF or β-MHC expression in verapamil-arrested myocytes. Data are means ± SEM for four different transfection experiments. ⋆, $p < 0.05$ vs. control + empty vector.

ANF mRNA levels, whereas daidzein had little effect. The downregulation of both genes was similar to that observed in verapamil-arrested cultures.

FAK overexpression transactivates β-MHC and ANF promoter activities

Finally, we examined whether overexpression of FAK influenced β-MHC and ANF promoter activity in contracting and arrested NRVMs. As seen in figure 5, cotransfection of wild-type FAK with either reporter gene in spontaneously contracting, control NRVMs significantly increased luciferase activity as compared to paired cultures cotransfected with the identical expression vector lacking the FAK coding region. As is evident from figure 5, "basal" expression of both reporter gene constructs in these high-density, contracting NRVMs was approximately five times higher than in arrested myocytes treated with the L-type Ca^{2+} channel blocker verapamil [23,24]. Overexpression of the empty vector had no effect on basal ANF or β-MHC promoter activity. However, as is evident from the figure, FAK overexpression increased β-MHC promoter activity approximately twofold and ANF promoter activity approximately fourfold in contracting NRVMs. However, FAK overexpression did not significantly increase either ANF or β-MHC expression in verapamil-arrested myocytes.

DISCUSSION

As indicated in this and in our previous report [5], the localization of cytoskeletal proteins within costameres and focal adhesions is markedly affected by the mechanical load placed upon the cell. Our previous study demonstrated that β_1-integrin and vinculin disappear from focal adhesions and costameres in response to contractile arrest. Restoration of contractile activity restored focal adhesions, which temporally preceded the reassembly of myofibrils. Similarly, FAK and paxillin, cytoskeletal proteins that are found in focal contacts of a variety of cultured nonmuscle cells, are readily detected in basilar structures of spontaneously contracting NRVMs. As seen in figure 1, their distribution, like that of vinculin and β_1-integrin, was markedly affected when spontaneous contractile activity was inhibited by L-type Ca^{2+} channel blockade.

Although these proteins are likely to play a structural role in maintaining myocyte adhesion, FAK activation has also been implicated in triggering the cell signaling events that directly lead to cytoskeletal reorganization and cellular growth. FAK has been shown to regulate the tyrosine phosphorylation of paxillin in vitro [25] and in vivo [26]. FAK also tyrosine-phosphorylates itself in response to integrin engagement, and thus provides a high-affinity binding site for Src-family protein kinases to localize to focal adhesions during integrin clustering [12]. The mechanisms whereby FAK and paxillin localization in focal adhesions and costameres are affected by mechanical load in NRVMs is not known, but may be related to the effects of actin–myosin cross-bridge formation on integrin clustering. Burridge and Chrzanowska-Wodnicka [27] have suggested that in nonmuscle cells, agonists that activate Rho lead to stress fiber formation and focal adhesion assembly. They propose that Rho-dependent activation of nonmuscle myosin cross-bridge cycling with actin "bundles" actin filaments to form stress fibers and "clusters" the integrins to which they are attached. In turn, the integrin clustering stimulates FAK activity, triggering the tyrosine phosphorylation of cytoskeletal proteins within focal adhesions leading to additional stress fiber formation. Interestingly, Rhee et al. [28] proposed a similar model for myofibrillogenesis in cardiac myocytes, which involves the initial localization of nonmuscle myosin to peripheral sites of newly forming myofibrils (so-called *premyofibrils*). Myofibril formation begins at the spreading edges of cardiomyocytes, which have characteristics of focal adhesions and are sites for basal membrane–actin cytoskeletal interaction. The actin-containing premyofibrils, which are decorated with nonmuscle myosin and α-actinin (but not sarcomeric myosin, titin, or zeugmatin), subsequently fuse at the level of the Z-bodies to form mature myofibrils. The results presented above in contracting, verapamil-arrested, and genistein-treated NRVMs are consistent with this model and provide a potential mechanism whereby FAK and paxillin are involved in the initiation and maintenance of sarcomeric assembly.

FAK activation by integrin clustering may also trigger cell signaling events that lead to alterations in gene expression and cellular growth. FAK activation by cell adhesion in nonmuscle cells induces the activation of a downstream signaling cascade involving the Ras–MAPK pathway (reviewed in [7]). This signaling cascade has been implicated in cardiac myocyte hypertrophy in response to both stretch [29] and neurohormonal stimuli [30]. Furthermore, Sadoshima et al. [31] have shown that hypotonic swelling of cardiac myocytes rapidly induced tyrosine kinase activity that was necessary for MAPK activation and c-fos gene expression. Nonreceptor PTKs are also activated in response to angiotensin II [32] and prostaglandin $F_{2\alpha}$ [33], both of which induce myocyte hypertrophy via activation of Gq-coupled receptors. A direct involvement of FAK (and/or other nonreceptor PTKs bound to FAK) is suggested by the fact that inhibitors of integrin clustering markedly attenuate ANF transcription in response to phenylephrine, another potent hypertrophic agonist [34]. Furthermore, Kuppuswamy et al. [35] have shown that FAK, Src, and β_3-integrin associate with the cytoskeleton following induction of acute pressure overload in vivo, where they are presumably involved in growth regulation via a load-activated, integrin-mediated signal transduction pathway. Studies currently under way in our laboratory hope to further define the role of FAK and other nonreceptor PTKs in signaling the hypertrophic phenotype in response to neurohormonal and mechanical factors.

ACKNOWLEDGMENTS

The authors thank M. Lisa Spragia and Alan G. Ferguson for excellent technical assistance in the performance of these experiments. These studies were supported by NIH RO1 HL34328, gifts to the Cardiovascular Institute from the Nalco Foundation, and the Ralph and Marian Falk Trust for Medical Research. Dr. Eble was a recipient of an NIH National Research Service Award (F32 HL09611) during the time these studies were performed.

REFERENCES

1. Terracio L, Rubin K, Gullberg D, Balog E, Carver W, Jyring R, Borg TK. 1991. Expression of collagen-binding integrins during cardiac development and hypertrophy. Circ Res 68:734–744.
2. Lu MH, DiLullo C, Schultheiss T, Holtzer S, Murray JM, Choi J, Fischman DA, Holtzer H. 1992. The vinculin/sarcomeric-α-actinin/α-actin nexus in cultured cardiac myocytes. J Cell Biol 117:1007–1022.
3. Hilenski KK, Xuehui MA, Vinson N, Terracio L, Borg TK. 1992. The role of β_1 integrin in spreading and myofibrillogenesis in neonatal rat cardiac myocytes in vitro. Cell Motil Cytoskel 21:87–100.
4. Simpson DG, Decker ML, Clark WA, Decker RS. 1993. Contractile activity and cell–cell contact regulate myofibrillar organization in cultured cardiac myocytes. J Cell Biol 123:323–336.
5. Sharp WW, Simpson DG, Borg TK, Samarel AM, Terracio L. 1997. Mechanical forces regulate focal adhesion and costamere assembly in cardiac myocytes. Am J Physiol 273:H546–H556.
6. Clark EA, Brugge JS. 1995. Integrins and signal transduction pathways: the road taken. Science 268:233–239.

7. Richardson A, Parsons JT. 1995. Signal transduction through integrins: a central role for focal adhesion kinase? BioEssays 17:229–236.
8. Schaller MD, Borgman CA, Cobb BS, Vines RR, Reynolds AB, Parsons JT. 1992. pp125[FAK], a structurally distinctive protein-tyrosine kinase associated with focal adhesions. Proc Natl Acad Sci USA 89:5192–5196.
9. Lev S, Moreno H, Martinez R, Canoll P, Peles E, Musacchio JM, Plowman GD, Rudy B, Schlessinger J. 1995. Protein tyrosine kinase PYK2 involved in Ca^{2+}-induced regulation of ion channel and MAP kinase functions. Nature 376:737–745.
10. Burridge K, Turner CE, Romer LH. 1992. Tyrosine phosphorylation of paxillin and pp125[FAK] accompanies cell adhesion to extracellular matrix: a role in cytoskeletal assembly. J Cell Biol 119:893–903.
11. Guan JL, Trevithick JE, Hynes RO. 1991. Fibronectin/integrin interaction induces tyrosine phosphorylation of a 120 kDa protein. Cell Regul 2:951–964.
12. Schaller MD, Hildebrand JD, Shannon JD, Fox JW, Vines RR, Parsons JT. 1994. Autophosphorylation of the focal adhesion kinase, pp125[FAK], directs SH2-dependent binding of pp60[Src]. Mol Cell Biol 14:1680–1688.
13. Samarel AM, Engelmann GL. 1991. Contractile activity modulates myosin heavy chain-β expression in neonatal rat heart cells. Am J Physiol 261:H1067–H1077.
14. Sharp WW, Terracio L, Borg TK, Samarel AM. 1993. Contractile activity modulates actin synthesis and turnover in cultured neonatal rat heart cells. Circ Res 73:172–183.
15. Samarel AM, Spragia ML, Maloney V, Kamal SA, Engelmann GL. 1992. Contractile arrest accelerates myosin heavy chain degradation in neonatal rat heart cells. Am J Physiol 263:C642–C652.
16. Chomczynshi P, Sacchi N. 1987. Single step method of RNA isolation by acid guanidinium thiocyanate phenol chloroform extraction. Anal Biochem 162:156–159.
17. Qi M, Ojamaa K, Eleftheriades EG, Klein I, Samarel AM. 1994. Regulation of rat ventricular myosin heavy chain expression by serum and contractile activity. Am J Physiol 267:C520–C528.
18. Maki M, Takayanagi R, Misono KS, Pandey KN, Tibbetts C, Inagami T. 1984. Structure of rat atrial natriuretic factor precursor deduced from cDNA sequence. Nature 309:722–724.
19. Chan YL, Gutell R, Noller HF, Wool IG. 1984. The nucleotide sequence of a rat 18S ribosomal ribonucleic acid gene and a proposed secondary structure of 18S ribosomal ribonucleic acid. J Biol Chem 259:224–230.
20. Knowlton KU, Braracchini E, Ross RS, Harris AN, Henderson SA, Evans SM, Glembotski CC, Chien KR. 1991. Co-regulation of the atrial natriuretic factor and cardiac myosin light chain-2 genes during α-adrenergic stimulation of neonatal rat ventricular cells. J Biol Chem 226:7759–7768.
21. Ojamaa K, Klemperer JD, MacGilvray SS, Klein I, Samarel AM. 1996. Thyroid hormone and hemodynamic regulation of β-myosin heavy chain promoter in heart. Endocrinology 137:802–808.
22. Byron KL, Puglisi JL, Holda JR, Eble DM, Samarel AM. 1996. Myosin heavy chain turnover in cultured neonatal rat heart cells: effects of $[Ca^{2+}]_i$ and contractile activity. Am J Physiol 271:C1447–C1456.
23. Qi M, Puglisi JL, Byron KL, Ojamaa K, Klein I, Bers DM, Samarel AM. 1997. Myosin heavy chain gene expression in neonatal rat heart cells: effects of $[Ca^{2+}]_i$ and contractile activity. Am J Physiol 273:C394–C403.
24. Eble DM, Cadre BM, Qi M, Bers DM, Samarel AM. 1998. Contractile activity modulates atrial natriuretic factor gene expression in neonatal rat ventricular myocytes. J Mol Cell Cardiol 30:55–60.
25. Bellis SL, Miller JT, Turner CE. 1995. Characterization of tyrosine phosphorylation of paxillin in vitro by focal adhesion kinase. J Biol Chem 270:17437–17441.
26. Schaller MD, Parsons JT. 1995. pp125[FAK]—dependent tyrosine phosphorylation of paxillin creates a high-affinity binding site for Crk. Mol Cell Biol 15:2635–2645.
27. Burridge K, Chrzanowska-Wodnicka M. 1996. Focal adhesions, contractility, and signaling. Annu Rev Cell Dev Biol 12:463–519.
28. Rhee D, Sanger JM, Sanger JW. 1994. The premyofibril: evidence for its role in myofibrillogenesis. Cell Motil Cytoskel 28:1–24.
29. Sadoshima J, Izumo S. 1997. The cellular and molecular response of cardiac myocytes to mechanical stress. Annu Rev Physiol 59:551–571.
30. Bogoyevitch MA, Sugden PH. 1996. The role of protein kinases in adaptational growth of the heart. Int J Biochem Cell Biol 28:1–12.
31. Sadishima J, Qiu Z, Morgan JP, Izumo S. 1996. Tyrosine kinase activation is an immediate and essential step in hypotonic cell swelling-induced ERK activation and c-fos gene expression in cardiac myocytes. EMBO J 15:5535–5546.

32. Sadoshima J, Izumo S. 1996. The heterotrimeric G_q protein-coupled angiotensin II receptor activates p21^{ras} via the tyrosine kinase-Shc-Grb2-Sos pathway in cardiac myocytes. EMBO J 15:775–787.
33. Adams JW, Sah VP, Henderson SA, Brown JH. 1998. Tyrosine kinase and c-Jun NH_2-terminal kinase mediate hypertrophic responses to prostaglandin $F_{2\alpha}$ in cultured neonatal rat ventricular myocytes. Circ Res 83:167–178.
34. Ross RS, Pham C, Shai SY, Goldhaber JI, Fenczik C, Glembotski CC, Ginsberg MH, Loftus JC. 1998. β_1 integrins participate in the hypertrophic response of rat ventricular myocytes. Circ Res 82:1160–1172.
35. Kuppuswamy D, Kerr C, Narishige T, Kasi VS, Menick DR, Cooper G IV. 1997. Association of tyrosine-phosphorylated c-Src with the cytoskeleton of hypertrophying myocardium. J Biol Chem 272:4500–4508.

N. Takeda, M. Nagano and N.S. Dhalla
(eds). The Hypertrophied Heart. Copyright
© 2000. pp. 109–121. Kluwer Academic
Publishers. Boston. All rights reserved.

MOLECULAR MECHANISM OF MECHANICAL STRESS-INDUCED CARDIAC HYPERTROPHY

ISSEI KOMURO

Department of Cardiovascular Medicine, University of Tokyo Graduate School of Medicine, 7-3-1 Hongo, Bunkyo-ku, Tokyo 113-8655, Japan

Summary. Mechanical stress is a major cause of cardiac hypertrophy. Although the mechanisms by which mechanical load induces cardiomyocyte hypertrophy have long been a subject of great interest for cardiologists, the lack of a good in vitro system has hampered the understanding of the biochemical mechanisms. For these past several years, however, an in vitro neonatal cardiocyte culture system has made it possible to examine the biochemical basis for the signal transduction of mechanical stress. Passive stretch of cardiac myocytes cultured on silicone membranes activates phosphorylation cascades of many protein kinases, including protein kinase C, Raf-1 kinase, and extracellular signal-regulated kinases, and induces the expression of specific genes as well as an increase in protein synthesis. During that process, secretion and production of vasoactive peptides such as angiotensin II and endothelin are increased, and these peptides play critical roles in the induction of these hypertrophic responses. However, we have recently obtained evidence suggesting that the vasoactive peptides are not indispensable for the development of mechanical stress-induced hypertrophic responses. The most important question—how mechanical stimulus is converted into biochemical signals—remains unknown.

INTRODUCTION

Cardiac hypertrophy is a very important issue for cardiologists, not only because it shows diastolic dysfunction and often leads to congestive heart failure but also because it is an independent risk factor for many cardiac diseases such as ischemic heart disease, arrhythmia, and sudden death [1]. Hemodynamic overload is a major cause of cardiac hypertrophy; however, the mechanism by which hemodynamic overload induces cardiomyocyte hypertrophy has long been elusive. An in vitro system by which mechanical stress is imposed on cultured neonatal cardiocytes has made it possible to examine the signal transduction of mechanical stress-induced cardiac hypertrophy [2]. Passive stretch of cardiac myocytes cultured on silicone membranes activates protein kinase cascades of phosphorylation and induces the expression of specific genes as well as an increase in protein synthesis [2–4]. During this process, secretion and production of vasoactive peptides such as angiotensin II

(Ang II) and endothelin-1 (ET-1) are increased, and these peptides play critical roles in the induction of these hypertrophic responses [5–7]. Although these in vitro studies are useful to identify molecules involved in the development of cardiac hypertrophy, it is even more important to test whether these molecules really play an important role in the development of cardiac hypertrophy in vivo. Mouse genetics is a very powerful strategy to elucidate the role of a molecule in the in vivo context.

MECHANICAL STRESS INDUCES CARDIAC HYPERTROPHY

A growing body of evidence has suggested that humoral factors in the circulating blood may have a marginal effect on the development of cardiac hypertrophy in response to hemodynamic overload and that mechanical stress induces cardiac hypertrophy by increasing the local production of humoral factors. How is mechanical stress perceived by a cardiomyocyte as a stimulus? With the use of Langendorf preparations, it has been shown that stretch of the ventricular wall as a consequence of increased aortic pressure is the mechanical parameter most closely related to an increase in protein synthesis [8]. This observation has been confirmed by experiments on cardiocytes cultured in vitro with serum-free media. When cardiocytes cultured on deformable silicone membranes were stretched, an increase in protein synthesis was observed [2]. Stretching cardiocytes also induced expression of specific genes, such as immediate early response genes (IEGs) and fetal type genes ([3,4]; for a review, see [9,10]). These observations suggest that mechanical stress (hemodynamic overload) induces cardiomyocyte hypertrophy by stretching.

MECHANICAL STRESS ACTIVATES A PROTEIN KINASE CASCADE OF PHOSPHORYLATION

Mitogen-activated protein kinase (MAPK) family (figure 1)

A number of intracellular signals are transduced into a nucleus through a protein kinase cascade of phosphorylation [11]. Once a mechanical stimulus is converted into biochemical signals involving phosphorylation events, how do these signals then regulate protein synthesis and gene expression in cardiac myocytes? A growing body of evidence has suggested that mitogen-activated protein kinase (MAPK) family plays a critical role in cell proliferation, differentiation, and death [11–13]. Several members of the MAPK family have been isolated to date, and three members in particular—extracellular signal-regulated kinases (ERKs), c-Jun N-terminal kinase/stress-activated protein kinase (JNK/SAPK), and p38MAPK—have been well characterized.

Extracellular signal regulated kinases (ERKs)

ERKs have been reported to be activated by a variety of growth factors, hormones, cytokines, and phorbol esters and play critical roles in cell proliferation and differentiation of many cell types, including cardiac myocytes [12,13]. ERKs have been reported to be important for the induction of hypertrophic responses, including

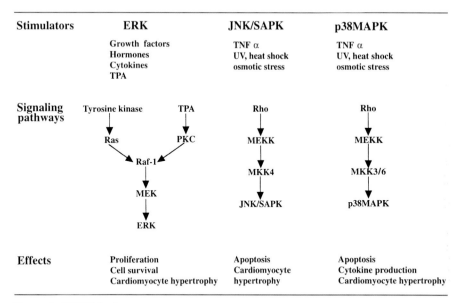

Stimulators	ERK	JNK/SAPK	p38MAPK
	Growth factors Hormones Cytokines TPA	TNF α UV, heat shock osmotic stress	TNF α UV, heat shock osmotic stress

Signaling pathways

Effects

Effects	Proliferation Cell survival Cardiomyocyte hypertrophy	Apoptosis Cardiomyocyte hypertrophy	Apoptosis Cytokine production Cardiomyocyte hypertrophy

Figure 1. MARK family.

specific gene expression and an increase in protein synthesis [14]. Although activation of ERKs is neither sufficient nor indispensable for the development of cardiomyocyte hypertrophy [15], antisense experiments showed that activated ERKs are critical to induce specific gene expression and sarcomere formation as well as an increase in protein synthesis [16]. Stretch of cultured cardiac myocytes by 20% for 10 minutes activated ERKs [17,18]. Stretch also activated its upstream kinases such as Raf-1 kinase and MAPK kinase (MEK; figure 1) [19]. Activation of PKC is known to increase the activity of Raf-1 kinase and ERKs in various cell types [20]. When PKC was depleted by preincubating myocytes with phorbol ester or when its activity was blocked by PKC inhibitors, stretch-induced ERK activity was decreased by more than 80%, suggesting that the stretch-induced increase in ERK activity occurs mainly through a PKC-dependent pathway. Although Ras exists upstream of ERKs in many cell types, and although it was reported that stretch activates Ras [17], inhibition of Ras had no effects on stretch-induced ERK activation [21]. These results suggest that, although it is not clear why activated Ras does not lead to activation of ERKs, stretch-induced ERK activation is dependent on PKC but not on Ras. Stretch also activated p90 S6 kinase as a downstream kinase of ERKs [17,18]. Although the signaling pathway remains to be determined, p70 S6 kinase was also activated by stretch. Stretch-induced activation of all these kinases, such as PKC, Raf-1, MEK, ERKs, and p90 and p70 S6 kinases, were partly suppressed by antagonists for Ang II and ET-1 receptors, suggesting the involvement of vasoactive peptides in stretch-induced activation of protein kinases (see Neuro-humoral Factors, below).

JNK/SAPK

JNK was first reported to be activated in response to cellular stresses such as osmotic stress, ultraviolet irradiation, oxidative stress, and heat shock [22]. JNK is not acti-vated by authentic growth factors such as EGF and basic FGF but is activated by proinflammatory cytokines, including tumor necrosis factor-α (TNFα). Since there are some similarities between osmotic stress and stretch, we examined whether mechanical stretch activates JNK in cardiac myocytes. Stretch by 20% for 10 minutes strongly activated JNK in cultured cardiac myocytes [23]. Of interest, unlike ERKs, stretch-induced JNK activation was not inhibited by Ang II receptor antagonists. Although vasoactive peptides such as Ang II and ET-1 could activate JNK in cul-tured cardiac myocytes [24], the degree of activation by stretch was severalfold stronger than that by Ang II. These results suggest that mechanical stress itself may activate JNK. JNK is activated by a dual protein kinase, JNK kinase (JNKK/SEK/MKK4 or 7). MEKK1 is one of the JNK kinase kinases and is also activated by stretch in cardiac myocytes [19]. Recently, Ask1 has been reported to be a JNK kinase kinase [25]. We have observed that stretch activates Ask1 and inhi-bition of Ask1 attenuates stretch-induced JNK activation (unpublished observation). The elucidation of the molecular mechanism by which stretch activates JNK may pave the way for an understanding how mechanical stress is converted into bio-chemical signals.

   JNK has been reported to be involved in gene regulation by phosphorylating transcription factors, such as c-Jun and ATF-2 [22]. Recently, JNK was reported to be involved in cardiomyocyte hypertrophy [26]. Wang et al. have reported that specific activation of the JNK pathway in cardiac myocytes induced characteristic features of hypertrophy, including an increase in cell size, elevated expression of atrial natriuretic peptide (ANP), and induction of sarcomere organization, and that co-activation of both JNK and p38MAPK in cadiomyocytes led to an induction of cytopathic responses and suppression of hypertrophic responses [26]. In contrast, Nemoto et al. have reported that expression of constitutive active p38MAPK stim-ulated the expression of ANP and that activation of p38MAPK was required for ANP expression induced by the hypertrophic agonists [27]. Activation of JNK led to inhibition of ANP expression induced by MEKK1 and the hypertrophic ago-nists. It remains unknown why contradictory results were obtained; however, the effects of JNK and p38MAPK may be dependent on how or how much the two kinases are activated or inhibited. Both papers [26,27] demonstrated that activation of either JNK or p38MAPK promotes cardiac hypertrophy and that both kinases have opposing effects to each other with references to the development of hyper-trophy. Since both JNK and p38MAPK are usually activated by many stimuli, it remains to be determined how JNK and p38MAPK are involved in the develop-ment of cardiac hypertrophy. Like ERKs, the precise role of JNK in the develop-ment of cardiac hypertrophy is still elusive.

p38MAPK

p38MAPK is usually activated by stimuli similar to those for JNK, namely, cellular stresses such as osmotic stress, ultraviolet irradiation, oxidative stress and heat shock, and anticancer agents [28]. p38MAPK has been reported to play important roles in the induction of apoptosis and the production of cytokines as well as in gene regulation [28]. Cytokines including interleukin-1β (IL-1β), IL-6, and TNFα attracted great attention in the cardiovascular field because they may cause cardiac dysfunction [29]. It has been reported that p38MAPK is activated by hypertrophic agonists such as ET-1, phenylephrine (PHE), and leukemia inhibitory factor (LIF) [30]. As mentioned above, p38MAPK may have effects opposite to JNK on cardiomyocyte hypertrophy, but the precise role of p38MAPK in cardiac hypertrophy is still controversial. Recently, Wang et al. have reported interesting results with reference to p38MAPK [31]. There are four different isoforms in p38MAPK [32]. Activation of p38MAPKα elicited apoptosis in cardiac myocytes, whereas overexpression of p38MAPKβ induces characteristic hypertrophic responses. It remains to be determined how two very similar isoforms elicit completely different effects on cardiac myocytes. A precise mapping of the region of p38MAPKα and β responsible for apoptosis and hypertrophy, respectively, may give us a clue.

p70 S6 protein kinase

There are many pathways by which stretch induces cardiomyocyte hypertrophy (see Future Directions, below). Among these, the phosphorylation of S6 protein in 40S ribosome is well correlated to the efficiency of protein synthesis, and p70 S6 protein kinase (p70^{S6K}) is reported to phosphorylate S6 protein in vivo [33]. Stretch by 20% for 15 minutes activated p70^{S6K} in cardiac myocytes, and inhibition of p70^{S6K} by a specific inhibitor, rapamycin, strongly suppressed stretch-induced increase in protein synthesis without affecting the activity of ERKs and the expression of c-fos [34]. These results suggest that p70^{S6K} is critically involved in stretch-induced cardiomyocyte hypertrophy and that the signaling pathway to p70^{S6K} activation is different from that of ERKs and c-fos. Phosphoinositide-3 kinase (PI3K) activates p70^{S6K} in many cell types; indeed, a PI3K-specific inhibitor, wortmannin, abolished stretch-induced activation of p70^{S6K}. However, activation of authentic PI3K could not be detected after stretch (unpublished observation), suggesting that atypical PI3K, including PI3-Kγ, may be activated by stretch or that p70^{S6K} may be activated through a PI3K independent pathway in cardiac myocytes.

NEUROHUMORAL FACTORS

The protein kinase cascade of phosphorylation activated by mechanical stress on cardiac myocytes is very similar to those evoked by the addition of growth factors and cytokines on many cell types. It is possible that cardiac myocytes and noncardiomyocytes such as fibroblasts, endothelial cells, and smooth muscle cells secrete some hypertrophy-promoting factors following stretch and that these factors induce cardiac hypertrophy by an autocrine or paracrine mechanism. Mechanical stress on myocardial cells has been reported to increase the synthesis of some growth-promoting factors [35].

Angiotensin II

A growing body of evidence has indicated that the local renin–angiotensin system plays a critical role in the development of cardiac hypertrophy (for a review, see [36]). All components of the renin–angiotensin system, such as angiotensinogen, renin, and angiotensin-converting enzyme (ACE), have been identified at both the mRNA and protein levels in the heart. Ang II stimulates protein synthesis in cultured cardiomyocytes [36]. Increases in angiotensinogen and ACE mRNAs have been reported in the hypertrophied left ventricle of rats [37]. Subpressor doses of ACE inhibitors can prevent or cause regression of cardiac hypertrophy with no change in systemic systolic blood pressure [38]. An increase in left ventricular mass that was produced by abdominal aortic constriction, without significant increase in plasma renin activity, was completely prevented with an ACE inhibitor, without any change in afterload [39]. These results strongly suggest that the local renin–angiotensin system, not the circulating one, may play a critical role in pressure overload-induced cardiac hypertrophy.

Ang II induces activation of ERKs and expression of the c-*fos* gene as well as an increase in protein synthesis in neonatal rat cardiocytes through the Ang II type 1 receptor (AT_1) [40]. Activation of ERKs and upregulation of c-*fos* gene expression by Ang II are blocked by PKC inhibitors, and Ang II actually increases production of inositol phosphates and activates PKC [40,41]. These signals elicited by Ang II in cardiac myocytes are very similar to those evoked by mechanical stress, as mentioned above. The involvement of Ang II in the stretch-induced hypertrophic responses was examined using AT_1-specific inhibitors. AT_1 antagonists partially but significantly suppressed all stretch-induced hypertrophic responses, such as an increase in amino acid incorporation, the induction of c-*fos* gene expression, and the activation of ERKs [5,6]. It was reported that Ang II is stored in secretory granules in neonatal ventricular myocytes and that mechanical stretch causes a release of Ang II from cultured cardiocytes [5]. Although it remains to be determined how stretch induces release of Ang II from the secretory granules in cardiac myocytes, these results suggest that Ang II is responsible at least in part for hypertrophic responses evoked by mechanical stress on cardiac myocytes.

Several studies have demonstrated that when the Ang II/AT_1 signals were inhibited, mechanical stress-induced hypertrophic responses were abolished in vivo [39] and in vitro [5]. We tested whether Ang II/AT_1 signals are indispensable for mechanical stress-induced cardiac hypertrophy using AT_{1a} knockout mice (KO mice) [42–44]. Reverse-transcriptase polymerase chain reaction analysis revealed that although the AT_2 gene was expressed at almost the same levels in the hearts of both types of mice, AT_1 mRNA levels were detected in the hearts of wild type (WT) mice but not in the hearts of KO mice. Acute pressure overload produced by constricting the transverse aorta induced expressions of IEG and activations of ERKs in the heart of KO mice as well as WT mice [42]. Both basal and activated levels of all these responses were significantly higher in KO mice than in WT mice. Chronic pressure overload for 40 days produced by constriction of the abdominal aorta markedly increased the ratio of heart weight to body weight and induced fetal gene expressions in both mice to almost the same degree [43]. These results suggest that cardiac hypertrophy could be induced by pressure overload in the in vivo heart with AT_{1a} signaling.

We next examined the molecular mechanism by which mechanical stress induces hypertrophic responses without Ang II/AT_1 signaling by using cultured cardiac myocytes prepared from AT_{1a} KO mice [44]. When cardiac myocytes were stretched by 20% for 10 minutes, ERKs were strongly activated in KO cardiomyocytes as well as in WT myocytes. Both basal and stimulated levels of ERKs were higher in cardiomyocytes of KO mice than in those of WT mice. An AT_1 antagonist attenuated stretch-induced ERK activation in WT myocytes but not in KO myocytes. Downregulation of protein kinase C inhibited stretch-induced ERK activation in WT cardiocytes, while a tyrosine kinase inhibitor, genistein, suppressed the ERK activation in KO cardiac myocytes. Tyrphostins (AG1478 and B42), inhibitors for EGF receptor kinase, also significantly attenuated stretch-induced activation of ERKs. Stretch for 8 minutes significantly enhanced phosphorylation of EGF receptor [44]. These results suggest that mechanical stretch could evoke hypertrophic responses in cardiac myocytes that lack AT_1 signaling, partly through tyrosine kinase activation. The clinical implication of this study is that, since there are multiple factors that mediate mechanical stress-induced cardiac hypertrophy, it is pivotal to suppress mechanical stress itself—but not to suppress a single mediator—to prevent the development of cardiac hypertrophy.

Intracellular signaling pathways evoked by Ang II are different among cell types. Ang II markedly activated ERKs in cardiac myocytes. Although Ang II activates Fyn, a Src family tyrosine kinase, and Ras [45], inhibition of these molecules had no effects on Ang II-induced ERK activation. Instead, downregulation of PKC or of a PKC inhibitor calphostin C abolished Ang II-induced ERK activation [46]. Ang II also activated Raf-1 kinase and MEK, and the activation of these kinases is also suppressed by the inhibition of PKC. Since PKC has been reported to directly activate Raf-1 kinase, Ang II activates ERKs possibly through PKC, Raf-1, and MEK. The signaling pathways from AT_1 to ERKs are divergent among cell types. In smooth muscle cells, pertussis toxin had no effects, but PLC, Ca^{2+}, and the Src family are critical for Ang II-induced activation of ERKs. Ang II activates ERKs possibly through Gq–PLCγ–Ca^{2+}–Ca^{2+}-dependent tyrosine kinase Pyk2 and Src–Shc–Grb2–Sos–Ras—ERKs [46]. Cardiac fibroblasts produce and secrete extracellular matrix proteins such as collagen and fibronectin in response to Ang II, which induces fibrosis of the heart. In cardiac fibroblasts, Ang II activates ERKs through pertussis toxin-sensitive G protein, possibly Gi protein. The $\beta\gamma$ subunit of Gi activates Src and then ERKs through Shc–Grb2–Sos–Ras [47]. It remains to be determined why signaling pathways are so divergent among cell types.

Endothelin-1 (ET-1)

ET-1 has been reported to be a strong inducer of cardiac hypertrophy [48]. Stretch-induced activation of ERKs is also suppressed by type A ET-1 (ETA) receptor antagonist [7], suggesting that ET-1 is also involved in mechanical stress-induced hypertrophic responses. Since ET-1-induced activation of ERKs is also inhibited by downregulation of PKC, ET-1 activates ERKs possibly through the same pathway as Ang II. Recently it was reported that Ang II does not have direct, potent, hypertrophy-promoting effects on cardiac myocytes and that Ang II may evoke hypertrophic responses in cardiac myocytes by inducing ET-1 secretion from cardiac fibroblasts [49]. Cross-talk among different cell types and among many molecules might be important not only for maintaining its highly differentiated phenotype but also for inducing cardiac hypertrophy. The beneficial effects of ET-1 receptor antagonists on myocardial infarction highlighted the importance of ET-1 on cardiovascular remodeling [50]. Recently, the importance of Gq protein in the development of pressure overload-induced cardiac hypertrophy was demonstrated using transgenic mice [51]. Class-specific inhibition of Gq-mediated signaling was produced in the hearts of transgenic mice by targeted expression of a carboxyl-terminal peptide of the α-subunit of Gq. When pressure overload was surgically produced, the transgenic mice developed significantly less ventricular hypertrophy than control mice. Although the prevention of cardiac hypertrophy was not complete in the transgenic mice, this study suggests that Gq-coupled receptors such as AT_1, ETA receptor, and seven other transmembrane receptors are important in the development of pressure overload-induced cardiac hypertrophy.

MECHANISMS BY WHICH MECHANICAL STRESS IS CONVERTED INTO BIOCHEMICAL SIGNALS

Stretch-sensitive ion channels and exchangers

Many cells respond to a variety of environmental stimuli by ion channels in the plasma membrane. Mechanosensitive ion channels have been observed with single-channel recordings in more than 30 cell types of prokaryotes, plants, fungi, and all animals so far examined (for a review, see [52]). The activation of stretch-sensitive channels has been proposed as the transduction mechanism between load and protein synthesis in cardiac hypertrophy [53]. The stretch-sensitive channels allow the passage of the major monovalent physiological cations, Na^+ and K^+, and the divalent cation, Ca^{2+}. With the use of a Ca^{2+}-binding fluorescent dye (fluo3) and the patch clamp technique, mechanically induced Ca^{2+} influx through stretch channels was shown to lead to waves of calcium-induced calcium release [54]. Therefore, stretch-sensitive ion channels are one good candidate for the initial responder for mechanical stress. Experiments using inhibitors of stretch-sensitive ion channels, however, failed to confirm this hypothesis. Gadolinium and streptomycin (inhibitors of stretch-sensitive cation channels), glibenclamide (ATP-sensitive K^+ channels), and CsCl (hyperpolarization-activated inward channels) did not inhibit activation of ERKs by stretching [55]. Although preincubation with Ca^{2+} channel blockers or short exposure to EDTA also did not change the induction of c-*fos* mRNA after stretching [56], preincubation with EGTA attenuated stretch-induced activation of ERKs. The result suggests that Ca^{2+} influx from extracellular space may be involved in stretch-induced activation of ERKs. Since the importance of Ca^{2+} in the development of cardiac hypertrophy was recently highlighted [57], it should be worth while to investigate the role of stretch-sensitive ion channels more extensively.

Highly selective inhibitors of the Na^+/H^+ exchanger significantly attenuated the activation of ERKs by stretch [55]. Although the actual activity of the Na^+/H^+ exchanger was not determined, the Na^+/H^+ exchanger may be activated by mechanical stress and function to convert mechanical stress into biochemical signals. It has been reported that alkalization is necessary for proliferation in many cell types and that alkalization may be also involved in stretch-induced activation of hypertrophic responses in cardiomyocytes.

Extracellular matrix and cytoskeleton

Many data have been accumulated indicating that mechanical stress is transduced into the cell from the sites at which cells attach to the extracellular matrix (ECM; for a review, see [58]). Therefore, transmembrane ECM receptors, such as the integrin family, are good candidates for mechanoreceptors. A large extracellular domain of the integrin receptor complex binds various ECM proteins, while a short cytoplasmic domain has been shown to interact with the cytoskeleton in the cell (for a review, see [59]). Since cytoskeleton proteins can potentially regulate plasma membrane proteins such as enzymes, ion channels, and antiporters, mechanical stress could modulate these membrane-associated proteins and stimulate second messenger systems through the cytoskeleton. Integrins can transmit signals not only by organizing the cytoskeleton but also by altering biochemical properties such as the extent of tyrosine phosphorylation of a complex of proteins including pp125[fak] [58]. Stretch of cultured mesangial cells actually enhanced phosphorylation of pp125[fak] [60].

The rho small G protein family, consisting of Rho, Rac, and Cdc42, is important for the function of integrins through regulating the actin cytoskeleton [61]. When functions of the Rho family were inhibited by C3 exoenzyme or by overexpression of Rho GDP dissociation inhibitor and dominant negative mutants, stretch-induced activation of ERKs and expression of IEG were strongly suppressed [21]. Recently, it has been reported that the C3 exoenzyme inhibits MEKK- and PHE-induced ANP expression but not actin organization, indicating that Rho regulates ANP gene expression but not sarcomere assembly [62]. Sah et al. also reported that Rho is involved in PHE- and $G\alpha q$-induced ANP expression but not in Ras-induced ANP expression [63]. Activated RhoA and Ras produced a synergistic effects on ANP gene expression, suggesting that Rho functions in a pathway separate from but complementary to Ras. Treatment of myocytes with Ang II caused a formation of nonstriated actin fiber (premyofibrils), which was abolished by C3 treatment [64]. The expression of constitutively active RhoA caused the formation of premyofibrils. These results suggest that RhoA is involved in premyofibril formation but not in mature myofibril formation.

FUTURE DIRECTIONS

Once mechanical stress is received and converted into biochemical signals, the signal transduction pathway leading to an increase in protein synthesis is similar to the pathway activated by various humoral factors such as growth factors, hormones, and cytokines in many other cells. Recently, yeast genes encoding members of the MAPK family have been isolated by complementary yeast mutations as essential proteins for restoring the osmotic gradient across the cell membrane in response to increased external osmolality [65]. This result suggests that mechanical stress-induced intracellular signal transduction pathways are highly conserved in evolution.

Although many biochemical events that occur in cardiac myocytes subsequent to mechanical stretch have been clarified, one central intriguing question remains unanswered. How is mechanical stress converted into biochemical signals? In other words, what is the mechanoreceptor or the transducer for mechanical stress in cardiac myocytes? It is conceivable that by stretching the plasma membrane, mechanical stress directly changes the conformations of the functional proteins in the membrane, such as enzymes and G proteins, or directly activates enzymes such as phospholipases by physically placing the enzymes close to phospholipid substances in the plasma membrane. As mentioned above, the integrin–cystoskeleton complex seems to be an alternate candidate structure for a mechanoreceptor and a transducer. Integrin–cytoskeleton proteins not only play a "passive" role, such as maintaining the cell structure, but also may play "active" roles in the regulation of cellular functions, such as protein phosphorylation and activation of an antiporter. Integrin was shown to activate the Na^+/H^+ antiporter by binding to fibronectin, suggesting that integrin can behave similarly to a growth factor receptor in activating signaling pathways [66]. The cytoskeleton has also been shown to play an important role in secretion. Mechanical stress may stimulate secretion of some cytokines, which generate multiple intracellular signals as a secondary event. Further studies are necessary to identify specific signaling molecules, including mechanoreceptors and mechanotransducers, and characterization of these molecules may pave the way to understand the definite mechanism of mechanical stress-induced cardiac hypertrophy and to finally clarify the mechanisms by which adaptive cardiac hypertrophy deteriorates into congestive heart failure.

REFERENCES

1. Levy D, Garrison RJ, Savage DD, Kannel WB, Castelli WP. 1990. Prognostic implications of echocardiographically determined left ventricular mass in the Framingham Heart Study. N Engl J Med 322:1561–1566.
2. Mann DL, Kent RL, Cooper G 4th. 1989. Load regulation of the properties of adult feline cardiocytes: growth induction by cellular deformation. Circ Res 64:1079–1090.
3. Komuro I, Kaida T, Shibazaki Y, Kurabayashi M, Katoch Y, Hoh E, Takaku F, Yazaki Y. 1990. Stretching cardiac myocytes stimulates protooncogene expression. J Biol Chem 265:3595–3598.
4. Komuro I, Katoh Y, Kaida T, Shibazaki Y, Kurabayashi M, Hoh E, Takaku F, Yazaki Y. 1991. Mechanical loading stimulates cell hypertrophy and specific gene expression in cultured rat cardiac myocytes. Possible role of protein kinase C activation. J Biol Chem 266:1265–1268.
5. Sadoshima J, Xu Y, Slayter HS, Izumo S. 1993. Autocrine release of angiotensin II mediates stretch-induced hypertrophy of cardiac myocytes in vitro. Cell 75:977–984.

6. Yamazaki T, Komuro I, Kudoh S, Zou Y, Shiojima I, Mizuno T, Takano H, Hiroi Y, Ueki K, Tobe K, Kadowaki T, Nagai R, Yazaki Y. 1995. Angiotensin II partly mediates mechanical stress-induced cardiac hypertrophy. Circ Res 77:258–265.

7. Yamazaki T, Komuro I, Kudoh S, Zou Y, Shiojima I, Hiroi Y, Mizuno T, Maemura K, Kurihara H, Aikawa R, Takano H, Yazaki Y. 1996. Endothelin-1 is involved in mechanical stress-induced cardiomyocyte hypertrophy. J Biol Chem 271:3221–3228.

8. Kira Y, Kochel PJ, Gordon EE, Morgan HE. 1984. Aortic perfusion pressure as a determinant of cardiac protein synthesis. Am J Physiol 246:C247–C258.

9. Komuro I, Yazaki Y. 1993. Control of cardiac gene expression by mechanical stress. Annu Rev Physiol 55:55–75.

10. Sadoshima J, Izumo S. 1997. The cellular and molecular response of cardiac myocytes to mechanical stress. Annu Rev Physiol 59:551–571.

11. Cantley LC, Auger KR, Carpenter C, Duckworth B, Graziani A, Kapeller R, Soltoff S. 1991. Oncogenes and signal transduction. Cell 64:281–302.

12. Blenis J. 1991. Growth-regulated signal transduction by the MAP kinases and RSKs. Cancer Cells 3:445–449.

13. Nishida E, Gotoh Y. 1993. The MAP kinase cascade is essential for diverse signal transduction pathways. Trends Biochem Sci 18:128–131.

14. Thoburn J, Frost JA, Thorburn A. 1994. Mitogen-activated protein kinases mediate changes in gene expression, but not cytoskeletal organization associated with cardiac muscle cell hypertrophy. J Cell Biol 126:1565–1572.

15. Post GR, Goldstein D, Thuerauf DJ, Glembotski CC, Brown JH. 1996. Dissociation of p44 and p42 mitogen-activated protein kinase activation from receptor-induced hypertrophy in neonatal rat ventricular myocytes. J Biol Chem 271:8452–8457.

16. Glennon PE, Kaddoura S, Sale EM, Sale GJ, Fuller SJ, Sugden PH. 1996. Depletion of mitogen-activated protein kinase using an antisense oligodeoxynucleotide approach downregulates the phenylephrine-induced hypertrophic response in rat cardiac myocytes. Circ Res 78:954–961.

17. Sadoshima J, Izumo S. 1993. Mechanical stretch rapidly activates multiple signal transduction pathways in cardiac myocytes: potential involvement of an autocrine/paracrine mechanism. EMBO J 12:1681–1692.

18. Yamazaki T, Tobe K, Hoh E, Maemura K, Kaida T, Komuro I, Tamemoto H, Kadowaki T, Nagai R, Yazaki Y. 1993. Mechanical loading activates mitogen-activated protein kinase and S6 peptide kinase in cultured rat cardiac myocytes. J Biol Chem 268:12069–12076.

19. Yamazaki T, Komuro I, Kudoh S, et al. 1995. Mechanical stress activates protein kinase cascade of phosphorylation in neonatal rat cardiac myocytes. J Clin Invest 96:438–446.

20. Kyriakis JM, App H, Zhang XF, Banerjee P, Brautigan DL, Rapp UR, Avruch J. 1992. Raf-1 activates MAP kinase-kinase. Nature 358:417–421.

21. Aikawa R, Komuro I, Yamazaki T, Zou Y, Kudoh S, Zhu W, Kadowaki T, Yazaki Y. 1999. Rho family small G proteins play critical roles in mechanical stress-induced hypertrophic responses in cardiac myocytes. Circ Res 84:458–466.

22. Ip YT, Davis RJ. 1998. Signal transduction by the c-Jun N-terminal kinase (JNK)—from inflammation to development. Curr Opin Cell Biol 10:205–219.

23. Komuro I, Kudo S, Yamazaki T, Zou Y, Shiojima I, Yazaki Y. 1996. Mechanical stretch activates the stress-activated protein kinases in cardiac myocytes. FASEB J 10:631–636.

24. Kudoh S, Komuro I, Mizuno T, Yamazaki T, Zou Y, Shiojima I, Takekoshi N, Yazaki Y. 1997. Angiotensin II stimulates c-Jun NH2-terminal kinase in cultured cardiac myocytes of neonatal rats. Circ Res 80:139–146.

25. Ichijo H, Nishida E, Irie K, ten Dijke P, Saitoh M, Moriguchi T, Takagi M, Matsumoto K, Miyazono K, Gotoh Y. 1997. Induction of apoptosis by ASK1, a mammalian MAPKKK that activates SAPK/JNK and p38 signaling pathways. Science 275:90–94.

26. Wang Y, Su B, Sah VP, Brown JH, Han J, Chien KR. 1998. Cardiac hypertrophy induced by mitogen-activated protein kinase kinase 7, a specific activator for c-Jun NH2-terminal kinase in ventricular muscle cells. J Biol Chem 273:5423–5426.

27. Nemoto S, Sheng Z, Lin A. 1998. Opposing effects of Jun kinase and p38 mitogen-activated protein kinases on cardiomyocyte hypertrophy. Mol Cell Biol 18:3518–3526.

28. New L, Han J. 1998. The p38 MAP kinase pathway and its biological function. Trends Cardiovasc Med 8:220–228.

29. Bozkurt B, Kribbs SB, Clubb FJ Jr, Michael LH, Didenko VV, Hornsby PJ, Seta Y, Oral H, Spinale FG, Mann DL. 1998. Pathophysiologically relevant concentrations of tumor necrosis factor-

alpha promote progressive left ventricular dysfunction and remodeling in rats. Circulation 97:1382–1391.

30. Clerk A, Fuller SJ, Michael A, Sugden PH. 1998. Stimulation of "stress-regulated" mitogen-activated protein kinases (stress-activated protein kinases/c-Jun N-terminal kinases and p38-mitogen-activated protein kinases) in perfused art hearts by oxidative and other stresses. J Biol Chem 273:7228–7234.

31. Wang Y, Huang S, Sah VP, Ross J Jr, Brown JH, Han J, Chien KR. 1998. Cardiac muscle cell hypertrophy and apoptosis induced by distinct members of the p38 mitogen-activated protein kinase family. J Biol Chem 273:2161–2168.

32. Jiang Y, Chen C, Li Z, Guo W, Gegner JA, Lin S, Han J. 1996. Characterization of the structure and function of a new mitogen-activated protein kinase (p38beta). J Biol Chem 271:17920–17926.

33. Erikson RL. 1991. Structure, expression, and regulation of protein kinases involved in the phosphorylation of ribosomal protein S6. J Biol Chem 266:6007–6010.

34. Sadoshima J, Izumo S. 1995. Rapamycin selectively inhibits angiotensin II-induced increase in protein synthesis in cardiac myocytes in vitro. Potential role of 70-kD S6 kinase in angiotensin II-induced cardiac hypertrophy. Circ Res 77:1040–1052.

35. Hammond GL, Wieben E, Markert CL. 1979. Molecular signals for initiating protein synthesis in organ hypertrophy. Proc Natl Acad Sci U S A 76:2455–2459.

36. Baker KM, Booz GW, Dostal DE. 1992. Cardiac actions of angiotensin II: role of an intracardiac renin–angiotensin system. Annu Rev Physiol 54:227–241.

37. Schunkert H, Dzau VJ, Tang SS, Hirsch AT, Apstein CS, Lorell BH. 1990. Increased rat cardiac angiotensin converting enzyme activity and mRNA expression in pressure overload left ventricular hypertrophy. Effects on coronary resistance, contractility, and relaxation. J Clin Invest 86:1913–1920.

38. Linz W, Scholkens BA, Ganten D. 1989. Converting enzyme inhibition specifically prevents the development and induces regression of cardiac hypertrophy in rats. Clin Exp Hypertens 11:1325–1350.

39. Baker KM, Chernin MI, Wixson SK, Aceto JF. 1990. Renin–angiotensin system involvement in pressure-overload cardiac hypertrophy in rats. Am J Physiol 259:H324–H332.

40. Sadoshima J, Izumo S. 1993. Molecular characterization of angiotensin II-induced hypertrophy of cardiac myocytes and hyperplasia of cardiac fibroblasts. Critical role of the AT1 receptor subtype. Circ Res 73:413–423.

41. Katoh Y, Komuro I, Shibasaki Y, Yamaguchi H, Yazaki Y. 1989. Angiotensin II induces hypertrophy and oncogene expression in cultured rat heart myocytes. Circulation 80:II–450.

42. Harada K, Komuro I, Shiojima I, Hayashi D, Kudoh S, Mizuno T, Kijima K, Matsubara H, Sugaya T, Murakami K, Yazaki Y. 1998. Pressure overload induces cardiac hypertrophy in angiotensin II type 1A receptor knockout mice. Circulation 97:1952–1959.

43. Harada K, Komuro I, Zou Y, Kudoh S, Kijima K, Matsubara H, Sugaya T, Murakami K, Yazaki Y. 1998. Acute pressure overload could induce hypertrophic responses in the heart of angiotensin II type 1a knockout mice. Circ Res 82:779–785.

44. Kudoh S, Komuro I, Hiroi Y, Zou Y, Harada K, Sugaya T, Takekoshi N, Murakami K, Kadowaki T, Yazaki Y. 1998. Mechanical stretch induces hypertrophic responses in cardiac myocytes of angiotensin II type 1a receptor knockout mice. J Biol Chem 273:24037–24043.

45. Sadoshima J, Izumo S. 1996. The heterotrimeric Gq protein-coupled angiotensin II receptor activates p21 ras via the tyrosine kinase–Shc-Grb2-Sos pathway in cardiac myocytes. EMBO J 15:775–787.

46. Zou Y, Komuro I, Yamazaki T, Kudoh S, Aikawa R, Zhu W, Shiojima I, Hiroi Y, Tobe K, Kadowaki T, Yazaki Y. 1998. Cell type-specific angiotensin II-evoked signal transduction pathways: critical roles of Gbetagamma subunit, Src family, and Ras in cardiac fibroblasts. Circ Res 82:337–345.

47. Zou Y, Komuro I, Yamazaki T, Aikawa R, Kudoh S, Shiojima I, Hiroi Y, Mizuno T, Yazaki Y. 1996. Protein kinase C, but not tyrosine kinases or Ras, plays a critical role in angiotensin II-induced activation of Raf-1 kinase and extracellular signal-regulated protein kinases in cardiac myocytes. J Biol Chem 271:33592–33597.

48. Ito H, Hirata Y, Adachi S, Tanaka M, Tsujino M, Koike A, Nogami A, Murumo F, Hiroe M. 1993. Endothelin-1 is an autocrine/paracrine factor in the mechanism of angiotensin II-induced hypertrophy in cultured rat cardiomyocytes. J Clin Invest 92:398–403.

49. Harada M, Itoh H, Nakagawa O, Ogawa Y, Miyamoto Y, Kuwahara K, Ogawa E, Igaki T, Yamashita J, Masuda I, Yoshimasa T, Tanaka I, Saito Y, Nakao K. 1997. Significance of ventricular myocytes and nonmyocytes interaction during cardiocyte hypertrophy: evidence for endothelin-1 as a paracrine hypertrophic factor from cardiac nonmyocytes. Circulation 96:3737–3744.

50. Sakai S, Miyauchi T, Kobayashi M, Yamaguchi I, Goto K, Sugishita Y. 1996. Inhibition of myocardial endothelin pathway improves long-term survival in heart failure. Nature 384:353–355.

51. Akhter SA, Luttreel LM, Rockman HA, Iaccarino G, Lefkowitz RJ, Koch WJ. 1998. Targeting the receptor-Gq interface to inhibit in vivo pressure overload myocardial hypertrophy. Science 28:574–577.
52. Morris CE. 1990. Mechanosensitive ion channels. J Membr Biol 113:93–107.
53. Bustamante JO, Ruknudin A, Sachs F. 1991. Stretch-activated channels in heart cells: relevance to cardiac hypertrophy. J Cardiovasc Pharmacol 17:S110–S113.
54. Sigurdson W, Ruknudin A, Sachs F. 1992. Calcium imaging of mechanically induced fluxes in tissue-cultured chick heart: role of stretch-activated ion channels. Am J Physiol 262:H1110–1115.
55. Yamazaki T, Komuro I, Kudoh S, Zou Y, Nagai R, Aikawa R, Uozumi H, Yazaki Y. 1998. Role of ion channels and exchangers in mechanical stretch-induced cardiomyocyte hypertrophy. Circ Res 82:430–437.
56. Komuro I, Katoh Y, Hoh E, Takaku F, Yazaki Y. 1991. Mechanisms of cardiac hypertrophy and injury—possible role of protein kinase C activation. Jpn Circ J 55:1149–1157.
57. Juliano RL, Haskill S. 1993. Signal transduction from the extracellular matrix. J Cell Biol 120:577–585.
58. Juliano RL, Haskill S. 1993. Signal transduction from the extracellular matrix. J Cell Biol 120:577–585.
59. Hynes RO. 1992. Integrins: versatility, modulation, and signaling in cell adhesion. Cell 69:11–25.
60. Hamasaki K, Mimura T, Furuya H, Morino N, Yamazaki T, Komuro I, Yazaki y, Nojima Y. 1995. Stretching mesangial cells stimulates tyrosine phosphorylation of focal adhesion kinase pp125FAK. Biochem Biophys Res Common 212:544–549.
61. Mackay DJ, Hall A. 1998. Rho GTPases. J Biol Chem 273:20685–20688.
62. Thorburn J, Xu S, Thorburn A. 1997. MAP kinase- and Rho-dependent signals interact to regulate gene expression but not actin morphology in cardiac muscle cells. EMBO J 16:1888–1900.
63. Sah VP, Hoshijima M, Chien KR, Brown JH. 1996. Rho is required for Galphaq and alpha1-adrenergic receptor signaling in cardiomyocytes. Dissociation of Ras and Rho pathways. J Biol Chem 271:31185–31190.
64. Aoki H, Izumo S, Sadoshima J. 1998. Angiotensin II activates RhoA in cardiac myocytes: a critical role of RhoA in angiotensin II-induced premyofibril formation. Circ Res 82:666–676.
65. Brewster JL, de Valoir T, Dwyer ND, Winter E, Gustin MC. 1993. An osmosensing signal transduction pathway in yeast. Science 259:1760–1763.
66. Schwartz MA, Lechene C, Ingber DE. 1991. Insoluble fibronectin activates the Na/H antiporter by clustering and immobilizing integrin alpha 5 beta 1, independent of cell shape. Proc Natl Acad Sci U S A 88:7849–7853.

N. Takeda, M. Nagano and N.S. Dhalla
(eds). The Hypertrophied Heart. Copyright
© 2000. pp. 123–129. Kluwer Academic
Publishers. Boston. All rights reserved.

POSSIBLE ROLES OF THE TENASCIN FAMILY DURING HEART DEVELOPMENT AND MYOCARDIAL TISSUE REMODELING

KYOKO IMANAKA-YOSHIDA, KAZUTO YOKOYAMA,
and TERUYO SAKAKURA

Department of Pathology, Mie University, School of Medicine, Tsu, Mie 514-8507, Japan

Summary. The tenascins are a family of extracellular matrix proteins. Tenascin-C (TNC) is expressed during embryogenesis or cancer invasion. Tenascin-X (TNX) is ubiquitously expressed, with the highest levels in the heart. To clarify the role of TNC and TNX in the heart, we analyzed TNC and TNX expression patterns in embryonic hearts of mice by immunohistochemistry and in situ hybridization. TNC was transiently expressed at four important steps of early heart development: (1) differentiation of cardiomyocytes from the mesoderm, (2) formation of endocardial cushion tissue, (3) development of the outflow tract, and (4) migration of the proepicardial cells (precursors of coronary vessels). After the expression of TNC was downregulated, TNX was expressed by epicardial cells invading the myocardial layer and forming vascular channels. In normal adult hearts, TNC was sparse but reappeared under pathological conditions. During tissue repair after electric injury to the ventricle of mice, TNC appeared at the border zone between intact and injured myocardium, the most active sites of tissue remodeling during the acute stage. These expression patterns strongly suggest the important roles of TNC in tissue remodeling of the myocardium as well as during early heart development. However, in TNC knockout mice, the heart developed normally, and the myocardial tissue repair seemed to proceed normally. Furthermore, our findings did not show that TNX compensates for the loss of TNC.

INTRODUCTION

Tenascins are a family of extracellular matrix glycoproteins. The first member, tenascin-C (TNC), appears transiently at restricted sites during active tissue remodeling such as wound healing, cancer invasion, or embryogenesis [1]. Findings have indicated that TNC counterbalances cell adhesion to the substrata, preventing cells from adhering too tightly to other extracellular matrix proteins [2]. A new member, tenascin-X (TNX), is ubiquitously expressed in various tissues but is most abundant in the heart and skeletal muscles. The expression of TNC and TNX is often reciprocal [3], although the biological function of TNX remains unclear.

In the heart, TNC is not expressed in normal adults but appears under various pathological conditions [4,5], suggesting that TNC is involved in tissue remodeling of the heart.

To elucidate the roles of the tenascin family in the heart, we analyzed the expression pattern of TNC and TNX during mouse heart development by *in situ* hybridization and immunohistochemistry. Then we studied the expression pattern of TNC and TNX in a mouse myocardial infarction model in mice. Furthermore, the myocardial tissue repair in TNC-deficient mice was compared to that in normal mice.

MATERIALS AND METHODS

Preparation of embryos

Embryos were removed from the uterus of timed pregnant ICR mice. The timed mating was carried out by assigning the morning vaginal plug identification as day 0.5.

Electric injury model

Eight-week-old C3H TNC-deficient mice and control mice were anesthetized with pentobarbital. The abdomen was entered through a midline incision, and electric injury of a portion of the left ventricular myocardium was induced across the intact diaphragm. Mice were sacrificed on days 1, 3, and 7 after injury. Their hearts were removed and fixed with 4% paraformaldehyde in PBS and embedded in paraffin.

Antibody

Antibodies used in this study were polyclonal rabbit anti-tenascin-C [6] and anti-tenascin-X [6].

Immunohistochemistry

Our procedure of whole-mount antibody staining followed that of Kataoka et al. [7]. The rabbit anti-TNC antibody was used at 1:1000 dilution, and the anti-TNX antibody was used at 1:1000. The secondary antibody was peroxidase-conjugated anti-rabbit IgG (MBL, Nagoya, Japan) and was used at 1:500. Immunostaining of tissue sections was performed as described previously [6,8].

In situ hybridization

Concerning the preparation of tissue sections, the in situ hybridization method and color development were previously described by Ishihara et al. [9].

RESULTS

Expression in normal embryos

TNC initially appeared in a presomite mouse embryo at the heart-forming region of a day-7.5 embryo. At this stage, the precardiac mesoderm is delineated from

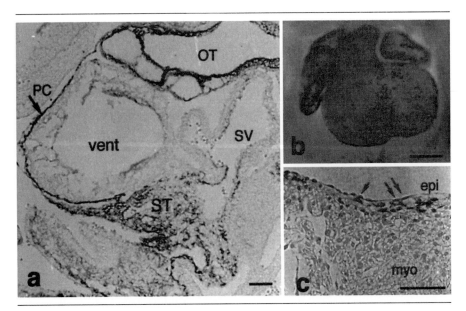

Figure 1. (a) Immunostaining for tenascin-C of a histological section of a 9.5-day-old mouse embryo. Positive staining is seen at the outflow, mesenchymal cells of the projections of the septum transversum and pericardium. (b) Whole-mount immunostaining of the hearts of a 11-day-old mouse embryo for tenascin-X. (c) Immunostaining for tenascin-X of the histological section. Positive staining is seen at the epicardial cells forming the vascular channel (arrows). OT, outflow tract; vent, ventricle; ST, septum transversum; PC, pericardium; SV, sinus venosus. Bars: in (a) and (c), 50 μm; in (b), 0.5 mm.

somatic mesoderm by formation of the pericardial cavity and differentiation into cardiomyocytes. The histological section demonstrated that the mesoderm cells forming the pericardial cavity were positive for TNC. When precardiomyocytes differentiated to express sarcomeric proteins, the expression of TNC was downregulated.

The differentiating precardiac mesoderm cells form a primitive single heart tube composed of the myocardium and endocardium, separated by a thick cell-free expanse of ECM termed *cardiac jelly*. A subset of the endocardium of the atrioventricular canal and proximal outflow tract undergo epithelial mesenchymal transformation and invade the cardiac jelly [10,11]. Endocardial cells that lined the endocardial tube and migrating cushion mesenchymal cells expressed TNC. During this stage, cardiomyocytes of the outflow tract also expressed TNC (figure 1a).

On day 9.5, when the heart tube forms an S-shaped loop, cells in the septum transversum form villous projections, adhere to the surface of the heart tube, and spread over the heart to become epicardium [12]. These epicardial cells are considered to be progenitors of coronary vessels or interstitial fibroblasts [13,14]. TNC expression was observed in the mesenchymal cells of the projections of the septum transversum (figure 1a); however, the expression was diminished in the proepicardial cells on the heart surface. TNX appeared as scattered small spots on the surface of the embryonic heart on day 11 (figure 1b). These spots increased in number and fused to each other to form a network pattern that covered the surface of the heart on day 12. Immunostaining of the histological sections of the heart demonstrated that the epicardial cells that form vascular channels and migrate into the myocardium expressed TNX (figure 1c).

Tenascin-C null embryos

In the TNC null embryo, the heart developed normally. Neither expression of mRNA nor TNC protein was seen in the TNC null embryos. The expression pattern of TNX was the same as that of the wild type.

Wound healing after electric injury

Electric injury resulted in myocardial lesions and subsequent wound healing. During the first day after the injury, edematous fluid and inflammatory cells began accumulating at the margin of the injured area. Within 2–3 days, granulation tissue started to develop at the edge of the intact myocardium toward the center of the lesion and to replace the necrotic mass. TNC appeared within 24 hours after injury, and intense immunostaining for TNC was localized at the border zone between injured and intact areas (figure 2b). *In situ* hybridization analysis demonstrated that the interstitial fibroblasts were the major source of TNC (figure 3). These findings were similar to those observed in experimental rat myocardial infarction by coronary ligation [15]. In contrast to TNC, the expression pattern of TNX did not show marked change. The immunostaining for TNX was ubiquitously seen in the extracellular space of intact myocardium (figure 2c). In TNC null animals, the healing process appeared to occur normally (figure 2d). Immunostaining for TNC confirmed the absence of TNC in our knockout mice (figure 2e). The anti-TNX staining pattern during myocardial healing of TNC null mice was the same as that of the wild type (figure 2f).

DISCUSSION

During early heart development, TNC was transiently expressed at four important steps: (1) differentiation of cardiomyocytes from the mesoderm, (2) formation of endocardial cushion tissue, (3) development of the outflow tract, and (4) migration of the proepicardial cells (precursors of coronary vessels).

   TNX appeared much later than TNC. TNX was expressed by epicardial cells after the expression of TNC was downregulated by proepicardial cells. This reciprocal expression pattern suggests that different functions and collaboration of tenascins are necessary for coronary vasculogenesis; TNC could play an important role in the initiation of migration of proepicardial cells (= precursors of coronary vessels) from the mesenchyme of the septum transversum to the surface of the primitive heart, while TNX could be involved in the formation of vascular channels by epicardial cells.

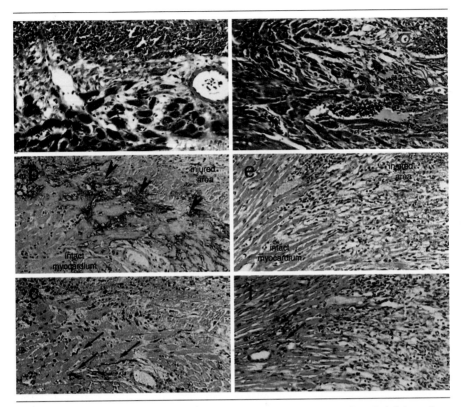

Figure 2. Myocardial repair 3 days after electric injury in control (**a**, **b**, **c**) and TNC-deficient mice (**d**, **e**, **f**). Hematoxilin/esosin staining (**a**, **d**) and immunostaining for tenascin-C (**b**, **e**) or tenascin-X (**c**, **f**). Immunostaining for tenascin-C is localized in the border zone of control mice (arrowheads in **c**), No positive staining for TNC is seen in TNC null mice (**e**). The immunostaining for TNX is seen in the extracellular space of intact myocardium (arrows in **c** and **f**). Bar indicates 50 μm.

When a primitive heart formed, the expression of TNC almost disappeared. In normal adult hearts, TNC is seen only at the coronary vascular wall but reappears in various pathological conditions. Interestingly, in a rat myocardial infarction model, TNC transiently appears during the acute stage and shows restricted distribution at the edge of the residual myocardium, where the tissue architecture should most actively change [15]. In normal hearts, cardiomyocytes are linked to connective tissue at costameres [16–19]. When they become disconnected from neighboring necrotic cells, they must remodel the cytoskeleton, cell arrangement, and cell–extracellular matrix attachment sites [18,20,21]. Counteradhesive activity of TNC may allow modulation of cell adhesion to the extracellular matrix. We observed here a very similar expression pattern of TNC during tissue myocardial repair after electric injury of the ventricle in mice. TNC appeared during the acute stage and was

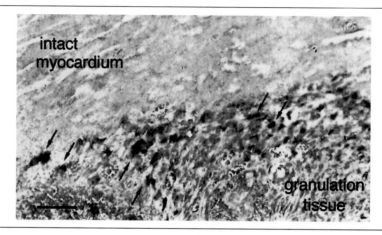

Figure 3. In situ hybridization for tenascin-C in a wild-type mouse myocardial tissue section 5 days after electric injury. Interstitial cells at the border zone are expressing TNC mRNA (arrows). Bar indicates 50 μm.

localized at the border zone of the intact myocardium and injured area (= granulation/scar tissue at the later stage).

These characteristic expression patterns strongly suggest the important roles of TNC in tissue remodeling of the myocardium as well as during early heart development; however, TNC knockout mice do not show a distinct phenotype [22,23]. Furthermore, our findings suggest that myocardial tissue repair seems to proceed normally.

A possible explanation for this finding is that another member of the family—for example, TNX—compensates for the lack of TNC. However, we did not note a difference in the expression pattern of TNX between TNC null mice and wild-type mice during heart development or myocardial repair. Another unidentified gene may substitute for TNC. Recently, Forsberg et al. reported that the expression of fibronectin is diminished in wounds of TNC-deficient mice [23]. Mammals likely have several compensatory pathways that effectively counterbalance deficits of matrix proteins.

ACKNOWLEDGMENTS

We thank S. Naota for her technical assistance. This research was supported by Grants-in-Aid from the Ministry of Education, Science and Culture of Japan and a Grant-in-Aid (1997) from Mie Medical Research Foundation to K. I.-Y.

REFERENCES

1. Chiquet-Ehrismann R, Mackie EJ, Pearson CA, Sakakura T. 1986. Tenascin interferes with fibronectin action. Cell 53:383–390.

2. Prieto AL, Anderson-Fisone C, Crossin KL. 1992. Characterization of multiple adhesive and coun-teradhesive domains in the extracellular matrix protein cytotactin. J Cell Biol 119:663–678.
3. Matsumoto K, Saga Y, Ikemura T, Sakakura T, Chiquet-Ehrismann R. 1994. The distribution of tenascin-X is distinct and often reciprocal to that of tenascin-C. J Cell Biol 125:483–493.
4. Tamura A, Kusachi S, Nogami K, Yamanishi A, Kajikawa Y, Hirohata S, Tsuji T. 1996. Tenascin expres-sion in endomyocardial biopsy specimens in patients with dilated cardiomyopathy: distribution along margins of fibrotic lesions. Heart 75:291–294.
5. Willems IE, Arends JW, Daemen MJ. 1996. Tenascin and fibronectin expression in healing human myocardial scars. J Pathol 179:321–325.
6. Hasegawa K, Yoshida T, Matsumoto K, Katsuta K, Waga S, Sakakura T. 1997. Differential expression of tenascin-C and tenascin-X in human astrocytomas. Acta Neuropathol 93:431–437.
7. Kataoka H, Takakura N, Nishikawa S, Tsuchida K, Kodama H, Kunisada T, Risau W, Kita T, Nishikawa SI. 1997. Expressions of PDGF receptor alpha, c-Kit and Flkl genes clustering in mouse chromo-some 5 define distinct subsets of nascent mesodermal cells. Dev Growth Differ 39:729–740.
8. Kalembey I, Yoshida T, Iriyama K, Sakakura T. 1997. Analysis of tenascin mRNA expression in the murine mammary gland from embryogenesis to carcinogenesis: an in situ hybridization study. Int J Dev Biol 41:569–573.
9. Ishihara A, Yoshida T, Tamaki H, Sakakura T. 1995. Tenascin expression in cancer cells and stroma of human breast cancer and its prognostic significance. Clin Cancer Res 1:1035–1041.
10. Markwald RR, Fitzharris TP, Smith A. 1975. Structural analysis of endocardial cytodifferentiation. Dev Biol 42:160–180.
11. Markwald RR, Fitzharris TP, Manasek FJ. 1977. Structural development of endocardial cushions. Am J Anat 148:85–119.
12. Komiyama M, Ito K, Shimada Y. 1987. Origin and development of the epicardium in the mouse embryo. Anat Embryol 176:183–189.
13. Poelmann RE, Gittenberger-de Groot AC, Mentink MMT, Bokenkamp R, Hogers B. 1993. Devel-opment of the cardiac coronary vascular endothelium, studied with antiendothelial antibodies in chicken quail chimeras. Circ Res 73:559–568.
14. Mikawa T, Fischman DA. 1992. Retroviral analysis of cardiac morphogenesis: discontinuous forma-tion of cardiac vessels. Proc Natl Acad Sci USA 89:9504–9508.
15. Imanaka-Yoshida K, Ishiyama S, Shimojo T, Hiroe M, Ohta T, Nishikawa T, Yoshida T, Sakakura T. 1997. A possible role of tenascin-C in tissue remodeling after myocardial infarction. J Mol Cell Cardiol 29:A291.
16. Imanaka-Yoshida K, Danowski BA, Sanger JM, Sanger JW. 1994. Vinculin-containing costameres: part of contraction force transmission sites of cardiomyocytes. In The Cardiomyopathic Heart. Ed. M. Nagano, N. Takeda, and N.S. Dalla, 245–255. New York: Raven Press.
17. Imanaka-Yoshida K, Danowski BA, Sanger JM, Sanger JW. 1996. Living adult rat cardiomyocytes in culture: evidence for dissociation of castameric distribution of vinculin from costameric distributions of attachments. Cell Motil Cytoskel 33:263–275.
18. Imanaka-Yoshida K, Enomoto-Iwamoto M, Yoshida T, Sakakura T. 1999. Vinculin, talin, integrin $\alpha6\beta1$ and laminin can serve as components of attachment complex mediating contraction force transmis-sion from cardiomyocytes to extracellular matrix. Cell Motil Cytoskel 42:1–11.
19. Danowski BA, Imanaka-Yoshida K, Sanger JM, Sanger JW. 1992. Costameres are sites of force trans-mission to the substratum in adult rat cardiomyocytes. J Cell Biol 118:1411–1420.
20. Imanaka-Yoshida K, Sanger JM, Sanger JW. 1993. Contractile protein dynamics of myofibrils in paired adult rat cardiomyocytes. Cell Motil Cytoskel 26:301–312.
21. Vracko R, Thorning D, Frederickson RG, Cunningham D. 1988. Myocyte reactions at the borders of injured and healing rat myocardium. Lab Invest 59:104–114.
22. Saga Y, Yagi T, Ikawa Y, Sakakura T, Aizawa S. 1992. Mice develop normally without tenascin. Genes Dev 6:1821–1831.
23. Forsberg E, Hirsh E, Frohlich L, Meyer M, Ekblom M, Aszodi A, Werner S, Fassler R. 1996. Skin wounds and nerves heal normally in mice lacking tenascin-C. Proc Natl Acad Sci USA 93:6594–6599.

N. Takeda, M. Nagano and N.S. Dhalla
(eds). The Hypertrophied Heart. Copyright
© 2000. pp. 131–141. Kluwer Academic
Publishers. Boston. All rights reserved.

CARDIAC CELL–ECM INTERACTIONS: A POSSIBLE SITE FOR MECHANICAL SIGNALING

SHALINI KANEKAR, WAYNE CARVER, THOMAS K. BORG, JOEL ATANCE, and LOUIS TERRACIO

Department of Developmental Biology and Anatomy, School of Medicine, University of South Carolina, Columbia, SC 29208, USA

Summary. The cardiac interstitium is a diverse system of extracellular matrix (EMC) components organized into a stress-tolerant three-dimensional network that interconnects the cellular components of the heart. At the molecular level, the ECM is attached to cells primarily via integrin receptors which in turn connect to the cytoskeleton. This ECM–integrin–cytoskeletal linkage is thought to be important in transducing extracellular mechanical forces to the cells. While it is generally believed that integrins are involved in the initial detection of mechanical signals by cells, the subsequent steps in the responses of cells to these signals have not been well elucidated. In this study, we demonstrate that stretch of cardiac fibroblasts results in a rapid but transient increase in MAPK phosphorylation. Blocking this pathway with a specific phamacological inhibitor resulted in a complete attenuation of the normally observed stretch-induced cytoskeletal and cellular realignment. The results support the notion that the MAPK pathway is involved in transducing mechanical stretch signals.

INTRODUCTION

During development of the heart, the various cellular components undergo commitment to their characteristic phenotypes, which are essential to establish proper cardiac form and function. At the cellular level, the shape of the cardiac myocyte changes from spherical to tubular in coordination with the formation of the contractile apparatus. During this metamorphosis, the contractile proteins undergo a precise association in a process known as myofibrillogenesis in order to form the contractile apparatus of the rod-shaped phenotype that is essential to myocyte contractility. As contractility increases, the fibroblasts also take on a characteristic elongated spindle shape and become the principal producers of the extracellular matrix, which forms the three-dimensional (3-D) connective tissue network of the myocardium.

The cardiac interstitium represents a system of diverse extracellular matrix (ECM) components organized into a complex, 3-D network that surrounds the cellular

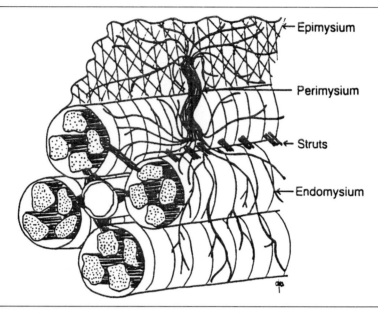

Figure 1. A schematic representation of the three-dimensional connective tissue network of the heart. The epimysial network beneath the epicardium connects thick spiral-shaped cables of collagen that constitute the perimysium. The perimysium is connected to the endomysial network that surrounds individual myocytes. The perimysial cables permit movement of the individual layers of myocytes. Myocyte–myocyte and myocyte–capillary struts are also shown attaching to specific sites on the myocyte. These sites are thought to be important in the transmission of mechanical signal and are further described in figure 2. Modified from [3], with permission of the authors.

components of the heart (figure 1) [1–4]. The interaction of the cellular components with the interstitium is dynamic and occurs in response to physiological signals during development, normal homeostasis, and disease [1,2]. Both the quantitative and qualitative expressions of ECM components play an important role in cardiac function; however, the mechanisms that regulate these parameters are not well understood.

The interactions between the cytoskeletal components, specific membrane receptors termed *integrins*, and the components of the ECM are fundamental during the growth of cardiac myocytes and fibroblasts (figure 2). The formation of the ECM–integrin–cytoskeletal complex has also been proposed to be a critical element in the transmission of mechanical signals to cardiac cells. Previously, we have shown that the in vitro composition and orientation of the ECM, the presence of integrins, and the proper alignment of cytoskeletal proteins are essential to the formation of the in vivo-like phenotype of cardiac myocytes [5]. These studies have demonstrated that when cardiac myocytes are plated on thin gels of collagen, they assume the rod-shaped phenotype and spatially express the essential components of the ECM–integrin–cytoskeletal complex [6].

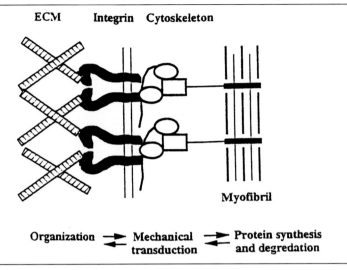

Figure 2. A schematic diagram of the ECM–integrin–cytoskeletal linkage showing that the organization of the ECM can transmit mechanical forces via the integrins to the cytoskeleton, which in turn can affect cell structure and function. This process may take place through the transmission of positional information or by triggering a chemical signal transduction cascade.

Extrinsic and intrinsic factors both act via chemical and mechanical pathways to modulate phenotype. While much is known concerning the chemical pathways, little is known concerning how mechanical information is transduced to the cell. The mechanical forces associated with cardiac function during various stages of development and disease have been implicated in regulating the expression [7–11], synthesis [12–16], and degradation [17–19] of a variety of contractile and regulatory proteins. In the presence of a sustained elevation in workload, these load-responsive elements precipitate an increase in cardiac protein content and cell mass [20]. Conversely, a chronic persistent reduction in cardiac workload initiates the loss of myofibrils and a regression in cell size. Thus, the mass and performance characteristics of heart cells are dynamically coupled to the mechanical forces that they experience during the contraction–relaxation cycle [21].

The basic organization of the myofibers, vasculature, and interstitium appear to be complete late in fetal development. During neonatal development, the interstitium undergoes rapid growth and establishes a pattern maintained throughout life (figure 1) [1]. Endothelial cells, smooth muscle cells, and myocytes appear to produce ECM components that are deposited in close proximity to that individual cell. An example of this type of deposition is laminin and collagen type IV in the basement membrane. It appears that the fibroblast is the principal cell type responsible for the production of the components of the ECM in the interstitium, especially fibrillar collagen types I and III, that interconnect the cellular components of the heart. Fibroblasts in the heart perform at least three essential functions: (1) synthesis and deposition of ECM components; (2) synthesis and release of enzymes responsible for the degradation and turnover of the ECM; and (3) generation of mechanical tension on the epimysial collagen network [1,2,22]. To perform these functions, fibroblasts must respond to and generate both chemical and mechanical signals unique to their particular environment. For example, cardiac fibroblasts may respond to increased contraction (pressure) during development by synthesizing and depositing interstitial collagens and integrins to attach the fibroblasts to the collagen [23–26]. Several studies have shown that mechanical stimulation can alter the production of the ECM by cardiac fibroblasts as well as affect their 3-D organization.

The transmission of physiological signals from the ECM to the cell takes place via specific transmembrane receptors (integrins) that connect with the cytoskeleton, which is important in determining cellular phenotype [27]. Thus, it is postulated that as the ECM changes, either during normal development or in response to disease, this information can cause changes in the shape of the cardiac cells—changes that are ultimately translated into changes in function. The spatial and temporal distribution of members of the β_1-integrin subfamily in the heart appears to be concomitant with morphogenesis and parallels the accumulation of ECM components, including laminin and interstitial collagen. In a wide variety of biological systems, including the heart, both in vivo and in vitro studies indicate that the β_1-integrin subfamily is important in basic processes such as adhesion, migration, phenotype regulation, and the generation of mechanical tension [26]. In the heart, the β_1-integrins have been shown to play roles in the cell–matrix interactions necessary for myofibrillogenesis [28,29] and matrix remodeling [30,31]. Fundamental to these functions are the interactions of the specific integrins with components of the ECM and with cytoskeletal elements of the cells. These investigations have documented that the clustering of the integrin receptors causes an activation of tyrosine kinase, in a manner similar to that of growth factors, and may act as an important regulatory messenger in eliciting a variety of physiological responses [32].

Mechanical stimulation has been proposed to be a major determinant of cellular function [19]. Numerous studies have been carried out indicating that cardiac cells undergo specific "downstream" responses following mechanical stimulation. These include changes in cell morphology, proliferation, and gene expression. However, the mechanisms whereby cells detect changes in mechanical forces have not been elucidated. It is now clear that mechanical stimulation works in concert with chemical signals [33,34]. Studies on stretch of cardiac myocytes and fibroblasts have shown that mechanical stimulation appears to be mediated by the autocrine release of angiotensin II, as evidenced by hypertrophy of the myocytes [33,34] and increased collagen expression in fibroblasts [35]. These mechanical forces that are inducing cellular growth of cardiac myocytes and ECM expression in fibroblasts are likely to be transmitted to the cell from its extracellular matrix environment and the cells surrounding it. The attachment of collagen fibrils at specific sites in both myocytes and fibroblasts make it highly probable that the mechanical forces are received by the cell from the ECM. Mechanical stimulation, either active or passive, can be derived by either the force of contraction of the myocytes and/or tension possibly applied by the interstitial cells on the endomysial collagenous network that surround the myocytes [1–4].

In this study, we have used uniaxial and equibiaxial stretch devices [36,37] to determine the effects of stretch on the morphology and collagen production in neonatal cardiac fibroblasts. We have also begun to investigate the possible signal transduction pathways involved in this response. These studies indicate that mitogen-activated protein kinase (MAPK) is rapidly phosphorylated in response to mechanical stretch. Experiments using pharmacological inhibitors indicate that the MAPK pathway plays a significant role in the reorganization of heart fibroblasts and their cytoskeletal filaments in response to stretch.

METHODS

Cell culture

Fibroblasts were isolated from neonatal hearts (3–5 days postpartum) and were maintained in Dulbecco's modified Eagle's medium containing 10% fetal bovine serum and 5% neonatal bovine serum. Distensible silicon membranes (Silicone Sheeting) were coated with monomeric collagen type I. These were then assembled on an equibiaxial-stretching device [36]. Neonatal cardiac fibroblasts were then grown on these membraness to subconfluency. Alternatively, fibroblasts on silastic membranes were assembled into a cyclic stretch apparatus [37]. These cultures were then subjected to varying degrees of stretch for 24 hours.

Northern analysis

At the end of the stretch period, total RNA was isolated using RNAzol (Tel Test Inc.) and subjected to Northern analysis using cDNA probes for collagen type I, collagen type III, β_1-integrin, and GAPDH.

MAPK activity assay

Neonatal cardiac fibroblasts were grown to subconfluency on distensible silicon membranes assembled on an equibiaxial-stretching device, as described above. These cultures were then serum starved for 24 hours in serum-free DMEM/F12 media (Sigma), after which they were subjected to 3% stretch for varying amounts of time. The cells were then washed in PBS and scraped in cell lysis buffer (20 mM Tris pH 7.5, 150 mM NaCl, 1 mM EDTA, 1 mM EGTA, 1 mM Na_3VO_4, 1% Triton, 2.5 mM sodium pyrophosphate, 1 mM β-glycerophosphate, 1 μg/mL leupeptin), and 200 μg of cell lysate was immunoprecipitated with phospho-MAPK antibody (New England Biolabs Inc.). The kinase assay was carried out as per the manufacturer's protocol. Briefly, the immunoprecipitated protein was incubated with Elk-1 fusion protein in kinase buffer (25 mM Tris pH 7.5, 5 mM β-glycerophosphate, 2 mM DTT, 0.1 mM Na_3VO_4, 10 mM $MgCl_2$) supplemented with APT, for 30 minutes at 30°C. This reaction was terminated with SDS gel loading buffer and then subjected to Western analysis on 12% SDS-PAGE, using phospho-specific Elk-1 antibody.

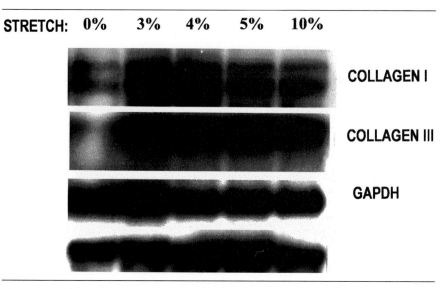

STRETCH: 0%   3%   4%   5%   10%

COLLAGEN I

COLLAGEN III

GAPDH

Figure 3. Northern analysis of total RNA extracted from neonatal cardiac fibroblasts subjected to varying degrees of stretch for 24 hours. Northern blots were probed with cDNAs specific for collagen type I, collagen type III, glyceraldehyde 3-phosphate dehydrogenase, or β_1-integrin. It is seen that collagen gene expression was induced maximally between 2% and 3% stretch.

Western analysis on the same cell extracts was carried out using p44 (ERK1) and p42 (ERK2) MAPK antibody (Santa Cruz Biotechnologies, Inc.) to demonstrate that the protein level of MAPK remained unchanged under the given conditions.

Analysis of cell organization

Cells were cultured on silastic membranes as described above, serum-starved for 24 hours, and subjected to cyclic uniaxial stretch [24,37]. Cells were stretched in the presence or absence of the MAPK pathway inhibitor PD 098059 (10 μM). Cells were subsequently fixed in 2% paraformaldehyde in phosphate-buffered saline. The membranes containing cells were incubated in rhodamine phalloidin (Molecular Probes) to stain the actin cytoskeleton. The cells were rinsed, coverslipped, and examined by laser scanning confocal microscopy (BioRad). One characteristic response of fibroblasts to mechanical stretch is the realignment of the cells and their cytoskeleton perpendicular to the direction of stretch. The effects of inhibition of the MAPK pathway on this realignment were determined.

RESULTS

Fibroblasts isolated from neonatal rat hearts were subjected to varying degrees of equibiaxial stretch for 24 hours and collagen mRNA levels examined by Northern blot analysis (figure 3). This set of experiments shows that mechanical stretch results in an increase in both collagen type I and type III mRNA levels (figure 3). These

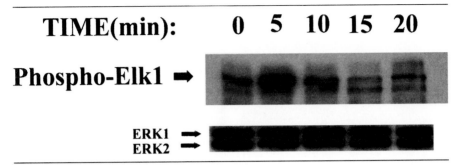

Figure 4. (a) MAPK activity assay from protein extracts derived from neonatal cardiac fibroblasts subjected to 3% stretch for different time points. Cell extracts were analyzed by IP/kinase assay, as described in the Methods section. Phosphorylation of Elk-1 was visualized by 12% SDS-PAGE followed by immunoblotting with phospho-Elk-1 antibody. It is seen that the MAPK activity was induced maximally after 5 minutes of stretch. (b) Western analysis of proteins derived as in (a), using p44/42 MAPK antibody. This figure shows that the amount of MAPK protein remains unchanged under the given conditions of stretch.

studies also indicate that the greatest increase in collagen mRNA levels is seen in response to 3% and 4% equibiaxial stretch. Increasing degrees of stretch above 5% resulted in a decrease in both type I and type II collagen mRNA levels.

To begin to determine the signal transduction pathways that are responsible for mediating the downstream responses of heart fibroblasts to mechanical stretch, cells were stretched and the activation of the MAPK pathway were examined (figure 4). A rapid and transient increase in MAPK activation was found in response to equibiaxial stretch. Activation of MAPK dramatically increased after 5 minutes of stretch and declined thereafter (figure 4). A similar increase in MAPK activation was found in response to cyclic, uniaxial stretch (not shown).

To determine the role of MAPK activation in mediating the downstream response of heart fibroblasts to mechanical stretch, cells were stretched in the presence of PD 098059, a pharmacological inhibitor of the MAPK pathway (figure 5). The ability of the fibroblasts to realign in response to cyclic, uniaxial stretch was then determined by confocal microscopy. Cyclic stretch of isolated fibroblasts in the presence of PD 098059 dramatically impaired the ability of the cells to realign. Most of the cells stretched in the presence of the MAPK pathway inhibitor remained randomly organized in response to stretch indicating that the MAPK pathway is, at least in part, responsible for mediating the realignment of these cells to cyclic stretch.

DISCUSSION

Sensing mechanical stimulation and responding to it is a fundamental property of all cells. It has been proposed that transmission of the mechanical stimuli in multi-cellular organisms is through the ECM receptors of the integrin family [27,38,39]. This response can either be through the physical interactions of the ECM–integrin–cytoskeletal linkage as proposed by Ingber [27,40] or a conversion of

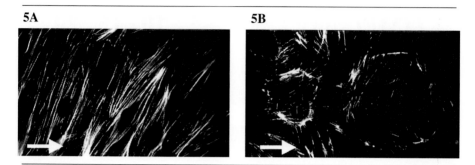

Figure 5. Confocal micrographs of fibroblasts that were subjected to 24 hours of cyclic uniaxial stretch in the absence (**a**) or presence (**b**) of 10 mM PD 098059. Following stretch, cells were stained with rhodamine phalloidin to visualize the orientation of the cells and their actin cytoskeleton. The arrows indicate the direction of stretch.

mechanical force to chemical signaling pathways inside the cell [41]. Integrins colocalize with cytoskeletal elements and kinases at specific sites on the membrane called *focal adhesions*. These sites contain abundant signaling molecules, including focal adhesion kinase or p125^{FAK} (FAK), Src-family kinases, Ras-family proteins, guanine nucleotide exchange factors, and MAPK [42,43]. Ligand binding of integrins has been shown to cause rapid and transient tyrosine phosphorylation of multiple signaling molecules. One of the signaling cascades that has been shown to be activated is the MAPK pathway [44,45]. This is achieved by activation of FAK, which in turn promotes its association with the GRB2 adaptor protein, finally leading to the activation of the MAPK pathway. The results presented here indicate that MAPK is rapidly activated in response to mechanical stretch of heart fibroblasts. The cellular realignment of these cells in response to stretch is, at least in part, dependent on MAPK activation.

It is not yet clear if the activation of MAPK is a direct response of cells to mechanical stimulation or if this requires a biochemical intermediary. Several studies have shown that downstream responses of heart myocytes to mechanical stretch are dependent on the release of angiotensin II in following mechanical stimulation [33,34]. This growth factor then has an autocrine/paracrine effect on these cells and mediates the stretch response. The fact that MAPK is activated after such a short duration of stretch in the present studies would suggest that this response is a direct result of mechanical stimulation and not mediated by autocrine/paracrine growth factor responsiveness. However, this possibility has not been directly tested in heart fibroblasts.

Numerous studies have shown increased expression of several growth factors, including angiotensin II, transforming growth factor-β, and insulin-like growth factor, in association with increased work load in the heart. The mechanistic similarity in the signaling initiated by growth factors and integrins points to the possibility of interactions between the two that can be collaborative or synergistic. Studies with an aorta organ culture model have shown that angiotensin II and mechanical forces act synergistically to induce ECM expression [46]. Recent studies have indicated that the responsiveness of cells to growth factors may be mediated, at least in part, through specific integrins. It has also been demonstrated that stimulation of integrins can induce PDGF-indepedent tyrosine phosphorylation of PDGFβ receptors [47]. Interactions between integrin- and growth factor-mediated signal transduction pathways are speculated to be either by direct physical interaction between the two [48–50] or by activation of common signaling pathways like MAPK. Determining how cells perceive and respond to the extracellular milieu is critical to understanding the underlying mechanisms of cardiovascular pathology.

The data presented here indicate that stretch of cardiac fibroblasts results in an increase in MAPK phosphorylation and that this increase is followed by a well-documented cellular response. The timing of the phosphorylation response is similar to that seen with administration of exogenous ligand. Thus, it is unlikely that the response we see is due to autocrine secretion of a growth factor or cytokine that in turn initiates receptor-mediated signaling; however, this possibility cannot be eliminated at this time. To further elucidate the mechanisms through which mechanical signals contribute to cardiovascular pathologies, it will be essential to determine the roles of the ECM-integrin interactions and subsequent signaling pathways in the response of cells to physical force.

REFERENCES

1. Borg TK, Caulfield JB. 1979. Collagen in the heart. Tex Rep Biol Med 39:321–333.
2. Robinson TF, Factor SM, Capasso JM, Wittenberg BA, Blumenfeld OO, Seifter S. 1987. Morphology and function of struts between cardiac myocytes of rat and hamster. Cell Tissue Res 249:247–255.
3. Borg TK, Terracio L. 1990. Interaction of the extracellular matrix with cardiac myocytes during development and disease. In Issues in Biomedicine. Ed. T. Robinson, 113–129. Basel: Karger Publishers.
4. Weber KT, Jalil JE, Janicki JS, Pick R. 1989. Myocardial collagen remodeling in pressure overload hypertrophy. A case for interstitial heart disease. Am J Hypertens 2:931–400.
5. Simpson DG, Terracio L, Terracio M, Price RL, Turner DC, Borg TK. 1994. Modulation of cardiac myocyte phenotype in vitro by the composition and orientation of the extracellular matrix. J Cell Physiol 161:89–105.
6. Simpson DG, Reaves T, Shih DT, Burgess W, Borg TK, Terracio L. 1998. Cardiac integrins: the ties that bind. Cardiovasc Pathol 7:135–143.
7. Yamazaki T, Komuro I, Kudoh S, Zou Y, Shiojima I. 1995. Angiotensin II partly mediates mechanical stress-induced cardiac hypertrophy. Circ Res 77:258–265.
8. Izumo S, Lompre AM, Matsuoka R, Koren G, Schwartz K, Nadal-Ginard B, Mahdavi V. 1987. Myosin heavy chain messenger RNA and protein isoform transitions during cardiac hypertrophy. Interaction between hemodynamic and thyroid-induced signals. J Clin Invest 79:979–997.
9. Samarel AM, Engelmann GL. 1991. Contractile activity modulates myosin heavy chain-beta expression in neonatal rat heart cells. Am J Physiol 261:H1067–H1077.
10. Sadoshima J, Jahn L, Takahashi T, Kulik TJ, Izumo S. 1992. Molecular characterization of the stretch-induced adaptation of cultured cardiac cells. J Biol Chem 267:10551–10560.
11. Sadoshima J, Izumo S. 1993. Mechanical stretch rapidly activates multiple signal transduction pathways in cardiac myocytes: potential involvement of an autocrine/paracrine mechanism. EMBO J 12:1681–1692.
12. Ojamma K, Petrie JF, Balkman C, Hong C, Klein I. 1994. Posttranscriptional modification of myosin heavy chain gene expression in the hypertrophied rat myocardium. Proc Natl Acad Sci USA 91:3468–3472.

13. Xenophontos XP, Gordon EE, Morgan HE. 1987. Effect of interventricular pressure on protein synthesis in arrested hearts. Am J Physiol 251:C95–C98.
14. Gordon EE, Kira Y, Morgan HE. 1987. Aortic perfusion pressure, protein synthesis and protein degradation. Circulation 75:178–180.
15. Klein I, Samarel AM, Welikson R, Hong C. 1991. Heterotopic cardiac transplantation decreases the capacity for rat myocardial protein synthesis. Circ Res 68:1100–1107.
16. Clark WA, Rudnick SJ, LaPres JJ, Anderson LC, Lapointe MC. 1993. Regulation of hypertrophy and atrophy in cultured adult heart cells. Circ Res 73:1163–1176.
17. Gordon EE, Kira Y, Demers LM, Morgan HE. 1986. Aortic pressure as a determinant of cardiac protein degradation. Am J Physiol 250:C932–C938.
18. Samarel AM, Spragia ML, Maloney V, Kamal SA, Engelmann GL. 1992. Contractile arrest accelerates myosin heavy chain degradation in neonatal rat heart cells. Am J Physiol 263:C642–C652.
19. Simpson DG, Carver W, Borg TK, Terracio L. 1994. The role of mechanical stimulation in the establishment of cardiac myofibrillar structure and protein turnover. In Mechanical Engineering of the Cytoskeleton in Developmental Biology. Ed. R. Gordon, 69–94. New York: Academic Press.
20. Beloussov LV, Saveliev SV, Naumidi II, Novoselov VV. 1994. Mechanical stresses in embryonic tissues: patterns, morphogenetic role, and involvement in regulatory feedback. In Mechanical Engineering of the Cytoskeleton in Developmental Biology. Ed. R. Gordon 1–34. New York: Academic Press.
21. Kent RL, Mann DL, Cooper G. 1991. Signals for cardiac muscle hypertrophy in hypertension. J Cardiovasc Pharm 17:S7–S13.
22. Borg TK, Burgess ML. 1993. Holding it all together. Organization and function(s) of the extracellular matrix in the heart. Heart Failure 8:230–238.
23. Hilenski LL, Terracio L, Sawyer R, Borg K. 1989. Effects of extracellular matrix on cytoskeletal and myfibrillar organization in vitro. Scan Microscopy 14:535–542.
24. Carver W, Nagpal ML, Nachtigal M, Borg TK, Terracio L. 1991. Collagen expression in mechanically stimulated cardiac fibroblasts. Circ Res 69:116–122.
25. Terracio L, Rubin K, Balog E, Jyring R, Carver W, Borg TK. 1991. Expression of collagen binding integrins during cardiac development and hypertrophy. Circ Res 68:734–743.
26. Carver W, Molano I, Reaves T, Borg TK, Terracio L. 1995. Role of the a1b1 integrin complex in collagen gel contraction in vitro by heart fibroblasts. J Cell Physiol 165:425–437.
27. Ingber DE, Dike L, Hansen L, Karp S, Liley H. 1994. Cellular tensegrity: exploring how mechanical changes in the cytoskeleton regulate cell growth, migration, and tissue pattern during morphogenesis. Int Rev Cytol 150:173–224.
28. Hilenski L, Terracio L, Borg TK. 1991. Myofibrillar and cytoskeletal assembly in neonatal rat cardiac myocytes cultured on laminin and collagen. Cell Tissue Res 264:577–587.
29. Fassler R, Rohwedel J, Maltsev V, Bloch W, Lentini S, Guan K, Gullberg D, Hescheler J, Addicks K, Wobus AM. 1996. Differentiation and integrity of cardiac muscle cells are impaired in the absence of beta 1 integrin. J Cell Sci 109:2989–2999.
30. Gullberg D, Tingstrom A, Thuresson A, Olsson L, Terracio L, Borg TK, Rubin K. 1990. Beta 1 integrin-mediated collagen gel contraction is stimulated by PDGF. Exp Cell Res 186:264–272.
31. Schiro JA, Chan BMC, Roswit WT, Kassner PD, Pentland AP, Hemler ME, Eisen AZ, Kupper TS. 1991. Integrin a2b1 (VLA-2) mediates reorganization and contraction of collagen matrices by human cells. Cell 67:403–410.
32. Sadoshima J, Izumo S. 1994. Roles of integrins in cell swelling-induced tyrosine phosphorylation in cardiac myocytes. Circulation 90:301–305.
33. Sadoshima J, Izumo S. 1993. Signal transduction pathways of angiotensin II induced c-fos gene expression in cardiac myocytes in vitro: roles of phospholipid-derived second messengers. Circ Res 73:424–438.
34. Sadoshima J, Qiu Z, Morgan JP, Izumo S. 1995. Angiotensin II and other hypertrophic stimuli mediated by G protein-coupled receptors activate tyrosine kinase, mitogen-activated protein kinase, and 90-kD S6 kinase in cardiac myocytes: the critical role of Ca^{2+}-dependent signaling. Circ Res 76:1–15.
35. Hori Y, Katoh T, Hirakata M, Joki N, Kaname S, Fukagawa M, Okuda T, Ohashi H, Fujita T, Miyazono K, Kurokawa K. 1998. Anti-latent TGF-beta binding protein-1 antibody or synthetic oligopeptides inhibit extracellular matrix expression induced by stretch in cultured rat mesangial cells. Kidney Int 53:1616–1625.
36. Gudi SR, Lee AA, Clark CB, Frangos JA. 1998. Equibiaxial strain and strain rate stimulate early activation of G proteins in cardiac fibroblasts. Am J Physiol 274:C1424–C1442.
37. Sharp WW, Simpson DG, Borg TK, Samarel AM, Terracio L. 1997. Mechanical forces regulate focal adhesion and costamere assembly in cardiac myocytes. Am J Physiol 273:H546–H556.

38. Vandenburgh HH, Shansky J, Karlisch P, Solerssi RL. 1993. Mechanical stimulation of skeletal muscle generates lipid-related second messengers by phospholipase activation. J Cell Physiol 155:63–71.
39. Wilson E, Mai Q, Sudhir K, Weiss RH, Ives HE. 1993. Mechanical strain induces growth of vascular smooth muscle cells via autocrine action of PDGF. J Cell Biol 123:741–747.
40. Ingber DE. 1997. Tensegrity: the architectural basis of cellular mechanotransduction. In Annual Review of Physiology. Ed. J.F. Hoffman, 575–599. Palo Alto: Annual Reviews Inc.
41. Juliano R. 1996. Cooperation between soluble factors and integrin-mediated cell anchorage in the control of cell growth and differentiation. BioEssays 18:911–917.
42. Plopper G, McNamee H, Dike L, Bojanowski K, Ingber D. 1995. Convergence of integrin and growth factor receptor signaling pathway within the focal adhesion complex. Mol Biol Cell 6:1349–1365.
43. Miyamoto S, Teramoto H, Coso O, Silvio G, Burbelo P, Akiyama S, Yamada K. 1995. Integrin function: molecular hierarchies of cytoskeletal and signaling molecules. J Cell Biol 131:701–805.
44. Chen Q, Kinch M, Lin T, Burridge K, Juliano R. 1994. Integrin mediated cell adhesion activates Mitogen-activated Protein Kinase. J Biol Chem 269:26602–26605.
45. Schaepfler D, Hanks S, Hunter T, van der Geer P. 1994. Integrin-mediated signal transduction linked to Ras pathway by GRB2 binding to focal adhesion kinase. Nature 372:786–791.
46. Bardy N, Merval R, Benessiano J, Samuel J-L, Tedgui A. 1996. Pressure and angiotensin II synergistically induce aortic fibronectin expression in organ culture model of rabbit aorta: evidence for a pressure-induced tissue renin–angiotensin system. Circ Res 79:70–78.
47. Sundberg C, Rubin K. 1996. Stimulation of $\beta1$ integrins on fibroblasts induces PDGF independent tyrosine phosphorylation of PDGF-β-receptors. J Cell Biol 132:741–752.
48. Hotchin N, Nobes C. 1996. Cell adhesion, signaling and thick skin. Trends Cell Biol 6:72–73.
49. Jones J, Gockerman A, Busby N, Wright G, Clemmons D. 1993. Insulin-like growth factor binding protein-1 stimulates cell migration and binds to the $\alpha5\beta1$ integrin by means of its Arg–Gly–Asp sequence. Proc Natl Acad Sci USA 90:10553–10557.
50. Sadoshima J, Izumo S. 1993. Mechanical stretch rapidly activates multiple signal transduction pathways in cardiac myocytes: potential involvement of an autocrine/paracrine mechanism. EMBO J 12:1691–1692.

N. Takeda, M. Nagano and N.S. Dhalla
(eds). The Hypertrophied Heart. Copyright
© 2000. pp. 143–164. Kluwer Academic
Publishers. Boston. All rights reserved.

INTEGRIN-DEPENDENT AND -INDEPENDENT SIGNALING DURING PRESSURE-OVERLOAD CARDIAC HYPERTROPHY

MARTIN LASER,[1] TOSHIO NAGAI,[1] VIJAYKUMAR S. KASI,[1]
CATALIN F. BAICU,[1] CHRISTOPHER D. WILLEY,[1]
CHARLENE M. KERR,[1] MICHAEL R. ZILE,[1,4] GEORGE COOPER IV,[1,2,4]
and DHANDAPANI KUPPUSWAMY[1,3]

[1] Cardiology Section of the Department of Medicine and [2] the Departments of Physiology and [3] Cell Biology,
Gazes Cardiac Research Institute, Medical University of South Carolina, Charleston, South Carolina 29425
and [4] the Veterans Administration Medical Center Charleston, South Carolina 29401, USA

Summary. In an attempt to uncover the linkage between hemodynamic load and cardiac hypertrophy, we focused on the cytoskeletal (CSK) assembly of signaling proteins in pressure-overloaded feline myocardium. Analysis showed CSK association of c-Src, β_3-integrin, FAK, PTP-1B, and p130Cas in 4 to 48 hour pressure overloaded (PO) myocardium. This assembly was accompanied by increased amounts of both total fibronectin (FN) and vitronectin (VN) and their attachment to the cardiocyte sarcolemma, indicating that a change in extracellular matrix (ECM) composition might be responsible for the CSK assembly of these signaling proteins. Furthermore, analysis with adult feline cardiocytes cultured in a three-dimensional (3-D) gel matrix made of either collagen containing FN and VN or of agarose alone for 12 hours revealed a CSK assembly of some of the signaling proteins only in collagen matrix, an event that could be blocked with RGD peptide. To investigate the role of CSK-assembled signaling proteins, activation of the two S6 kinase (S6K) isoforms, p70^{S6K} and p85^{S6K}, that are involved in translational and transcriptional activation was measured in PO myocardium. While both isoforms are activated substantially, p70^{S6K} activation occurred maximally at 1 hour of pressure overload prior to the CSK assembly of signaling proteins. The activation of both isoforms of S6K was found to be mediated by a PI 3-kinase-independent pathway with the possible involvement of protein kinase C. Furthermore, studies performed in vitro by embedding adult cardiocytes either in collagen or in agarose gels and stimulating them electrically to contract showed S6K activation in both types of gels, although CSK association of signaling proteins was present only in the collagen gel matrix. Therefore, these studies demonstrate that pressure overload activates both integrin-dependent and -independent signaling, which results, respectively, in cytoskeletal recruitment of signaling proteins and in S6K activation. Both may play critical roles in hypertrophic growth regulation.

INTRODUCTION

Cardiac hypertrophy is an adaptive mechanism by which the heart compensates for a sustained increase in hemodynamic loading. Hemodynamic overload of the heart is one of the common causes that leads to the development of cardiac hypertrophy. Conditions such as systemic hypertension, myocardial infarction, or valvular defects contribute to an increased mechanical load that eventually leads to the onset of heart failure. The signaling mechanisms that mediate the hypertrophic response of the heart are poorly understood, and this could be partly because several stress factors can combinatorially interplay and respond to hemodynamic overload. Such stresses include systemic neurohumoral factors, autocrine/paracrine factors, and other load-induced local changes occurring at the cardiocyte level, which include the activation of membrane-stretch-sensitive ion channels and cytoskeletal reorganization, as observed during extracellular matrix (ECM)[1] remodeling [1]. Previous studies from these laboratories have shown that increased load itself is directly linked to the changes occurring at the cardiocyte level, which include both a quantitative increase in cardiac mass and qualitative changes in the cardiac phenotype [1].

To investigate signaling events that result predominantly in a local response of the cardiocyte during a mechanical stress of the heart, we have chosen a feline right ventricular pressure overload (RVPO) model. In this model, the right ventricle is pressure overloaded by partial pulmonary artery occlusion, whereas the left ventricle is normally loaded and serves as a same-animal control. Thus, this model allows us to attribute changes seen in the right ventricle as exclusively due to the consequences of pressure overloading and not due to neurohumoral factors, which will be accounted for by using the same-animal LV control. The adaptive response of the heart to the load consists of both quantitative changes in the total amount of protein and qualitative changes in the expression of specific proteins (for reviews, see [1,2]).

It is well established that growth stimulation is often triggered when transmembrane cell surface receptors are occupied by their specific ligands, which results in the activation of either their intrinsic or associated tyrosine kinases. Subsequent events involving tyrosine phosphorylation of cellular proteins are important not only for the growth response but also for cellular morphological changes. In addition to these receptor-mediated pathways, there is growing evidence that integrin-mediated signaling via nonreceptor tyrosine kinases could contribute similarly to growth stimulation. Integrins are transmembrane proteins that provide tight adhesion of cells to ECM proteins at sites referred to as *focal adhesions* and that connect the ECM proteins to intracellular actin cytoskeleton [3–9]. There are 20 or more known integrin isoforms that are heterodimers of a specific combination of α- and β-subunits (for reviews, see [10,11]. Two of the major β-subunits of integrins that are known to be expressed in the adult heart include β_1 [12] and β_3 [13,14]. The β_1-integrin-containing heterodimers in the heart include α_1, α_3, α_5, α_6, or α_{7B} [12,15], and fibronectin and laminin serve as their primary ligands, whereas β_3-integrin forms heterodimers mostly with α_v, and vitronectin serves as its primary ligand [13]. In addition, increased expression of these integrins and of ECM proteins has been reported in the hypertrophying heart [15–17]. Binding of ECM proteins to integrins has been shown to trigger a variety of intracellular signaling events in several cell types and tissues [18,19], including the hypertrophying heart [14] and cardiocytes [20]. Although integrins are transmembrane proteins bearing short cytoplasmic domains, they do not exhibit intrinsic tyrosine kinase activity. Therefore, they transmit signaling via their interaction with nonreceptor tyrosine kinases, including focal adhesion kinase (FAK) and Src-family kinases such as c-Src and c-Fyn [21]. Since integrins are known to interact with cytoskeletal components [22,23], it is suggested that integrins transmit signals by organizing the cytoskeleton and regulating cell shape. It is believed that such a change in cell shape and cytoskeletal organization might regulate the biosynthetic capabilities of the cell, thereby controlling cell growth and differentiation [24,25]. Cytoskeletal assembly of nonreceptor tyrosine kinases, in particular c-Src and FAK, has been demonstrated in several agonist-induced cell types [26,27], and ligation of integrins with extracellular matrix proteins has been shown to be necessary for the activation and translocation of these signaling proteins. Although integrin-mediated signaling is widely studied in several cell types, its role in hypertrophying myocardium is beginning to emerge.

TYROSINE PHOSPHORYLATION IN PRESSURE-OVERLOADED MYOCARDIUM

It is well established that the activation of tyrosine kinases and the associated protein phosphorylation are important both for hyperplastic and hypertrophic cell growth. As reviewed recently [28], integrins could play a critical role in mediating mechanical stresses via the activation of tyrosine kinases and the formation of focal assembly of signaling proteins to promote cell growth. Activation of tyrosine kinases has been shown in many models of cardiac hypertrophy [29,30]. Although angiotensin-mediated signaling is suggested to be important for cardiac hypertrophy, recent studies indicate that hypertrophic growth can proceed independent of angiotensin II stimulation, although these pathways are still dependent on tyrosine kinases [31].

Since in terminally differentiated cells, such as platelets, mechanical stirring has been shown to cause cytoskeletal recruitment of nonreceptor tyrosine kinases, resulting in tyrosine phosphorylation of several cytoskeletal proteins [26], we undertook a similar approach to analyze changes in the tyrosine phosphorylation pattern in pressure-overloaded myocardium. For subcellular fractionation, ventricular tissue was detergent extracted and centrifuged to obtain the following three fractions [14,26]: Triton X-100-soluble, Triton X-100-insoluble low spin fraction (cytoskeleton), and Triton X-100-insoluble high spin fraction (membrane skeleton). When these fractions were analyzed for load-induced protein tyrosine phosphorylation in a 48 hour pressure-overloaded right ventricle and compared with normally loaded left ventricle, several cytoskeleton-bound proteins were found to be newly tyrosine phosphorylated in substantial amounts in pressure-overloaded myocardium (figure 1). As will be discussed later, several of these newly phosphorylated proteins appeared to be recruited to the cytoskeleton as a response to pressure overload. These changes in the tyrosine phosphorylation pattern were observed during a period of 4 to 48 hours of pressure overload and were absent at an earlier time point of 1 hour pres-

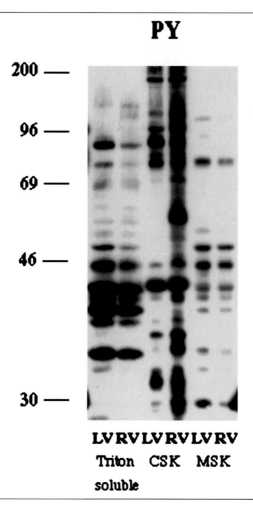

Figure 1. Tyrosine phosphorylation of cytoskeletal proteins in 48-hour pressure-overloaded myocardium. Normally loaded LV and pressure overloaded RV samples were obtained from a 48 hour RVPO feline heart and used for preparing Triton X-100-lysed subfractions, namely, soluble (Triton soluble) and insoluble (cytoskeleton and membrane skeleton) fractions, as we described previously [14]. After resolving the proteins on SDS-PAGE, tyrosine phosphorylated proteins were detected by Western blotting with anti-phosphotyrosine antibody (Transduction Lab.). The figure was obtained from our previous studies published in the *Journal of Biological Chemistry* 272:4500–4508 (1997), with the permission of the publisher.

sure overload [14]. At least two major differences between growth factor-stimulated tyrosine phosphorylation of cellular proteins and pressure overload-induced tyrosine phosphorylation of cardiac proteins appear to exist: (1) growth factor-stimulated tyrosine phosphorylation is rapid (occurring usually within minutes) when compared to load-induced phosphorylation, which occurs mostly between 4 and 48 hours of pressure overload and (2) whereas phosphorylation of several new proteins is readily seen in the Triton X-100-soluble fraction of growth factor-stimulated cells, most of the newly tyrosine phosphorylated proteins in the load-induced hypertrophying myocardium are found in the detergent-insoluble cytoskeletal fraction. Therefore, these studies indicate that unlike the growth factor-stimulated tyrosine phosphorylation, which is important for mitogenic stimulation, load-induced tyrosine phosphorylation appears to be playing a major role in the structural changes associated with cardiac hypertrophy.

ANALYSIS OF CYTOSKELETON-ASSEMBLED PROTEINS

A potential important candidate for mediating both the assembly and phosphorylation of cytoskeletal proteins is cell surface integrins. In addition to playing both structural and adhesive roles, integrins function as cell surface receptors and mediate multiple cellular functions like proliferation, migration, differentiation, and apoptosis (for reviews, see [10,11,19]). They are composed of α- and β-heterodimers, which are expressed in a tissue- or cell type-specific manner. Although several α- and β-isoforms and their combination for specialized functions have been described [10,11], previous studies [12–17] (including ours) that involve coimmunoprecipitation combined Western blot analyses indicate that there are predominantly three different integrin heterodimers, namely, $\alpha_5\beta_1$, $\alpha_v\beta_3$, and $\alpha_v\beta_5$, present in the adult heart. Subcellular fractionation of the normal adult myocardium using detergent containing buffers indicates that under normal conditions, these integrins are usually present in the Triton X-100-soluble compartment; however, in 4- to 48-hour pressure-overloaded myocardium, part of the cellular β_3-integrin was found to become detergent insoluble due to its association with the cytoskeleton [14]. Such changes were not observed for other integrins. These findings suggest that a β_3-integrin containing focal adhesion might be important for the cytoskeletal recruitment and phosphorylation of several cytoskeleton-bound proteins.

There are two broad views towards integrin-mediated signaling (for a review, see [23]). Since the cytoplasmic domains of integrins interact with several cytoskeletal proteins, one view suggests that integrins are linked to the regulation of cell shape and cytoskeletal reorganization [24,32]. In the second view, integrins are expected to mediate signaling similar to growth factor receptors [25]. In platelets, activation of glycoprotein IIb–IIIa (a major form of platelet integrins, structurally similar to $\alpha_v\beta_3$) by fibrinogen binding has been shown to result in the cytoskeletal binding of this glycoprotein [26] accompanied by a similar association of nonreceptor tyrosine kinases, such as c-Src and FAK. Assembly and activation of these kinases have been suggested to be responsible for cytoskeletal structural changes and for overall platelet-shape changes. Interestingly, our studies in the pressure-overloaded myocardium for 48 hours also show cytoskeletal recruitment of β_3-integrin, c-Src, and FAK, resulting in the phosphorylation of several cytoskeletal proteins [14]. In order to understand the importance of this assembly of proteins, we explored for additional signaling proteins that associate with the cytoskeleton in response to pressure overload. Analysis revealed that in addition to c-Src and FAK, as we

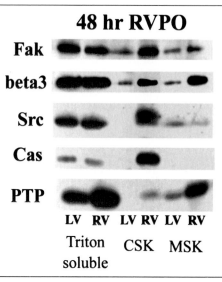

48 hr RVPO

Fak

beta3

Src

Cas

PTP

LV RV LV RV LV RV

Triton   CSK   MSK
soluble

Figure 2. Cytoskeletal associations of signaling proteins during RVPO for 48 hours. Normally loaded LV and pressure overloaded RV samples were obtained from a 48 hour RVPO feline heart and used for preparing Triton X-100-lysed subfractions, namely, soluble (Triton-soluble) and insoluble (cytoskeleton and membrane skeleton) fractions, as we described previously [14]. The samples were resolved on SDS-PAGE and analyzed for the presence of β_3-integrin, FAK, c-Src, p130Cas, and PTP-1B. The following antibodies were commercially obtained; β_3-integrin (monoclonal, Transduction Lab.), FAK (monoclonal, Transduction Lab.), c-Src (monoclonal, Upstate Biotech.), p130Cas (polyclonal, Santa Cruz), and PTP-1B (monoclonal, Calbiochem). The figures for β_3-integrin, FAK, and c-Src were obtained from our previous studies published in the *Journal of Biological Chemistry* 272:4500–4508 (1997), with the permission of the publisher.

described previously [14], the adapter protein p130Cas and the tyrosine phosphatase PTP-1B were also present in the detergent-insoluble cytoskeletal fraction of 48-hour pressure-overloaded myocardium (figure 2). Confocal microscopic analyses were performed using some of these antibodies, which show colocalization of FAK, Cas, and PTP-1B along the cardiocyte plasma membrane in the 48-hour pressure-overloaded right ventricle (figure 3). All these studies showing the cytoskeletal assembly of tyrosine kinases, tyrosine phosphatases, and adapter proteins during pressure overloading is intriguing in the sense that a spatial organization or scaffolding of signaling proteins might be a requirement for efficient signal transduction and/or structural remodeling of the cells during their active growth. It has been pointed out recently that the scaffolding of signaling proteins could play an important role in signal transmission [33], and an increasing number of adapter proteins have been identified as scaffolding molecules. The presence of multiple SH2, SH3, or pleckstrin homology domains and/or tyrosine and proline motifs enables them to interact with several cellular proteins, including structural cytoskeletal proteins, receptors, and other signaling proteins such as kinases and phosphatases. Overall, these studies show that several signaling proteins are immobilized on the cytoskeletal structures during pressure overloading following integrin activation.

48 hr RVPO

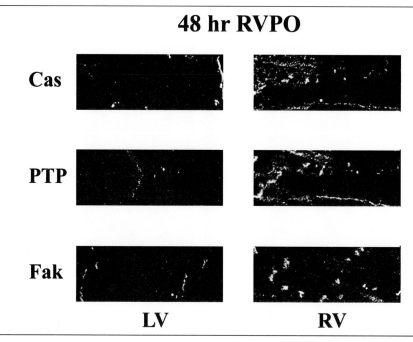

Figure 3. Immunofluoresence confocal micrographs showing focal accumulation of signaling proteins on the cardiocyte surface of pressure-overloaded myocardium. Normally loaded left ventricles and 48 hour pressure-overloaded right ventricles were used to prepare fresh-frozen tissue sections and were processed for confocal microscopy [44]. These sections were fixed with either methanol/acetone (for Cas and PTP-1B) or formaldehyde solution (for FAK), as we described previously [56], and were incubated with primary antibodies. Cy3 donkey anti-rabbit IgG was used as the secondary antibody.

What triggers the cardiocyte integrins to mediate the assembly of signaling proteins and form focal adhesion complexes in response to pressure overload? It is known that during the development of cardiac hypertrophy and heart failure, a remodeling of the affected myocardium occurs with changes in the ECM composition. Increased levels of ECM proteins such as collagen, fibronectin, and osteopontin during cardiac hypertrophy have been described [17,34,35]. Furthermore, several binding motifs on the ECM proteins have been shown to interact not only with integrins but also with a variety of cell surface receptors, growth factors, and ECM proteins themselves. The arginine–glycine–aspartate (RGD) motif, found in many ECM proteins, makes them specific ligands for integrins. We, therefore, asked whether a change in the level of one or more of the ECM proteins and/or in their interaction with integrins in pressure-overloaded myocardium is responsible for the cytoskeletal assembly of signaling. Specifically, we analyzed for the secretion and assembly of two ECM proteins, fibronectin and vitronectin. Both these proteins contain the RGD motif and could serve as ligands for $\alpha_5\beta_1$ and $\alpha_v\beta_3$ integrins. Interestingly, pressure overloading resulted in an increase in the levels of these two ECM proteins as well as their assembly on the 48-hour RVPO cardiocyte surface

48 hr RVPO

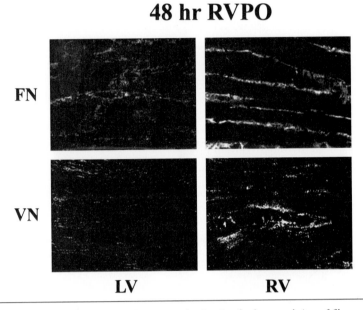

Figure 4. Immunofluoresence confocal micorographs showing focal accumulation of fibronectin and vitronectin on the cardiocyte surface of pressure-overloaded myocardium. Normally loaded left ventricles and 48 hour pressure-overloaded right ventricles were used to prepare fresh-frozen tissue sections and were processed for confocal microscopy [44]. These sections were fixed with formaldehyde solution, as we described previously [56], and were incubated with primary antibodies. Cy3 donkey anti-rabbit IgG was used as the secondary antibody.

(figure 4), colocalized along the cardiocyte membrane (confocal microscopic analyses), as observed for FAK, Cas, and PTP-1B (figure 3). Furthermore, Western blot analysis showed the presence of both fibronectin and vitronectin, mostly in the cytoskeletal fraction of pressure-overloaded myocardium (data not shown). Taken together, these studies strongly indicate that during pressure overloading, increased levels of ECM proteins and their interaction with integrins are responsible for the cytoskeletal recruitment of signaling proteins.

INTEGRIN-DEPENDENT SIGNALING

Several integrin-mediated signaling cascades have been described previously (for a review, see [36]). The activation of the mitogen-activated protein kinase (MAPK) signaling cascade via integrins has been described [37] and has been shown to occur by both FAK-dependent [37] and -independent [38] mechanisms. Furthermore, integrin ligation has been shown to activate small GTP binding proteins, such as Rac, Cdc-42, and Rho, resulting in the activation of PAK, p38MAPK, and JNK (for a review, see [39]). $\alpha_v\beta_3$-integrin has been shown recently to mediate a c-Src-dependent signaling cascade, which leads to NFκB translocation into the nucleus for protecting cells from apoptosis [40]). Another well-characterized pathway downstream of integrins includes a PI-3-kinase-mediated signaling cascade. Integrin interaction with ECM proteins has been shown to result in the activation of PI-3-kinase (PI-3-K) via FAK phosphorylation and activation [41]. Furthermore, PI-3-K activation results in the activation of $p70/85^{S6K}$ (S6K), and a serine/threonine kinase, AKT, has been shown to act as an intermediate kinase [42]. Although we could observe activation of PAK, p38MAPK, and p42/44MAPK in our pressure-overload model, the most prominent activation was found for S6K, a serine/threonine kinase important for translational and transcriptional regulation. Overall, multiple pathways can mediate signaling events subsequent to the integrin activation, although some of these signaling cascades are rather cell type specific and need not necessarily apply to terminally differentiated cells like adult cardiocytes.

INTEGRIN-INDEPENDENT ACTIVATION OF P70/85 S6 KINASE IN PRESSURE OVERLOAD HYPERTROPHY

A hallmark of cardiac hypertrophy is enhanced protein synthesis resulting in an increase in cardiac mass. $p70/85^{S6K}$ has been shown to play an important role in the control of both translational and transcriptional activation, and by phosphorylating the 40S ribosomal protein, it is involved in the translational control of mRNA transcripts that contain a polypyrimidine tract at their transcriptional start site [43]. Since our studies show that integrin engagement is responsible for the cytoskeletal assembly of signaling proteins in the pressure-overloaded myocardium and since previous reports show that integrin engagement can result in the activation of $p70/85^{S6K}$, we initiated a study to determine whether $p70/85^{S6K}$ is activated in response to pressure overload via integrin-mediated signaling. To determine the activation profile, we performed a time course of load-induced $p70/85^{S6K}$ activation and phosphorylation. Pressure-overloaded right ventricles and normally loaded same-animal control left ventricles were used to prepare total lysates with Triton X-100 buffer [14,44]. After resolving the proteins on SDS-PAGE, Western blotting was performed with anti-$p70/85^{S6K}$ antibody (Santa Cruz). A 70 kDa protein doublet representing $p70^{S6K}$ could be readily detected in all the normally loaded control ventricles (figure 5). Analysis of pressure-overloaded right ventricular samples revealed a shift in the mobility of this isoform (i.e., lower band of the doublet disappears with the appearance of a new band on top of the upper band), which is indicative of phosphorylated species of $p70^{S6K}$ [44,45]. This change in SDS gel migration of $p70^{S6K}$ was observed as early as 1 hour RVPO, persisted up to 4 hours, declined substantially at 48 hours, and returned to the basal level in 1 week pressure-overloaded right ventricle. In the case of $p85^{S6K}$, a similar trend showing retarded mobility was also observed at 1 and 4 hours RVPO; however, unlike the $p70^{S6K}$, this isoform did not decline appreciably at 48 hours RVPO and was found to reach the control levels only at a later time point of 1 week RVPO. All these data indicate that both isoforms of $p70/85^{S6K}$ exhibit a mobility band shift on SDS-PAGE in response to pressure overloading in as little as 1 hour. Such a mobility change for these isoforms has been reported to be indicative of kinase activation [44]. Analysis of the $p70^{S6K}$

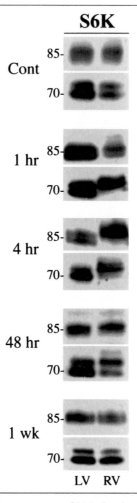

Figure 5. Western blot showing the time course of S6K phosphorylation during RVPO. Left ventricles and right ventricles obtained from sham-operated control feline hearts (Cont) and from 1 hour, 4 hour, 48 hour, and 1 week RVPO feline hearts were extracted with Triton X-100 buffer, as we described previously [15,41], and were used for Western blot analysis with anti-s6K antibody (C-18 polyclonal, Santa Cruz). The molecular sizes of p70[S6K] and p85[S6K] are indicated in the figure. The figure was obtained from our previous studies published in the *Journal of Biological Chemistry* 273:24610–24619 (1998), with the permission of the publisher.

activity in the cytosolic samples obtained from these pressure-overloaded ventricles showed an activation time course similar to the time course of band shifting shown in the figure (data not shown).

Interestingly, the activation of p70/85[S6K], which occurs between 1 and 4 hours of RVPO, precedes the integrin-mediated cytoskeletal assembly of signaling proteins, which is observed profoundly between 4 and 48 hours RVPO. Therefore, load-induced activation of one or more signaling pathways occurs prior to the integrin-mediated cytoskeletal assembly of signaling proteins. As mentioned before, in a typical receptor-mediated S6K activation pathway, a tyrosine kinase-dependent pathway with the involvement of PI3K activation and AKT phosphorylation has been described. However, our studies [44] clearly rule out the possible involvement of this pathway, since neither the PI3K activation nor AKT phosphorylation was observed during pressure overload. These observations strongly suggest that integrin-mediated cytoskeletal assembly of signaling proteins and the associated tyrosine phos-phorylation, which are occurring at a later time point of pressure overload, do not contribute to the activation of S6K.

Since $p70/85^{S6K}$ activation can also occur via a PI3K-independent pathway mediated by PKC [46,47], we analyzed this possibility in the pressure-overloaded myocardium. Our results show load-induced activation of PKC isoforms (α, γ, and ε) whose time courses of activation were similar to that of $p70/85^{S6K}$ [44]. Furthermore, treatment of adult cardiocytes with TPA, which is well known to activate PKC, mim-icked our in vivo observations on the activation of $p70/85^{S6K}$. Interestingly, our study clearly shows that c-Raf, which could potentially serve as a downstream target of PKC, is activated during pressure overload [44]. c-Raf is one of the key serine/threo-nine protein kinases involved in the transmission of mitogenic signals generated by receptor and nonreceptor tyrosine kinases (for a review, see [48]). The expression of constitutively active c-Raf has been shown to result in the activation of $p70/85^{S6K}$ [49]. Therefore, we analyzed both localization and activation of c-Raf using Triton X-100 lysed subfractions prepared from normal and pressure-overloaded cat ventricles (soluble, insoluble cytoskeleton, and insoluble membrane skeleton), as we described previously [14]. Pressure overloading for 1 to 4 hours resulted in retarded mobility of c-Raf on SDS-PAGE in all the Triton X-100 lysed-subfractions [44], suggesting that the kinase had undergone phosphorylation, which is indicative of kinase activation [50]. These studies show that an initial wave of integrin-independent signaling events is triggered during pressure overload for the activation of PKC isoforms and c-Raf, which might mediate the activation of $p70/85^{S6K}$.

Our studies show that the early phase of S6K activation might contribute to the acute phase of adaptation to an increased work load via increased protein synthe-sis. Phosphorylation of the ribosomal S6 protein by $p70/85^{S6K}$ leads to a selective increase in the translational efficiency of polypyrimidine tract containing mRNAs. Those RNAs are known to encode predominantly ribosomal proteins and cofac-tors important for the translational machinery, which lead ultimately to an increase in the translational capacity [43]. The role of the nuclear isoform of S6K ($p85^{S6K}$) is not as well characterized as the cytoplasmic S6K ($p70^{S6K}$). However, several transcription factors, such as c-AMP response-element binding proteins (CREB/CREM), appear to have a consensus sequence for phosphorylation and could serve as potential substrates for $p85^{S6K}$ [51]. Indeed, both transcriptional factors, CREB and CREM, have been shown to be directly phosphorylated by $p85^{S6K}$, resulting in enhanced gene expression [51]. Whether or not CREB/CREM could serve as targets for nuclear S6K remains speculative, although these transcriptional factors have been shown to activate immediate early genes (IEGs) and delayed response genes. We have reported previously the activation of these transcriptional factors in pressure-overloaded myocardium [52]. The finding that some of the IEG products are integrins as well as ECM proteins such as fibronectin [53] makes this pathway even more attractive in pressure-overloaded hypertrophy, since this initial wave of signaling via p70/85[S6K] might prime the cardiocytes for a second wave of integrin-mediated signaling.

In summary, these in vivo studies of actively hypertrophying myocardium show the existence of at least two waves of signaling in response to pressure overload: (1) an initial wave of integrin-independent signaling in the window of 1 to 4 hour pressure overload that appears to be responsible for the activation of certain PKC isoforms, c-Raf and p70/85[S6K], which in turn might be related to the overall increase in cardiac protein synthesis and mass, and (2) a subsequent integrin-dependent signaling that occurs in the window of 4 to 48 hour pressure overload, resulting in the cytoskeletal assembly and tyrosine phosphorylation of signaling proteins. Based on the available evidence, this latter pathway might be responsible for the structural changes associated with cardiac hypertrophy.

THREE-DIMENSIONAL COLLAGEN MATRIX AS AN IN VITRO MODEL FOR CULTURING AND STIMULATING ISOLATED ADULT CARDIOCYTES

One of our major research efforts was to establish an in vitro cardiocyte culture model that would enable us to reproduce most, if not all, of our in vivo findings on the cytoskeletal assembly of signaling proteins. In this context, a three-dimensional (3-D) matrix model, in which freshly isolated adult feline cardiocytes were embedded in a type I collagen matrix [54,55], was found to be attractive. It was anticipated that in the 3-D environment, the integrins would interact uniformly on the cardiocyte surface with their given ECM ligands. This model differs from the conventional 2-D culture models, in which only a part of the cardiocyte surface is in contact with the ECM proteins coated on the culture dishes. Also, in 3-D models, mechanical stress can be imposed uniformly on the entire surface of the cardiocyte, whereas in the 2-D models, the stress is imposed only at the attached area of the cardiocytes.

We performed experiments to establish a 3D model for adult cardiocytes [56] and then initiated a series of experiments to determine the localization of focal adhesion proteins in the cardiocyte. For this, freshly isolated cardiocytes were embedded in 0.1% collagen gel matrix [56], maintained in the tissue culture incubator for various time periods and processed for both confocal microscopy and Western blot analyses, as we described recently [44,56]. When cardiocytes embedded in collagen matrix were processed immediately for the presence of signaling proteins, β_{1D}-integrin (a muscle-specific isoform of β_1-integrin [57]), β_3-integrin, FAK, Cas, and PTP-1B were present on the sarcolemma (figure 6). Since none of the commercially available antibodies was found to be suitable for c-Src, we were unable to analyze c-Src. Western blot analysis of the 3-D embedded cardiocytes revealed a

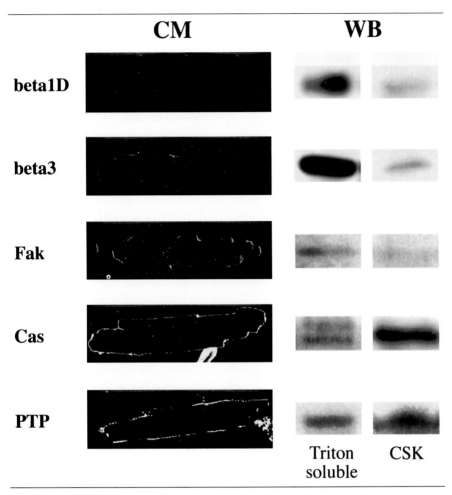

Figure 6. Focal assembly of signaling proteins in freshly isolated cardiocytes embedded three-dimensionally in collagen matrix. Freshly isolated adult feline cardiocytes were embedded in 0.1% collagen, as we described previously [56]. For confocal microscopy (CM), then section of collagen gel matrix were made at 90 minutes after collagen polymerization, fixed with either methanol/acetone or formaldehyde solution, as we described previously [56], and incubated with primary antibodies. Cy3 donkey anti-mouse IgM was used as the secondary antibody for β_3-integrin, and Cy3 donkey anti-rabbit IgG was used for β_{1D}-integrin and FAK. For Western blot analysis (WB), cardiocytes from the collagen matrix were recovered by digesting with collagenase and were then used for preparing Triton X-100 soluble and insoluble fractions, as we described previously [14]. The samples were resolved on SDS-PAGE and analyzed for the presence of β_{1D}- and β_3-integrins, FAK, c-Src, p130Cas, and PTP-1B using commercially obtained antibodies.

strong signal for cytoskeleton-assembled Cas and PTP-1B, whereas FAK showed only a weak association (figure 6). However, β_1- and β_3-integrins were not present in detectable levels in the cytoskeletal factions. These results suggest that although aggregation of integrins and a few other signaling proteins (Cas, PTP-1B, and FAK)

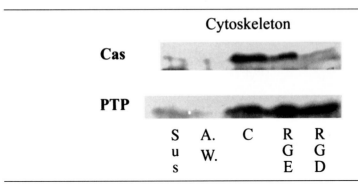

Figure 7. Effect of "RGD" peptide on the cytoskeleton-bound p130Cas and PTP-1B. Adult cardiocytes were isolated from a feline heart. Part of the cell preparations was maintained in suspension at 37°C for 90 minutes while the remaining cardiocytes were used for embedding in collagen matrix gel. For collagen matrix, both acid washed (A.W.) or unwashed cardiocytes were embedded in 0.1% collagen matrix, as we described previously [56]. In the case of unwashed cardiocytes, they were embedded either in the absence (control, C) or in the presence of 5 mM RGE or RGD peptides. After a 90 minute incubation at 37°C in the tissue culture incubator, cardiocytes from the collagen matrix were recovered by digesting with collagenase. Both suspended (Sus) and collagen-embedded cardiocytes were then used for preparing Triton X-100-soluble and -insoluble fractions, as we described previously [15]. The samples were resolved on SDS-PAGE and analyzed for the presence of p130Cas and PTP-1B using commercially obtained antibodies.

can be visualized on the cardiocyte sarcolemma, only some of them (Cas and PTP-1B) show cytoskeletal assembly upon embedding cardiocytes in collagen matrix.

To demonstrate that the cytoskeletal binding of p130Cas and PTP-1B occurs in an integrin-dependent manner, the following studies were performed (figure 7). We have shown recently that freshly isolated cardiocytes from feline hearts possess a preexisting integrin complex on the cardiocyte surface that consists of components like laminin and β_{1D}-integrin. We also demonstrated that this complex can be removed by acid washing the cardiocytes [56]. Therefore, in order to prove that the cytoskeleton-bound Cas and PTP-1B in 3-D collagen gel could be due to a preexisting integrin–ECM complex, we acid washed freshly isolated cardiocytes at pH 4.0 mildly for 1 minute before embedding them in collagen gel. Interestingly, the acid washing led to the disappearance of Cas and PTP-1B from the cytoskeletal fractions (figure 7), suggesting that the ligation of laminin and/or other unidentified ECM proteins on the freshly isolated cardiocyte surface might be responsible for the cytoskeletal association of Cas and PTP-1B. Although the acid-wash experiments indicate that a preexisting integrin complex might be responsible for the cytoskeletal binding of Cas and PTP-1B, persistence of this complex requires immediate embedding of isolated cardiocytes in the 3-D collagen matrix. That is, when freshly isolated cardiocytes were kept in suspension (Sus), they did not exhibit the cytoskeleton-bound Cas and PTP-1B.

To directly test whether the cytoskeletal binding of Cas and PTP-1B is integrin mediated, we included RGD peptides to alter the cytoskeletal assembly of signaling proteins. Inclusion of RGD peptide, which could compete with preexisting ECM proteins on the cardiocyte surface, blocked the association of Cas (figure 7), although such blocking was only partially observed for PTP-1B. Under these conditions, a nonspecific peptide, RGE, did not show such blocking. Taken together, these studies indicate that one or more specific preexisting integrin complexes on the cardiocyte surface might be responsible for the cytoskeletal assembly of Cas, and we suspect it is β_{1D}/laminin. However, PTP-1B association could be either via integrin engagement with a binding motif different from the RGD sequence [58] or via integrin-independent mechanisms as suggested for cadherins (for a review, see [59]). Unlike Cas and PTP-1B, freshly isolated cells, when embedded in 3-D matrix, did not show cytoskeletal assembly of c-Src (data not shown) and FAK (figure 6). These observations reveal three possibilities: (1) Cas, which has been shown to be a substrate for c-Src, does not depend on c-Src for its recruitment to the cytoskeleton; (2) the integrins and/or the ECM proteins needed for the cytoskeletal assembly of c-Src and Cas may be different; and (3) Immobilization of cardiocytes in 3-D collagen matrix is a prerequisite for the cytoskeletal assembly of Cas and PTP-1B.

We suspect β_3-integrin might be a potential candidate for mediating the cytoskeletal assembly of c-Src and FAK, based on the following observations: (1) our in vivo studies show that the cytoskeletal assembly of c-Src and FAK is accompanied by a similar association of β_3-integrin; (2) our in vitro studies show absence of all these members when freshly isolated cardiocytes are embedded in collagen matrix; and (3) previous studies of platelets [26] demonstrate that the engagement of α_{IIB}-β_3-integrin (which is similar to $\alpha_v\beta_3$ integrin) is responsible for the cytoskeletal binding of c-Src and FAK. We are currently exploring such possibilities by including in the collagen matrix gels several ECM proteins that contain the RGD binding motifs. However, to identify precise integrin isoform(s), specific blocking antibodies need to be employed in these studies. Furthermore, to test whether mechanical stimulation is required for the cytoskeletal assembly, these cardiocytes embedded in collagen matrix could be stimulated electrically to contract. In summary, the 3-D collagen cell culture model appears to be a useful model to explore the cytoskeletal assembly of signaling proteins and to identify the specific integrin isoform and its ECM proteins. Additionally, this model seems to provide an environment for cardiocytes to immobilize their integrins with specific ECM proteins for the formation of focal adhesions and/or their cytoskeletal assembly, thus allowing one to study the paradigm of integrin ligation, aggregation, and focal adhesion, as has been described recently by Miyamoto et al. [60].

Our next goal with the collagen 3-D model was to establish S6K activation as we observed in vivo during pressure overloading and to demonstrate that such activation was integrin independent. Although we observe preexisting complexes of integrin and signaling molecules on the cardiocyte sarcolemma [56] (figure 6) as well as cytoskeletal assembly of p130Cas and PTP-1B upon embedding freshly isolated cardiocytes in collagen matrix gel (figures 6 and 7), we did not see activation of S6K under these conditions (data not shown). Therefore, we stimulated the collagen-embedded cardiocytes mechanically by electrical pacing (1 Hz). Electrical

A

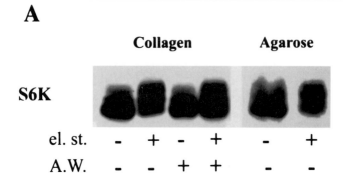

Collagen   Agarose

S6K

el. st.	-	+	-	+	-	+
A.W.	-	-	+	+	-	-

B   Collagen

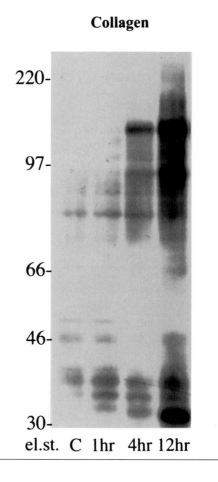

220-

97-

66-

46-

30-

el.st. C 1hr 4hr 12hr

Figure 8. p70S6K activation and tyrosine phosphorylation during contraction by electrical stimulation of cardiocytes embedded three-dimensionally in collagen matrix. Freshly isolated cardiocytes were embedded three-dimensionally in collagen matrix, in agarose, or were acid washed (A.W) and then embedded in collagen matrix, as we described previously [56]. After culturing for 12 hours in the tissue culture incubator at 37°C, cardiocytes were stimulated to contract by electrical stimulation (el. st.) for various time periods. Both control and stimulated cardiocytes were used for preparing Triton X-100-soluble fractions, and the samples were resolved on SDS-PAGE for Western blot analyses with anti-S6K antibody and anti-phosphotyrosine antibody. For the p70S6K experiment, cardiocytes were stimulated for 1 hour and compared with unstimulated quiescent cells. For the detection of phosphotyrosine containing proteins, cardiocytes were stimulated for various time periods (1, 4 and 12 hours) and compared with unstimulated control (C) cardiocytes.

stimulation of both adult and neonatal cardiocytes has been shown to enhance the protein synthesis rate and induce hypertrophic growth [61,62]. Electrical stimulation of the 3-D-collagen-embedded adult cardiocytes for 1 hour resulted in the activation of S6K, as observed by a mobility band shift on SDS-PAGE similar to our in vivo observations in pressure-overloaded myocardium (figure 5). To analyze whether any of the preexisting focal adhesion proteins was responsible for this activation process, we repeated these experiments with acid-washed cardiocytes embedded in collagen matrix or by embedding unwashed cardiocytes three-dimensionally in agarose. While both conditions showed no aggregation of integrins on the cardiocyte surface [56], electrical stimulation still resulted in S6K activation (figure 8A). Therefore, these studies clearly suggest that S6K activation in response to mechanical stimulation occurs independent of integrins and supports our in vivo observations. Interestingly, whereas S6K activation could be observed as early as 1 hour after electrical stimulation, a change in tyrosine phosphorylation could be observed only between a period of 4 to 12 hours of stimulation (figure 8B), supporting our hypothesis that S6K activation can occur independently from tyrosine kinases. We are currently using this model to confirm our in vivo findings that S6K activation, in response to a mechanical stimulation, occurs via an integrin-independent pathway with the involvement of PKC.

CONCLUSIONS

Our studies suggest that the activation of an integrin-independent pathway during the early phase of pressure-overload induced cardiac hypertrophy leads to the activation of PKC isoforms, c-Raf, and S6K isoforms. Although we and others have identified the activation of these kinases, several intermediate serine/threonine kinases of the signaling cascade that translates the mechanical load into biochemical signaling cascades have yet to be identified. However, the activation of these kinases appears to be independent of tyrosine kinases, suggesting that the receptor and nonreceptor tyrosine kinases may not be required for their activation. Our studies also indicate a second wave of signaling during the later phase of pressure overload. In this pathway, integrin-ECM interactions appear to play a major role in the cytoskeletal assembly of signaling molecules, such as c-Src, FAK, Cas, and

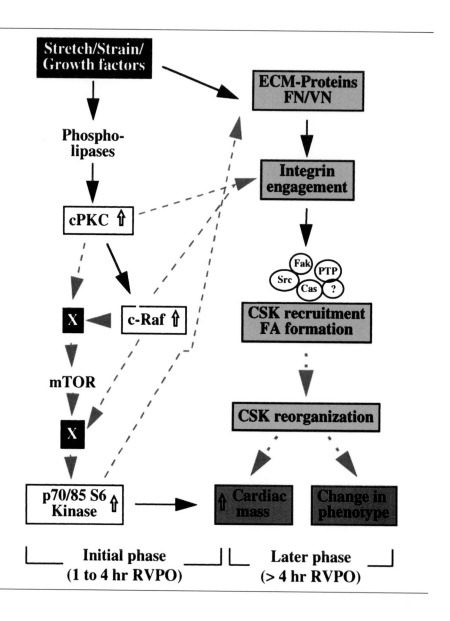

PTP-1B. In this second phase of signaling, integrin–ECM interaction and focal adhesion complex formation are triggered by the upregulation of ECM proteins, such as fibronectin and vitronectin. Yet these two waves of signaling could be functioning in a sequential manner. As depicted in figure 9, activation of PKC isoforms may participate in inside-out signaling, resulting in an increase in the affinity of integrins for ECM proteins [63]. In addition, of the two isoforms of the p70/85[S6K]

◄ ──

Figure 9. Model for load-induced signaling during hypertrophic cardiac growth. Based on our studies, we propose that there are two waves of signaling in pressure overload-induced hypertrophying myocardium. In the initial phase of signaling, which occurs as early as in 1 hour of pressure overload, there is a remarkable activation of p70S6K, accompanied by the activation of c-Raf and PKC isoforms. We speculate that the PKC activation might occur via phospholipases, which are likely to be independent of tyrosine kinases. The activation of this pathway leads to the activaton of p70S6K, with the probable involvement of c-Raf. Since rapamycin blocks the activation of p70S6K during electrical stimulation of cardiocytes, this initial phase of PKC-mediated signaling is expected to act via mTOR (mammalian target of rapamycin) on p70S6K. During this initial phase of signaling, activation of p70S6K, which plays an important role in the translational control, might be important for the increase in cardiac mass of hypertrophying heart. A second wave (latter phase) of signaling occurs during 4 to 48 hour pressure overloading. This signaling appears to be triggered due to a change in the ECM composition and integrin engagement. As a result, focal adhesion formation occurs (FA), and several signaling proteins, such as c-Src, FAK, p130Cas, and PTP-1B, are recruited to the pressure-overloaded cardiocyte cytoskeleton. Since several phenotypic changes are encountered during hypertrophic cardiac growth, we speculate that the cytoskeletal association of signaling proteins might contribute to these changes and to the overall hypertrophic cardiac growth. The activation of this second wave of signaling might be positively regulated by the initial signaling cascade in several different ways (see text). In the figure, solid arrows indicate pathways that have been well established, and dotted arrows indicate the probable pathways that might also be triggered during cardiac hypertrophy.

that are known to play a major role in the translational control, the p85 isoform can activate transcriptional factors such as CREM/CREB. Activation of these factors could result in the secretion of ECM proteins. Therefore, activation of PKC and S6K could lead to the engagement of integrins and ECM proteins. Furthermore, our studies show that c-Raf not only undergoes activation but also associates with the cytoskeleton of pressure-overloaded myocardium. The role of cytoskeleton-bound c-Raf is largely unknown at the present time. One possible role might be to prime the cytoskeleton for the later recruitment of signaling proteins. Therefore, the initial phase of signaling might also participate in the integrin-mediated cytoskeletal assembly of signaling proteins. The critical question that remains is what role these cytoskeleton-bound signaling proteins might have in transducing cardiac load into a hypertrophic growth response. Whether the signaling pathway mediated by the cytoskeleton-bound proteins is beneficial for compensatory growth in response to load or rather contributes to deterioration of cardiac function and the development of heart failure still needs to be explored.

ACKNOWLEDGMENTS

This study was supported by Program Project Grant HL-48788 from the National Heart, Lung, and Blood Institute, by research funds from the Department of Veterans Affairs, and by the Deutsche Forschungsgemeinschaft (M. Laser). The authors thank Mary Barnes for her excellent technical assistance.

REFERENCES

1. Cooper G. 1987. Cardiocyte adaptation to chronically altered load. Annu Rev Physiol 49:501–518.
2. Chien KR, Zhu H, Knowlton KU, Miller-Hance W, van-Bilsen M, O'Brien TX, Evans SM. 1993. Transcriptional regulation during cardiac growth and development. Annu Rev Physiol 55:77–95.

3. Miyamoto S, Teramoto H, Coso OA, Gutkind JS, Burbelo PD, Akiyama SK, Yamada KM. 1995. Integrin function: molecular hierarchies of cytoskeletal and signaling molecules. J Cell Biol 131:791–805.

4. Haimovich B, Lipfert L, Brugge JS, Shattil SJ. 1993. Tyrosine phosphorylation and cytoskeletal reorganization in platelets are triggered by interaction of integrin receptors with their immobilized ligands. J Biol Chem 268:15868–15877.

5. Chen WT, Singer SJ. 1982. Immunoelectron microscopic studies of the sites of cell–substratum and cell–cell contacts in cultured fibroblasts. J Cell Biol 95:205–222.

6. Burridge K, Fath K, Kelly T, Nuckolls G, Turner C. Focal adhesions: transmembrane junctions between the extracellular matrix and the cytoskeleton. Annu Rev Cell Biol 4:487–525.

7. Turner CE,, Burridge K. 1991. Transmembrane molecular assemblies in cell–extracellular matrix interactions. Curr Opin Cell Biol 3:849–853.

8. Schaller MD, Parsons JT. 1994. Focal adhesion kinase and associated proteins. Curr Opin Cell Biol 6:705–710.

9. Shattil SJ, Haimovich B, Cunningham M, Lipfert L, Parsons JT, Ginsberg MH, Brugge JS. 1994. Tyrosine phosphorylation of pp125FAK in platelets requires coordinated signaling through integrin and agonist receptors. J Biol Chem 269:14738–14745.

10. Hynes RO. 1992. Integrins: versatility, modulation, and signaling in cell adhesion. Cell 69:11–25.

11. Hughes PE, Pfaff M. 1998. Integrin affinity modulation. Trends cell Biol 8:359–364.

12. Collo G, Starr L, Quaranta V. 1993. A new isoform of the laminin receptor integrin alpha 7 beta 1 is developmentally regulated in skeletal muscle. J Biol Chem 268:19019–19024.

13. Ashizawa N, Graf K, Do YS, Nunohiro T, Giachelli CM, Meehan WP, Tuan TL, Hsueh WA. 1996. Osteopontin is produced by rat cardiac fibroblasts and mediates A(II)-induced DNA synthesis and collagen gel contraction. J Clin Invest 98:2218–2227.

14. Kuppuswamy D, Kerr C, Narishige T, Kasi VS, Menick DR, Cooper G. 1997. Association of tyrosine-phosphorylated c-Src with the cytoskeleton of hypertrophying myocardium. J Biol Chem 272:4500–4508.

15. Terracio L, Rubin K, Gullberg D, Balog E, Carver W, Jyring R, Borg TK. 1991. Expression of collagen-binding integrins during cardiac development and hypertrophy. Circ Res 68:734–744.

16. Samuel JL, Barrieux A, Dufour S, Dubus I, Contard F, Koteliansky V, Farhadian F, Marotte F, Thiery JP, Rappaport L. 1991. Accumulation of fetal fibronectin mRNAs during the development of rat cardiac hypertrophy induced by pressure overload. J Clin Invest 88:1737–1746.

17. Villarreal FJ, Dillmann WH. 1992. Cardiac hypertrophy-induced changes in mRNA levels for TGF-beta 1, fibronectin, and collagen, Am J Physiol 262(6, Pt 2):H1861–H1866.

18. Clark EA, Brugge JS. 1995. Integrins and signal transduction pathways: the rod taken. Science 268:233–239.

19. Schlaepfer DD, Hunter T. 1998. Integrin signalling and tyrosine phosphorylation: just the FAKs? Trends Cell Biol 8:151–157.

20. Ross RS, Pham C, Shai SY, Goldhaber JI, Fenczik C, Glembotski CC, Ginsberg MH, Loftus JC. 1998. Beta1 integrins participate in the hypertrophic response of rat ventricular myocytes. Circ Res 82:1160–1172.

21. Schaller MD, Hildebrand JD, Shannon JD, Fox JW, Vines RR, Parsons JT. 1994. Autophosphorylation of the focal adhesion kinase, pp125FAK, directs SH2-dependent binding of pp60src. Mol Cell Biol 14:1680–1688.

22. Horwitz A, Duggan K, Buck C, Beckerle MC, Burridge K. 1986. Interaction of plasma membrane fibronectin receptor with talin: a transmembrane linkage. Nature 320:531–533.

23. Juliano RL, Haskill S. 1993. Signal transduction from the extracellular matrix. J Cell Biol 120:577–585.

24. Ingber DE. 1993. Cellular tensegrity: defining new rules of biological design that govern the cytoskeleton. J Cell Sci 104(Pt 3):613–627.

25. Schlaepfer DD, Hanks SK, Hunter T, van der Geer P. 1994. Integrin-mediated signal transduction linked to Ras pathway by GRB2 binding to focal adhesion kinase. Nature 372:786–791.

26. Fox JE, Lipfert L, Clark EA, Reynolds CC, Austin CD, Brugge JS. 1993. On the role of the platelet membrane skeleton in mediating signal transduction. Association of GP IIb–IIIa, pp60c-src, pp62c-yes, and the p21ras GTPase-activating protein with the membrane skeleton. J Biol Chem 268:25973–25984.

27. Weernink PA, Rijksen G. 1995. Activation and translocation of c-Src to the cytoskeleton by both platelet-derived growth factor and epidermal growth factor. J Biol Chem 270:2264–2267.

28. Shyy JY, Chien S. 1997. Role of integrins in cellular responses to mechanical stress and adhesion. Curr Opin Cell Biol 9:707–713.

29. Rabkin SW, Damen JE, Goutsouliak V, Krystal G. 1996. Cardiac hypertrophy in the Dahl rat is associated with increased tyrosine phosphorylation of several cytosolic proteins, including a 120 kDa protein. Am J Hypertens 9:230–236.

30. Melillo G, Lima JA, Judd RM, Goldschmidt-Clermont PJ, Silverman HS. 1996. Intrinsic myocyte dysfunction and tyrosine kinase pathway activation underlie the impaired wall thickening of adjacent regions during postinfarct left ventricular remodeling. Circulation 93:1447–1458.

31. Kudoh S, Komuro I, Hiroi Y, Zou Y, Harada K, Sugaya T, Takekoshi N, Murakami K, Kadowaki T, Yazaki Y. 1998. Mechanical stretch induces hypertrophic responses in cardiac myocytes of angiotensin II type 1a receptor knockout mice. J Biol Chem 273:24037–24043.

32. Ben-Ze'ev A, Robinson GS, Bucher NL, Farmer SR. 1988. Cell–cell and cell–matrix interactions differentially regulate the expression of hepatic and cytoskeletal genes in primary cultures of rat hepatocytes. Proc Natl Acad Sci USA 85:2161–2165.

33. Pawson T, Scott JD. 1997. Signaling through scaffold, anchoring, and adaptor proteins. Science 278:2075–2080.

34. Graf K, Do YS, Ashizawa N, Meehan WP, Giachelli CM, Marboe CC, Fleck E, Hsueh WA. 1997. Myocardial osteopontin expression is associated with left ventricular hypertrophy. Circulation 96: 3063–3071.

35. Boluyt MO, Bing OH. 1995. The lonely failing heart: a case for ECM genes. Cardiovasc Res 30: 836–840.

36. Howe A, Aplin AE, Alahari SK, Juliano RL. 1998. Integrin signaling and cell growth control. Curr Opin Cell Biol 10:220–231.

37. Schlaepfer DD, Jones KC, Hunter T. 1998. Multiple Grb2-mediated integrin-stimulated signaling pathways to ERK2/mitogen-activated protein kinase: summation of both c-Src- and focal adhesion kinase-initiated tyrosine phosphorylation events. Mol Cell Biol 18:2571–2585.

38. Lin TH, Aplin AE, Shen Y, Chen Q, Schaller M, Romer L, Aukhil I, Juliano RL. 1997. Integrin-mediated activation of MAP kinase is independent of FAK: evidence for dual integrin signaling pathways in fibroblasts. J Cell Biol 136:1385–1395.

39. Van Aelst L, D'Souza-Schorey C. 1997. Rho GTPases and signaling networks. Genes Dev 11:2295–2322.

40. Scatena M, Almeida M, Chaisson ML, Fausto N, Nicosia RF, Giachelli CM. 1998. NF-kappaB mediates alphavbeta3 integrin-induced endothelial cell survival. J Cell Biol 141:1083–1093.

41. Malik RK, Parsons JT. 1996. Integrin-dependent activation of the p70 ribosomal S6 kinase signaling pathway. J Biol Chem 271:29785–29791.

42. Khwaja A, Rodriguez-Viciana P, Wennstrom S, Warne PH, Downward J. 1997. Matrix adhesion and Ras transformation both activate a phosphoinositide 3-OH kinase and protein kinase B/Akt cellular survival pathway. EMBO J 16:2783–2793.

43. Jefferies HB, Reinhard C, Kozma SC, Thomas G. 1994. Rapamycin selectively represses translation of the "polypyrimidine tract" mRNA family. Proc Natl Acad Sci USA 91:4441–4445.

44. Laser M, Kasi VS, Hamawaki M, Cooper G 4th, Kerr CM, Kuppuswamy D. 1998. Differential activation of p70 and p85 S6 kinase isoforms during cardiac hypertrophy in the adult mammal. J Biol Chem 273:24610–24619.

45. Ferrari S, Pearson RB, Siegmann M, Kozma SC, Thomas G. 1993. The immunosuppressant rapamycin induces inactivation of p70s6k through dephosphorylation of a novel set of sites. J Biol Chem 268:16091–16094.

46. Homma T, Akai Y, Burns KD, Harris RC. 1992. Activation of S6 kinase by repeated cycles of stretching and relaxation in rat glomerular mesangial cells. Evidence for involvement of protein kinase C. J Biol Chem 267:23129–23135.

47. Monfar M, Lemon KP, Grammer TC, Cheatham L, Chung J, Vlahos CJ, Blenis J. 1995. Activation of pp70/85 S6 kinases in interleukin-2-responsive lymphoid cells is mediated by phosphatidylinositol 3-kinase and inhibited by cyclic AMP. Mol Cell Biol 15:326–337.

48. Morrison DK. 1995. Mechanisms regulating Raf-1 activity in signal transduction pathways. Mol Reprod Dev 42:507–514.

49. Lenormand P, McMahon M, Pouyssegur J. 1996. Oncogenic Raf-1 activates p70 S6 kinase via a mitogen-activated protein kinase-independent pathway. J Biol Chem 271:15762–15768.

50. Stokoe D, McCormick F. 1997. Activation of c-Raf-1 by Ras and Src through different mechanisms: activation in vivo and in vitro. EMBO J 16:2384–2396.

51. de Groot RP, Ballou LM, Sassone-Corsi P. 1994. Positive regulation of the cAMP-responsive activator CREM by the p70 S6 kinase: an alternative route to mitogen-induced gene expression. Cell 79:81–91.

52. Rozich JD, Barnes MA, Schmid PG, Zile MR, McDermott PJ, Cooper G. 1995. Load effects on gene expression during cardiac hypertrophy. J Mol Cell Cardiol 27:485–499.
53. Nahman NS Jr, Rothe KL, Falkenhain ME, Frazer KM, Dacio LE, Madia JD, Leonhart KL, Kronenberger JC, Stauch DA. 1996. Angiotensin II induction of fibronectin biosynthesis in cultured human mesangial cells: association with CREB transcription factor activation. J Lab Clin Med 127:599–611.
54. Eschenhagen T, Fink C, Remmers U, Scholz H, Wattchow J, Weil J, Zimmermann W, Dohmen HH, Schafter H, Bishopric N, Wakatsuki T, Elson EL. 1997. Three-dimensional reconstitution of embryonic cardiomyocytes in a collagen matrix: a new heart muscle model system. FASEB J 11:683–694.
55. VanWinkle WB, Snuggs MB, Buja LM. 1996. Cardiogel: a biosynthetic extracellular matrix for cardiomyocyte culture. In Vitro Cell Dev Biol Anim 32:478–485.
56. Nagai T, Laser M, Baicu CF, Zile MR, Cooper G IV, Kuppuswamy D. In press. β_3-integrin-mediated focal adhesion complex formation: studies of adult cardiocytes embedded in a three-dimensional collagen matrix. Am J Cardiol.
57. Belkin AM, Retta SF, Pletjushkina OY, Balzac F, Silengo L, Fassler R, Koteliansky VE, Burridge K, Tarone G. 1997. Muscle beta1D integrin reinforces the cytoskeleton–matrix link: modulation of integrin adhesive function by alternative splicing. J Cell Biol 139:1583–1595.
58. Pasqualini R, Koivunen E, Ruoslahti E. 1996. Peptides in cell adhesion: powerful tools for the study of integrin-ligand interactions. Braz J Med Biol Res 29:1151–1158.
59. Daniel JM, Reynolds AB. 1997. Tyrosine phosphorylation and cadherin/catenin function. Bioessays 19:883–891.
60. Miyamoto S, Teramoto H, Coso OA, Gutkind JS, Burbelo PD, Akiyama SK, Yamada KM. 1995. Integrin function: molecular hierarchies of cytoskeletal and signaling molecules. J Cell Biol 131:791–805.
61. Ivester CT, Tuxworth WJ, Cooper G IV, McDermott PJ. 1995. Contraction accelerates myosin heavy chain synthesis rates in adult cardiocytes by an increase in the translational initiation. J Biol Chem 270:21950–21957.
62. Wada H, Zile MR, Ivester G, Cooper G, McDermott PJ. 1996. Comparative effects of contraction and angiotensin II on growth of adult feline cardiocytes in primary culture. Am J Physiol 271: H29–H37.
63. Kolanus W, Seed B. 1997. Integrins and inside-out signal transduction: converging signals from PKC and PIP3. Curr Opin Cell Biol 9:725–731.

N. Takeda, M. Nagano and N.S. Dhalla
(eds). The Hypertrophied Heart. Copyright
© 2000. pp. 165–178. Kluwer Academic
Publishers. Boston. All rights reserved.

ROLE OF G PROTEINS IN HYPERTENSION AND HYPERTROPHY

MADHU B. ANAND-SRIVASTAVA and FRANCESCO DI FUSCO

*Department of Physiology, and Groupe de recherche sur le système nerveux autonome, Faculty of Medicine,
University of Montreal Succ. Centre-ville, Montreal, Quebec, Canada H3C 3J7*

Summary. We have recently shown an enhanced expression of $Gi\alpha$-2 and $Gi\alpha$-3 protein and mRNA levels in heart and aorta from spontaneously hypertensive rats (SHRs) and DOCA-salt hypertensive rats with established hypertrophy, whereas the levels of $Gs\alpha$ were unaltered in SHRs and decreased in DOCA-salt hypertensive rats. The present studies were undertaken to investigate if the enhanced expression of Gi and decreased expression of Gs observed in DOCA-salt hypertensive rats is due to hypertension or hypertrophy. $N\omega$-nitro-L-arginine methyl ester (L-NAME)-treated rats and aortocaval Fistula (AV shunt) rats were used for these studies. L-NAME-treated rats showed an enhanced blood pressure and no hypertrophy, whereas AV shunt rats did not have increased blood pressure but exhibited cardiac hypertrophy. The stimulatory effects of $GTP\gamma S$, isoproterenol, NaF, and forskolin on adenylyl cyclase were diminished in L-NAME-treated and AV shunt rats, whereas the inhibitory effect of low concentrations of guanosine $5'$-[γ-thio]triphosphate ($GTP\gamma S$) on forskolin-stimulated enzyme activity was significantly enhanced in L-NAME and not in AV shunt rats. In addition, the inhibitions exerted by inhibitory hormones on adenylyl cyclase were abolished in L-NAME hypertensive rats and were unaltered in AV shunt rats. The levels of $Gi\alpha$-2 and $Gi\alpha$-3 proteins and mRNA as determined by immunoblotting and Northern blotting were significantly augmented in L-NAME-treated rats and not in AV shunt rats; however, the levels of $Gs\alpha$ were decreased in AV shunt rats and not in L-NAME treated rats. These results suggest that the enhanced expression of $Gi\alpha$ proteins may be attributed to hypertension, decreased expression of $Gs\alpha$ may be associated with hypertrophy, and the changes in Gi and Gs may be responsible for the diminished hormonal stimulation of adenylyl cyclase in hypertension and hypertrophy, respectively.

INTRODUCTION

Adenylyl cyclase/cAMP signal transduction system has been implicated in the regulation of various physiological functions such as vascular tone and reactivity, cardiac functions, platelet functions, etc. [1]. Adenylyl cyclase system consists of three distinct components: receptor, catalytic subunit, and guanine nucleotide regulatory proteins (G proteins). The stimulatory and inhibitory responses of hormones on adenylyl cyclase are mediated via the stimulatory (Gs) and inhibitory (Gi) proteins, respectively [2–4]. G proteins are heterotrimeric proteins composed of α-, β-, and γ-subunits, and the specificity of G proteins is attributed to the α-subunit [3]. Molecular cloning has revealed four different isoforms of Gsα resulting from the differential splicing of one gene [5–7] and three distinct isoforms of Giα: Giα-1, Giα-2, and Giα-3, encoded by three different genes [8–10]. All three forms of Giα have been shown to be implicated in adenylyl cyclase inhibition [11] and the activation of ACh-K^+ channels [12]. Five different β-subunits of 35–36 KDa and seven γ-subunits of 8–10 KDa have been identified by molecular cloning [13,14]. The G$\beta\gamma$ subunit has been shown to regulate various effectors, including adenylyl cyclase, phospholipase Cβ, and K^+ channels [13,15,16]. Of the eight types of adenylyl cyclase that have been cloned and expressed [17], only two types, namely, types V and VI, have been identified in the heart, aorta, and brain [18,19]. Adenylyl cyclase types II and IV are activated by G$\beta\gamma$ in the presence of Gsα; type I is inhibited by G$\beta\gamma$; and types III, V, and VI do not appear to be directly regulated by G$\beta\gamma$ [20,21].

Alterations in G-protein levels and adenylyl cyclase activity and its responsiveness to various hormones have been documented in cardiovascular tissues from genetic (spontaneously hypertensive rats, SHRs) and various experimental models of hypertension [22–27]. We have recently shown an increased expression of Giα-2 and Giα-3 at protein and mRNA levels and an altered hormonal inhibition and stimulation of adenylyl cyclase in heart and aorta from SHR as well as in DOCA-salt hypertensive rats [23,25–28], whereas an unaltered expression of Giα and Gsα proteins has also been reported in hearts from SHR and other models of hypertension [29,30]. However, due to the expression of cardiac hypertrophy with hypertension, it is not known whether these changes are due to the expressed hypertrophy or hypertension. To exclude one conflicting parameter from the other, we employed an Nω-nitro-L-arginine methyl ester (L-NAME) rat model with sustained, established arterial hypertension without cardiac hypertrophy [31] and AV shunt (volume overload) rats that exhibit cardiac hypertrophy without hypertension [32], and we have determined the expression of G proteins and adenylyl cyclase activity in hearts from these rats.

MATERIALS AND METHODS

Animals

Male Sprague-Dawley rats (200–250 g) purchased from Charles-River Canada (St. Constant, Quebec, Canada) were used in the present studies. Hypertension in these rats was induced by the oral administration of L-NAME (100 mg/kg/day) in their drinking tap water for a period of 4 weeks, whereas the control group received plain tap water only. The arterial blood pressure (mmHg), was measured after 4 weeks of treatment by the tail-cuff method without anesthesia. After 4 weeks of treatment, the rats were sacrificed by decapitation, and the hearts were removed for adenylyl cyclase activity determination and mRNA and protein quantification.

Preparation of heart particulate fraction

Heart particulate fraction was prepared as described previously [33]. Frozen hearts were quickly pulverized to a fine powder using mortar and pestle cooled in liquid N_2. The powder was stored at $-80°C$ until assayed. The powder was homogenized (12 strokes) in a Teflon glass homogenizer, in a buffer containing 10 mM Tris-HCl, 1 mM EDTA (pH 7.5). The homogenate was centrifuged at $1000 \times g$ for 10 minutes. The supernatant fraction was discarded and the pellet was finally resuspended and homogenized in a buffer containing 10 mM Tris HCl and 1 mM EDTA, pH 7.5, and used for adenylyl cyclase activity determination and immunoblotting studies.

Cholera-toxin (CT) treatment of heart particulate fraction

Heart particulate fraction was treated with CT as described earlier [23,24]. CT (500 μg/mL) was preactivated for 20 minutes at 37°C in a mixture containing 20 mmol/L dithiothreitol, 1 μg/mL bovine serum albumin, and 25 mmol/L KH_2PO_4 (pH 8.0). To study the effect of CT on adenylyl cyclase activity, heart particulate fraction was pretreated with and without CT for 30 minutes at 30°C in a reaction mixture containing 250 mM KH_2PO_4 (pH 6.8), 1 mM $MgCl_2$, 0.5 mM EDTA (pH 8.0), 5 mM ATP, 15 mM thymidine, 0.15 mM GTP, 20 mM dithiothreitol, and 1 mM NAD. The particulate fractions were washed twice with buffer containing 10 mM Tris and 1 mM EDTA (pH 7.5) and finally suspended in the same buffer for adenylyl cyclase activity determination.

Adenylyl cyclase activity determination

Adenylyl cyclase activity was determined by measuring (^{32}P)-cAMP formation from $(\alpha\text{-}^{32}P)$ATP, as described previously [23,24]. The assay medium containing 50 mM glycylglycine, pH 7.5, 0.5 mM MgATP, $(\alpha\text{-}^{32}P)$ATP $(1\text{--}1.5 \times 10^6$ CPM), 5 mM $MgCl_2$, 100 mM NaCl, 0.5 mM cAMP, 1 mM 3-isobutyl-1-methylxanthine (IBMX), 0.1 mM EGTA, 10 μM guanosine 5′ (γ-thio)triphosphate (or otherwise as indicated), and an ATP regenerating system consisting of 2 mM phosphocreatine, 0.1 mg of creatine kinase/mL, and 0.1 mg of myokinase/mL in a final volume of 200 μL. Incubations were initiated by addition of the heart particulate fraction (50–100 μg) to the reaction mixture, which had been thermally preequilibrated for 2 minutes at 37°C. The reactions conducted in triplicate for 10 minutes at 37°C were terminated by the addition of 0.6 mL of 120 mM zinc acetate. cAMP was purified by coprecipitation of other nucleotides with $ZnCO_3$, by addition of 0.5 mL of 144 mM Na_2CO_3, and by subsequent chromatography that used the double column system, as described by Salomon et al. [34]. Under the assay conditions used, adenylyl cyclase activity was linear with respect to protein concentration and time of incubation.

Protein was determined essentially as described by Lowry et al. [35], with crystalline bovine serum albumin (BSA) as standard.

Immunoblotting

Immunoblotting of G proteins was performed as described previously [23]. After SDS-PAGE, the separated proteins were electrophoretically transferred to a nitro-cellulose sheet (Schleicher and Schuell) with a semidry transblot apparatus (Bio-Rad) at 15V for 45 minutes. After transfer, the membranes were washed twice in phosphate-buffered saline (PBS) and were incubated in PBS containing 3% skim milk at room temperature for 2 hours. The blots were then incubated with anti-bodies against G proteins in PBS containing 1.5% skim milk and 0.1% Tween-20 at room temperature overnight. The antigen–antibody complexes were detected by incubating the blots with goat anti-rabbit IgG (Bio-Rad) conjugated with horse-radish peroxidase for 2 hours at room temperature. The blots were then washed three times with PBS before reaction with enhanced-chemiluminescence (ECL) Western-blotting detection reagents (Amersham).

Northern analysis

Total RNA was isolated by the guanidinium thiocyanate-phenol-chloroform method described by Chomczynski et al. [36]. cDNA inserts encoding for $Gi\alpha$-2, $Gi\alpha$-3, $Gs\alpha$, and catalytic subunit V of adenylyl cyclase were radiolabeled with $(\alpha$-^{32}P)dCTP by random priming essentially described by Feinberg et al. [37].

DMSO/glyoxal-treated total RNA was resolved on 1% agarose gels and trans-ferred to nylon membrane as described by Sambrook et al. [38]. Filters, after pre-hybridization at 65°C for 6 hours in hybridization solution [600mM NaCl, 8mM EDTA, 120mM Tris, pH 7.4) containing 0.1% sodium pyrophosphate, 0.2% SDS and heparin (500U/mL), were hybridized overnight in hybridization solution con-taining 10% dextran sulfate (w:v) and cDNA probe (1–3×10^6 ct/min/mL). Filters were then rinsed at 65°C for 2×30 minutes in 300mM NaCl, 4mM EDTA, 60mM Tris, pH 7.4, and 0.1% SDS. Autoradiography was performed with X-ray films at −70°C. In order to assess the possibility of any variations in the amounts of total RNA in individual samples applied to the gel, each filter was hybridized with the ^{32}P end-labeled oligonucleotide, which recognizes a highly conserved region of 28S ribosomal RNA. The blots that had been probed with the G-protein cDNA were dehybridized by washing for 1 hour at 65°C in 50% formamide, 300mM NaCl, 4mM EDTA, and 60mM Tris, pH 7.4, and rehybridized overnight at room temperature with the oligonucleotide. Quantitative analysis of the hybridization of probes bound was performed by densitometric scanning of the autoradiographic film employing the enhanced laser densitometer, LKB Utroscan XL and quantified using the gel scan XL evaluation software (v. 2.1) from Pharmacia (PQ, Canada).

Data analysis

Results are expressed as mean ± S.E.M. Comparisons between groups (control and L-NAME-treated rats) were made with Student's t-test for unpaired samples. Results were considered significant at a value of $p < 0.05$.

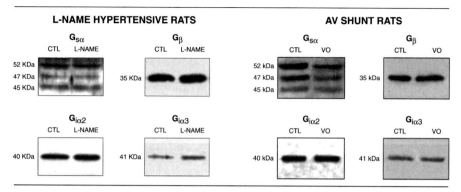

Figure 1. Quantification of G proteins by immunoblotting in hearts from control, L-NAME-hypertensive, and AV shunt rats. The membrane proteins (50 µg) from control, L-NAME-hypertensive, and AV shunt rats were separated by sodium dodecyl sulphate-polyacrylamide gel electrophoresis and transferred to nitrocellulose, which was then immunoblotted using antibody AS/7 for Giα-1 and Giα-2, antibody EC/2 for Giα-3, antibody RM/1 for Gsα, and antibody SW/1 for Gβ, as described in Materials and Methods. The autoradiogram is representative of three separate experiments. The detection of different G proteins was performed by using chemiluminescence (ECL) Western blotting detection reagents from Amersham.

RESULTS

The arterial systolic blood pressure was significantly increased in hypertensive rats (control 121.0 ± 6.4 mmHg, L-NAME hypertensive rats 190.0 ± 9.2 mmHg) but not in AV shunt rats (control 110.2 ± 8.3 mmHg AV shunt rats 107.7 ± 4.6 mmHg) whereas heart/body weight ratio was increased in AV shunt rats as compared to control rats (3.51 ± 0.10 versus 2.97 ± 0.08 mg/g) but not in L-NAME hypertensive rats (2.80 ± 0.36 versus 2.71 ± 0.26 mg/g).

G-protein levels

To investigate if the increased levels of Giα proteins observed in SHR and DOCA salt hypertensive rats [23,25] were attributed to hypertension and not to hypertrophy, the levels of Gi proteins were determined in hearts from L-NAME hypertensive rats and AV shunt rats by immunoblotting techniques using specific antibodies AS/7 against Giα-1 and Giα-2, and antibodies EC/2 against Giα-3. The results depicted in figure 1 show that the AS/7 and EC/2 antibodies recognized a single protein of M_r 40 kDa referred to as Giα-2 (Giα-1 has been shown to be absent in heart [39]) and 41 kDa referred to as Giα-3, respectively, in control, hypertensive, and AV shunt rats; however, the amounts of immunodetectable Giα-2 and Giα-3 protein were increased in hypertensive rats by about 30% and 200% ($n = 4$), respectively, and were unaltered in AV shunt rats as compared to control rats, as determined by densitometric scanning. In addition, the levels of Gsα and Gβ were also determined by using antibodies RM/1 and SW/1 against Gsα and Gβ (common), respectively. The RM/1 antibody recognized three isoforms of Gsα—Gsα$_{45}$, Gsα$_{47}$, and Gsα$_{52}$—in hearts from control, L-NAME hypertensive rats, and AV shunt rats;

however, the amount of immunodetectable $Gs\alpha_{45}$ and $Gs\alpha_{52}$ were significantly decreased in AV shunt rats but were not altered in L–NAME hypertensive rats. In addition, SW/1 antibody detected a single band of 35 kDa (Gβ) in all the groups; however, no differences in the amounts of immunodetectable Gβ protein were detected in L–NAME hypertensive and AV shunt rats as compared to control rats.

We extended our studies further to investigate if mRNA levels of G proteins change concomitantly with protein levels and determined the mRNA content of G proteins from hearts from control, L–NAME-induced hypertensive rats, and AV shunt rats using cDNA probes encoding for Giα-2, Giα-3, and Gsα. The results depicted in figure 2 shows that the Giα-2 and Giα-3 probes detected a message of 2.3 and 3.5 kilobases, respectively, in hearts from control, L–NAME hypertensive, and AV shunt rats; however, the Giα-2 and Giα-3 mRNA levels were increased by $31.5 \pm 1.2\%$ ($n = 4$) and $211.5 \pm 10.5\%$ ($n = 4$), respectively, in hearts from L–NAME hypertensive rats and not in AV shunt rats as compared to control rats, as determined by densitometric scanning. On the other hand, the cDNA probe encoding Gsα detected a message of 1.8 kilobases in control, L–NAME-induced hypertensive, and AV shunt rats; however, no difference in Gsα mRNA levels was detected between the groups. The alterations in Giα-2 and Giα-3 mRNA in L–NAME hypertensive hearts as compared to control rats may not be attributed to the variation in the amounts of total RNA applied to the gels, because hybridization with 32-mer oligonucleotide that recognizes a highly conserved region of 28S rRNA showed a similar amount of 28S rRNA loaded from control and L–NAME hypertensive rats onto the gels (data not shown).

Gi protein functions

In order to investigate the relationship between the levels and functions of G proteins, the effect of low concentrations of GTPγS on FSK-stimulated adenylyl cyclase activity was examined in hearts from L–NAME and AV shunt rats, and the results are shown in figure 3. GTPγS inhibited FSK-stimulated adenylyl cyclase activity in a concentration-dependent manner in L–NAME and in AV shunt rats and their respective control rats; however, the inhibition of FSK-stimulated adenylyl cyclase by GTPγS was significantly enhanced in L–NAME hypertensive rats and not in AV shunt rats as compared to their control rats. For example, GTPγS at 1 nM inhibited FSK-stimulated enzyme activity by about 20% in control rats and about 50% in L–NAME hypertensive rats.

Since Gi proteins couple the inhibitory hormone receptors to adenylyl cyclase and mediate the inhibitory responses of hormones on adenylyl cyclase activity, it was of interest to determine whether enhanced expression and functions of Giα were also associated with enhanced inhibition of adenylyl cyclase by inhibitory hormones. To explore this, the effects of inhibitory hormones on adenylyl cyclase activity was examined in hearts from control, L–NAME-induced hypertensive, and AV shunts rats. The inhibitory effects of inhibitory hormones on adenylyl cyclase were completely attenuated in L–NAME hypertensive rats and were unaltered in hearts from AV shunt rats (data not shown).

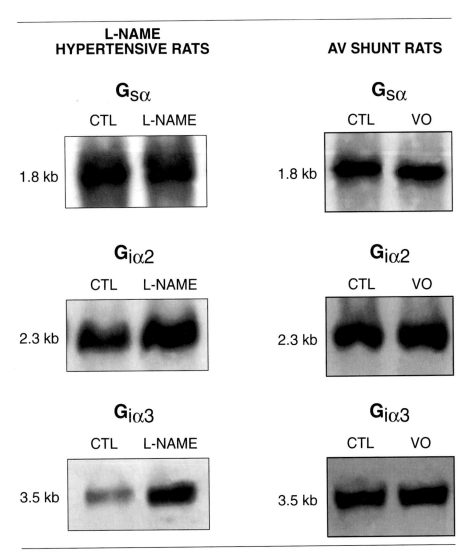

Figure 2. mRNA expression of G proteins by Northern blot in hearts from control, L-NAME-hypertensive and AV shunt rats. Total RNA (10 μg) extracted from heart from control, L-NAME-hypertensive, and AV shunt rats was separated on 1% agarose and transferred to nylon membranes, which were then hybridized with full-length cDNA probe encoding Gsα, Giα-2, and Giα-3 as described in Materials and Methods. The autoradiogram is representative of three to four separate experiments.

Gs protein functions

To corroborate our results of Gsα levels with Gsα-mediated functions, the effect of some hormones were examined on adenylyl cyclase activity from control, L-NAME hypertensive, and AV shunt rats. Figure 4 shows that isoproterenol,

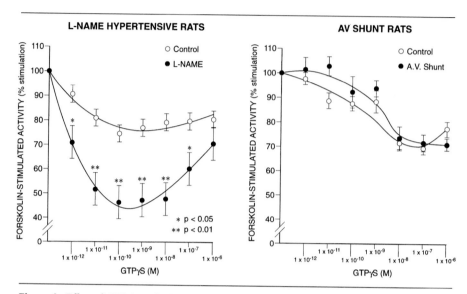

Figure 3. Effect of GTPγS on forskolin-stimulated adenylyl cyclase activity in heart membranes from control, L-NAME hypertensive, and AV shunt rats. Adenylyl cyclase activity was determined in the absence (basal) or presence of 100 μM FSK alone or in the presence of increasing concentration of GTPγS in control (O), L-NAME hypertensive, and AV shunt rats (●) as described in Material and Methods. Basal adenylyl cyclase activities in control and L-NAME hypertensive rats in the absence of GTPγS were 40.0 ± 3.1 and 46.8 ± 5.2 pmol cAMP (mg protein/10 min), respectively, and in control and AV shunt rats were 49.9 ± 2.7 and 47.8 ± 3.4 pmol cAMP (mg protein/10 min), respectively. Values are means ± SEM of three separate experiments. ⋆, $p < 0.05$.

N-Ethylcarboxamide adenosine (NECA), and glucagon stimulated adenylyl cyclase activity to various degrees in heart membranes from control and L-NAME hypertensive groups; however, the extent of stimulation of adenylyl cyclase was significantly diminished in L-NAME hypertensive rats as compared to control rats. Similarly, isoproterenol and glucagon stimulated adenylyl cyclase activity to various extent in control and AV shunt rats; however, isoproterenol stimulation, but not glucagon-mediated stimulation, was significantly diminished in AV shunt rats. In addition, GTPγS stimulated adenylyl cyclase activity in L-NAME hypertensive and AV shunt rats and their respective control rats in a concentration–dependent manner; however, the extent of stimulation was significantly decreased in both L-NAME hypertensive and AV shunt rats as compared to their respective control rats (figure 5).

FSK and NaF-stimulated adenylyl cyclase activity

Forskolin stimulates adenylyl cyclase activity by interacting directly with the catalytic subunit of adenylyl cyclase. In order to investigate whether the catalytic subunit of adenylyl cyclase is impaired in L-NAME hypertensive and AV shunt rats, the effect of forskolin was investigated in hearts from both groups of rats. Figure 6

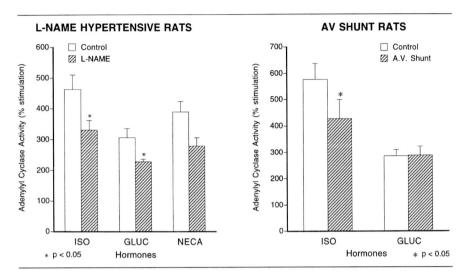

Figure 4. Effect of stimulatory hormones on adenylyl cyclase activity in heart membranes from control, L-NAME hypertensive, and AV shunt rats. Adenylyl cyclase activity in heart membranes from control (□), L-NAME hypertensive, and AV shun rats (▨) was determined in the presence of 10 μM GTP alone (basal) or in combination with 50 μM isoproterenol (ISO), 1 μM glucagon (GLU), and 10 μM 5′-N-Ethylcarboxamideadenosine (NECA) as described in Materials and Methods. Basal adenylyl cyclase activities in control and L-NAME hypertensive rats in the presence of 10 μM GTP were 66.6 ± 1.4 and 68.3 ± 2.8 pmol cAMP (mg protein/10 min), respectively, and in control and AV shunt rats were 58.2 ± 1.3 and 52.7 ± 2.1 pmol cAMP (mg protein/10 min), respectively. Values are means ± SEM of three separate experiments. $p < 0.05$.

shows that FSK stimulated adenylyl cyclase activity to various extents in both groups; however, the percent stimulations over basal were significantly attenuated in L-NAME hypertensive rats but not in AV shunt rats as compared to their respective control rats. Similarly, NaF, which stimulates adenylyl cyclase by a receptor-independent mechanism but requires Gs protein, stimulated adenylyl cyclase activity to a lower extent in L-NAME hypertensive rats but not in AV shunt rats as compared to control rats (figure 6).

DISCUSSION

The present studies demonstrate that hearts from L-NAME hypertensive rats that exhibit arterial hypertension exhibited an increased expression of Gi proteins as compared to control rats, whereas the levels of Gi were unaltered in hearts from AV shunt rats expresing only cardiac hypertrophy. In addition, the levels of Giα-2 and Giα-3 mRNA were also enhanced in hearts from L-NAME hypertensive rats as compared to control rats. These data suggest that the increased expression of Giα protein is attributed to hypertension and not to hypertrophy. This is further substantiated by our earlier studies showing that hearts from spontaneously hypertensive rats exhibited increased levels of Giα-2 and Giα-3 at early ages when there

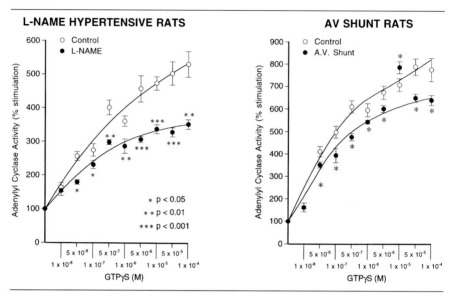

Figure 5. Effect of GTPγS on adenylyl cyclase activity in hearts from control, L-NAME hypertensive and AV shunt rats. Adenylyl cyclase activity was determined in the presence and absence of increasing concentrations of GTPγS in control (O), L-NAME hypertensive, and AV shunt rats (●) as described in Materials and Methods. Basal adenylyl cyclase activities in control and L-NAME hypertensive rats were 40.1 ± 3.9 and 46.6 ± 6.6 pmol cAMP (mg protein/10 min), respectively, and in control and AV shunt rats were 60.6 ± 1.5 and 58.4 ± 0.62 pmol cAMP (mg protein/10 min), Values are means ± SEM of three separate experiments. ★, $p < 0.05$; ★★, $p < 0.01$; ★★★, $p < 0.001$.

were no signs of hypertrophy [33]. However, on the other hand, the levels of Gsα proteins as well as Gsα mRNA levels were unaltered in L-NAME hypertensive rats but were significnatly decreased in AV shunt rats. These results are in agreement with the studies reported earlier in SHR, that did not exhibit hypertrophy [33]. However, the hearts from DOCA-salt hypertensive rats [25,26] and 1K1C hypertensive rats [40] with established hypertrophy exhibited decreased levels of Gsα protein and Gsα mRNA. Our results are in agreement with the studies reported in pigs with volume-overload hypertrophy, where the levels of Gsα were shown to be decreased in hearts and the levels of pertussis toxin substrates were unaltered [41]. When these findings are taken together, it can be suggested that Gsα may not be implicated in the regulation of blood pressure and may be associated with hypertrophy.

The unaltered expression of Giα protein in AV shunt rats and an increased expression of Giα-2 and Giα-3 in L-NAME hypertensive rats were correlated with Giα functions, as was shown by unaltered inhibition of adenylyl cyclase by oxotremorine and FSK-stimulated adenylyl cyclase activity by GTPγS in AV shunt rats and increased inhibition of FSK-stimulated adenylyl cyclase activity by GTPγS in L-NAME hypertensive rats respectively as compared to control rats. These results are

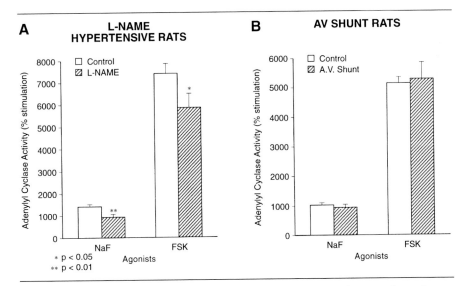

Figure 6. Effect of NaF and forskolin (FSK) on adenylyl cyclase activity in heart membranes from control, L-NAME hypertensive, and AV shunt rats. Adenylyl cyclase activity was determined in the absence (basal) or presence of 10 mM NaF or 50 μM FSK in the absence of GTP or GTPγS in heart membranes from control (□), L-NAME hypertensive, and AV shunt rats (▨) as described in Materials and Methods. Basal adenylyl cyclase activities in control and L-NAME hypertensive rats were 40.0 ± 3.1 and 40.8 ± 5.2 pmol cAMP (mg protein/10 min), respectively, and in control and AV shunt rats were 49.9 ± 2.7 and 47.8 ± 3.5 pmol cAMP (mg protein/10 min), respectively. Values are means ± SEM of three separate experiments. *, $p < 0.05$; **, $p < 0.01$.

in agreement with the previous studies reported in SHRs and other models of hypertension [23,25–28]. However, a complete attenuation of adenylyl cyclase inhibition by inhibitory hormones in hearts from L-NAME hypertensive rats is in contrast with other studies conducted in genetic and DOCA-salt hypertensive rats, where a correlation between the enhanced levels of Gi protein and receptor-dependent functions of Gi have been reported [23,25,26]. These apparent discrepencies may be attributed to the differences in the hypertensive rat model used in the present studies. It may be possible that the hormone receptors are downregulated by increased activity of the renin–angiotensin system in this model of hypertension [42]. In this regard, an increased expression of Giα proteins and attenuation of C-ANP-$_{4-23}$ and AII-mediated inhibitions of adenylyl cyclase by AII treatment in A10 smooth muscle cells has recently been shown [43].

On the other hand, the decreased stimulations exerted by NECA, glucagon, isoproterenol, and GTPγS in L-NAME hypertensive rats and isoproterenol and GTPγS in AV shunt rats as compared to control rats may be attributed to downregulation of hormone receptors [44] or decreased levels of Gsα. In this regard, the levels of plasma catecholamines have been shown to be enhanced by L-NAME [45], which may be responsible for the desensitization of β-adrenergic receptors in L-NAME hypertensive rats. However, Laflamme et al. [46] did not observe any changes in density and affinity of cardiac β-adrenergic receptors in L–NAME-induced hypertensive rats as compared to sham-operated control rats. Since no alterations in Gsα levels were observed in L–NAME hypertensive rats, it appears that Gsα may not be responsible for the observed attenuated responsiveness of adenylyl cyclase to stimulatory hormones. On the other hand, decreased levels of Giα in AV shunt rats may be responsible for the decreased sensitivity of adenylyl cyclase to GTPγS as well as to NECA stimulation. The modulation of Gsα functions by Giα has been reported by several investigators [47,48]. An increased expression of Giα-2 and Giα-3 has been shown to be associated with attenuated responsiveness of adenylyl cyclase to stimulatory hormones [23,26], whereas a decreased expression of Giα-2 resulted in the augmentation of responsiveness of adenylyl cyclase to stimulatory hormones [24]. Taken together, it may be possible that the enhanced levels of Giα-2 and Giα-3 in hearts from L–NAME hypertensive rats and not from AV shunt rats may be responsible for the diminished sensitivity of adenylyl cyclase to hormonal stimulations.

The decreased stimulation of adenylyl cyclase by FSK in L–NAME hypertensive rats as compared to control rats is also in accordance with the previous results reported in other models of hypertension [23,26], which may be due to the defective catalytic subunit per se or to the overexpression of Giα or both. On the other hand, because of the fact that FSK stimulated adenylyl cyclase activity to a similar extent in hearts from AV shunt rats and control rats, it appears that the catalytic subunit of adenylyl cyclase may not be impaired in AV shunt rats.

In conclusion, we have demonstrated that L–NAME-induced hypertensive rats that do not have cardiac hypertrophy exhibit increased expression of Giα-2 and Giα-3 genes and translated proteins, whereas the levels and functions of Gsα are not altered. On the other hand, AV shunt rats that exhibit cardiac hypertrophy show decreased expression of Gsα proteins and Gsα-mediated functions without any changes in the expression of Gi proteins. It may thus be suggested that the increased expression of Giα proteins reported in various models of hypertension may be due to hypertension per se and not to expressed hypertrophy, whereas decreased expression of Gsα is associated with hypertrophy and not with hypertension.

ACKNOWLEDGMENTS

We are grateful to Drs. Randall Reed and Hiroshi Itoh for their kind gift of cDNAs of G proteins. We would like to thank Christiane Laurier for her valuable secretarial help. This work was supported by grants from Quebec Heart Foundation and the Medical Research Council of Canada. M.B.A-S was a recipient of the Medical Research Council Scientist Award from the Medical Research Council of Canada, during the course of these studies.

REFERENCES

1. Triner L, Vullienoz Y, Verosky H, Habif DV, Nahas VV. 1992. Adenylyl cyclase phosphodiesterase system in arterial smooth muscle. Life Sci 11:817–824.
2. Gilman AG. 1984. G proteins and dual control of adenylyl cyclase. Cell 36:577–579.

3. Stryer L, Bourne HR. 1986. G-proteins: a family of signal transducers. Annu Rev Cell Biol 2:391–419.
4. Spiegel AM. Signal transduction by guanine nucleotide binding proteins. 1987. Mol Cell Endocrinol 49:1–6.
5. Murakami T, Yasuda H. 1988. Rat heart cell membranes contain three substrate for cholera toxin-catalyzed ADP-ribosylation and a single substrate for pertussis toxin-catalyzed ADP-ribosylation. Biochem Biophys Res Commun 138:1355–1361.
6. Robishaw JD, Smigel MD, Gilman AG. 1986. Molecular basis for two forms of the G protein that stimulates adenylate cyclase. J Biol Chem 261:9587–9590.
7. Bray P, Carter A, Simons C, Guo V, Puckett C, Hamholz J, Spiege A, Nirenberg M. 1986. Human cDNA clones for four species of G alpha's signal transduct protein. Proc Natl Acad Sci USA 83:8893–8897.
8. Itoh H, Lozasa T, Nagata S, Nakamura S, Katada T, Ui M, Iwai S, Ohtsuka E, Kawasaki H, Suzuki K. 1986. Molecular cloning and sequence determination of cDNA s for alpha of the guanine nucleotide-binding proteins Gs, Gi and Go from rat brain. Proc Natl Acad Sci USA 83:37776–37786.
9. Jones DT, Reed RR. 1987. Molecular cloning of five GTP-binding protein cDNA species from rat olfactory neuroepithelium. J Biol Chem 262:14241–14249.
10. Itoh H, Toyama RI, Kozasa TI, Tsukamoto TI, Matsuoka M, Kazirory. 1988. Presence of three distinct molecular species of G protein: a subunit structure of rat cDNA and human genomic DNAs. J Biol Chem 263:6656–6664.
11. Wong YH, Conklin BB, Bourne HR. 1992. Gz-mediated hormonal inhibition of cyclic AMP accumulation. Science 255:339–342.
12. Brown AM, Birnbaumer L. 1988. Direct G protein gating of ion channels. Am J Physiol 254:H401–H410.
13. Simon MI, Strathmannn MP, Gautam N. 1991. Diversity of G proteins in signal transduction. Science 252:802–808.
14. Cali JJ, Balcueva EA, Rybalkin I, Robishaw JD. 1992. Selective tissue distribution of G protein gamma subunits, including a new form of the gamma subunits identified by cDNA cloning. J Biol Chem 267:24023–24027.
15. Tang WJ, Gilman G. 1991. Type-specific regulation of adenylyl cyclase by G protein beta gamma subunits. Science 254:1500–1503.
16. Wickman KD, Iniguez Lluhl JA, Davenport PA, Taussig R, Krapivisky GB, Linder ME, Gilman AG, Clapham DE. 1994. Recombinant G-protein beta gamma-subunits activate the muscarinic-gated atrial potassium channel. Nature 368:255–257.
17. De Vivo M, Iyengar RG. 1994. G-protein pathways: signal processing by effectors. Mol Cell Endocrinol 100:65–70.
18. Katsushika S, Chen LJ, Nilakantan R, Halnon NJ, Homcy CJ, Ishikawa Y. 1992. Cloning and characterization of sixth adenylyl cyclase isoform: types V and VI constitute a subgrap within the mammalian adenylyl cyclase family. Proc Natl Acad Sci USA 89:8774–8778.
19. Premont RT, Chen J, Ma HW, Ponnapalli M, Iyengar R. 1992. Two members of a widely expressed subfamily of hormone-stimulated adenylyl cyclases. Proc Natl Acad Sci USA 89:9809–9813.
20. Toro MJ, Montoya E, Bimbaumer L. 1987. Inhibitory regulation of adenylyl cyclases. Evidence inconsistent with beta gamma-complexes of Gi proteins mediating hormonal effects by interfering with activation of Gs. Mol Edocrinol 1:669–676.
21. Taussig R, Quarnby LM, Gilman AG. 1993. Regulation of purified type I and type II adenylyl cyclases by a G protein beta gamma subunits. J Biol Chem 268:9–12.
22. Anand-Srivastava MB. 1988. Altered responsiveness of adenylate cyclase to adenosine and other agents in the myocardial sarcolemma and aorta of spontaneously hypertensive rats. Biochem Pharmacol 37:3017–3022.
23. Anand-Srivastava MB. 1992. Enhanced expression of inhibitory guanine nucleotide regulatory protein in spontaneously hypertensive rats: relationship to adenylate cyclase inhibition. Biochem J 288:79–85.
24. Anand-Srivastava MB. 1993. Platelets from spontaneously hypertensive rats exhibit decreased expression of inhibitory guanine nucleotide regulatory protein: relation with adenylyl cyclase activity. Circ Res 73:1032–1039.
25. Anand-Srivastava MB, de Champlain J, Thibault C. 1993. DOCA-salt hypertensive rat hearts exhibit altered expression of G-proteins. Am J Hypertens 6:72–75.
26. Marcil J, de Champlain J, Anand-Srivastava MB. 1998. Overexpression of Gi-proteins precedes the development of DOCA-salt-induced hypertension: relationship with adenylyl cyclase. Cardiovasc Res 39:492–505.

27. Bohm M, Gierschik P, Knorr A, Larisch K, Weismann K, Erdmann E. 1992. Desensitization of adenylate cyclase and increase of Giα in cardiac hypertrophy due to acquired hypertension. Hypertension 20:103–112.

28. Anand-Srivastava MB, Picard S, Thibault C. 1991b. Altered expression of inhibitory guanine nucleotide regulatory proteins (Giα) in spontaneously hypertensive rats. Am J Hypertens 4:840–843.

29. McLellan AR, Milligan G, Houslay MD, Connell MC. 1993. G-protein in experimental hypertension. J Hypertens 11:365–372.

30. Michel MC, Broodde OE, Insel PA. 1993. Are cardiac G-proteins altered in rat models of hypertension. J Hypertens 11:355–363.

31. Arnal JF, elAmrani AI, Chatellier G, Menard J, Michel JB. 1993. Cardiac weight in hypertension induced by nitric oxide synthase blockade. Hypertension 22:380–387.

32. Garcia R, Debold S. 1990. Simple rapid and effective method of producting aortocaval shunts in rats. Cardiovasc Res 24:430–432.

33. Marcil J, Thibault C, Anand-Srivastava MB. 1997. Enhanced expression of Gi-protein precedes the development of blood pressure in spontaneously hypertensive rats. J Mol Cell Cardiol 29:1009–1022.

34. Salomon Y, Londos C, Rodbell M. 1974. A highly sensitive adenylyl cyclase assay. Anal Biochem 58:541–548.

35. Lowry OM, Rosebrought NJ, Farr AL, Randall RJ. 1951. Protein measurement with the folin phenol reagent. J Biol Chem 193:265–275.

36. Chomczynski F, Sacchi N. 1987. Single-step method of RNA isolation by acid guanidium thiocyanate-phenol-chloroform extraction. Anal Biochem 162:156–159.

37. Feinberg AP, Vogelstein B. 1983. A technique for radiolabelling DNA restriction-endonuclease fragment to high specific activity. Anal Biochem 132:6–13.

38. Sambrook J, Fritsch EF, Maniatis T. 1989. Labeling the 5′ terminus of DNA with bacteriophage T4 polynucleotide kinase. In Molecular Cloning. A Laboratory Manual, 10.59–10.61. Cold Spring Harbor, NY; Cold Spring Harbor Laboratory.

39. Jones DT, Reed R. 1987. Molecular cloning of five GTP-binding protein cDNA species from rat olfactory neuroepithelium. J Biol Chem 262:14241–14249.

40. Chang GE, Anand-Srivastava MB. 1997. Altération des protéines G et de l'activité adénylyl cyclase dans le coeur du rat hypertendu par champagne d'une artère rénale. Médecine-Sciences 13:18.

41. Hammond HK, Roth DA, Insel PA, Ford CE, White FC, Maisel AS, Ziegler MG, Bloor CM. 1992. Myocardial beta adrenergic receptor expression and signal transduction after chronic volume-overload hypertrophy and circulatory congestion. Circulation 85:269–280.

42. Ribeiro MO, Antunes E, de Nucci G, Lovisolo SM, Zatz R. 1992. Chronic inhibition of nitric oxide synthesis: a new model of arterial hypertension. Hypertension 20:298–303.

43. Palaparti A, Ge C, Anand-Srivastava MB. In press. Angiotensin II enhances the expression of Giα-2 in A10 cells (smooth muscle): relationship with adenylyl cyclase activity. Arch Biochem Biophys.

44. Limas C, Limans CJ. 1978. Reduced number of β-adrenergic receptors in the myocardium of spntaneously hypertensive rats. Biochem Biophys Res Commun 83:710–714.

45. Zanchi A, Schad NC, Osterheld MC, Growzmann E, Nussberger J, Brunner HR, Waeber B. 1995. Effect of NO synthase inhibition in rats on renin–angiotensin system and sympathetic nervous system. Am J Physiol 37:H2267–H2273.

46. Laflamme AK, Foucart S, Moreau P, Lambert C, Cardinal R, de Champlain J. 1998. Sympathetic functions in N^G-nitro-L-arginine-methyl-ester-induced hypertension: modulation by the renin–angiotensin system. J Hypertens 16:63–76.

47. Cerione RA, Staniszewski C, Caron MG, Lefkowitz RJ, Codina J, Birnbaumer L. 1985. A role for Ni in the hormonal stimulation of adenylate cyclase. Nature 318:293–295.

48. Feldman AM, Cates AE, Veazey WB, Hershberger RE, Bristow MR, Baughman KL, Baumgartner WA, Dop CV. 1988. Increase of the 40,000 mol wt pertussis toxin substrate (G-protein) in the failing human heart. J Clin Invest 82:189–197.

N. Takeda, M. Nagano and N.S. Dhalla
(eds). The Hypertrophied Heart. Copyright
© 2000. pp. 179–186. Kluwer Academic
Publishers. Boston. All rights reserved.

THREE-DIMENSIONAL NUCLEAR SIZE AND DNA CONTENT IN HYPERTENSIVE HEART DISEASE

ATSUSHI TAKEDA, YUUSAKU HAYASHI, CHIHIRO SHIKATA, YASUYUKI TANAKA, and NOBUAKIRA TAKEDA

Department of Internal Medicine, Aoto Hospital, Jikei University School of Medicine, Aoto 6-41-2, Katsushika-ku, Tokyo 125-8506, Japan

Summary. Cardiac myocyte hypertrophy is commonly observed histologically in the hypertensive heart. Hypertrophic nuclei of myocytes are also detected in myocardial tissue. However, it is not clear whether an increase of nuclear size in myocytes indicates high DNA synthesis in hypertensive hearts. A total of 20 human hearts obtained at autopsy were studied. Following preparation of the hearts, the myocardium was weighed and total DNA content was determined biochemically. The DNA content was calculated by flow cytometry, and the structural changes of myocyte nuclei were visualized by three-dimensional (3-D) reconstruction. The percentage of myocytes in the G2M phase of the cell cycle was significantly increased in hypertensive hearts, compared with control hearts. The number of S-phase myocytes in hypertensive hearts was approximately twice that in control hearts. The 3-D myocardial nuclear size was bigger in hypertensive hearts than in control hearts. In conclusion, there were no dramatic changes of the DNA content and 3-D nuclear size, and such changes depended on remodeling of the intranuclear matrix in hypertrophic myocytes.

INTRODUCTION

Extensive evidence supports the concept that cardiac hypertrophy and normal cardiac growth occur in response to an increased hemodynamic load that causes abnormal systolic and diastolic stresses at the myocardial fiber level. Cardiac hypertrophy may be regarded as a useful adaptation to a hemodynamic load [1–3].

It is well known that the mode of left ventricular hypertrophy varies in accordance with hemodynamic conditions, such as volume or pressure overload, as well as with the underlying disease, e.g., aortic or mitral valvular heart failure. In hypertensive heart disease (HHD), an increase in myocardial wall tension results in additional oxygen consumption, and a series of biochemical events leads to left ventricular hypertrophy [2–5].

In the Framingham study [6], the left ventricular wall thickness at autopsy showed a better correlation with premorbid systolic than with diastolic blood pressure. Recent clinical investigations have suggested that long-standing HHD can some-times resemble hypertrophic cardiomyopathy in the elderly with respect to macro-scopic observations and microscopic histopathological findings. In the present study, we investigated whether nuclear hypertrophy of cardiac myocytes indicated equally high DNA synthesis, and assessed the 3-D nuclear size in HHD [7,8].

We used flow cytometry for DNA analysis of myocytes, and we also investigated the 3-D size of myocyte nuclei (Vol%) in HHD.

MATERIALS AND METHODS

Materials

Twenty hearts from elderly autopsy patients were studied. Fresh tissues from the left ventricle were obtained at autopsy within 6 hours of death of patients with HHD and control patients who had died of cancer, cerebral infarction, or bleeding. The HHD group was composed of four men and six women with a mean age of 61 ± 10 years (heart weight: 470 ± 79 g, mean ± SD). The age-matched control group was composed of eight men and two women, with a mean age of 66 ± 11 years (heart weight: 263 ± 68 g).

Methods

Myocardial tissue from the left ventricular free wall was obtained at autopsy from the patients with HHD as well as from the age-matched controls without cardio-vascular disease. Three myocardial sections were studied with hematoxylin-eosin and Masson trichrome stains after routine fixing in 10% formalin, embedding in paraffin, and sectioning.

Myocardial DNA synthesis

The myocardial cell cycle was automatically assessed by flow cytometry (FACScan, Becton Dickinson Co., USA). A piece of tissue was cut from each heart for flow cytometric analysis. After fixation, several 60 μm sections were cut from paraffin blocks [9–12], placed in a small tube with xylene for 20 minutes, and gradually rehydrated with distilled water. These sample tubes were then incubated for 1 hour at 37°C in a hot water bath after adding 1 mL of 0.5% pepsin solution, and the nuclei of cardiac myocytes were purified by filtering through 30–60 μm Teflon mesh to remove interstitial cell nuclei and debris (modified Hedley method) [12–15]. Then the nuclei were stained with 50 μg/mL propidium iodide (PI) and 0.1% Triton X-100 solution in 4 mmol/L sodium citrate (Vindelov method). The nuclei mixture was centrifuged (4°C, 400 × g, 10 min), the supernatant was discarded, 0.5 mL of PI solution was added, and then flow cytometric analysis was done [2,12,16–19]. In the typical DNA fluorescence histogram of cardiac myocytes, the first high peak indicates the G0–G1 phase of the cell cycle, the second peak is the G2M phase, and the valley between the G0–G1 and the G2M phase represents the S phase [17,18]. DNA frequency histograms were generated, and the results were analyzed by computer using Multi-cycle software (Phoenix Flow System, San Diego, CA,

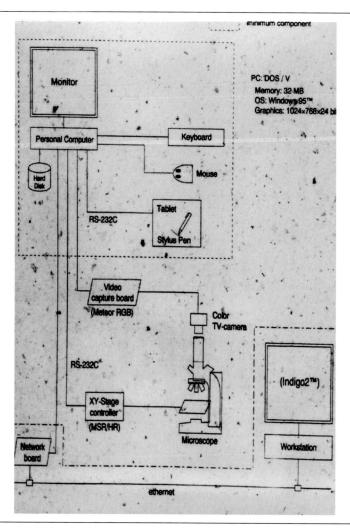

Figure 1. Three-dimensional image reconstruction system. Three-dimensional myocardial images were reconstructed using a TRI software system (TRI; Ratoc System Engineering, Tokyo, Japan).

USA) [20] (figure 1). Results are presented as mean ± SD (Table 1). Comparisons between the HHD and control groups were performed using Student's *t*-test for the data from 150 myocytes. The *p* values of less than 0.05 were considered statistically significant.

3-D image reconstruction

Several sections (4 μm thick) were prepared from the left ventricular free wall after paraffin embedding in a routine manner. Each of the 20 serial sections was subjected to Masson trichrome staining. The 3-D size of nucleus per myocyte (N/C ratio) (Volume%) was measured on the reconstructed serial sections using a 3-D reconstruction system (figure 1). Images obtained by light microscopy were traced in detail with a fine pencil and digitized automatically using a computer (Gateway 2000 Co., USA) with the Windows 95 operating system. The 3-D myocardial images were reconstructed using TRI software system (TRI; Ratoc System Engineering Co., Tokyo, Japan), and reconstructed images were displayed on a monitor (1024 × 768 × 24 bit) [20].

RESULTS

Histopathological study

The myocytes were hypertrophied in HHD patients (figure 2) and possessed large nuclei. There were also regular interconnections between myocytes as in control myocardial tissue (figure 3).

Myocardial DNA synthesis

The myocardial cell cycle was assessed by flow cytometry. In the HHD group, S-phase cells were more prominent than in the control group (11.5 ± 6.2 vs. $6.5 \pm 2.1\%$, mean $\pm$ SD, $p < 0.05$; table 1). G2M phase cells were also increased in the HHD group compared with the control group (7.7 ± 2.6 vs. $4.9 \pm 1.8\%$, mean $\pm$ SD, $p < 0.05$; table 1).

3-D imaging of myocytes

Table 2 shows the nucleocytoplasmic ratio (Vol%) in HHD and control hearts. The nuclei of hypertrophic myocytes in the HHD group (figures 4 and 5) were slightly bigger than in the controls (figures 6 and 7).

DISCUSSION

Generally speaking, mammalian cardiac myocytes cannot regenerate. Knowledge of the mechanism that controls the cell cycle of cardiac myocytes would allow us to design agents to promote regeneration of the adult myocardium following injury. Linzbach [21] has reported that if the heart weight was over a critical level of 500 g, hyperplasia could occur along with myocardial hypertrophy in hypertensive hearts. In this study, the mean heart weight of the HHD group was about 500 g

Table 1. Cell cycle of myocytes in hypertensive and control hearts

	Hypertensive hearts	Control hearts
G0–G1 phase	$80.9 \pm 7.5\%$[a]	$88.6 \pm 3.2\%$
S phase	$11.5 \pm 6.2\%$[a]	$6.5 \pm 2.1\%$
G2M phase	$7.7 \pm 2.6\%$[a]	$4.9 \pm 1.8\%$

[a] $p < 0.05$ vs. control, mean $\pm$ SD ($n = 10$).

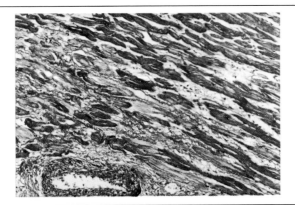

Figure 2. Myocardium in hypertensive heart disease. Hypertrophic myocytes with perivascular and interstitial fibrosis. Masson trichrome stain; original magnification ×200.

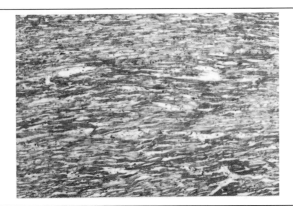

Figure 3. Myocardium of a control heart. There is a regular myofiber arrangement without hypertrophy. Masson trichrome stain; original magnification ×100.

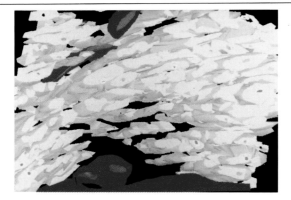

Figure 4. Three-dimensional view of the myocardium in hypertensive heart disease. Blue, nucleus; pink, myocyte; red, small artery.

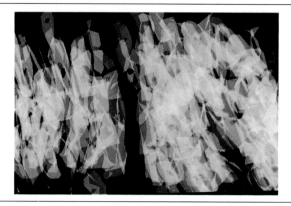

Figure 5. Three-dimensional view of the myocardium in hypertensive heart disease. Blue, nucleus; pink, myocyte; red, small artery.

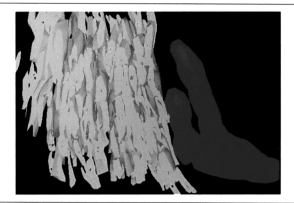

Figure 6. Three-dimensional view of control myocardium. Blue, nucleus; pink, myocyte; red, small artery.

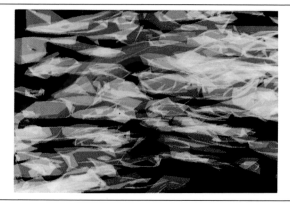

Figure 7. Three-dimensional view of control myocardium. Blue, nucleus; pink, myocyte; red, small artery.

Table 2. Nucleocytoplasmic ratio in hypertensive and control hearts

	Hypertensive hearts	Control hearts
N/C (%)	1.22 ± 1.05	1.16 ± 0.77

NS: HHD vs. control, mean ± SD, n = 150; N/C: nucleocytoplasmic ratio (Vol%).

(470 ± 79 g, mean ± SD), so hyperplasia might have been present. However, it may be difficult for hypertrophic myocytes to actually divide in hypertensive hearts because of the tight interconnections between myocytes [9–11]. In fact, hyperplasia may actually be very rare in HHD, since most myocytes remain in the G2 phase under genetic restriction. According to the present cell cycle analysis (table 1), G2M phase cells were increased in the HHD group. However, the 3-D nuclear size was almost the same in hypertensive and control hearts. This discrepancy may be related to the duration of hypertension and may depend on remodeling of the intranuclear matrix of hypertrophic myocytes under physical restrictions.

ACKNOWLEDGMENTS

This study was partly supported by the Research Committee for Epidemiology and Etiology of Idiopathic Cardiomyopathy of the Ministry of Health and Welfare of Japan. We thank Miss Isoko Arasaki and Mr. Yukihiro Takeuchi of the Pathological Laboratory for their skill in cutting serial sections and Mr. Toshiyuki Iizuka of Ratoc System Engineering Co. in Tokyo for his technical advice.

REFERENCES

1. Grossman W. 1980. Cardiac hypertrophy: useful adaptation or pathologic process? Am J Med 69:576–580.
2. Baba HA, Takeda A, Schmid C, Nagano M. 1996. Early proliferative changes in hearts of hypertensive Goldblatt rats: an immunohistochemical and flow-cytometrical study. Basic Res Cardiol 91:275–282.
3. Komuro I, Kurabayashi M, Shibazaki Y, Katoh Y, Hoh E, Kaida T, Ikeda K, Takaku F, Yazaki Y. 1990. Molecular mechanism of cardiac hypertrophy. Jpn Circ J 54:526–534.
4. Badeer HS. 1972. Development of cardiomegaly. A unifying hypothesis explaining the growth of muscle fiber, blood vessels and collagen of heart. Cardiology 57:247.
5. Hollander W. 1976. Role of hypertension in atherosclerosis and cardiovascular disease. Am J Cardiol 38:786.
6. Kannel WB, Castelli WP, McNamara PL, McKee PA, Feinleib M. 1972. Role of blood pressure in the development of congestive heart failure. N Engl J Med 287:784.
7. Geisterfer-Lowrance AA, Kass S, Tanigawa G, Vosberg HP. 1990. A molecular basis for hypertrophic cardiomyopathy. Cell 62:999–1006.
8. Tanigawa G, Jarcho JA, Kass S, Solomon SD, Vosberg HP, Seidman JG, Seidman CE. 1990. A molecular basis for familial hypertrophic cardiomyopathy. Cell 62:991–998.
9. Takeda A, Takeda N. 1997. Different pathophysiology of cardiac hypertrophy in hypertension and hypertrophic cardiomyopathy. J Mol Cardiol 29:2961–2965.
10. Takeda A, Chiba S, Iwai T, Tanamura A, Yamaguchi Y, Takeda N. 1998. Cell cycle of myocytes of cardiac and skeletal muscle in mitochondrial myopathy. Jpn Circ J 62:695–699.
11. Tezuka F. 1975. Muscle fiber orientation in normal and hypertrophied hearts. Tohoku J Exp Med 117:289–297.

12. Stephenson RA, Gay H, Fair WR. 1986. Effect of section thickness on quality of flow cytometric DNA content determinations in paraffin-embedded tissue. Cytometry 7:41–44.
13. David W, Hedley ML, Friedlander IW, Taylor LW. 1983. Method for analysis of celluar DNA content of paraffin-embedded pathological materials using flow cytometry. J Histochem Cytochem 31:1333–1335.
14. David W, Hedley ML, Friedlander IW, Taylor LW. 1985. Application of DNA flow cytometry to paraffin-embedded archival material for the study of aneuploid and its clinical significance. Cytometry 6:327–333.
15. Hedley DW, Friedlander ML, Taylor LW. 1985. Application of DNA flowcytometry to paraffin-embedded archival materials for the study of aneuploid and clinical significance. Cytometry 6:327–333.
16. Reynder SB, Bosman MJ. 1985. Flow cytometric determination of DNA ploid level in nuclei isolated from paraffin-embedded tissue. Cytometry 6:26–30.
17. Fried J. 1976. Method for the quantitative evaluation of data from microfluorometry. Comput Biomed Res 9:263.
18. Dean PN, Jett JH. 1974. Mathematical analysis of DNA distribution derived from flow microfluorometry. J Cell Biol 60:523.
19. Vindelov LL, Christensen IJ, Nissen NI. 1983. A detergent-trypsin method for the preparation of nuclei for flow cytometric DNA analysis. Cytometry 3:323–327.
20. Takeda A, Kawai S, Okada R, Nagai M, Takeda N, Nagano M. 1993. Three-dimensional distribution of myocardial fibrosis in the new J-2-N cardiomyopathic hamster: comparison with electrocardiographic findings. Heart Vessels 8:186–193.
21. Linzbach AJ. 1976. Hypertrophy, hyperplasia and structural dilatation of the human heart. Adv Cardiol 18:1–14.

N. Takeda, M. Nagano and N.S. Dhalla
(eds). The Hypertrophied Heart. Copyright
© 2000. pp. 187–196. Kluwer Academic
Publishers. Boston. All rights reserved.

AGE-RELATED ANISOTROPIC CHANGES IN CARDIOCYTE CONNECTIONS IN SPONTANEOUSLY HYPERTENSIVE RATS

MAKOTO OKABE, KEISHIRO KAWAMURA, FUMIO TERASAKI, TETSUYA HAYASHI, YUMIKO KANZAKI, and HARUHIRO TOKO

Third Division, Department of Internal Medicine, Osaka Medical College, 2-7, Daigaku-machi, Takatsuki City, Osaka, Japan 569-8686

Summary. An individual cardiocyte connects to adjacent cells at the ends and the sides of the cell in various ways. In this scanning electron microscopic (SEM) study, we compared the number and the mode of cardiocyte connections in the left ventricular myocardium between spontaneously hypertensive rats (SHR) and Wistar Kyoto rats (WKY) at 8, 15, and 63 weeks of age. Each rat group consisted of five rats. The number of cardiocytes connected to an individual cell was counted in 100 cells in each heart of each rat group. Among the 8-week-old rats hearts, the number of cardiocytes connected to an individual cardiocyte did not differ between the SHR (4.98 ± 0.11/cell) and the WKY (4.99 ± 0.02/cell). From 8 to 63 weeks of age, the number of cardiocyte connections in series significantly increased by 22% in the SHR and by 10% in the WKY, the number of lateral cardiocyte connections significantly decreased by 48% in the SHR and by 24% in the WKY, and the number of all cardiocytes connected to an individual cell significantly decreased by 15% in the SHR and by 8% in the WKY. Furthermore, all three indices were significantly different between the SHR and WKY at 63 weeks of age. These findings suggest that the number of lateral cardiocyte connections selectively reduced with age and that the reduction was more marked in the SHR. In the 63-week-old SHRs, SEM revealed that the hypertrophied myocardium contained some foci of replacement fibrosis in which several cardiocytes had undergone atrophy and some of them were dissociated at cell junctions. The decreased number of lateral cardiocyte connections may be associated with an enhanced propensity for the anisotropic electrical properties that may be more prominent in aged SHR. The age-related anisotropic change of the cardiocyte connections associated with cardiocytic hypertrophy and interstitial fibrosis may be one of the important mechanism of cardiac dysfunction and arrhythmia in hypertrophied myocardium as structural heart disease.

INTRODUCTION

An individual cardiocyte connects to other cardiocytes through intercalated disks at the ends and the sides of the cells. With many of these intercellular connections, the contraction of a single cell can be integrated for the optimal systolic function of the heart. Although the intercellular connections have a profound influence on electrical propagation and force generation of cardiocytes, the structural features of intercellular connections between cardiocytes in normal and hypertrophied hearts have not yet fully elucidated [1,2].

The spontaneously hypertensive rat (SHR) represents an animal model of essential hypertension, with hypertensive heart disease characterized by concentric hypertrophy [3,4] and dysfunction [5] of the left ventricle and potential arrhythmias that may develop with increasing age [6]. In our study by scanning electron microscopy (SEM) on SHR and WKY ventricles, side-to-side junctions and step-to-step junctions were commonly seen between parallel neighboring cells in the young animals, and these junctions apparently diminished in number with age even in normotensive WKY [7,8]. These lateral cell junctions always contained gap junctions so that they may facilitate lateral transmission between cardiocytes. These findings suggest the effects and interactions of aging and hypertension on the development of left ventricular (LV) hypertrophy in SHR and warrant a further quantitative analysis on intercellular connections of the hypertrophied cardiocytes.

The purpose of this study was to evaluate the remodeling of intercellular connections of cardiocytes. We examined structural features of connected cardiocytes by SEM and compared the number of cardiocytes connected to an individual cardiocyte in the left ventricle between SHR and normotensive WKY at various ages.

MATERIALS AND METHODS

Male SHR and WKY were studied at 8, 15, and 63 weeks of age. Each rat group consisted of five rats. Systolic blood pressure and body- and LV weight were measured as described elsewhere [3–5,8,9]. After measurement of LV weight, tissue specimens (each approximately $2 \times 2 \times 2\,mm$ in size) were excised from the epicardial side of the lateral wall of the left ventricle and fixed in 3% glutaraldehyde in 0.1 M phosphate buffer (pH 7.2). The tissue preparations for scanning electron microscopy (SEM) and conventional transmission electron microscopy (TEM) were processed as described elsewhere [3,4,8,9]. The tissue specimens were studied in a Hitachi S-800 SEM at an accelerating voltage of 20 KV at direct magnification of 40–10,000X. On SEM micrographs of en face views of the subepicardial portion of the left ventricular lateral wall, the size (width and length) of the cardiocytes was measured. As will be detailed later, series and lateral connections of cardiocytes were defined, and the number of cardiocytes connected to any individual cardiocyte was counted; the total number of all cardiocytes and separate numbers of each type of cardiocyte connected to an individual cardiocyte were counted.

Statistical analysis

All quantitative data were expressed as mean ± standard error of the mean. Student's t-test was used to compare systolic blood pressure, body weight, LV weight, and LV weight to body weight ratio between the age-matched SHR and WKY groups.

Morphometric data regarding cardiocytes were obtained from 100 cells arbitrarily selected in scanning electron micrographs from each ventricle and averaged for each group of five rats. Statistical analyses of these data among the six groups of rats were made by one-way analysis of variance (ANOVA). If ANOVA revealed significant differences, multiple comparisons were made using Scheffe's method. Probability values of less than 0.05 were considered to be significant.

RESULTS

Systolic blood pressure, body weight, and left ventricular weight (table 1)

In SHR, systolic blood pressure increased from 147 to 226 mmHg between 8 and 63 weeks of age and was always significantly higher than in age-matched WKY. In WKY, blood pressure remained between 109 and 130 mmHg throughout the experiment.

Body weight increased between 8 and 63 weeks of age in both rat strains with no significant difference between age-matched SHR and WKY. In SHR, LV weight and the LV weight/body weight ratio increased between 8 and 63 weeks of age, and both values were always significantly larger than in WKY at 8 weeks of age and thereafter.

Qualitative scanning electron microscopy

In this study, the intercellular connections between cardiocytes were classified into the series connection and the lateral-connection. The series connection is defined as an end-to-end connection at the axial end, when the overlap at the cell end between cardiocytes is 50% or more. The lateral connection is defined as a connection between two parallel neighboring cells. Even when two cells connect at the cell ends, it is defined as a lateral connection when their end-to-end overlap is less than 50%.

Table 1. Systolic blood pressure, body weight, left ventricular weight, and left ventricular weight/body weight ratio of SHR and WKY

	Systolic blood pressure (mmHg)	Body weight (BW) (g)	Left ventricular weight (LVW) (g)	LVW/BW ratio (mg/g)
8 weeks				
SHR	146.9 ± 4.8[a]	217.8 ± 3.6	0.60 ± 0.01[a]	2.78 ± 0.01[a]
WKY	109.2 ± 2.3	207.6 ± 3.1	0.52 ± 0.02	2.50 ± 0.05
15 weeks				
SHR	194.4 ± 4.7[a]	320.8 ± 1.9	0.94 ± 0.01[a]	2.93 ± 0.02[a]
WKY	119.6 ± 2.4	320.2 ± 1.0	0.71 ± 0.01	2.22 ± 0.02
63 weeks				
SHR	226.0 ± 2.5[a]	404.0 ± 4.2	1.29 ± 0.01[a]	3.18 ± 0.04[a]
WKY	130.0 ± 3.2	407.8 ± 8.9	1.03 ± 0.03	2.54 ± 0.05

[a] Significantly different from age-matched WKY ($p < 0.01$).
Values represent the mean ± SEM.

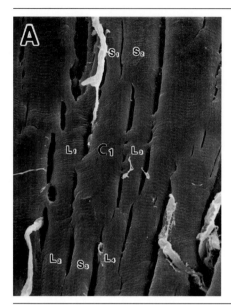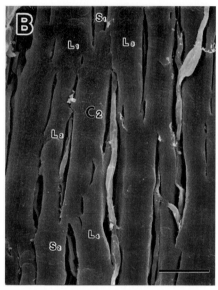

Figure 1. Comparative SEM photographs of LV cardiocytes at the same magnification in WKY (**A**) and SHR (**B**) at 8 weeks of age. In WKY (**A**), the cardiocyte C1 connects to three cardiocytes in series at both axial ends (S1–3). C1 also connects to four lateral neighboring cardiocytes (L1–4). Cardiocyte C1 connects to seven cardiocytes in all. In SHR (**B**), the cardiocyte C2 connects to two cardiocytes in series at both axial ends (S1–2). C2 also connects to four lateral neighboring cardiocytes (L1–4). Cardiocyte C2 connects with six cardiocytes in all. Scale indicates 20 μm.

In growing 8-week-old SHR and WKY, the general features of cardiocyte arrangements were similar; cell branchings were rarely seen, and step-to-step junctions and side-to-side junctions were occasionally seen in succession, like stepping stones, between parallel neighboring cells (figure 1).

In matured 15-week-old SHR, cardiocytes were apparently more thickened and elongated with more prominent lateral and series branches, and step-to-step and side-to-side junctions were apparently less in number than in age-matched WKY (figure 2).

In aged 63-week-old WKY (figure 3A), the general features of cardiocyte arrangements were similar to those in 15-week-old WKY (figure 2A) except for slightly broadened intermyofiber spaces. In aged 63-week-old SHR (figure 3B), cardiocytes were hypertrophied and lateral branches, step-to-step junctions, and side-to-side junctions were rarely seen. The extracellular space was often widened to some extent, reflecting an increase in connective tissues. In addition, in the 63-week-old SHR, some other cardiocytes appeared to have undergone atrophy, and some of them were dissociated at cell junctions (figure 4). In some largely widened spaces were seen disrupted free ends of cardiocyte trunks, which represent debris of connective tissue (figure 4C).

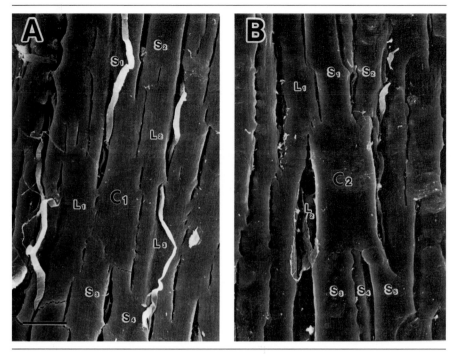

Figure 2. Comparative SEM photographs of LV cardiocytes at the same magnification in WKY (**A**) and SHR (**B**) at 15 weeks of age. In WKY (**A**), cardiocyte C1 connects to four cardiocytes in series (S1–4) and three lateral neighboring cardiocytes (L1–3). In SHR (**B**), C2 connects to five cardiocytes in series (S1–5) and two cardiocytes in lateral (L1–2). Scale indicates 20 μm.

Quantitative scanning electron microscopy

LV cardiocytes (table 2)

At 8 weeks of age, cells were much the same in size between the SHR and WKY groups; cells were significantly longer in SHR but the difference was so small that the ratio of the length to width of the cells was not different between the two animal strains. At 15 weeks of age, cells were more thickened and elongated in the SHR than in the WKY group, and the length-to-width ratio was significantly reduced in SHR. At 63 weeks of age, in SHR, cells were much more thickened and elongated than in WKY and the length-to-width ratio was significantly reduced.

The number of cardiocytes connected to an individual cell (figure 5)

THE NUMBER OF SERIES CARDIOCYTES CONNECTION PER CELL (FIGURE 5A). At 8 weeks of age, the number of series-connected cardiocytes per cell did not differ between the SHR (2.30 ± 0.03) and WKY (2.25 ± 0.03) groups. In both rat strains, the number increased with age. In SHR, the number of series-connected cardiocytes per cell increased by 22% (2.81 ± 0.06/cell), whereas in the WKY, it increased

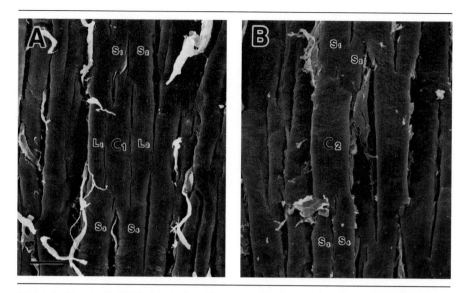

Figure 3. Comparative SEM photographs of LV cardiocytes at the same magnification in WKY (**A**) and SHR (**B**) at 63 weeks of age. In WKY rats (**A**), cardiocyte C1 connects to four cardiocytes in series (S1–4) and two cardiocytes in lateral (L1–2). In SHR (**B**), C2 connects to four cardiocytes in series (S1–4). There is no lateral cardiocyte connection in C2. Scale indicates 20 μm.

Table 2. Width, length, and length/width ratio of left ventricular cardocytes in SHR and WKY

	Width (μm)	Length (μm)	Length/width ratio
8 weeks			
SHR	13.5 ± 0.3	64.8 ± 0.9^a	5.01 ± 0.07
WKY	12.9 ± 0.3	61.3 ± 0.8	4.95 ± 0.05
15 weeks			
SHR	17.9 ± 0.3^a	76.4 ± 0.7^a	4.52 ± 0.11^a
WKY	15.4 ± 0.2	71.4 ± 1.0	4.93 ± 0.10
63 weeks			
SHR	20.5 ± 0.3^a	83.5 ± 0.8^a	4.23 ± 0.05^a
WKY	16.2 ± 0.3	75.8 ± 0.7	4.85 ± 0.08

[a] Significantly different from age-matched WKY ($p < 0.01$).
Values represent the mean ± SEM.

by 10% (2.47 ± 0.03/cell) at 63 weeks of age. Thus, the number in the SHR was significantly higher than that in the WKY at 63 weeks of age.

THE NUMBER OF LATERAL CARDIOCYTES CONNECTION PER CELL (FIGURE 5B). At 8 weeks of age, the number of lateral connected cardiocytes per cell did not differ between the SHR (2.68 ± 0.09/cell) and WKY (2.74 ± 0.03) groups. In both rat strains, the number decreased with age. In the SHR, the number of lateral con-

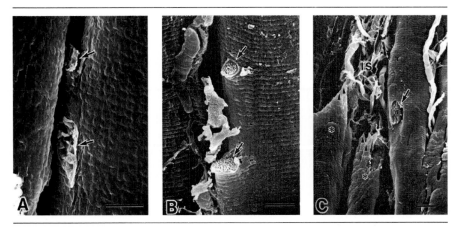

Figure 4. Panels illustrate dissociated intercellular junctions of LV cardiocytes in 63–week-old SHR. (**A–C**) Note the "plicate structure" of dissociated intercalated disks (arrows). (**A**) Intercellular junctions are separated without cell injury between two cardiocytes. Scale indicates 5 μm. (**B**) Dissociated intercalated disks of cell steps are observed (arrows). Scale indicates 5 μm. (**C**) In a largely widened intercellular space (IS), there are connective tissue remnants, and the trunks of cardiocytes (*) have dissociated free ends (arrowheads). Scale indicates 20 μm.

nected cardiocytes per cell decreased by 48% (1.39 ± 0.07/cell), whereas in the WKY, it decreased by 24% (2.08 ± 0.06/cell) at 63 weeks of age. The number in the SHR was significantly less than that in WKY at 63 weeks of age.

THE NUMBER OF ALL CARDIOCYTES CONNECTED TO AN INDIVIDUAL CELL (FIGURE 5C). At 8 weeks of age, the number of all cardiocytes connected to an individual cardiocytes did not differ between the SHR (4.98 ± 0.11/cell) and WKY (4.99 ± 0.02) groups. In both rat strains, the number decreased with age. In the SHR, the number decreased by 15% (4.20 ± 0.08/cell), whereas in the WKY, it was decreased by 9% (4.55 ± 0.07/cell) at 63 weeks of age. Thus, the number in the SHR was significantly less than that in the WKY at 63 weeks of age.

DISCUSSION

During the period between 8 and 63 weeks in SHR, marked hypertension and LV hypertrophy developed, and cardiocytes thickened and elongated more than those in WKY. In both strains, an individual cardiocyte connected to 2~10 other cells through intercalated disks, and the number of cardiocytes connected an individual cell decreased with age. The decrease was more marked in the SHR. In addition, the decrease was primarily found in the form of lateral connections.

In aged 63-week-old SHR, SEM has revealed that the hypertrophied myocardium contained some foci of replacement fibrosis in which several cardiocytes had undergone marked deformations and/or loss, with dissociation of intercellular junctions (figure 4). These findings suggest that increased mass of connective tissue widened

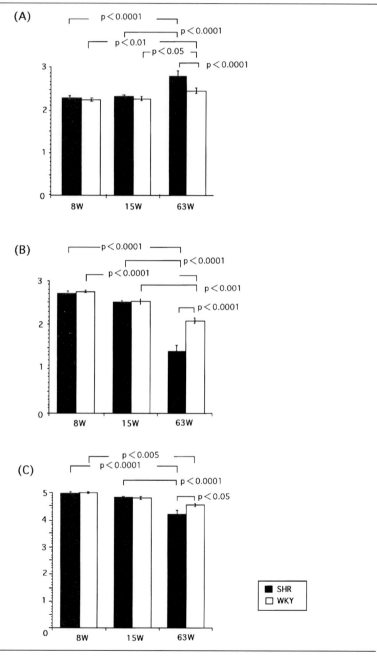

Figure 5. Bar graphs showing age-related changes of the number of cardiocytes connected to an individual cell in SHR (black bars) and WKY (open bars) at 8, 15, and 63 weeks of age. Results are presented as the mean ± SD of five rats per group. (**A**) The number of cardiocytes connections in series per cell; (**B**) the number of cardiocytes connections in lateral per cell; (**C**) the number of all cardiocyte connections per cell. See the text for discussion.

intercellular spaces and that cell junctions may be dissociated. Therefore, the decrease of connected cardiocytes may have more relevance to the dissociation of intercellular junctions and/or loss of cardiocytes.

A decrease in the number of neighbor cells connected to any single cardiocyte may signify a loss of the gap junction that couples the cells and may distort the normal pattern of electrical activation. A selective decrease of lateral cell connections may disproportionately increase resistance to propagation in a direction transverse to the long cardiocytic axis. It may cause disproportionately enhanced axial resistivity in the transverse direction and may potentially contribute to development of reentrant arrhythmias based on anisotropic discontinuous conduction [10].

Together with the problem of electrical activation, this numerical reduction of intercellular connections may also have mechanical disadvantages. The decreased number of cardiocytic connections of an individual cell may impair the contraction of the LV. A lateral cellular connection may serve to resist an intercellular force in a direction transverse to the cardiocytic axis. In this sense, the decrease number of lateral connections may cause a slippage between the cardiocytes in situated in parallel, predisposing to the ventricular dilatation.

Thus the decrease in number of connected cardiocytes during the process of LV hypertrophy may present a disadvantage to the electrical and mechanical communication between cardiocytes. Our observation concerning an age-related decrease in the number of cardiocytes connected to an individual cell in SHR may suggest the structural basis for an age-related increase in the incidence of ventricular dysfunction and arrhythmias.

ACKNOWLEDGMENTS

This study was supported in part by the Vehicle Racing Commemorative Foundation.

REFERENCES

1. Sawada K, Kawamura K. 1991. Architecture of myocardial cells in human cardiac ventricles with concentric and eccentric hypertrophy as demonstrated by quantitative scanning electron microscopy. Heart Vessels 6:129–142.
2. Yamamoto S, James TN, Sawada K, Okabe M, Kawamura K. 1996. Generation of new intercellular junctions between cardiocytes. A possible mechanism compensating for mechanical overload in the hypertrophied adult myocardium. Circ Res 78:362–370.
3. Imamura K. 1978. Ultrastructural aspect of left ventricular hypertrophy in spontaneously hypertensive rats: a qualitative and quantitative study. Jpn Circ J 42:979–1002.
4. Kawamura K, Imamura K, Uehara H, Nakayama Y, Sawada K, Yamamoto S. 1984. Architecture of hypertrophied myocardium: scanning and transmission electron microscopy. In Regulation of Cardiac Function. Ed. H Abe, Y Ito, M Tada, LH Opie, 81–105. Tokyo: Japan Scientific Press.
5. Nishimura H, Kubo S, Nishioka A, Imamura K, Kawamura K, Hasegawa M. 1985. Left ventricular diastolic function of spontaneously hypertensive rats and its relationship to structural components of the left ventricle. Clin Sci 69:571–580.
6. Pahor M, Giudice PL, Bernabei R, Gennaro MD, Pacifici L, Ramacci MT, Carbonin PU. 1989. Age-related increase in the incidence of ventricular arrhythmias in isolated hearts from spontaneously hypertensive rats. Cardiovasc Drugs Ther 3:163–169.
7. Okabe M, Kimpara T, Terasaki F, Hayashi T, Sawada K, Nishimura H, Nakayama Y, Kawamura K. 1988. Scanning electron microscopic study of ventricular cardiocytes of spontaneously hypertensive rats (SHR). J Clin Electron Microsc 21:568–569.

8. Okabe M, Kawamura K, Terasaki F, Hayashi T. 1999. Remodeling of cardiomyocytes and their branches in juvenile, adult and senescent spontaneously hypertensive rats and Wistar Kyoto rats: comparative morphometric analyses by scanning electron microscopy. Heart Vessels 14:15–28.
9. Kimpara T, Okabe M, Nishimura H, Hayashi T, Imamura K, Kawamura K. 1997. Ultrastructural changes during myocardial hypertrophy and its regression: long-term effects of nifedipine in adult spontaneously hypertensive rats. Heart Vessels 12:143–151.
10. Spach MS. 1997. Discontinuous cardiac conduction: Its origin in cellular connectivity with long-term adaptive changes that cause arrhythmias. In Discontinuous Conduction in the Heart. Ed. PM Spooner, RW Joyner, J Jolife (pp. 5–51). New York: Futura, Armonk.

N. Takeda, M. Nagano and N.S. Dhalla
(eds). The Hypertrophied Heart. Copyright
© 2000. pp. 197–206. Kluwer Academic
Publishers. Boston. All rights reserved.

STIMULATION OF MITOGEN-ACTIVATED PROTEIN KINASES ERK-1 AND ERK-2 BY H_2O_2 IN VASCULAR SMOOTH MUSCLE CELLS

ASHOK K. SRIVASTAVA and SANJAY K. PANDEY

Department of Medicine, University of Montreal Research Center-Centre hospitalier de l'Université de Montréal (CHUM), Campus Hôtel-Dieu, 3840 St. Urbain Street, Montreal, Quebec H2W 1T8, Canada

Summary. The possible roles of the mitogen-activated protein kinases (MAPKs) ERK-1 and ERK-2 in mediating growth-promoting and hypertrophic responses were investigated by examining the effect of H_2O_2 on ERK-1 and ERK-2 phosphorylation and activation in an established vascular smooth muscle cell (VSMC) line (A10). H_2O_2 treatment of VSMCs stimulated the phosphorylation of both ERK-1 and ERK-2 in a concentration-dependent manner with maximal impact at the dose level of $2\,mM$ H_2O_2. Treatment of cells with aminotriazole, an inhibitor of catalase, potentiated the effect of H_2O_2 and reduced the H_2O_2 concentration required to elicit the maximum response. In addition, PD98059, an inhibitor of MAPK kinase (MEK), and wortmannin, an inhibitor of phosphatidylinositol 3-kinase (PI3K), attenuated the H_2O_2-induced activation of ERK-1 and ERK-2. H_2O_2 was also found to stimulate PI3K activity, which was inhibited by wortmannin. Taken together, these data demonstrate that oxidative stress-induced ERK activation is mediated, at least in part, through a PI3K-dependent pathway and suggest a role of this pathway in eliciting growth-promoting and hypertrophic responses to H_2O_2 in VSMCs.

INTRODUCTION

In recent years, evidence has accumulated that indicates a potential role of oxidant-derived by-products, commonly known as reactive oxygen species (ROS) or free radicals, in the pathogenesis of several disorders, including cardiovascular diseases such as hypertension and atherosclerosis [1,2]. NADH/NADPH oxidase-derived generation of ROS in angiotensin II (Ang II)-induced hypertrophy has also been suggested [3–5]. Furthermore, oleic acid-induced formation of H_2O_2 has been linked to vascular smooth muscle cell (VSMC) mitogenesis [6], and ROS have been shown to stimulate growth and expression of oncogenes in VSMCs [7]. The cellular mechanism responsible for eliciting growth-promoting responses to ROS remains poorly characterized in VSMCs. However, there is a growing body of evidence suggesting that oxidative stress activates the protein kinase signaling cascade [8,9]. Important components of this cascade are mitogen-activated protein kinases (MAPKs) [8–11] and phosphatidylinositol 3-kinase (PI3K) [12,13].

Mammalian MAPKs are serine/threonine protein kinases that can be subdivided into five broad families: MAPK$^{erk1/2}$, MAPK^{p38}, MAPK^{jnk}, MAPK$^{erk3/4}$, and MAPK^{erk5} (reviewed in [10]). Among these, MAPK$^{erk1/2}$ is activated in response to various stimuli, including growth factors, phorbol esters, ionophores, heat shock, etc., and play a key role in cell growth and development [11]. The activity of MAPK$^{erk1/2}$ is regulated by its dual phosphorylation in threonine and tyrosine residues catalyzed by MAPK kinase, also known as MEK (for **m**itogen and **e**xtracellular signal-regulated kinase **k**inase). MEK is, in turn, activated by phosphorylation in serine/threonine residues by an upstream kinase, C-raf, while p21-ras (ras), a low-molecular-weight GTP-binding protein that cycles between active GTP-bound and inactive GDP-bound forms, has been attributed to the activation of C-raf. The activated form of MAPK$^{erk1/2}$ mediates the phosphorylation of downstream cytosolic targets and nuclear transcription factors, leading to growth, mitogenesis, and gene expression [11].

PI3Ks are heterodimeric enzymes composed of a 85 kDa (p85) regulatory subunit and a 110 kDa (p110) catalytic subunit. The p85 subunit contains the src homology-2 (SH-2) domain and is able to interact with phosphorylated tyrosine residues on receptor or other docking proteins. This interaction eventually stimulates the activity of the 110 kDa catalytic subunit. The catalytic subunit catalyzes the phosphorylation of phosphatidylinositol (PI), PI4 phosphate and PI4,5 bisphosphate in the 3' position of the inositol ring to generate PI3 phosphate, PI3,4 bisphosphate, and PI3,4,5 trisphosphate, respectively [13]. PI3Ks are activated in response to growth factors and other agents, including vasoactive peptides, and have been suggested to regulate a variety of cellular responses such as proliferation, differentiation, growth, and cell survival [13–15]. The lipid products of the PI3K reaction have downstream targets such as phosphatidylinositol phosphate-dependent kinases (PDK 1/2) and protein kinase B, which are involved in mediating the end-point biological effects of PI3K activation [16,17]. In several studies, inhibition of PI3K by a potent inhibitor, wortmannin, has been shown to block activation of the MAPK ERK-1 and ERK-2 by various agonists [18–22], indicating a role of PI3K in their stimulation.

Oxidative stress by H_2O_2 has been demonstrated to activate ERK-1 and ERK-2 in neutrophils [23], HeLa, Rat1, NIH 3T3, PC12, VSMC [24], and neurons [25]. However, despite data supporting the involvement of ERK-1 and ERK-2 in Ang II-stimulated protein synthesis and hypertrophy in VSMCs [26,27], activation of ERK-1 and ERK-2 by H_2O_2 in VSMCs remains controversial. Some reports indicate that H_2O_2 has no effect on ERK-1 and ERK-2 [27–29], whereas significant stimulation of ERK-1 and ERK-2 in VSMCs has been observed by Guyton et al. [24]. Therefore, the present study was initiated to clarify the effect of H_2O_2 on ERK-1 and ERK-2 activation in A10 cells, which are derived from rat embryonal thoracic aortic smooth muscles and have characteristics similar to VSMCs [30–33]. In addition, we also investigated the role of PI3K in H_2O_2-stimulated ERK-1 and ERK-2 activation.

MATERIALS AND METHODS

Materials

Phospho-ERK antibodies, which detect the active forms of ERK-1 and ERK-2 phosphorylated in Thr^{202}/Tyr^{204} residues, were obtained from New England Biolabs (Beverly, MA, USA). Regular MAPK antibodies, which recognize both phospho- and dephospho-ERK-1/2, were a generous gift from Drs. A. Sorokin and M.J. Dunn, Medical College of Wisconsin (Milwaukee, WI, USA). Antibody against the p85 regulatory subunit of PI3K was purchased from Santa Cruz Biotechnology (Santa Cruz, CA, USA). PD98059 and wortmannin were obtained from Calbiochem (La Jolla, CA, USA). Aminotriazole (ATZ) was procured from the Sigma Chemical Co. (St. Louis, MO, USA). All other reagents were from commercial sources, as described earlier [34].

Cell culture

VSMCs were maintained in DMEM containing 10% fetal bovine serum and passaged twice a week by harvesting with trypsin/EDTA. The cells were grown to 80–90% confluence in 100 mm culture plates and incubated in serum-free DMEM for 20 hours prior to the experiment [35].

Detection of ERK-1/2 by immunoblotting

VSMCs at 80–90% confluency in 100 mm dishes were stimulated with H_2O_2 or other agents. The cells were lysed on ice in 400 μl of buffer A (25 mM Tris-HCl, pH 7.5, 25 mM NaCl, 1 mM Na orthovanadate, 10 mM Na fluoride, 10 mM Na pyrophosphate, 20 nM okadaic acid, 0.5 mM EGTA, 1 mM phenylmethyl-sulphonyl fluoride, 10 μg/mL aprotinin, 1% Triton X-100, and 0.1% SDS). The clarified lysates containing equal amounts of protein, as determined by Bradford assay, were electrophoresed on 12% SDS-polyacrylamide gels and transferred to polyvinylidine difluoride membranes [34]. The membranes were incubated with phosphospecific or regular ERK-1/2 antibodies. The signal was detected by horseradish peroxidase-conjugated goat anti-rabbit antibody and the enhanced chemiluminescence method.

PI3K assay

The clarified cell lysates were subjected to immunoprecipitation with 5 μg of p85 antibody for 2 hours at 4°C, followed by incubation with protein A sepharose for an additional 2 hours. The immunoprecipitates were washed and subjected to in vitro PI3K assay, as described earlier [34]. Phosphorylated lipid products were extracted and separated by ascending thin layer chromatography [34]. Radioactivity in the spots corresponding to PI3-phosphate (PIP) was quantified by Phosphor Imager (Molecular Dynamics, Sunnyvale, CA, USA).

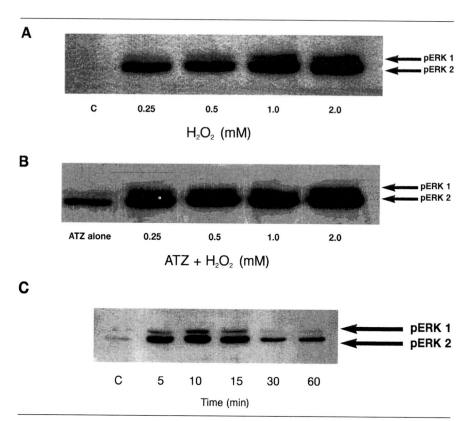

Figure 1. Effect of H_2O_2 on ERK-1 and ERK-2 phosphorylation by H_2O_2. Serum-starved, quiescent VSMCs were stimulated under different experimental conditions. (**A**) Stimulation was induced in the absence (C) or presence of the indicated H_2O_2 concentrations for 10 minutes. (**B**) Cells were pretreated with 50 mM ATZ for 30 minutes, then stimulated in the absence (ATZ alone) or presence of the indicated H_2O_2 concentrations for 10 minutes. (**C**) Cells were incubated in the absence (C) or presence of 2 mM H_2O_2 for the indicated time periods. Cell lysates were prepared, and equal amounts of proteins were separated on 12% SDS-PAGE. Active and phosphorylated ERK-1/2 (pERK-1 and pERK-2) were detected by immunoblot analysis with phospho-ERK antibody, as described in Materials and Methods. Representative immunoblots from three experiments with similar results are shown.

RESULTS

Effect of H_2O_2 on phosphorylation of the MAPKs ERK-1 and ERK-2

As shown in figure 1A, H_2O_2 caused a dose-dependent increase of ERK-1 and ERK-2 phosphorylation. Since ERK-1 and ERK-2 phosphorylation is associated with their activation [11], it was taken routinely as a measure of stimulation of catalytic activity. A clear rise in ERK phosphorylation was evident at the lowest dose (0.25 mM) of H_2O_2, which elicited more than a 25-fold elevation compared to the controls. However, under these conditions, we noted higher activation of ERK-2 compared to ERK-1 due to higher expression of this protein in VSMCs (data not shown).

Since an unusually high concentration of H_2O_2 was required to achieve a significant level of ERK phosphorylation (figure 1A), the possibility was considered that a highly active endogenous catalase present in VSMCs might degrade exogenous H_2O_2 and result in underestimation of the stimulatory effect of H_2O_2 on ERK activation. To address this issue, we examined the effect of ATZ, an inhibitor of catalase [23], on H_2O_2-induced activation of ERK-1 and ERK-2. As shown in figure 1B, prior treatment of cells with ATZ (50 mM) for 30 minutes, followed by stimulation with H_2O_2, potentiated the effect of H_2O_2 and reduced the amount of H_2O_2 required to elicit the maximum response compared to cells not treated with ATZ. Interestingly, incubation of cells with ATZ alone caused more than a 10-fold increase of ERK phosphorylation relative to untreated cells (compare the control (C) and ATZ-alone lanes in figures 1A and 1B, respectively). These data indicate that inhibition of endogenous catalase by ATZ allowed H_2O_2, produced by constitutive activation of oxidant-generating systems in VSMCs, to attain a concentration sufficient to induce phosphorylation of cellular ERK-1 and ERK-2 in the absence of any exogenous stimulus.

Figure 1C shows the time dependence of H_2O_2-induced ERK-1 and ERK-2 phosphorylation in VSMCs. H_2O_2 treatment enhanced ERK-1 and ERK-2 phosphorylation within 5 minutes, which reached peak value at 10 minutes, followed by a rapid decline thereafter. It should be noted, however, that even after 60 minutes, significant ERK-2 phosphorylation was clearly detectable.

Effect of pharmacological inhibitors of MEK and PI3K on H_2O_2-induced ERK-1 and ERK-2 phosphorylation

MEK, a dual-specificity kinase, catalyzes ERK-1 and ERK-2 phosphorylation, resulting in their activation [11]. Recently, a highly specific inhibitor of MEK, PD98059, was used to demonstrate a role of MEK in ERK activation [36]. Therefore, the involvement of MEK in H_2O_2-induced phosphorylation of ERK-1 and ERK-2 in VSMCs was investigated by pretreatment of cells with different concentrations of PD98059 for 30 minutes, followed by stimulation with H_2O_2 (2 mM) for 10 minutes. As shown in figure 2A, PD98059 pretreatment attenuated H_2O_2-stimulated ERK-1 and ERK-2 phosphorylation in a dose-dependent manner, with near total inhibition observed at the 40 µM dose level. These data indicate a role of MEK in mediating H_2O_2-induced ERK-1 and ERK-2 phosphorylation in VSMCs.

A requirement of PI3K in the activation of ERK-1/2 has been demonstrated in response to several agonists [18–22,37,38] by using wortmannin, a potent and specific inhibitor of PI3K [39]. Therefore, a role of PI3K in H_2O_2-induced ERK-1 and ERK-2 phosphorylation was examined by treating VSMCs with wortmannin for 30 minutes, followed by stimulation with H_2O_2. As seen in figure 2B, wortmannin pretreatment resulted in partial but significant inhibition of ERK-1 and ERK-2 phosphorylation compared to wortmannin-untreated cells.

A

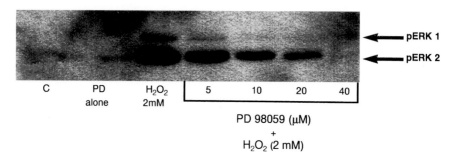

| C | PD | H₂O₂ | 5 | 10 | 20 | 40 |

$$\text{C} \quad \text{PD alone} \quad \text{H}_2\text{O}_2 \text{ 2mM} \quad \boxed{5 \quad 10 \quad 20 \quad 40}$$

PD 98059 (μM)
+
H₂O₂ (2 mM)

B

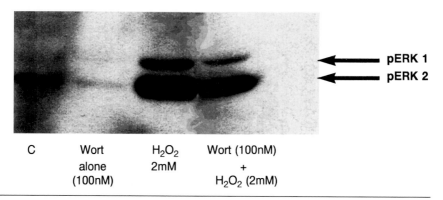

C   Wort   H₂O₂   Wort (100nM)
         alone   2mM   +
        (100nM)   H₂O₂ (2mM)

Figure 2. Effect of the MEK inhibitor PD98059 and the PI3K inhibitor wortmannin on H_2O_2-induced ERK phosphorylation. (**A**) Serum-starved, quiescent VSMCs were treated without or with the indicated PD98059 concentrations for 30 minutes, followed by incubation in the absence (C) or presence of 2 mM H_2O_2 for 10 minutes. Cell lysates were prepared and equal amounts of protein were separated on 12% SDS-PAGE. Active and phosphorylated forms of ERK-1/2 (pERK-1 and pERK-2) were detected as described in figure 1. A representative immunoblot from two separate experiments with identical results is shown. (**B**) Serum-starved, quiescent VSMCs were treated without or with 100 nM wortmannin for 30 minutes, followed by incubation in the absence (C) or presence of 2 mM H_2O_2 for 10 minutes, and active phosphorylated forms of ERK-1/2 (pERK-1 and pERK-2) were detected as described above. A representative immunoblot from two experiments with identical results is shown.

The participation of PI3K in H_2O_2-stimulated responses was confirmed by directly determining the effect of H_2O_2 on PI3K activity. H_2O_2 was found to stimulate PI3K activity in PI3K immunoprecipitates by more than threefold compared to unstimulated VSMCs (data not shown).

DISCUSSION

In this study, we report that oxidative stress by H_2O_2 results in ERK-1 and ERK-2 phosphorylation in VSMCs, which is dependent on MEK and PI3K activation. Our observations with regard to ERK-1 and ERK-2 stimulation in response to H_2O_2 are in agreement with those of Guyton et al. [24], who documented a marked increase of MAPK activation in VSMCs, but are at variance with the findings of Ushio-Fukai et al. [27], Bass and Berk [28], and Abe et al. [29], who failed to demonstrate any effect of H_2O_2 on MAPK activity. H_2O_2 has been shown to stimulate MAPK activity in other systems, such as neurons [25], rat hearts [40], cultured cardiac myocytes [41], and bovine tracheal myocytes [42], consistent with our data in VSMCs. The reason for the conflicting observations in VSMCs is not known at this time but may be attributed to the different experimental conditions employed.

The potentiating effect of ATZ on H_2O_2-stimulated ERK-1 and ERK-2 phosphorylation indicates that a highly active catalase present in VSMCs is able to degrade exogenously added H_2O_2. This suggestion is confirmed by our observations, where ATZ treatment alone, in the absence of exogenously-added H_2O_2, was sufficient to phosophorylate ERK-1 and ERK-2. The presence of a highly active catalase may also explain the failure of low concentrations of H_2O_2 to activate MAPK in earlier studies [27–29].

The finding that PD98059, a pharmacological inhibitor of MEK, blocked H_2O_2-stimulated ERK-1 and ERK-2 phosphorylation indicates that MEK is the putative upstream kinase catalyzing their phosphorylation. In cultured rat cardiac myocytes [41] and bovine tracheal myocytes [42], H_2O_2 was shown to activate MEK. Partial inhibition of H_2O_2-induced ERK phosphorylation by wortmannin and stimulation of PI3K activity by H_2O_2 clearly demonstrated that at least some of the effects of H_2O_2 on ERK phosphorylation are mediated by a PI3K-dependent pathway.

The precise mechanism leading to the activation of PI3K, ERK-1, and ERK-2 by H_2O_2 as well as its direct targets remains unknown. However, a potential target could be protein tyrosine phosphatase (PTPase). PTPases possess a cysteine residue in their active site, and its mutation or deletion inhibits their catalytic activity [43]. Moreover, H_2O_2 has also been shown to oxidize the cysteine residue in PTB1B [44] and to directly inhibit PTPase activity [45]. PTPase inhibition would, thus, allow enhancement of tyrosine phosphorylation of relevant signaling molecules by protein tyrosine kinases in a ligand-independent manner, leading to the activation of downstream signaling molecules such as PI3K and ras/raf/MEK/MAPK.

In summary, we have demonstrated that the oxidant H_2O_2 activates ERK-1 and ERK-2 in VSMCs via the mediation of MEK, an immediate upstream regulator of ERK-1 and ERK-2. Most importantly, this study provides the first evidence of PI3K activation by H_2O_2 and its partial involvement as an upstream modulator of ERK-1 and ERK-2 phosphorylation in response to H_2O_2 in VSMCs. Since PI3K, ERK-1, and ERK-2 play critical roles in a variety of cellular responses, it is possible that hypertrophic and hyperproliferative responses to H_2O_2 are mediated by activation of these pathways in VSMCs.

ACKNOWLEDGMENTS

This study was supported by a grant from the Heart and Stroke Foundation of Quebec to A.K.S. We are grateful to Dr. Madhu B. Anand-Srivastava for kindly providing A10 VSMCs. We thank also Carmen Sabu for her technical assistance, Claude Dufour for producing the illustrations, Ovid Da Silva for editing, and Susanne Bordeleau-Chénier for preparing this manuscript.

REFERENCES

1. Ames BN, Shigenaga MK, Hagen TM. 1993. Oxidant, antioxidants and the pathogenesis of degenerative diseases of aging. Proc Natl Acad Sci USA 90:7915–7922.
2. Alexander RW. 1995. Hypertension and the pathogenesis of atherosclerosis: oxidative stress and the mediation of arterial inflammatory response: a new perspective. Hypertension 25:155–161.
3. Griendling KK, Mineri CA, Ollerenshaw JD, Alexander RW. 1994. Angiotensin II stimulates NADH and NADPH oxidase activity in cultured vascular smooth muscle cells. Circ Res 74:1141–1148.
4. Ushio-Fukai M, Zafari AM, Fukui T, Ishizaka N, Griendling KK. 1996. P22 phox is a critical component of the superoxide generating NADH/NADPH oxidase system and regulates angiotensin II-induced hypertrophy in vascular smooth muscle cells. J Biol Chem 271:23317–23322.
5. Fukui T, Ishizaka N, Rajagopalan S, Laursen JB, Capers Q, Taylor WR, Harrison DG, de Leon H, Wilcox JN, Griendling KK. 1997. P22 phox mRNA expression and NADPH oxidase activity are increased in aortas from hypertensive rats. Circ Res 80:45–51.
6. Lu G, Greene EL, Nagui T, Egan BM. 1998. Reactive oxygen species are critical in the oleic acid-mediated signaling pathway in vascular smooth muscle cells. Hypertension 32:1003–1010.
7. Rao GN, Berk BC. 1992. Active oxygen species stimulate vascular smooth muscle cell growth and protooncogene expression. Circ Res 70:593–599.
8. Chakraborti S, Chakraborti T. 1998. Oxidant-mediated activation of mitogen-activated protein kinases and nuclear transcription factors in cardiovascular system: a brief overview. Cell Signal 10:675–683.
9. Kamata H, Hirata H. 1999. Redox regulation of cellular signaling. Cell Signal 11:1–14.
10. Widmann C, Gibson S, Jarpe MB, Johnson GL. 1999. Mitogen-activated protein kinase: Conservation of a three-kinase module from yeast to human. Physiol Rev 79:143–180.
11. Seger R, Krebs EG. 1995. The MAPK signaling cascade. FASEB J 9:726–735.
12. Toker A, Cantley LC. 1997. Signaling through the lipid products of phosphoinositide-3-OH-kinase. Nature (Lond) 387:673–676.
13. Fruman DA, Meyers RE, Cantley LC. 1998. Phosphoinositide kinase. Annu Rev Biochem 67:481–507.
14. Vanhaesebroeck B, Stein RC, Waterfield MD. 1996. The study of phosphoinositide function. Cancer Surv 27:249–270.
15. Saward L, Zahradka P. 1997. Angiotensin II activates phosphatidylinositol 3-kinase in vascular smooth muscle cells. Circ Res 81:249–257.
16. Cotter PJ, Woodgett JR. 1998. Protein kinase B (c-Akt): a multifunctional mediator of phosphatidylinositol 3-kinase activation. Biochem J 335:1–13.
17. Cohen P, Alessi DR, Cross DAE. 1997. PDK1, one of the missing links in insulin signal transduction. FEBS Lett 410:3–10.
18. Cross DAE, Alessi DR, Vandenheede JR, McDowell HE, Hundal HS, Cohen P. 1994. The inhibition of glycogen synthase kinase-3 by insulin or insulin-like growth factor 1 in the rat skeletal muscle cell line L6 is blocked by wortmannin but not repamycin: Evidence that wortmannin blocks activation of the mitogen-activated protein kinase pathway between ras and raf. Biochem J 303:21–26.
19. Hurel SJ, Rochford JJ, Borthwick AC, Wells AM, Vandenheede JR, Turnbull DM, Yeaman SJ. 1996. Insulin action in cultured human myoblasts: contribution of different signaling pathways to regulate glycogen synthesis. Biochem J 320:871–877.
20. Welsh GI, Foulstone EJ, Young SW, Tavare JM, Proud CG. 1994. Wortmannin inhibits the effects of insulin and serum on the activities of glycogen synthase kinase-3 and mitogen-activated protein kinase. Biochem J 303:15–20.
21. Uehara T, Tokumitsu Y, Nomura Y. 1995. Wortmannin inhibits insulin-induced ras and mitogen-activated protein kinase activation related to adipocyte differentiation in 3T3-L1 fibroblasts. Biochem Biophys Res Commun 210:574–580.

22. Standaert ML, Bandyopadhayay G, Farese RV. 1995. Studies with wortmannin suggest a role for phosphatidylinositol 3-kinase in the activation of glycogen synthase and mitogen-activated protein kinase by insulin rat adipocytes: comparison of insulin and protein kinase C modulators. Biochem Biophys Res Commun 209:1082–1088.

23. Fialkow L, Chan CK, Rotin D, Grinstein S, Downey GP. 1994. Activation of mitogenactivated protein kinase signaling pathway in neutrophils: role of oxidants. J Biol Chem 269:31234–31242.

24. Guyton KZ, Liu Y, Gorospe M, Xu Q, Holbrook NJ. 1996. Activation of mitogen-activated protein kinase by H_2O_2. Role in cell survival following oxidant injury. J Biol Chem 271:4138–4142.

25. Samanta S, Perkinton MS, Morgan M, Williams RJ. 1998. Hydrogen peroxide enhances signal-responsive arachidonic acid release from neurons: role of mitogen-activated protein kinase. J Neurochem 70:2082–2090.

26. Servant MJ, Giasson E, Meloche S. 1996. Inhibition of growth factor induced protein synthesis by a selective MEK inhibitor in aortic smooth muscle cells. J Biol Chem 271:16047–16052.

27. Ushio-Fukai M, Alexander RW, Akers M, Griendling KK. 1998. P^{38} mitogen-activated protein kinase is a critical component of the radox-sensitive signaling pathways activated by angiotensin II. Role in vascular smooth muscle cell hypertrophy. J Biol Chem 273:15022–15029.

28. Baas AS, Berk BC. 1995. Differential activation of mitogen-activated protein kinases by H_2O_2 and O_2 in vascular smooth muscle cell. Circ Res 77:29–36.

29. Abe J-I, Kusuhara M, Ulevitch RJ, Berk BC, Lee J-D. 1996. Big mitogen-activated protein kinase 1 (BMK1) is a redox-sensitive kinase. J Biol Chem 271:16586–16590.

30. Kimes BW, Brandt BL. 1976. Characterization of two putative smooth muscle cell lines from rat thoracic aorta. Exp Cell Res 98:349–366.

31. Lutz W, Sanders M, Salisbury J, Kumar R. 1990. Internalization of vasopressin analogs in kidney and smooth muscle cells: evidence for receptor-mediated endocytosis in cells with V2 and V1 receptors. Proc Natl Acad Sci USA 87:6507–6511.

32. Muldoon LL, Rodland KD, Forsythe ML, Magun BE. 1989. Stimulation of phosphatidylinositol hydrolysis, diacylglycerol release, and gene expression in response to endothelin, a potent new agonist for fibroblasts and smooth muscle cells. J Biol Chem 264:8529–8536.

33. Tan CM, Xenoyannis S, Feldman RD. 1995. Oxidant stress enhances adenylyl cyclase activation. Circ Res 77:710–717.

34. Pandey SK, Anand-Srivastava MB, Srivastava AK. 1998. Vanadyl sulfate-stimulated glycogen synthesis is associated with activation of phosphatidylinositol 3-kinase and is independent of insulin receptor tyrosine phosphorylation. Biochemistry 37:7006–7014.

35. Palaparti A, Anand-Srivastava MB. 1996. Modulation of ANF-R2/ANP-C receptors by angiotensin II in vascular smooth muscle cells. Am J Hypertens 9:930–934.

36. Alessi DR, Cuenda A, Cohen P, Dudley DT, Saltiel AR. 1995. PD98059 is a specific inhibitor of the activation of mitogen activated protein kinase kinase in vitro and in vivo. J Biol Chem 270:27489–27494.

37. Knall C, Young S, Nick JA, Buhl AM, Worthen GS, Johnson GL. 1996. Interleukin-8 regulation of the ras/raf/mitogen-activated protein kinase pathway in human neutrophils. J Biol Chem 271:2832–2838.

38. Karnitz LM, Burns LA, Sutor SL, Blenis J, Abraham RT. 1995. Interleukin-2 triggers a novel phosphatidylinositol 3-kinase-dependent MEK activation pathway. Mol Cell Biol 15:3049–3057.

39. Ui M, Okada T, Hazeki K, Hazeki O. 1995. Wortmannin as a unique probe for an intracellular signaling protein, phosphoinositol 3-kinase. Trends Biochem Sci 20:303–307.

40. Clerk A, Fuller SJ, Michael A, Sugden PH. 1998. Stimulation of "stress-regulated" mitogen-activated protein kinases (stress-activated protein kinases/c-Jun N-terminal kinases and p^{38} mitogen-activated protein kinases) in perfused rat hearts by oxidative and other stresses. J Biol Chem 273:7228–7234.

41. Aikawa R, Komuro I, Yamazaki T, Zou Y, Kudoh S, Tanaka M, Shiojima I, Hiroi Y, Yazaki Y. 1997. Oxidative stress activates extracellular signal regulated kinases through src and ras in cultured cardiac myocytes of neonatal rats. J Clin Invest 100:1813–1821.

42. Abe MK, Kartha S, Karpova AY, Li J, Liu PT, Kuo W-L, Hershenson MB. 1998. Hydrogen peroxide activates extracellular signal-regulated kinase via protein kinase C, raf-1 and MEK-1. Am J Respir Cell Mol Biol 18:562–569.

43. Stone RL, Dixon JE. 1994. Protein tyrosine phosphatases. J Biol Chem 269:31323–31326.

44. Wu Y, Kwon K-S, Rhe SG. 1998. Probing cellular protein targets of H_2O_2 with fluorescein-conjugated iodoacetamide and antibodies to fluorescein. FEBS Lett 440:111–115.

45. Hecht D, Zick Y. 1992. Selective inhibition of protein tyrosine phosphatase activity by H_2O_2 and vanadate in vitro. Biochem Biophys Res Commun 188:773–778.

N. Takeda, M. Nagano and N.S. Dhalla
(eds). The Hypertrophied Heart. Copyright
© 2000. pp. 207–216. Kluwer Academic
Publishers. Boston. All rights reserved.

EFFECTS OF RENIN–ANGIOTENSIN SYSTEM INHIBITION ON CARDIAC HYPERTROPHY AND FIBROSIS IN SPONTANEOUSLY HYPERTENSIVE RATS

NAOKI MAKINO, MASAHIRO SUGANO, and SACHIYO TAGUCHI

Department of Bioclimatology and Medicine, Medical Institute of Bioregulation, Kyushu University, 4546 Tsurumihara, Beppu, 874

Summary. The present study examined whether the inhibition of the renin–angiotensin system can change the cardiac remodeling process in spontaneously hypertensive rats (SHR). First, we administered AT_1 blockade (losartan), AT_2 blockade (PD123319), or ACE inhibitor (enalapril) to SHR from 10 to 20 weeks of age. Both losartan and enalapril reduced the arterial systolic blood pressure (BP) as well as the collagen concentration compared with the untreated SHR (U-SHR) to the level of Wistar Kyoto rats (WKY). Both agents also reduced both the left ventricular (LV) weight and the ratio of LV to body weight (BW) compared with the untreated SHR, although these measures were still larger than those of WKY. However, PD123319 was without effect. Second, to inhibit the plasma angiotensinogen (ATN) in SHR, we intravenously injected antisense oligodeoxynucleotides (ODNs) against rat ATN coupled to asialoglyco-protein carrier molecules into SHR (A-SHR) from 10 to 20 weeks via their tail veins twice a week. Both the ATN and Ang II concentrations in plasma decreased in A-SHR compared with those of the sense-treated SHR (S-SHR) or U-SHR. The BP in A-SHR was reduced in comparison with those of S-SHR or U-SHR, although BP in A-SHR was still higher than that in WKY. Both LV weight and the ratio of LV to BW also decreased in A-SHR compared with S-SHR or U-SHR. No difference in the LV collagen concentrations was observed among all SHR groups. These findings showed that ATN inhibition, ACE, and AT_1 blockade could reduce the hypertrophy of myocytes in SHR. However, since the partial BP reduction did not produce changes in the remodeling of matrix tissue, it may be that both the reduction of BP and the inhibition of RAS play a crucial role in cardiac hypertrophy in SHR.

INTRODUCTION

The renin–angiotensin system (RAS) plays an important role in cardiac and vascular development and the process of cardiac hypertrophy [1]. In spontaneously hypertensive rats (SHR), both left ventricular hypertrophy and characteristic vascular resistance properties are already present early in life, based on the results of a comparison with normotensive Wistar-Kyoto rats (WKY), thus suggesting that they play a role in the pathogenesis of hypertension [2,3]. Angiotensin-converting enzyme (ACE) inhibitors can lower the blood pressure in SHR by reducing angiotensin II (Ang II) production and decreasing bradykinin degradation [4,5], but it is thought that most of the observed actions, affecting both blood pressure and cardiovascular hypertrophy, are caused by Ang II generation [6,7].

Specific Ang II receptor antagonists have been developed, including those blocking the AT_1 and AT_2 receptor subtypes, with the aim of affecting the RAS more specifically [8]. The antihypertensive action of losartan is based on the blockade of AT_1 receptors, which are believed to mediate most of the cardiovascular actions of Ang II [9]. AT_2 receptors are also thought to have some role in the maintenance of systemic blood pressure and responsiveness of the cardiovascular system to Ang II [10,11]. However, there is little information regarding the interaction among mRNAs for AT_1 and AT_2 receptors and ACE to the extracellular matrix and the cardiac AT_1 myocyte.

Angiotensinogen (AGT) has also been suggested to be an important determinant of both blood pressure and electrolyte homeostasis [12]. The potential contribution of AGT in the pathogenesis of hypertension has been suggested by genetic approaches [12,13]. AGT is mainly synthesized in the liver and released into the blood. It is cut by renin, which is produced by the kidneys and then becomes Ang I [14]. Ang I is cleaved by ACE into Ang II, which is an active presser substance. Ang II is thus considered to act as a growth-promoting factor in the cardiovascular system [1,6], while it also increases collagen synthesis in the interstitium of the heart [15,16]. The role of AGT in cardiac remodeling has not been determined. We have already showed that intravenous injection with antisense ODNs against AGT coupled to asialoglycoprotein carrier molecules targeted to the liver could inhibit the plasma AGT and Ang II and induce a decrease in the systolic blood pressure in SHR [17]. The present study was therefore undertaken to determine whether the administration of the ACE inhibitor enalapril, the AT_1 receptor losartan, or antisense ODNs against AGT could affect cardiac remodeling in SHR.

METHODS

Animals and experimental protocols

Male SHR at 5 weeks of age ($n = 60$) and age-matched male WKY (each group: $n = 12$) as genetically normotensive control strains were used in this study. All animals were housed in a temperature-humidity-, and light-controlled room, and a standard rat diet plus water was provided ad libitum. Systolic blood pressure and heart rate were measured once a week using the tail-cuff method, and body weight was also checked. The AT_1 receptor antagonist losartan or the AT_2 receptor antagonist PD123319 [18] was administered daily to SHR from 10 weeks of age, when cardiac hypertrophy had not yet developed, administration of the agent was continued until 20 weeks of age. The doses of losartan were administered at 40 mg/kg/day ($n = 11$), and PD123319 was given at 100 mg/kg/day ($n = 10$). Other

SHR were treated with the ACE inhibitor enalapril (30 mg/kg/day, $n = 10$) or vehicle ($n = 10$) from 10 weeks of age. All drugs were administered daily to SHR in water. The 18 other eighteen SHR were divided into three groups (six animals in each group) at 10 weeks of age, among which the systolic blood pressure did not significantly change. The control group was injected with saline, the sense group was injected with asialoglycoprotein (ASOR)-poly(L)lysine-sense ODNs complex, and the antisense group was injected with ASOR-poly(L)lysine-antisense ODNs complex, and all animals were fed until 20 weeks. Five WKY were also injected with saline from 10 to 20 weeks of age (Standard group). ASOR-poly(L)lysine-antisense ODNs complex were injected via the tail veins twice a week. The amount of ODNs injected was 20 μg for each rat. The sequences of oligodeoxynucleotides (ODNs) against rat AGT and asialoglycoprotein–poly(L)lysine–ODN complex used in this study were same as described previously [17]. At the end of the treatment with each drug, the body weight and the blood pressure were measured.

Biochemical assays

ACE activity was measured by the modified method of Hayakari et al. [19]. Myocardial collagen content was measured by the hydroxyproline concentration of tissue, as described by Bergman and Loxley [20]. Plasma AGT and Ang II concentrations were measured as described previously [17].

Measurement of mRNAs

Total RNA was isolated from the LV tissues with an RNAzolB solution (Biotex, Friendswood, TX) according to the manufacturer's procedure. ACE, AT_1, and AT_2 mRNAs were measured by the reverse transcription polymerase chain reaction (RT-PCR) as described previously [17,21], except for the fact that in the present study, fluorescent 11-dUTP (Boehringer, Japan) was used to label the PCR product. The amplification profile involved denaturation at 95°C for 1 minute, annealing at 58°C for 1 minute, and extension at 72°C for 1 minute. After we examined the relation between the amount of RT-PCR products and the PCR cycles (after determining the efficiency of amplification) in each mRNA, the PCR cycles for determining the amount of each mRNA were determined. For ACE, the sense primer was 5′-CACCCTCTCGCTACAACTACG-3′, the antisense primer was 5-′CCTCGCCATTCCGCTGATTCT-3′, and the PCR product size was 408 bp for 27 cycles. For the AT_1-receptor, the sense primer was 5′-GCCAAAGTCACCTG-CATCAT-3′, the antisense primer was 5′-AATTTTTTCCCCAGAAAGCC-3′, and the PCR product size was 494 bp for 27 cycles. For the AT_2 receptor, the sense primer was 5′-TGAGTCCGCATTTAACTGC-3′, the antisense primer was 5′-ACCACTGAGCATATTTCTCAG-3′, and the PCR product size was 436 bp for 28 cycles. For glyceraldehyde-3-phosphate-dehydrogenase (GAPDH) as an inner control, the sense primer was 5′-GGTCTACATGTTCCAGTATG-3′, the antisense primer was 5′-TAAGCAGTTGGTGGTGCAGG-3′, and the PCR product size was 343 bp for 16 cycles. The abundance of hepatic AGT mRNA was determined by a

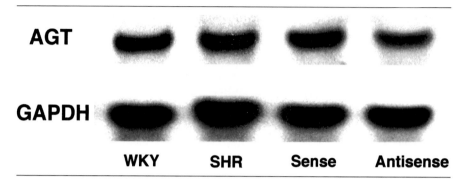

Figure 1. Representative Northern blot analyses of angiotensinogen mRNA in the liver from WKY, untreated SHR, and SHR injected with sense or antisense ODNs at the end of study. GAPDH mRNA is an internal control.

Northern blot analysis using the DIG detection system (Boehringer, Japan) after poly (A+) RNA was isolated from the total RNA with Oligotex Super (Rosche, Japan). The rat cDNA probes for AGT and GAPDH mRNA were produced by the reverse transcription polymerase chain reaction (RT-PCR) according to the rat sequence, as described previously [17]. The labeled cDNA probes were produced using the DIG random prime labeling system (Boehringer, Japan).

Statistical analysis

The data are given as the mean ± SEM. Comparisons among three or more groups were made using a one-way ANOVA followed by Dunnetts' modified t-test. A value of $p < 0.05$ was considered to be statistically significant.

RESULTS

Figure 1 shows a typical example of Northern blot analyses of hepatic mRNAs in each group. When the amount of hepatic AGT mRNA was measured by scanning and was expressed as a ratio to GAPDH mRNA, a significant reduction of hepatic AGT mRNA was observed only in the SHR injected with antisense ODNs compared with WKY, the untreated SHR, and the SHR injected with sense ODNs.

Table 1 summarizes the characteristics of WKY and SHR at the end of the treatment with losartan, PD123319, enalapril, the sense ODN, or the antisense ODN against AGT. In the untreated SHR, both the left ventricular (LV) weight and the LV-to-body weight (BW) ratios were significantly ($p < 0.05$) higher than those of WKY aged 20 weeks. The systolic blood pressure (BP) in the 20-week-old SHR was also higher than that in WKY. The administration of losartan or enalapril to SHR normalized BP, which was brought to the levels of WKY. However, both the LV weight and the LV/BW ratio in the treatment were significantly reduced compared with the untreated SHR, but remained well above the level of WKY. The administration of PD123319 had no effect on the LV weight or the LV/BW ratio. Thus, AT$_2$ blockade did not reduce BP and did not decrease the LV weight in SHR.

Table 1. Left ventricular weight, left ventricle to body
weight ratio, and systolic blood pressure in the experimental groups

Group	LV weight (mg)	LV/body weight ratio (mg/g)	SBP (mmHg)
WKY	932 ± 40	2.48 ± 0.05	141 ± 4.1
SHR (untreated)	1082 ± 63[a]	2.87 ± 0.06[a]	218 ± 7.1[a]
SHR + losartan	954 ± 23[b]	2.61 ± 0.071[a,b]	152 ± 5.7[b]
SHR + PD	997 ± 19[a]	2.79 ± 0.072[a]	189 ± 7.5
SHR + enalapril	948 ± 21[b]	2.64 ± 0.048[a,b]	150 ± 6.7[b]
Sense ATN	1061 ± 40[a]	2.78 ± 0.07[a]	220 ± 4.7[a]
Antisense ATN	957 ± 35[a,b]	2.60 ± 0.05[a,b]	177 ± 4.5[a,b]

[a] $p < 0.05$ compared with WKY.
[b] $p < 0.05$ compared with the untreated SHR.
Each value represents the mean ± SE of six experiments. The administration dosages of losartan, PD123319 (PD), and enalapril were 40, 100, and 30 mg/kg/day, respectively. The sense or antisense ODNs for angiotensinogen (ATN) were injected in 10- to 20-week-old SHR. LV, left ventricle; SBP, systolic blood plessure.

Table 2. Plasma angiotensin converting enzyme (ACE) activity and plasma levels of
angiotensinogen and angiotensin II at the end of treatment in the experimental groups

	ACT activity (nmol/mim/mL)	Angiotensinogen (pmol/mL)	Angiotensin II (pmol/mL)
WKY	53 ± 2.8	442 ± 20.8	22.3 ± 1.9
SHR (untreated)	94 ± 4.4[a]	456 ± 21.4	38.7 ± 2.0[a]
SHR + losartan	87 ± 4.2[a]	428 ± 24.2	44.5 ± 2.2[a,b]
SHR + PD	91 ± 3.6[a]	441 ± 19.5	39.4 ± 2.1[a]
SHR + enalapril	19 ± 0.8[a,b]	435 ± 20.2	36.6 ± 2.4[a]
Sense ATN	88 ± 4.2[a]	448 ± 22.3	37.9 ± 2.2[a]
Antisense ATN	89 ± 3.7[a]	266 ± 18.1[a,b]	19.0 ± 2.1[b]

[a] $p < 0.05$ vs. WKY.
[b] $p < 0.05$ vs. untreated SHR.
The values are the mean ± SE of six experiments. The administration dosage of losartan, PD123319 (PD), and enalapril were 40, 100, and 30 mg/kg/day, respectively. The sense or antisense ODNs for angiotensinogen (ATN) were injected into 10- to 20-week-old SHR.

The LV weight and the LV/BW ratio were significantly reduced in SHR injected with antisense ODNs compared with untreated SHR or with SHR injected with sense ODNs, but were not reduced to the levels of WKY. The administration of antisense ODNs to SHR significantly reduced BP, which was still higher than that of WKY. However, the administration of sense ODNs had no effect on BP.

Table 2 shows the ACE activity and AGT and Ang II concentrations from the plasma in the experimental animals. The ACE activity in the untreated SHR was significantly increased by 77% in the plasma when compared with WKY. These activities were not significantly different among the untreated SHR and the SHR treated with losartan, PD12377, or sense or antisense injected ODNs. However, the ACE activity in the enalapril-treated SHR significantly decreased in both plasma levels (79%) compared with the untreated SHR. The plasma AGT levels were only

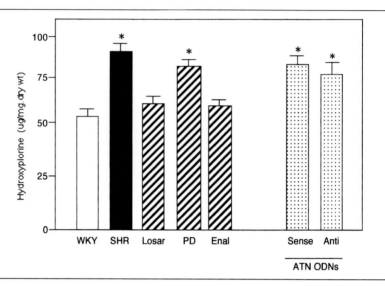

Figure 2. The bar graphs show the hydroxyproline concentration in the left ventricle from WKY or the experimental SHR. Each values is the mean ± SE of six experiments. Losar, losartan; PD, PD123319; Enal, enalapril. ★, $p < 0.05$ vs WKY.

reduced in the SHR injected with antisense ODNs compared to WKY, untreated SHR, and the sense-injected SHR. On the other hand, in the losartan-treated SHR, these levels were significantly increased compared with the untreated SHR. The plasma Ang II levels were more elevated in the untreated SHR than those of WKY. These levels in the antisense-injected SHR significantly decreased to the level of WKY compared to the untreated SHR or the sense-injected SHR.

The hydroxyproline concentration in LV tissue from each group was also studied (figure 2). This concentration significantly increased in SHR in comparison to WKY and significantly decreased in the samples obtained from SHR treated with losartan or enalapril to the same extent (20%), compared with the untreated SHR. The administration of PD12377 did not affect this concentration. There were no significant difference among the untreated, sense-injected, and antisense-injected SHR.

The levels of AT_1, AT_2, and ACE mRNA expression were detected in the left ventricles in each experimental group by the RT-PCR method. The GAPDH signals used as internal controls appeared to be unchanged in these experimental rats. An apparent higher level in AT_1 mRNA was also seen in the myocardium of SHR (figure 3), whereas with a high dose of losartan (40 mg/kg/day), the mRNA level of the SHR was significantly restored to the level of WKY. Although the levels of AT_1 mRNA did not change in the SHR treated with enalapril, this gene expression was significantly reduced with PD123319 in compared with untreated SHR. The AT_2 mRNA was not significantly different between the WKY and the untreated SHR. However, the administration of losartan or PD123319 to the SHR reduced

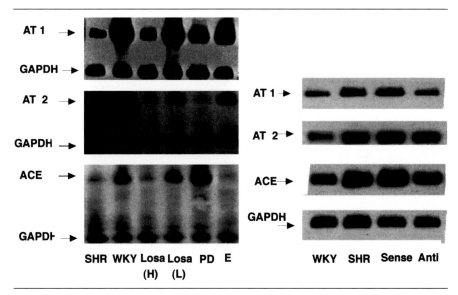

Figure 3. Detection of AT_1, ACE, and AT_2 mRNA expressions by RT-PCR. GAPDH mRNA is an internal control. Losa (high) and Los (low) indicate the SHR group treated with a high concentration of losartan (40 mg/kg/day) and a low concentration of losartan (10 mg/kg/day), respectively. PD, PD123319; E, enalapril; sense, SHR injected with sense ODNs for angiotensinogen; Anti, SHR injected with antisense ODNs for angiotensinogen.

the level of AT_2 mRNA compared with the untreated SHR. The ACE mRNA increased in the untreated SHR compared with WKY. The level of ACE mRNA also significantly decreased in SHR after being treated with losartan or enalapril. The ACE mRNA expression by PD12377 treatment was also more enhanced than that in the untreated SHR. Those three expressions were not significantly different among the untreated SHR and the SHR injected with sense or antisense ODNs.

DISCUSSION

The present study demonstrates that chronic treatment with losartan and enalapril normalized BP. An injection of antisense ODN complex for ATN also induced the reduction of BP. Those treatments attenuated both LV weight and LV/BW in SHR, which were still above the corresponding levels in WKY. In contrast, the hydrox-yproline concentration in the heart was nearly normalized by losartan and enalapril, but not by an injection of antisense ODN complex. These observations suggest that the RAS has a more important effect on cardiac remodeling in SHR and indicate that cardiac remodeling is different at the site of RAS inhibition.

It is well known that ACE inhibitors induce the regression of hypertrophied hearts both in experimental studies and in humans through either a blood pressure-dependent or a blood pressure-independent mechanism [1,4,6]. In the renovascular hypertensive rat model, ramipril treatment was associated with a complete inhibition of cardiac fibrosis. This antifibrotic effect was also present with low doses of ramipril that did not lower BP [22]. Thus, there are several studies in which the effects of ACE inhibitors on cardiac and vascular functions were independent of their antihypertensive and antihypertrophic actions [23,24].

In the present study, regression of both cardiac hypertrophy and fibrosis was found in SHR treated with enalapril or losartan. Treatment with AT_1 receptor antagonists was associated with a regression of cardiac hypertrophy and fibrosis in animal models of SHR and with a decrease in renovascular hypertension as well in hypertensive patients [7,9]. AT_1 blockade induced cardiac regression and a fall in blood pressure in SHR, in contrast to hydralazine, despite the greater blood pressure reduction with the latter drug [25]. These observations thus suggested that the regression of cardiac hypertrophy was mainly carried out by the inhibition of the effects of Ang II in cardiac tissue. PD123319 did not affect either the systolic blood pressure or the LV weight and collagen concentration in the present study. These results thus indicate that the AT_1 receptor rather than the AT_2 receptor may be more important in cardiac growth and the development of hypertrophy. These findings mean that Ang II taken up through the AT_1 receptor in the heart is important for the extracellular matrix and for collagen accumulation and regulation of blood pressure. It was recently reported that the AT_2 receptor modulates antigrowth effects in vascular smooth muscle [26], endothelial cells [27], and programmed cell death [28]. The present study showed that AT_2 mRNA was similar in 20-week-old SHR and WKY. However, AT_1 blockade by losartan significantly reduced the expression of AT_1 and AT_2 mRNA in the present study.

Our findings also suggest that plasma AGT has an important effect on myocyte hypertrophy and the extracellular matrix in the heart. The asialoglycoprotein carrier moiety used in the present study was efficiently targeted to the asialoglycoprotein receptor on hepatocytes [29,30]. Although we did not evaluate either the transfection efficacy or the stability of this antisense–protein conjugate in the present study, Lu et al. [31] demonstrated that the biodistribution pattern is consistent with the mechanism of specific uptake of the conjugate by the liver. The plasma AGT levels presented here did not differ between adult SHR and WKY, as was already described by Lodwiick et al. [32], but the plasma ACE and Ang II levels were more elevated in SHR than in WKY. The plasma AGT levels in the antisense-injected SHR were reduced in spite of the high plasma ACE activity, while the plasma Ang II levels decreased to the level of WKY rats. AGT is cut by renin and then becomes angiotensin I [14], which is cleaved by ACE into Ang II. Although the plasma Ang II concentration was reduced in antisense-injected SHR or enalapril-treated SHR, this concentration was increased in losartan-treated SHR. We cannot therefore explain the regression of hypertrophy by Ang II alone. The antisense therapy did not affect the hydroxyproline concentration in the LV tissue of SHR but did induce the reduction of collagen, although this measure remained well above the level in WKY rats. Also, BP reduction by antisense therapy was not to the levels of WKY; on the other hand, the addition of enalapril or losartan to SHR completely reduced

BP to the level of WKY and inhibited the production of cardiac fibrosis. Thus, the antisense therapy produced incomplete BP reduction, and therefore this therapy may not exert an inhibitory action on collagen metabolism and growth of cardiac fibroblasts. From our results, when the suppression of hypertension was insufficient in SHR, cardiac regression was partially shown, even though plasma Ang II levels decreased to the level of WKY.

ACKNOWLEDGMENT

This work was supported in part by a Grant-in-Aid from the Ministry of Education, Science and Culture of Japan.

REFERENCES

1. Baker KM, Booz GW, Dostal DE. 1992. Cardiac actions of angiotensin II: role of an intracardiac renin–angiotensin system. Annu Rev Physiol 54:227–241.
2. Adams MA, Bobik A, Korner PI. 1989. Differential development of vascular and cardiac hypertrophy in genetic hypertension: relation to sympathetic function. Hypertension 14:191–202.
3. Korner P, Bobik A, Oddie C, Friberg P. 1993. Sympathoadrenal system is critical for structural changes in genetic hypertension. Hypertension 22:243–252.
4. Gohlke P, Linz W, Scholkens BA, Kuwer I, Bartenbach S, Schnell A, Unger T. 1994. Angiotensin-converting enzyme inhibitions improves cardiac function: role of bradykinin. Hypertension 23:411–418.
5. Johnson CI. 1994. Tissue angiotensin converting enzyme in cardiac and vascular hypertrophy, repair, and remodeling. Hypertension 23:258–268.
6. Schunkert H, Sadoshima J, Cornelius T, Kagaya Y, Weinberg EO, Izumo S, Riegger G, Lorell BH. 1995. Angiotensin II-induced growth responses in isolated adult rat hearts: evidence for load-independent induction of cardiac protein synthesis by angiotensin II. Circ Res 76:489–497.
7. Suzuki J, Matsubara H, Urakami M, Inada M. 1993. Rat angiotensin II (type 1A) receptor mRNA regulation and subtype expression in myocardial growth and hypertrophy. Circ Res 73:439–447.
8. Yoshida H, Kakuchi J, Guo DF, Furuta H, Iwai N, Jong R, Inagami T, Ichikawa I. 1992. Analysis of the evolution of angiotensin II type 1 receptor gene in mammals (mouse, rat, bovine and human). Biochem Biophys Res Commun 186:1042–1049.
9. Gottlieb SS, Dickstein K, Fleck E, Kostis J, Levine B, LeJemtel T, DeKock M. 1993. Hemodynamic and neurohumoral effects of the angiotensin II antagonist losartan in patients with congestive heart failure. Circulation 88(pt 1):1602–1609.
10. Ichiki T, Labosky PA, Shiota C, Okuyama S, Inagawa Y, Fogo A, Niimura F, Ichikawa I, Hogan BLM, Inagami T. 1995. Effects on blood pressure and exploratory behavior of mice lacking angiotensin II type-2 receptor. Nature 377:748–750.
11. Hei L, Barsh GS, Pratt RE, Dzau VJ, Koblika BK. 1995. Behavioural and cardiovascular effects of disrupting the angiotensin II type-2 receptor gene in mice. Nature 377:744–747.
12. Jeunemaitre X, Soubrier F, Kotelevetsev YV, Lifton RP, Williams CS, Charru A, Hunt SC, Hopkins PN, Williams RR, Lalouel JM, Corvol P. 1992. Molecular basis of human hypertension: role of angiotensinogen. Cell 71:169–180.
13. Caulfield M, Lavender P, Farrall M, Munroe P, Lawson M, Turner P, Clark A. 1994. Linkage of the angiotensinogen gene to essential hypertension. N Engl J Med 330:1629–1633.
14. Lynch KR, Peach MJ. 1991. Molecular biology of angiotensinogen. Hypertension 17:263–269.
15. Panizo A, Pardo J, Hernandez M, Galindo MF, Cenarruzabeitia E, Diez J. 1995. Quinapril decreases myocardial accumulation of extracellular matrix components in spontaneously hypertensive rats. Am J Hypertens 8:815–822.
16. Keeley FW, Elmoselhi A, Leenen FHH. 1992. Enalapril supresses normal accumulation of elastin and collagen in cardiovascular tissues of growing rats. Am J Physiol 262:H1013–H1021.
17. Makino N, Sugano M, Ohtsuka S, Sawada S. 1998. Intravenous injection with antisense oligodeoxynucleotides against angiotensinogen decreases both the blood pressure and plasma angiotensin II levels. Hypertension 31:1166–1170.

18. Widdop RE, Gardiner SM, Kemp PA, Benett T. 1993. Central administration of PD123319 or EXP-3174 inhibits effects of angiotensin II. Am J Physiol 264(Heart Circ Physiol 33):H117–H125.
19. Hayakari M, Kondoh Y, Ihumi H. 1978. A rapid and simple spectrophotometric assay of angiotensin-converting enzyme. Anal Biochem 84:361–369.
20. Bergman I, Loxley R. 1961. Two improved and simplified methods for the spectrophotometric determination of hydroxyproline. Anal Chem 35:1961–1965.
21. Makino N, Sugano M, Otsuka S, Hata T. 1997. Molecular mechanism of angiotensin II type I and type II receptors in cardiac hypertrophy of spontaneously hypertensive rats. Hypertension 30:796–802.
22. Nagasawa K, Zimmermamm R, Munkel B, Linz W, Scholkens B, Schaper J. 1995. Extracellular matrix deposition in hypertensive hearts: antifibrotic effects of ramipril. Eur Hear J 16(Suppl C):33–37.
23. Makino N, Sugano M, Hata T, Yanaga T. 1996. Chronic low dose treatment with enalapril induced cardiac regression of left ventricular hypertrophy. Mol Cell Biochem 164:239–245.
24. Gohlke P, Lamberty V, Kuwer I, Bartenbach S, Schnell A, Linz W, Scholkens BA, Wiemer G, Unger T. 1993. Long-term low-dose angiotensin-converting enzyme inhibition treatment increases vascular cyclic guanine 3′,5′-monophospate. Hypertension 22:682–687.
25. Kojima M, Shiojima I, Yamazaki T, Komuro I, Yunzeng Z, Ying W, Mizuni T, Ueki K, Tobe K, Kadowaki T, Nagai R, Yazaki Y. 1994. Angiotensin II receptor antagonist TCV-116 induces regression of hypertensive left ventricular hypertrophy in vivo and inhibits the intracellular signaling pathway of stretch-mediated cardiomyocytes hypertrophy in vitro. Circulation 89:2204–2211.
26. Nakajima M, Hutchinson HG, Fujinaga M, Hayashida W, Morishita R, Zhang L, Horiuchi M, Pratt RE, Dzau VJ. 1995. The angiotensin II type 2 (AT_2) receptor antagonizes the growth effects of the AT_1 receptor: gain-of-function study using gene transfer. Proc Natl Acad Sci USA 92:10663–10667.
27. Stoll M, Steckelings M, Paul M, Bottari SP, Metzger R, Unger T. 1995. The angiotensin AT_2-receptor mediates inhibition of cell proliferation in coronary endothelial cells. J Clin Invest 95:651–657.
28. Yamada T, Horiuchi M, Dzau V. 1996. Angiotensin II type 2 receptor mediates programmed cell death. Proc Natl Acad Sci USA 93:156–160.
29. Wu GY, Wilson JM, Shalaby F, Grossman M, Shafritz DA, Wu CH. 1991. Receptor-mediated gene delivery in vivo. J Biol Chem 266:14338–14342.
30. Chowdhury NR, Wu CH, Wu GY, Yerneni PC, Bormmineni VR, Chowdhury JR. 1993. Fate of DNA targeted to the liver by asialoglycoprotein receptor-mediated endocytosis in vivo. J Biol Chem 268:11265–11271.
31. Lu XM, Fischman AJ, Jyawook SL, Hendricks K, Tompkins RG, Yarmush ML. 1994. Antisense DNA delivery in vivo: liver targeting by receptor-mediated uptake. J Nucl Med 35:269–275.
32. Lodwick D, Kaiser MA, Harris J, Cumin F, Vincent M, Samani NJ. 1995. Analysis of the role of angiotensinogen in spontaneous hypertension. Hypertension 25:1245–1251.

N. Takeda, M. Nagano and N.S. Dhalla
(eds). The Hypertrophied Heart. Copyright
© 2000. pp. 217–226. Kluwer Academic
Publishers. Boston. All rights reserved.

ADAPTATION OF THE POIKILOTHERMIC HEART TO CATECHOLAMINE-INDUCED OVERLOAD

BOHUSLAV OSTADAL,[1] **VACLAV PELOUCH,**[1] **ARNOST BASS,**[1] **PAVEL PUCELIK,**[2] **and OLGA NOVAKOVA**[3]

[1] *Institute of Physiology, Academy of Sciences of the Czech Republic, Videnska 1083, 142 20 Prague 4;*

[2] *Institute of Physiology, Faculty of Medicine, Charles University, Pilsen, Czech Republic; and* [3] *Department of Physiology and Developmental Biology, Faculty of Science, Charles University, Prague, Czech Republic*

Summary. Excessive release or administration of beta-mimetic catecholamines may induce cardiomegaly, necrotic lesions, and accumulation of connective tissue in the heart of adult homeotherms. The aim of our studies was to analyze whether similar changes can also be observed in the heterogenous heart of poikilothemic animals. Their ventricular myocardium is formed by two different layers: the inner spongious musculature supplied by diffusion from ventricular lumen is covered by an outer compact layer with coronary supply. Sensitivity of the poikilothermic hearts (carp, frog, turtle) to necrogenic doses of isoproterenol (IPRO, 2 × 40 mg/kg/48 h) was significantly lower than in homeotherms. Necrotic lesions, if present, were localized in the inner spongious musculature, which exhibits higher activities of enzymes connected with aerobic oxidation. Repeated administration of lower doses of IPRO (5 mg/kg/day, for 10 days) did not influence the total weight of the fish heart (*Cyprinus carpio*) but significantly increased the absolute weight of the outer compact layer and thus also its proportion (from 33% to 43%) in the whole ventricle. In both layers, the changes were accompanied by a higher water content, an increase of isomyosin with a lower ATPase activity, and an increase of collagenous proteins (types I and III). It may be concluded that the response of the poikilothermic heart to catecholamine-induced overload differs significantly from that in the mammalian myocardium: it results in the remodeling of the cardiac structure without development of cardiac hypertrophy. Whether the described increase of the compact/spongious ratio is the first step or the only mechanism of the adaptation of the poikilothermic heart to overload remains a matter of speculation.

INTRODUCTION

Excessive release or administration of beta-mimetic catecholamines may induce necrotic lesions, cardiomegaly, and accumulation of connective tissue in the heart of adult homeotherms (for reviews, see [1,2]). Since their discovery by Rona et al. [3], isoproterenol (IPRO)-induced cardiac lesions have been demonstrated not only

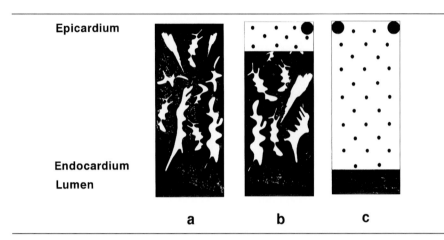

Figure 1. Different types of the myocardial blood supply: (**a**) spongious musculature supplied from the ventricular lumen; (**b**) the inner spongious layer is covered by an outer compact musculature with vascular supply; (**c**) compact musculature supplied from coronary vessels. Data from [20].

in a number of adult mammals, such as dogs [4], hamsters [5], rabbits [6], cats [7], monkeys [8], and mice [9], but also in adult birds [10]. The pathogenesis of catecholamine-induced myocardial lesions is multifactorial; the major hypotheses include a relative hypoxia, coronary microcirculatory effects, altered membrane permeability, myofilament overstimulation, high-energy phosphate deficiency, catecholamine-induced formation of oxidation products, and calcium overload [2].

Whereas abundant data are available concerning the adverse effects of beta-mimetic catecholamines on the heart of adult homeotherms, much less is known about the possible response of the heterogenous heart of poikilotherms, i.e., at a different period of evolution of the cardiovascular system. The aim of this short review is, therefore, (1) to characterize the heterogeneity of the poikilothermic heart, with particular attention to its remodeling due to adaptation to increased work load, and (2) to summarize some of experimental data on the effect of IPRO on the compact and spongious ventricular myocardium of the cold-blooded heart.

HETEROGENEITY OF THE POIKILOTHERMIC HEART

Differences between compact and spongious musculature

While the heart of adult homeotherms consists entirely of a compact musculature with coronary blood supply, the ventricular myocardium of most species of cold-blooded vertebrates is formed by two different muscular layers: the inner avascular spongious musculature, supplied by diffusion from the ventricular lumen, is covered by an outer compact layer with a coronary blood supply ([11–13]; figure 1).

Whereas the water content as well as the protein composition of the two layers is not different [14], the layers differ in many other aspects. The activities of enzymes, connected with aerobic oxidation (citrate synthase, malate dehydrogenase) and

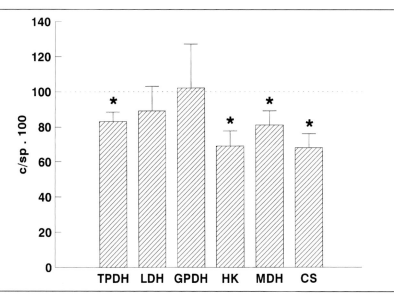

Figure 2. Enzyme activities in the compact layer of the carp heart (expressed as the percentage of the spongious musculature). TPDH, triosephosphate dehydrogenase; LDH, lactate dehydrogenase; GPDH, glycerol-3-phosphate dehydrogenase; HK, hexokinase; MDH, malate dehydrogenase; CS, citrate synthase. *, $p < 0.01$. Data from [14].

glucose phosphorylation (hexokinase), are higher in the spongious musculature as compared with the compact layer [14] (figure 2). Furthermore, Maresca et al. [15] and Greco et al. [16] have demonstrated that differences in enzyme activities are accompanied by different mitochondrial populations in the two layers. Similarly, the content of phopholipids is higher in the spongious musculature, the greatest difference being in the content of diphospatidylglycerol [17]. On the other hand, the myosin ATPase activity (Ca^{2+}-activated) is significantly higher in the compact musculature as compared with the spongious layer of the carp heart [14]. From the basic membrane electrophysiological parameters in the carp heart, resting membrane potential and maximal velocity of depolarization were significantly higher in the compact musculature. On the other hand, the duration of repolarization was significantly longer in the spongious layer at all voltage levels. The administration of tetraethylammonium bromide, which blocks the delayed rectifier potassium current, has revealed that the compact layer is more TEA sensitive [18] (figure 3).

It may be concluded that the structural differences between the compact and spongious ventricular myocardium in the carp heart are accompanied by significant metabolic and electrophysiological changes. The heterogenous heart of cold-blooded animals thus offers a unique opportunity to compare the sensitivity of two defined types of musculature to injury and increased load.

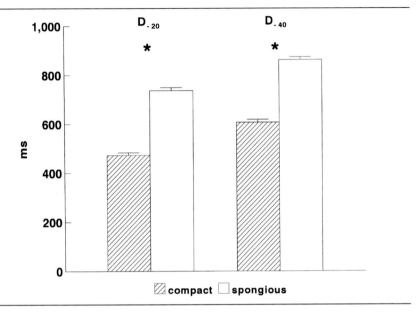

Figure 3. Duration of repolarization at different voltage level in the compact and spongious layer of the carp heart. *, $p < 0.01$. Data from [18].

Growth of the compact layer

In this connection, a question arises about the main determinants of the cardiac transformation from the avascular spongy-like to the compact type with vascular supply. The exclusively spongious type can be observed not only in cyclostomes and some teleost fish but also in some amphibians. On the other hand, the mixed types (compact + spongious) are present in fish (for a review, see [19]), amphibians [20], and reptiles [13,21–23]. It seems, therefore, that the presence of the compact layer is not related to the phylogenetic position of the poikilothermic animals.

More than 25 years ago, an attempt was made to relate the growth of the compact layer to the physiological factors that determine overall oxygen consumption [12,13,20,24]. These factors are body mass, muscular activity, capacity of oxidative metabolism, and maintenance of body temperature. It had been found that the myocardium of fish and amphibians with low body weight is spongious; the thickness of the compact layer increases with increasing heart and body weight. This relation is valid also within the same species investigated, carp and turtle [14] (figure 4). The suggestion that the total amount of the compact layer might be related more to the physiological demand of the species than to its phylogenetic classification has been further supported by an extensive survey by Santer and Greer

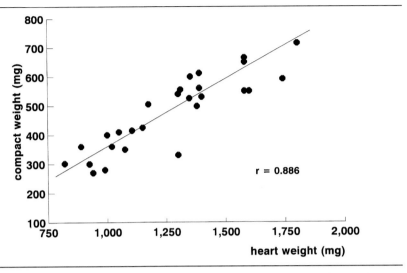

Figure 4. Relation between the weight of the total heart and its compact layer in the carp. Data from [14].

Walker [25]. The proportion of the cardiac wall occupied by coronary supplied compact myocardium varies considerably—e.g., in fish, between 7% and 37% [13,26,27], with the highest proportion in very active species (e.g., tuna, mackerel, sprat, herring, etc.). Moreover, Poupa et al. [28] observed an increase in the thickness of the fish (salmonids) compact myocardium in the course of ontogenetic development. In the turtle, the compact layer composes 55% of the total cardiac weight [14].

Agnisola and Tota [29] analyzed the relationship between the ventricular myoarchitecture and hemodynamic conditions in cold-blooded animals. They compared the stroke volume and afterload in different species with various degree of development of the compact musculature with vascular supply. The entirely spongious frog heart moves relatively large volumes against small pressures; the entirely compact rat left ventricle moves relatively small volumes against high pressures. A similar relationship can be observed among different species of fish; from the spongious heart of icefish with a "volume" pump chamber to that of tuna with mixed (arterial and lacunar) blood supply, as a prototype of a "pressure" pump. The sedentary icefish living in polar seas are characterized by the evolutionary loss of hemoglobin and the lack of functionally significant amounts of myoglobin. This fact is compensated for by a high blood volume, low systemic resistance, and high cardiac output by means of a very large stroke volume at low rate (approximately 16 beats per minute). On the other hand, athletic tuna living in warm tropical water have a cardiovascular system designed to generate a high pressure in high-resistance systemic circulation. The high values are attained, in contrast with icefish, at a heart rate as high as 120 beats per minute. On the basis of these observations, it may be concluded that generation of higher blood volume requires a higher level of ventricular wall stress, which can be better attained by the development and/or thickening of the compact musculature.

All these findings provide additional support for the hypothesis that an increase of the compact layer is necessary for the maintenance of higher blood pressure in the larger hearts (application of the law of Laplace to poikilothermic hearts). This hypothesis also means, however, that the primary evolutionary step is not the development of arterial blood supply but the development of the compact layer, necessary for hemodynamic adaptations, i.e., for higher blood pressure generation. Vascularization is thus the consequence of this evolution, since coronary arteries are the only way to supply the compact musculature with blood.

EFFECT OF BETA-MIMETIC CATECHOLAMINES

Necrotic lesions

The administration of large doses of IPRO ($2 \times 80\,mg/kg$) induced similar myocardial lesions as in adult homeotherms in adult fish [10] and reptiles [30]. The changes typically included myolysis of the muscle fibers, accompanied by marked inflammatory cell infiltration, mainly of a mononuclear character. Unlike reptiles and homeotherms, the fish react to the action of IPRO with some delay, as demonstrated by the fact that necrotic lesions were not observed unless the observation period was extended to 7 days. It is necessary to emphasize that in poikilothermic animals, the IPRO-induced lesions were localized exclusively in the inner spongy-like musculature, which has no vascular supply but which has higher activities of enzymes connected with aerobic oxidation (see above). This suggests that the formation of pathological changes is independent of the presence of vascularization and that the catecholamines act directly on the myocardium. The sensitivity of the poikilothermic heart to the cardiotoxic effect of IPRO was, however, significantly lower as compared with homeotherms: the incidence of necrotic lesions was 100% in rats, pigeons, and chicken, 30% in turtles, and 3% in tench [10].

Frog cardiac muscle was found to be resistant to the necrogenic effect of IPRO [10,31]. This resistance could be abolished by increasing the environmental temperature from +8°C to +25°C; the character of the changes was, however, significantly different. Gross lesions appeared in the form of multiple small aneurysms with paradoxical movements during the heart cycle [32]. For an explanation of this interesting finding, the fact that the predominant neural transmitter in the frog heart is adrenaline and not noradrenaline [33] has to be taken into the consideration. Furthermore, it has been found that catecholamine-induced injury in the frog heart does not affect the sarcolemmal Na^+/Ca^{2+} exchange and is not associated with passive leakage of Ca^{2+} from the extracellular to the intracellular space [34].

Administration of large doses of IPRO in adult homeotherms leads to a change in the phospholipid metabolism, suggesting that the alteration in heart membranes in catecholamine-induced lesions is of crucial importance in determining the functional and structural status of the myocardium (35–37). Okumura et al. [38] found a decrease of total phospholipid content in the rat heart 24 hours after a single (40 mg/kg) dose of IPRO. In contrast to the rat heart, the carp ventricle does not respond to the same high dose of IPRO by diminishing the total phopholipid content 24 hours after treatment [39]. However, a significant (40%) decrease of phosphatidylinositol occurred in the spongious layer, whereas no differences were found in the compact musculature. This observation confirms the above results that spongious musculature is more sensitive to IPRO than the compact musculature.

Adaptation to IPRO-induced overload

The administration of a single or two consecutive doses of IPRO (40 mg/kg) did not affect either the total heart weight or weight proportions of the compact and spongious layer of the poikilothermic (carp) myocardium. Repeated administration of lower doses (15 × 5 mg/kg) did not influence the total weight of the fish heart, but the proportion of the outer compact layer was significantly higher (from 33% to 43%; [39–41]) (figure 5). In both layers, the changes were accompanied by a higher water content, an increase of isomyosin with a lower ATPase activity, and increase of concentration of collagenous proteins (type I and III). This effect, observed both in homeotherms [42] and poikilotherms, may be partly explained by the direct effect of IPRO on collagen synthesis and partly by the development of connective tissue scars [43,44]. A transient decrease of the mitochondrial phospholipid diphosphatidylglycerol (DPG) was more pronounced in the spongious musculature [39].

The response of the poikilothermic heart to catecholamine-induced overload thus differs significantly from homeotherms, where IPRO induces a significant increase of the absolute right and left ventricular weight (rat; [42,45,46]). As described above, the size of the compact layer increased even in intact poikilotherms with increasing body weight, both during ontogeny and in different species. All these results brought forth another piece of evidence that the development of the compact musculature is, in accordance with the law of Laplace, necessary for the maintenance of balanced blood pressure conditions in larger hearts.

CONCLUSIONS

The sensitivity of the heterogenous poikilothermic heart to beta-mimetic catecholamines differs significantly from that of the mammalian myocardium: (1) the poikilothermic heart is less sensitive to the cardiotoxic effect of catecholamines, and the spongious avascular layer is more sensitive than the compact one, and (2) adaptation to catecholamine-induced overload results in the remodeling of the cardiac structure without development of cardiac hypertrophy. Whether the observed

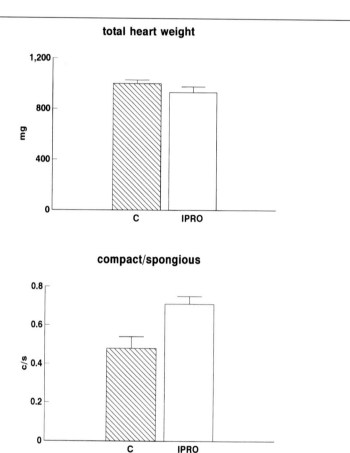

Figure 5. Total heart weight and the ratio of compact weight/spongious weight in controls (C) and isoproterenol (IPRO)-treated (15 × 5 mg/kg) carps. Data from [40,41].

increase of the compact/spongious ratio is the first step or the only mechanism of adaptation of the poikilothermic heart to an overload remains a matter of speculation.

REFERENCES

1. Rona G. 1985. Catecholamine toxicity. J Mol Cell Cardiol 17:291–306.
2. Dhalla NS, Yates JC, Naimark B, Dhalla KS, Beamish RE, Ostadal B. 1992. In Cardiovascular Toxicology. Ed. D Acosta, 239–283. New York: Raven Press.
3. Rona G, Chappel C, Balasz T, Gaudry R. 1959. An infarct-like myocardial lesion and other toxic manifestations produced by isoproterenol in the rat. Arch Pathol 67:443–455.
4. Rona G, Zsoter T, Chappel C, Gaudry R. 1959. Myocardial lesions, circulatory and electrographic changes produced by isoproterenol in the dog. Rev Can Biol 18:83–94.
5. Handforth CP. 1962. Myocardial infarction and necrotizing arteritis in hamsters, produced by isoproterrenol (Isuprel). Med Serv J Can 18:506–512.

6. Amelin AZ, Anshelevich JV, Malzobar MJ. 1963. Experimentalnyje izmenenija miokarda pri vozdějstvii izadrinom (isopropylnoradrenalinom). Arkh Pathol 25:25–30.
7. Rosenblum I, Wohl A, Stein AA. 1965. Studies in cardiac necrosis. I. Production of cardiac lesion with symphathomimetic amines. Toxicol Appl Pharmacol 7:1–8.
8. Maruffo CA. 1967. Fine structural study of myocardial changes induced by isoproterenol in Rhesus monkeys (Macaca mulatta). Am J Pathol 50:27–37.
9. Zbinden G, Moe RA. 1969. Pharmacological studies on heart muscle lesions induced by isoproterenol. Ann NY Acad Sci 156:294–308.
10. Ostadal B, Rychterova V. 1971. Effect of necrogenic doses of isoproterenol on the heart of tench (Tinca tinca—Osteoichthyes), the frog (Rana temporaria—Anura) and the pigeon (Columbia livia—Aves). Physiol Bohemoslov 20:541–547.
11. Benninghoff A. 1933. Herz. In Handbuch vergleich. Anat. Wirbeltiere. Ed. L Bolk, E Göppert, E Killius, W Lubosch, Anat Wirbeltiere, VI Band. Wien, Berlin: Springer Verlag.
12. Poupa O, Ostadal B. 1969. Experimental cardiomegalies and "cardiomegalies" in free living animals. Ann NY Acad Sci 156:445–468.
13. Ostadal B, Schiebler TH. 1971. Über die terminale Strombahn in Fischherzen. Z Anat Entwicklungsgesch 133:288–304.
14. Bass A, Ostadal B, Pelouch V, Vitek V. 1973. Differences in weight parameters, myosin-ATPase activity and the enzyme pattern of energy supplying metabolism between the compact and spongious cardiac musculature of carp (Cyprinus carpio) and turtle (Testudo Horsfieldi). Pflügers Arch 343:65–77.
15. Maresca B, Modigh M, Servillo L, Tota B. 1976. Different temperature dependences of oxidative phosphorylation in the inner and outer layers of tuna heart ventricle. J Comp Physiol 105:167–172.
16. Greco G, Martino G, Tota B. 1982. Further characterization of two mitochondrial populations in tuna heart ventricle. Comp Biochem Physiol 71B:71–75.
17. Drnkova J, Novakova O, Pelouch V, Ostadal B, Kubista V. 1985. Phospholipid content in the compact and spongious musculature of the carp heart (Cyprinus carpio). Physiol Bohemoslov 34:381–384.
18. Ostadal B, Pucelik P, Bass A, Novakova O. In press. Comparison of basic metabolic and electrophysiological parameters in the compact and spongious layer of the carp ventricular myocardium. J Physiol.
19. Santer RM. 1985. Morphology and innervation of the fish heart. Adv Anat Embryol Cell Biol 89:••.
20. Ostadal B, Rychter Z, Poupa O. 1970. Comparative aspects of the development of the terminal vascular bed in the myocardium. Physiol Bohemoslov 19:1–7.
21. Juhasz-Nagy A, Szentivany M, Vamosi B. 1965. Coronary circulation of the tortoise heart. Acta Physiol Hung 23:33–48.
22. Brady AJ, Dubkin Ch. 1964. Coronary circulation in the turtle ventricle. Comp Biochem Physiol 13:119–128.
23. Ostadal B, Schiebler TH. 1971. Die terminale Strombahn im Herzen der Schildkröte (Testudo Hermanni). Z Anat Entwicklungsgesch 134:111–116.
24. Poupa O, Rakusan K, Ostadal B. 1970. The effect of physical activity upon the heart of vertebrates. Med Sport 4:202–233.
25. Santer RM, Greer Walker M. 1980. Morphological studies on the ventricle of teleost and elasmobranch hearts. J Zool (Lond) 190:259–272.
26. Santer RM, Greer Walker M, Emerson L, Witthames PR. 1983. On the morphology of the heart ventricle in marine teleost fish (Teleostei). Comp Biochem Physiol 76[A]:453–459.
27. Sanchez-Quintana D, Hurle JM. 1987. Ventricular myocardial architecture in marine fishes. Anat Record 217:263–273.
28. Poupa O, Gesser H, Jonsson S, Sullivan L. 1974. Coronary-supplied compact shell of ventricular myocardium in salmonids: growth and enzyme pattern. Comp Biochem Physiol 48[A]:85–95.
29. Agnisola C, Tota B. 1994. Structure and function of the fish cardiac ventricle: flexibility and limitations. Cardioscience 5:145–153.
30. Ostadal B, Rychterova V, Poupa O. 1968. Isoproterenol-induced acute experimental cardiac necrosis in the turtle (Testudo Horsfieldi). Am Heart J 76:645–649.
31. Carlsten A, Poupa O, Volkman R. 1983. Cardiac lesions in poikilotherms by catecholamines. Comp Biochem Physiol 76A:567–581.
32. Poupa O, Carlsten S. 1969. Experimental aneurysms of frog heart observed in vivo. In Drugs and Metabolism of Myocardium and Striated Muscle. Ed. M Lamarche and R Royer. 93–98. Nancy.
33. Angelakos ET, King MP, MillardI RW. 1969. Regional distribution of catecholamines in the hearts of various species. Ann NY Acad Sci 156:219–240.

34. Volkmann R. 1983. Electrical activity in frog heart after isoproterenol. Comp Biochem Physiol 76A:593–600.
35. Vorbeck ML, Malewski FF, Erhart LS, Martin AP. 1975. Membrane phospholipid metabolism in the isoproterenol-induced cardiomyopathy in the rat. In Recent Advances in the Study of Cardiac Structure and Metabolism. Ed. A Fleckenstein and G Rona (pp. 175–181). Baltimore: University Press.
36. Dhalla NS, Dzurba A, Pierce GN, Tregaskis MG, Panagia V, Beamish RE. 1983. Membrane changes in myocardium during catecholamine-induced pathological hypertrophy. In Perspectives in Cardiovascular Research. Ed. NR Alpert, 527–534. New York: Raven Press.
37. Dhalla NS, Ganguly PJ, Panagia V, Beamish RE. 1987. Catecholamine-induced cardiomyopathy: alterations in Ca transport systems. In Pathogenesis of Myocarditis and Cardiomyopathy. Ed. C Kawai, WH Abelman, 135–147. Tokyo: University of Tokyo Press.
38. Okumura K, Ogawa K, Satake T. 1983. Pretreatment with chlorpromazine prevents phospholipid degradation and creatine kinase depletion in isoproterenol-induced myocardial damage in rats. J Cardiovasc Pharmacol 5:983–988.
39. Drnkova J, Novakova O, Pelouch V, Ostadal B, Kubista V. 1988. The effect of isoprenaline on the phospholipid content of the compact and spongious musculature of the carp ventricular myocardium. Comp Biochem Physiol 90C:257–261.
40. Pelouch V, Ostadal B, Cerveny M, Prochazka J. 1983. Isoprenaline-induced cardiac enlargement in fish. J Moll Cell Cardiol 15:221.
41. Ostadal B, Pelouch V, Ostadalova I, Novakova O. 1995. Structural and biochemical remodeling in catecholamine-induced cardiomyopathy: comparative and ontogenetic aspects. Mol Cell Biochem 147:83–88.
42. Cihak R, Kolar F, Pelouch V, Prochazka J, Ostadal B, Widimsky J. 1992. Functional changes in the right and left ventricle during the development of cardiac hypertrophy and after its regression. Cardiovasc Res 26:845–850.
43. Collins P, Billings CG, Doly JJ, Jolly A. 1975. Quantitation of isoprenaline induced changes in the ventricular myocardium. Cardiovasc Res 9:797–806.
44. Jalil JE, Doering CW, Janicki JS, Pick R, Shroff SG, Weber KT. 1989. Fibrillar collagen and myocardial stiffness in the intact hypertrophied rat left ventricle. Circ Res 64:1041–1050.
45. Rakusan K, Tietzova H, Turek Z, Poupa O. 1965. Cardiomegaly after repeated application of isoprenaline in the rat. Physiol Bohemoslov 14:456–459.
46. Stanton HC, Brenner G, Mayfield ED. 1969. Studies on isoproterenol-induced cardiomegaly in rats. Am Heart J 77:72–80.

N. Takeda, M. Nagano and N.S. Dhalla
(eds). The Hypertrophied Heart. Copyright
© 2000. pp. 227–241. Kluwer Academic
Publishers. Boston. All rights reserved.

ANGIOGENESIS AND FIBROSIS DURING RIGHT VENTRICULAR HYPERTROPHY IN HUMAN TETRALOGY OF FALLOT

HARI S. SHARMA,[1] ERIK T.H.F. PETERS,[1,2] and AD J.J.C. BOGERS[2]

[1] Department of Pharmacology and [2] Department of Thoracic Surgery, Dijkzigt Hospital, Erasmus University Medical Center Rotterdam, Dr. Molewaterplein 50, 3015 GE Rotterdam, The Netherlands

Summary. Right ventricular hypertrophy (RVH) due to pressure as well as volume overload caused by (sub) pulmonary stenosis and ventricular septal defect is one of the main features in human tetralogy of Fallot (TF). Currently, primary correction at a very young age is the treatment of choice. However, it is not yet known to what extent RVH in TF patients regresses after corrective surgery. The aim of our study was to evaluate the changes in magnitude of the myocardial fibrosis and angiogenesis during RVH in patients undergoing corrective surgery. For this purpose, we examined endomyocardial biopsies for the expression of extracellular matrix proteins such as collagens, fibronectin, and an angiogenic growth factor, vascular endothelial growth factor (VEGF), in TF patients with RVH and compared the expression with patients without RVH. Myocardial tissue biopsies were obtained from patients undergoing primary correction (TF-1 group, mean age 0.4 ± 0.1 years, $n = 8$), from those undergoing secondary surgery (TF-2 group, mean age 38.1 ± 3.7 years, $n = 6$), and from control patients with normal right ventricle (control group, mean age 36.4 ± 1.8 years, $n = 12$). Picro-sirius red staining depicting total collagens and fibronectin staining were semiquantitatively analyzed. Interstitial levels for total collagens were significantly increased in the TF-2 group as compared to the TF-1 group ($p < 0.04$) and control ($p < 0.05$) groups. Immunolocalization of fibronectin showed the expression in the interstitium and perivascular areas. Semiquantitative analysis of fibronectin staining revealed that the expression levels were not significantly different in the TF-2 group as compared to the TF-1 and control groups. Angiogenesis, assessed by the increased number of small ($p < 0.05$) vessels, was observed in both TF groups as compared to the control group. Densitometric analysis of mRNAs encoding VEGF showed significantly enhanced expression in TF-1 ($p < 0.02$) and TF-2 ($p < 0.05$) groups as compared to control. Immunoreactive VEGF was localized mainly in the myocytes and smooth muscle cells and not in fibrotic areas in the case of TF groups. Our results show an increased degree of myocardial fibrosis and angiogenesis during RVH in TF patients. This information leaves room for the improvement in contemporary clinical treatment of patients with TF by allowing an assessment of timing for surgery and possibly supports long-term postoperative prognosis.

INTRODUCTION

With an incidence of 5 per 10,000 live births, tetralogy of Fallot (TF) is a fairly common congenital cardiac anomaly [1]. TF is characterized by overriding of the aorta, a ventricular septal defect, (sub)valvular pulmonary stenosis, and right ventricular hypertrophy (RVH) resulting in hypoxemia due to diminished pulmonary flow [1,2]. Without appropriate treatment, TF ultimately results in cyanotic complications and cardiac failure. For this reason, nearly 70% of patients with TF require an operation during the first year of life. Due to improved perioperative care, the results of primary repair have increased dramatically in the past decade, and such repair is now the surgical treatment of choice [3,4]. Nowadays, most TF patients usually are operated during their first year of life by primary repair. The aim of early primary repair, by closing the ventricular septal defect and removing the right ventricular outflow tract obstruction, is to relieve the hypoxemia and to eliminate the stimulus for the adaptive right ventricular hypertrophy (RVH) as well as to preserve right ventricular function [2–4]. However, some patients suffer from pulmonary regurgitation after primary correction, causing right ventricular failure due to volume overload. For these patients, further secondary corrective surgery later in life is performed by implanting a pulmonary allograft heart valve between the right ventricle and the pulmonary artery [5,6].

Most attention in research on human TF so far has been focused on clinical treatment and surgical methods. In addition, histopathological data on TF myocardial tissue showed a reduction of the myocardial cell diameter in patients after corrective surgery [7]. This would indicate a diminishing degree of RVH. But to what extent the RVH in TF patients finally regresses is still uncertain. Only very limited information is available concerning the complex molecular phenotype of (right ventricular) myocardium in the different stages of TF. In this regard, we have developed strategies to evaluate whether different forms and stages of disease could be correlated with histopathological and molecular biological data. To elucidate the myocardial phenotype and fate of RVH after corrective surgery in patients with TF, we examined the degree of fibrosis and angiogenesis in endomyocardial biopsies obtained during corrective surgery. We investigated the total collagens and fibronectin contents and the expression pattern of an angiogenic glycopeptide, vascular endothelial growth factor (VEGF), and compared the data with those of age-matched patients with a normal right ventricle.

Myocardial hypertrophy

Cellular hypertrophy is an adaptive mechanism in response to chronic hemodynamic overload, leading to remodeling of the myocardium with an increased risk of ultimately developing cardiac failure [8,9]. Histopathological alterations in TF myocardium in patients under 3 years of age have been reported, but data on regression of RVH in the later postoperative period are scarce [10,11]. Recently, a histopathological study on TF myocardial tissue biopsies reported that the myocardial cell diameter was reduced in postoperative patients as compared to preoperative patients with TF, but postoperative cellular diameter was still larger than that in the age-matched normal subjects [7,12]. These findings suggest that RVH after corrective surgery of TF can regress to some extent, provided that residual pulmonary stenosis can be avoided. Until now, no data on molecular markers or their dynamics in RVH in human TF have been available. Several animal models of ventricular hypertrophy [9,13–15] have been described, but none can approximate the TF situation in humans. Experimental animal studies have mainly focused on the morphological and cellular changes in the hypertrophic myocardium in response to volume or pressure overload. A battery of genes, including immediate early genes (such as proto-oncogenes, c-fos, c-jun, c-myc, c-fos) and genes from the foetal period (such as ANF, β-MHC, α-skeletal actin) have been implicated in the cellular alterations leading to ventricular hypertrophy [9,14,15]. It is believed that alterations in gene expression play an important role in myocardial adaptation in response to increased work load [14]. Employing molecular biological methods, we have shown in experimental animal work that a number of genes get induced and reprogrammed during the adaptive phase of myocardium after an ischemic or a hypertrophic stimulus [15–18]. Exploring molecular mechanisms contributing to cardiac hypertrophy, we have recently shown that angiotensin II, a potent vasoconstricting octapeptide, induces expression of transcription factors that precedes an increase in TGF-β_1 in cultured rat cardiac fibroblasts [19]. The information on the complex cascade of molecular mechanisms contributing to right ventricular hypertrophy in humans is very limited and warrants further investigation.

Myocardial fibrosis in TF

Progressive myocardial fibrosis due to cardiac hypertrophy is an important cause of myocardial dysfunction, clinical deterioration, and cardiac death. One of the major contributing factors to myocardial fibrosis is a disproportionate accumulation, either reactive or reparative, of collagens [20–23]. Collagen fibers are organized in the collagen network found in the extracellular space of the myocardium [21,23]. In a morphometrical study, increased fibrosis in TF was associated with an increased diameter of myocytes and an increase in myocardial disarray [11]. In rats, types I and III collagen mRNA were associated with fibroblasts and type IV collagen mRNA with interstitium as well as myocytes [23]. The levels of mRNA encoding for collagen and fibronectin were found to be increased in experimental models of pressure-overloaded cardiac hypertrophy [24]. Studying the expression and localization of genes encoding for fibronectin, collagens, and collagenases at all stages of RVH in TF may further elucidate the dynamics of the collagen network and myocardial fibrosis. Right ventricular hypertrophy with expansion of cardiomyocytes in human TF is an adaptive response to the increased pressure overload caused by (sub) pulmonary stenosis in combination with the ventricular septal defect. This response requires a proportionate increase of coronary flow or growth of the coronary vasculature and leads to remodeling of the myocardium and to development of fibrosis [8,9,25]. Collagens and fibronectin play an important role in myocardial fibrosis. The collagen network, in the extracellular space of the myocardium, consists of collagen fibers, which support the myocardial strength and stiffness [21,22]. When this network is damaged, the myocyte support is compromised and allows tissue expansion [26]. Disproportionate accumulation of collagen, either reactive or reparative, has been observed during myocardial fibrosis. Experimental [27] and clinical data [28] show that a rise in the collagen content increases the myocardial stiffness and promotes abnormalities of cardiac function during hypertrophy. In a morphometrical study, an increase in fibrosis in TF was associated with an increased diameter of myocytes and an increase of myocardial disarray [11].

Fibronectin located in the extracellular matrix of most tissue serves as a bridge between cells and the interstitial collagen mesh network. If further influences diverse processes, including cell growth, adhesion, migration, and wound repair [29]. During the development of cardiac hypertrophy due to pressure overload, fetal fibronectin has been shown to accumulate in rats [24]. In a hypertrophied heart, a significant change in the expression pattern, qualitative as well as quantitative, for several genes has been observed. Focused on fibronectin and collagen, animal studies show an increased level of mRNA during cardiac hypertrophy.

Myocardial angiogenesis

Cardiac hypertrophy, being an adaptive response of cardiomyocytes to increased work load, requires proportionate increase of coronary flow or growth of the coronary vasculature (angiogenesis) [13,30,31]. It has been suggested that mechanical factors such as stretch, shear stress, and wall tension may provide an initial stimulus for capillary angiogenesis during cardiac hypertrophy [13]. A number of peptide growth factors, which are widely attributed to angiogenesis in vivo and in vitro, could play a role in modulating the angiogenesis during cardiac hypertrophy. An increase in mRNA for TGF-β_1 has been reported in cardiac hypertrophy [13]. Virtually nothing is known regarding the molecular mechanisms and role of specific endothelial cell mitogens in cardiac angiogenesis particularly during right ventricular hypertrophy in TF.

MATERIALS AND METHODS

Patient selection and biopsies

The present study was approved by the Medical Ethical Committee of the University Hospital, Erasmus University, Rotterdam. The group operated upon for primary correction of TF (TF-1) consisted of eight patients. The mean age of the TF-1 group at the time of operation was 0.4 ± 0.1 years. The group of patients operated upon for pulmonary allograft implantation late after correction of TF (TF-2) consisted of six patients, with a mean age of 38.1 ± 3.7 years. Their age-matched control group (Control) consisted of 12 patients who were operated upon for a pulmonary autograft replacement and who had a mean age of 36.4 ± 1.8 years. All patients operated upon for a pulmonary autograft procedure showed clinically normal right ventricular function.

All operations were done with the use of cardiopulmonary bypass with moderate hypothermia using bicaval cannulation. In selected cases of both Control and TF-2, single right atrial cannulation was used. The St. Thomas hospital cardioplegic solution was applied except in some of the TF-2 patients, in whom the pulmonary allograft was implanted in the beating heart. In primary correction of TF (TF-1), the aim of preserving pulmonary valve function was met in five patients; a transannular patch was necessary in the remaining three patients. In those with preserved pulmonary valve function, the biopsies consisted of removed endomyocardial tissue from the right ventricular outflow tract. In those patients with a transannular patch, the biopsies consisted of a transmural sample from the incision level of anterior right ventricular wall. In late secondary surgery after correction of TF (TF-2), pulmonary allografts were implanted as previously described [32,33]. Biopsies consisted of tissue from the anterior free wall of the right ventriculotomy. All autograft procedures were done as previously described [34,35]. In harvesting the pulmonary autograft, the main pulmonary artery was transacted just proximal to its bifurcation and through the right ventricular outflow tract, leaving a ridge of supporting myocardial cuff. From the area of the free right ventricular wall of this cuff, the control biopsies were taken as a transmural sample. There was no operative or other early mortality. There were no complications that could be attributed to taking the biopsies.

Part of the myocardial tissue biopsy was immediately frozen in liquid nitrogen for mRNA expression studies, and the other part was fixed in 4% paraformaldehyde in PBS for at least 24 hours and further processed for dehydration and embedding in paraffin for histological and immunohistochemical studies.

Total RNA isolation and Northern blot analysis

Right ventricular tissue biopsies (50–100 mg) were homogenized in guanidinium isothiocyanate buffer and processed for the extraction of total cellular RNA according to the methods described elsewhere [16,17]. The RNA concentration was measured by spectrophotometry, and the quality of RNA was tested on a denatured formaldehyde agarose gel. For Northern hybridization, 15 μg of total RNA was electrophoresed on 1% agarose gel containing 2.2 M formaldehyde, and subsequently, RNA was transferred to hybond-N membrane (Amersham Nederland, Den Bosch, The Netherlands). Thereafter, filters were air dried and UV cross-linked in a gene linker (Bio-Rad Laboratories, Veenendaal, The Netherlands), and ribosomal RNA bands were marked under UV light. Blots were hybridized with a radioactively labeled cDNA probe encoding human VEGF [36] at 42°C in a buffer containing 50% deionized formamide, 1.0 M sodium chloride, 1% sodium dodecylsulfate (SDS), 0.2% polyvinyl pyrrolidone, 0.2% ficoll, 0.2% bovine serum albumin, 50 mM Tris-HCl (pH 7.5), 0.1% sodium pyrophosphate, 10% dextran sulfate and denatured salmon sperm DNA (100 μg/mL). Filters were washed at room temperature for 5 minutes in 2×SSC (1×SSC = 150 mM NaCl, 15 mM trisodium citrate) containing 0.1% SDS and at 55°C in 0.1×SSC containing 0.1% SDS for 20 minutes. Subsequently, filters were wrapped in household plastic wrap and exposed to Kodak X-

OMAT AR films (Kodak Nederland, Odijk, The Netherlands) at −80°C for 1–3 days. A glyceraldehyde-3-phosphate dehydrogenase (GAPDH) cDNA probe encoding human enzyme (ATCC, Rockville, MD, USA) was used to rehybridize membranes for references purposes. Hybridization signals on autoroadiographs were quantified by video scanning in optical density mode using a densitometer (LKB-Pharmacia Biotech, Roosendaal, The Netherlands). For normalization, the optical density (OD) of the hybridization signal for VEGF was divided by the OD of the corresponding GAPDH signal, and relative percentages of mRNA levels were calculated in each group relative to control.

Picro-sirius Red staining

The total collagen in myocardial tissue specimens was stained with Picro-sirius Red F3BA [21,37]. Tissue sections of 6 μm thickness were treated with 0.2% aqueous phosphomolybdic acid and incubated in 0.1% Prico-sirius Red. Before dehydration, the slides were treated with 0.01 N HCl and mounted. Slides were visualized under a light microscope using a polarized filter, and eventually collagen contents were quantified.

Immunohistochemistry

Expression of fibronectin

Paraffin sections (6 μm thickness) of the myocardial tissues were cut and mounted on 3-amino-propyl-trioxysilane (Sigma, St. Louis, MO, USA) coated glass slides. Immunohistochemistry using a multiple-step avidin–biotin complex (ABC) method was performed, essentially following the supplier's instructions. In brief, after deparaffinization in xylene and rehydration through graded alcohol, the slides were rinsed with water and phosphate buffered saline and were quenched for endogenous peroxidase by 2% hydrogen peroxide in methanol. The slides were placed in Sequeza Immunostaining Workstation (Shandon Scientific Ltd, Astmoor, Runcorn). Slides were preincubated for 15 minutes with 10% normal goat serum to block nonspecific binding. Specific human-preabsorbed polyclonal antibodies, against human fibronectin in 1:1000 dilution (Life Technologies, Breda, The Netherlands), were applied as primary antiserum, and the sections were incubated at room temperature for 30 minutes. The supraoptimal dilution was obtained by examining the intensity of staining obtained with a series of dilutions of the antisera from 1:100 to 1:2500 and selecting the dilution that gave specific, weak, but easily visible signals [37]. Negative controls were performed by omission of the primary antibody. After washing in 0.5% tween-20 in PBS solution, the sections were incubated with mouse biotinylated anti-rabbit IgG (BioGenex, San Ramon, CA, USA) for 30 minutes and, subsequently, with peroxidase conjugated streptavidin. Color was developed using DAB (3,3′-diaminobenzidine tetrahydrochloride dehydrate), and then sections were counterstained with hematoxyline. Sections were mounted and visualized under the light microscope and photographed.

Expression of VEGF

Immunohistochemistry was performed using a standard avidin–biotin complex (ABC) method, as described earlier [38,39]. In brief, after deparaffinization in xylene and rehydration through graded alcohol, the slides were rinsed with water and phosphate buffered saline (PBS) and placed in a Sequeza Immunostaining Workstation (Shandon Scientific Ltd, Astmoor, Runcorn). Slides were preincubated for 15 minutes with normal goat serum to block nonspecific binding, then incubated for 30 minutes at room temperature with affinity-purified rabbit polyclonal antibodies in a dilution of 1 : 200. The anti-VEGF antiserum used was raised against a 20-amino-acid synthetic peptide corresponding to residues 1–20 of the amino terminus of human VEGF [40] (Santa Cruz Biotechnology, Inc., Santa Cruz, CA, USA). The optimal dilution was identified by examining the intensity of staining obtained with a series of dilutions of the antiserum from 1 : 50 to 1 : 500. The dilution (1 : 200) resulted in specific and easily visible signals in paraffin sections of a capillary hemangioma. The hemangioma sections served as a positive control in the study. After washing with PBS, the test and control slides were incubated for 30 minutes with biotinylated secondary antibody (Multilink, 1 : 75 dilution, Biogenex, San Ramon, MO, USA). After two washes in PBS, slides were incubated for 30 minutes with alkaline phosphatase-conjugated strep-tavidin (Biogenex) in a dilution of 1 : 50. Finally, the slides were rinsed with 0.2 M TRIS-HCl pH 8.0, Levamizole (Sigma) was used to block the endogenous alkaline phosphatase activity, and then the slides were stained for 30 minutes with 0.3% New Fuchsin/TRIS-HCl (Sigma) as a color enhancement system. Negative controls were prepared by omission of the primary antiserum. Slides were lightly counterstained with Mayer's hematoxylin for 10 seconds.

Expression of CD31 and α-SMA

Immunolocalization of VEGF in endothelial cells as well as in vascular smooth muscle cells was verified by staining these cells with specific markers. Endothelial cells were identified by CD31 immunostaining [38,39]. Staining was done by the ABC method, but using 0.025% 3,3-diaminobenzidine (DAB) as chromogen. Slides were incubated for 20 minutes in methanol with 0.3% H_2O_2 to block the endogenous peroxidase activity. Slides were incubated with the primary anti-human CD 31 monoclonal antibody in dilution of 1 : 80 (Dako Corporation, Glostrup, Denmark) at room temperature for 30 minutes and subsequently visualized after developing the color using 0.025% 3,3-diaminobenzidine (DAB) (Sigma). Employing the DAB-based color development method, consecutive tissue sections were stained with anti-human mouse monoclonal alpha-smooth muscle actin (α-SMA) antibody (clone 1A4: Biogenex) in a dilution of 1 : 1000.

Semiquantitative analysis

Prior to screening, sections were coded, so the observers were unaware of the clinical details of the case under study. The expression VEGF, fibronectin, and collagens was analyzed semiquantitatively, using a visual scale that ranged from 0–4: grade 0 = no staining, grade 1 = focal staining, grade 2 = diffuse faint staining, grade 3 = diffuse moderate staining, and grade 4 = diffuse strong staining [38]. The entire surface area of the tissue section on the slides was visualized and scored at the same magnification by three independent observers. The interstitial staining for collagens and fibronectin was quantified. The average of the three scores was used for subsequent analysis. This scoring method has previously been shown to allow the detection of differences in expression level as small as 1.5 times [38,41].

Statistical analysis

The expression of collagens and the fibronection staining score were calculated for the three different groups, and the results are expressed as mean ± SEM. Statistical analysis was performed after ranking using a nonparametric test–either the Mann–Whitney test or Fisher's exact test, according to what was appropriate to the compared groups. Interobserver variability was analyzed by linear regression and analysis of agreement. Densitometric values for VEGF mRNA expression were statistically tested. Results were accepted as statistically significant with $p \leq 0.05$.

RESULTS AND DISCUSSION

Collagens and fibronectin expression

Myocardial Picro-sirius Red staining patterns from both the TF groups showed extensive staining for collagens in the interstitium as well as around the blood vessels in all patients. Semiquantitative analysis revealed an increased interstitial staining for total collagens in the TF-2 group as compared to the TF-1 group (scoring: 3.1 ± 0.2 vs. 2.4 ± 0.2, $p < 0.04$; figure 1). Furthermore, collagen contents in the TF-2 group were also significantly higher than those in the age-matched controls (scoring: 3.1 ± 0.2 vs. 2.6 ± 0.1, $p < 0.05$; figure 1). Statistically, interobserver agreement was high ($r = 0.9$, $p < 0.05$).

Myocardial localization of fibronectin showed that the expression is confined to the interstitial perivascular region, as well as to the cytoplasm of some cardiomyocytes in all groups. Semiquantitative analysis revealed that fibronectin expression was not increased in the TF-1 group (figure 2) as compared to controls (3.2 ± 0.4 vs. 3.1 ± 0.4, $p =$ ns). There were no significant differences in fibronectin expression in patients from the TF-2 group when compared either with the TF-1 group (3.1 ± 0.4 vs. 3.2 ± 0.6, $p =$ ns) or with age-matched controls (3.1 ± 0.4 vs. 3.2 ± 0.6, $p =$ ns). Interobserver agreement was high ($r = 0.9$, $p < 0.05$).

Despite the fact that data are lacking on normal myocardium regarding the amount of collagens and fibronectin in children, our results indicate an increased amount of myocardial extracellular matrix deposition in RVH in patients with TF, with an apparent increase of total collagen at a young age. The extracellular matrix deposition is a sign of fibrosis during RVH in patients with TF. The apparent development of cardiac hypertrophy is induced by changes in cardiac gene expression that provide a means of compensation for increased hemodynamic load. In this

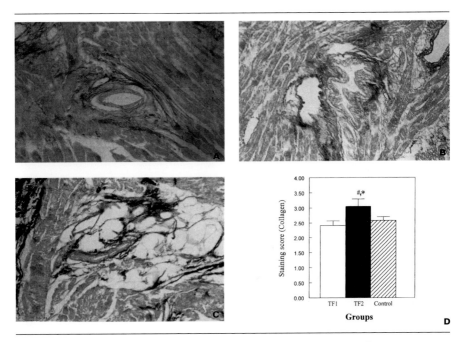

Figure 1. Right ventricular total collagen content in patients with tetralogy of Fallot Microphotographs (200 × magnification) of the human right ventricular tissue obtained from patients undergoing surgery (**A**) for autograft aortic root replacement (Control), (**B**) for primary repair of tetralogy of Fallot (TF-1), and (**C**) for secondary surgery (TF-2). Tissue sections were prepared and stained with the collagen-specific stain Picro-sirius Red. Collagen fibers appear red and are localized in interstitial and perivascular areas. Note the interstitial fibrosis in the case of TF patients. (**D**) Bar diagram depicting significantly enhanced interstitial collagen content in the TF-2 group as compared to the Control group. Distribution of collagen fibers in tissue was visualized under normal light microscopy. Red positive interstitial collagen in the tissue area was analyzed semiquantitatively by three independent observers using a staining score ranging from 0 (no staining) to 4 (strong red staining) to assess the levels of staining. Values are shown as mean ± SEM.

regard, our data are in agreement with the histopathologic findings from the RV myocardium in preoperative TF that show interstitial fibrosis, myofibrillar disorganization, disarray, and degenerative changes in addition to myocardial cell hypertrophy [15,21].

The changes as found in our study for collagen, along with an altered structure or function of the myocardium, may induce the findings of fibronectin expression. It is believed that changes in gene expression accompanying cardiac hypertrophy are the result of a multifactorial process. The observed changes may therefore be concomitant phenomena. The alteration in ventricular gene expression might be an indicator of cardiac hypertrophy and may result from a number of different stimuli. We assume that the changes in the right ventricular collagen expression in TF patients could be a result of increased hemodynamic load, with a parallel increase

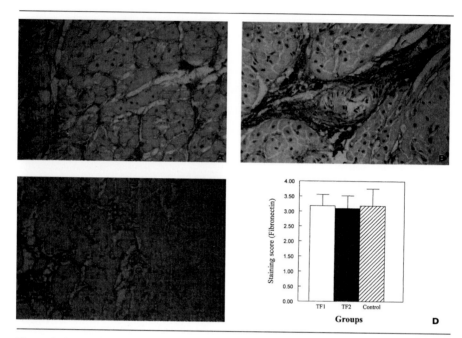

Figure 2. Immunohistochemical localization of fibronectin in right ventricular tissue of patients with tetralogy of Fallot. Microphotographs (200 × magnification) showing human right ventricular tissue immunostained with fibronectin as described in Materials and Methods from patients who underwent surgery (**A**) for antograft aortic root replacement (Control), (**B**) for primary repair of tetralogy of Fallot (TF-1), and (**C**) for secondary surgery (TF-2). (**D**) Bar diagram depicting semiquantitative analysis of interstitial fibronectin staining in the three groups. Values are shown as mean ± SEM.

in ventricular mass [42,43]. We have as yet no adequate explanation for the finding of fibronectin expression, the need for young control biopsies being obvious. Nevertheless, it is clear from our results that fibronectin levels are already high in patients with TF at a very young age (TF-1) and remain elevated later in life (TF-2).

The early increase of collagen deposition in the right ventricle as found at primary correction may occur because the original myocardial extracellular matrix has been expanded and weakened due to the hemodynamic overload. The myocardium will compensate until enough new collagen has been produced to restore tensile strength and to resist the distending forces. Our findings in the TF-1 and TF-2 groups fit into this concept, since the TF-2 group shows a more prominent increase in the amount of collagen as compared to the TF-1 group. Corrective surgery limits myocardial overload and may therefore limit the amount of damage to the myocardial collagen matrix [26].

VEGF expression and angiogenesis

At clinical analysis, all patients from the TF-1 group showed RVH, and all TF-2 patients showed RVH as well as right ventricular dilatation. All control patients had a normal right ventricle at clinical analysis. VEGF expression was evaluated employing Northern blot analysis. Using a human-specific cDNA insert encoding VEGF, we detected two mRNA species of 3.9 and 1.7 kb, respectively, expressed in the human RV tissue. Densitometric analysis of the mRNAs bands encoding VEGF on the autoradiographs showed significantly enhanced (1.8 ± 0.3-fold) expression in the TF-1 group as compared to the control group (figure 3D). VEGF expression was not significantly altered in the TF-2 group when compared to the control group [41]. To immunolocalize VEGF, we incubated tissue sections with affinity-purified anti-human rabbit polyclonal antibody and processed the tissue specimens for color development. A clear cytoplasmic staining pattern was observed in myocytes and in smooth muscle cells around the blood vessels but not in the fibrotic area in the case of the TF groups (figure 3B,C). In order to assess angiogenesis in the myocardial tissue from patients with TF and controls, tissue section were immunostained with anti-α-smooth muscle actin (figure 3A) and CD31 antibodies. CD31 antibody stained all endothelial cells in both small (<200 μm) and large vessels (>200 μm), whereas vascular smooth muscle cells were stained intensely with α-smooth muscle actin antibodies. Qualitatively, the tissue obtained from TF patients showed an enhanced number of vessels as compared to the controls [39].

In order to assess myocardial angiogenesis in the tissue specimens obtained from TF patients, VEGF, a potent angiogenic molecule, was examined at the mRNA and protein levels. At the mRNA level, VEGF showed significantly enhanced expression in the TF-1 group as compared to the control group. Immunohistochemical localization of VEGF indicates that cardiac myocytes and vascular smooth muscle cells produce this mitogen, which could be secreted from these cells to act on endothelial cells in a paracrine manner, resulting in cardiac angiogenesis. Experimental animal studies from our research group as well as from others have shown that myocardial ischemia is a strong inducer of VEGF gene expression [17,31,36]. It is very likely in the TF situation that RV tissue experiences hypoxia, which in term could be responsible for inducing the expression of VEGF. At this juncture, we think that the enhanced expression of VEGF mRNA could contribute to the angiogenesis in the right ventricle of TF patients. The increased number of blood vessels as observed by light microscopy could explain this finding of enhanced VEGF expression in the RV myocardium from patients with TF. Furthermore, a detailed morphometric analysis of existing blood vessels would allow us to validate this point.

CONCLUSION

In conclusion, we have shown that RVH in patients with TF was accompanied with enhanced myocardial collagen deposition in the interstitium and around the blood vessels, giving rise to abnormal myocardial architecture. Though we did not measure

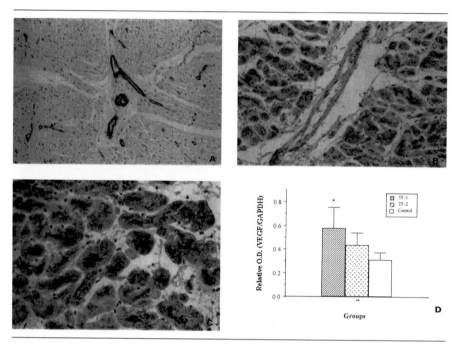

Figure 3. Myocardial expression of vascular endothelial growth factor and angiogenesis during RVH in TF patients. (**A**) Myocardial tissue sections (6 μm thick) obtained from TF patients were immunostained using human-specific monoclonal antibody raised against α-smooth muscle actin, and all the blood vessels in the range of more than 200 μm were counted. The blood vessel counts were also assessed using CD31 immunostaining and compared with the above staining values. Note several small and large blood vessels stained for smooth muscle-specific actin. (**B,C**) Immunohistochemical localization of VEGF was performed on 6 μm-thick paraffin sections of myocardial tissue from a control patient (**B**, ×200 magnification) and from a patient derived from group TF-1 (**C**, ×400 magnification). Sections were incubated with a monospecific polyclonal anti-VEGF antibody followed by immunoalkaline phosphatase color reaction and visualization under light microscope as described in Materials and Methods. Immunoreactive VEGF is seen in the smooth muscle cells and in the cardiomyocytes. (**D**) Line diagram showing densitometric analysis of VEGF mRNA expression. Total RNA (10 μg) from right ventricular biopsies obtained from the control as well as from the TF-1 and TF-2 groups of patients were subjected to Northern hybridization with radiolabeled cDNA probes encoding VEGF and GAPDH as described in Materials and Methods. Scanning densitometric values for VEGF were normalized with respective GAPDH values and expressed as relative optical density (O.D.). Results represent the mean values from three different blots. $\star$, $p < 0.05$ vs. control group.

the cell size, our data correspond with the finding that after early primary correc-tive surgery, RVH appears to regress and eventually leads to less collagen contents, as observed in the TF-2 group. Our study provides further evidence that myocar-dial architecture in patients with TF depicts increased fibrosis at the expression level of extracellular matrix components such as collagens. However, the lack of data on normal myocardium in young patients limits the interpretation of data. Addition-ally, the hypertrophic state of the myocardium seems to be correlated with increased angiogenesis. This is evident by enhanced levels of VEGF mRNAs in the children with TF at the time of primary surgery. Furthermore, histochemical examination of tissue biopsies showed increased number of blood vessels in patients with TF as compared to the control group. Thus, our results as presented here clearly indicate an increased degree of fibrosis and ongoing angiogenesis during RVH in patients with TF. This information leaves room for the improvement of contemporary clinical treatment of patients with TF by allowing an assessment of timing for surgery and possibly supports long-term postoperative prognosis.

ACKNOWLEDGEMENTS

Financial support from the Netherlands Heart Foundation (NHS 96.082) is gratefully acknowledged. The authors thank Mrs. E. Yilmaz for her technical assistance.

REFERENCES

1. Jordan SC, Scott O. 1989. Heart Disease in Paediatrics, 3rd ed. Oxford: Butterworth Heinneman.
2. Bogers AJJC, van der Laarse A, Vliegen HW. 1988. Assessment of hypertrophy in myocardial biopsies taken during correction of congenital heart disease. Thorac Cardiovasc Surgeon 36:137–140.
3. Starnes VA, Luciani GB, Latter DA, Griffin ML. 1994. Current surgical management of tetralogy of Fallot. Ann Thorac Surg 58:211–215.
4. Castaneda AR, Jonas RA, Mayer JE Jr, Hanley FL. 1994. Cardiac Surgery of the Neonate and Infant. Philadelphia: W.B. Saunders Company.
5. Murphy JG, Gersh BJ, Mair DD, Fuster V, McGoon MD, Ilstrup DM, McGoon DC, Kirklin JW, Danielson GK. 1993. Long-term outcome in patients undergoing surgical repair of tetralogy of Fallot. N Engl J Med 329:593–599.
6. Warner KG, Anderson JE, Fulton DR, Payne DD, Geggel RL, Marx GR. 1993. Restoration of the pulmonary valve reduces right ventricular volume overload after previous repair of tetralogy of Fallot. Circulation 88:II189–II197.
7. Seliem SA, Wu YT, Glenwright K. 1995. Relation between age and surgery and regression of right ventricular hypertrophy in tetralogy of Fallot. Pediatr Cardiol 16:53–55.
8. van Bilsen M, Chien KR. 1993. Growth and hypertrophy of the heart: towards an understanding of cardiac specific and inducible gene expression. Cardiovasc Res 27:1140–1149.
9. Schwartz K, Carrier L, Mercadier JJ, Lompre AM. 1993. Molecular phenotype of hypertrophied and failing myocardium. Circulation 87:VII-5–VII-10.
10. Kato M. 1976. Right ventricular hypertrophy in tetralogy of Fallot, a pathohistologic study. Jpn Ass Thorac Surg 24:1436–1445.
11. Kawai S, Okada R, Kitamura K, Suzuki A, Saito S. 1984. A morphometrical study of myocardial disarray associated with right ventricular outflow tract obstruction. Jpn Circ J 48:445–456.
12. Mitsuno M, Nakano S, Shimazaki Y. 1993. Fate of right ventricular hypertrophy in tetralogy of Fallot after corrective surgery. Am J Cardiol 72:694–698.
13. Tomanek RJ, Torry RJ. 1994. Growth of the coronary vasculature in hypertrophy: mechanisms and model dependence. Cell Mol Biol Res 40:129–136.
14. Boheler KR, Schwartz K. 1992. Gene expression in cardiac hypertrophy. Trends Cardiovasc Med 2:176–182.
15. Brand T, Sharma HS, Schaper W. 1993. Expression of nuclear proto-oncogenes in isoproterenol-induced cardiac hypertrophy. J Mol Cell Cardiol 25:1325–1337.
16. Brand T, Sharma HS, Fleischmann KE, Duncker DJ, McFalls EO, Verdouw PD, Schaper W. 1992. Proto-oncogene expression in porcine myocardium subjected to ischemia and reperfusion. Circ Res 71:1351–1360.
17. Sharma HS, Wünsch M, Brand T, Schaper W. 1992. Molecular biology of the coronary vascular and myocardial responses to ischemia. J Cardiovasc Pharmacol 20:S23–S31.
18. Sharma HS, Verdouw PD, Lamers JMJ. 1994. Involvement of sarcoplasmic reticulum calcium pump in myocardial contractile dysfunction: comparison between chronic pressure-overload and stunning. Cardiovasc Drugs Ther 8:461–468.

19. Sharma HS, van Heugten HAA, Goedbloed MA, Lamers JMJ. 1994. Angiotensin II induced expression of transcription factors precedes increase in Transforming Growth Factor-β1 mRNA in neonatal cardiac fibroblasts. Biochem Biophys Res Commun 205:105–112.
20. Volders PGA, Willems IEMG, Cleutjens JPM. 1993. Interstitial collagen is increased in the noninfarcted human myocardium after myocardial infarction. J Mol Cell Cardiol 25:1317–1323.
21. Weber KT, Sun Y, Tyagi SC, Cleutjens JP. 1994. Collagen network of the myocardium: function, structural remodeling and regulatory mechanisms. J Mol Cell Cardiol 26:279–292.
22. Bishop JE, Rhodes S, Laurent GJ, Low RB, Stirewalt WS. 1994. Increased collagen synthesis and decreased collagen degradation in right ventricular hypertrophy induced by pressure overload. Cardiovasc Res 28:1581–1585.
23. Chapman D, Weber KT, Eghbali M. 1990. Regulation of fibrillar collagen types I and III and basement membrane type IV collagen gene expression in pressure overloaded rat myocardium. Circulation Res 67:787–794.
24. Samuel JL, Barrieux A, Dufour S, Dubus I, Contard F, Koteliansky V, Farhadian F, Marotte F, Thiery JP, Rappaport L. 1991. Accumulation of fetal fibronectin mRNAs during the development of rat cardiac hypertrophy induced by pressure overload. J Clin Invest 88:1737–1746.
25. Boluyt MO, O'Neill L, Meredith AL, Bing OH, Brooks WW, Conrad CH, Crow MT, Lakatta EG. 1994. Alterations in cardiac gene expression during the transition from stable hypertrophy to heart failure. Marked upregulation of genes encoding extracellular matrix components. Circ Res 75:23–32.
26. Whittaker P. 1997. Collagen and ventricular remodeling after acute myocardial infarction: concepts and hypotheses. Basic Res Cardiol 92:79–81.
27. Jalil JE, Doering CW, Janicki JS, Pick R, Shroff SG, Weber KT. 1989. Fibrillar collagen and myocardial stiffness in the intact hypertrophied rat left ventricle. Circ Res 64:1041–1050.
28. McLenachan JM, Dargie HJ. 1990. Ventricular arrhythmias in hypertensive left ventricular hypertrophy. Relationship to coronary artery disease, left ventricular dysfunction, and myocardial fibrosis. Am J Hypertens 3:735–740.
29. Farhadian F, Contard F, Corbier A, Barrieux A, Rappaport L, Samuel JL. 1995. Fibronectin expression during physiological and pathological cardiac growth. J Mol Cell Cardiol 27:981–990.
30. Villarreal FJ, Dillmann WH. 1992. Cardiac hypertrophy-induced changes in mRNA levels for TGF-β1, fibronectin and collagen. Am J Physiol 262:H1861–H1866.
31. Sharma HS, Preters E, Yilmaz E, Hokken R, Bogers AJJC. 1997. Right ventricular hypertrophy in human tetralogy of Fallot is associated with increased myocardial fibrosis and vascularization. Circulation 96(8):I.17–I.18.
32. Bogers AJJC, Roofthooft M, Pisters H, Spitaels SEC, Bos E. 1994. Longterm follow-up of gamma irradiated transannular homograft patch in surgical treatment of tetralogy of Fallot. Thorac Cardiovasc Surgeon 42:337–339.
33. Hokken RB, Bogers AJJC, Spitaels SEC, Hess J, Bos E. 1995. Pulmonary homograft insertion after repair of pulmonary stenosis. J Heart Valve 4:182–186.
34. Schoof PH, Cromme-Dijkhuis AH, Bogers AJJC, Thijssen EJM, Witsenburg M, Hess J, Bos E. 1994. Aortic root replacement with pulmonary autograft in children. J Thorac Cardiovasc Surg 107:367–373.
35. Hokken RB, Bogers AJJC, Taams MA, Willems TP, Cromme-Dijkhuis AH, Witsenburg M, Spitaels SEC, van Herwerden LA, Bos E. 1995. Aortic root replacement with a pulmonary autograft. Eur J Cardiothorac Surg 9:378–383.
36. Sharma HS, Tang ZH, Gho BC, Verdouw PD. 1995. Nucleotide sequence and expression of the porcine vascular endothelial growth factor. Biochim Biophys Acta 1260:235–238.
37. Peters THF, Sharma HS, Yilmaz E, Bogers AJJC. 1999. Quantitative analysis of collagens and fibronectin expression in human right ventricular hypertrophy. Ann N Y Acad Sci 874:278–285.
38. Shehata SMK, Mooi WJ, Okazaki T, El-Banna I, Sharma HS, Tibboel D. 1999. Enhanced expression of vascular endothelial growth factor in lungs of newborns with congenital diaphragmatic hernia and pulmonary hypertension. Thorax 54(5):427–431.
39. Sharma HS, Hokken RB, Bosman FT, Bogers AJJC. 1995. Myocardial expression and immunohistochemical localisation of vascular endothelial growth factor in human tetralogy of Fallot. Eur Heart J 16:353.
40. Ferrara N, Houck KA, Jakeman LB. 1991. The vascular endothelial growth factor family of polypeptides. J Cell Biochem 47:211–218.

41. Giaid A, Michel RP, Stewart DJ, Sheppard M, Corrin B, Hamid Q. 1993. Expression of endothelin-1 in lungs of patients with cryptogenic fibrosing alveolitis. Lancet 341:1550–1554.
42. Schwartz SM, Gordon D, Mosca RS, Bove EL, Heidelberger KP, Kulik TJ. 1996. Collagen content in normal, pressure, and pressure–volume overloaded developing human hearts. Am J Cardiol 77:734–738.
43. Vikstrom KL, Bohlmeyer T, Factor SM, Leinwand LA. 1998. Hypertrophy, pathology, and molecular markers of cardiac pathogenesis. Circ Res 82:773–778.

N. Takeda, M. Nagano and N.S. Dhalla
(eds). The Hypertrophied Heart. Copyright
© 2000. pp. 243–249. Kluwer Academic
Publishers. Boston. All rights reserved.

MOLECULAR MECHANISMS OF PHENOTYPIC MODULATION OF VASCULAR SMOOTH MUSCLE CELLS

MASAHIKO KURABAYASHI and RYOZO NAGAI

Second Department of Internal Medicine, Gunma University School of Medicine, 3-39-15 Showa-machi, Maebashi, Gunma 371-8511, Japan

Summary. Phenotypic modulation plays a pivotal role in the development of vascular disease, such as atherosclerosis and restenosis after angioplasty. We have identified zinc finger protein BTEB2 as a DNA binding protein that regulates the nonmuscle myosin heavy chain (SMemb) promoter. BTEB2 is expressed in the fetal aorta but not in the adult aorta and is induced in neointima in response to vascular injury. BTEB2 activates a number of vascular disease-associated genes, such as tissue factor and PAI-1 (plasminogen activator inhibitor-1), as well as the SMemb gene. We have isolated and characterized human BTEB2 genomic clone. Functional studies using 5′-deletion and site-directed mutation constructs localized the major phorbol ester-responsive motifs to Egr-1 consensus binding site located at −32 from the transcription start site. These results suggest that BTEB2 functions as a transcription factor for phenotypic modulation of vascular smooth muscle cells. Furthermore, given that Egr-1 expression is induced in response to vascular injury, BTEB2 may play a role in the development of vascular disease.

INTRODUCTION

Vascular smooth muscle cells (SMCs) displays two distinct phenotypes depending upon the growth condition both in vivo and in vitro [1,2]. Phenotypic modulation of vascular SMCs plays a critical role in the development of vascular disease, such as atherosclerosis and restenosis after percutaneous transcatheter coronary angioplasty (PTCA) [3,4]. Among many different characteristics between these two phenotypes are their cytoskeletal organization, ability to synthesize growth factors, and receptors and extracellular matrix [5,6]. Since phenotypic modulation of SMCs is thought to involve a cascade of events in which different genes are turned on and off in a precisely regulated manner, one approach to studying SMC differentiation or dedifferentiation is to analyze the regulatory mechanisms of gene expression that clearly differs between the two phenotypes [4].

Smooth muscle myosin heavy chain is one of the most extensively characterized molecules that distinguish neointimal SMCs from medial SMCs [7–12]. We and other laboratories have identified at least three different isoforms of myosin heavy chains expressed in vascular SMCs [13]. SM1 and SM2 are generated from a single gene by an alternative splicing of the 3' exons and represent a differentiated marker of contractile phenotype. SMemb, also known as NMHC-B, is encoded by a distinct gene and represents an undifferentiated marker of vascular SMCs [7].

In this study, we address the question as to the mechanisms that allow the SMemb gene to be transcriptionally active in a cetain set of tissues and to be regulated in a characteristic manner in vascular SMCs.

MATERIALS AND METHODS

Cell culture

C2/2 cells, an established cell line derived from rabbit aortic smooth muscle cells, were cultured in Dubecco's modified Eagle's medium (DMEM, GIBCO) with 5% fetal calf serum. COS-7 cells were cultured in DMEM with 10% fetal calf serum.

Southwestern screening of C2/2 cDNA library

The C2/2 cell cDNA library constructed in the expression vector 1 gt11 was screened with the five-times-repeated fragment of −115 to −85 SMemb promoter as a probe, using the procedure of Singh et al. [14] and Vinson et al. [15]. One of the positive clones selected was used as a probe of second screening with a rabbit fetal aortic cDNA library. The probe was radiolabeled using a random primed DNA labeling kit (Amersham). The insert cDNA was sequenced by using the dideoxy-chain termination method in denatured double-stranded plasmid.

DNA transfection and luciferase assay

Reporter plasmids for luciferase assay by deletion effects in SMemb promoter were prepared through a wild-type 5'-deletion constructs at −105 bp, −89 bp, −62 bp, and −32 bp of SMemb promoter sequence, which were named Del-105, Del-89, Del-62, and Del-32. DNA transfection was performed by the modified calcium phosphate–DNA coprecipitation method. Transfected cell cultures were harvested for extract preparation at 48 hours after transfection. Cell extracts were prepared by luciferase assay kit (PicaGeneTM system, Nippon Gene), and levels of luciferase activity were measured by the Lumat LB9501 luminometer (Berthold). Protein concentration was measured by using BCA Protein Assay Reagent (PIERCE) with bovine serum albumin as standard. The luciferase activity was normalized to the protein concentration (mg/mL) of the cell lysate.

Immunohistochemistry

Balloon injury of the aorta was performed in adult male Wister rats (300–350 g) under general anesthesia. A 2-French balloon embolectomy catheter was introduced via the femoral artery and advanced to the level of the thoracic aorta. The balloon was then inflated and the catheter withdrawn along the length of the thoracoabdominal aorta. The balloon was deflated, and the procedure was repeated three times. Rats were sacrificed at 2 weeks after injury. The aorta was fixed in 10% formalin

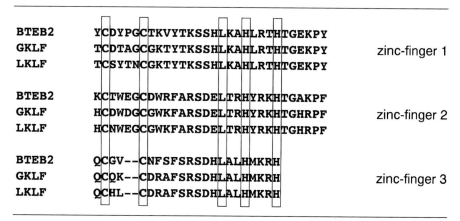

BTEB2	YCDYPGCTKVYTKSSHLKAHLRTHTGEKPY	
GKLF	TCDTAGCGKTYTKSSHLKAHLRTHTGEKPY	zinc-finger 1
LKLF	TCSYTNCGKTYTKSSHLKAHLRTHTGEKPY	
BTEB2	KCTWEGCDWRFARSDELTRHYRKHTGAKPF	
GKLF	HCDWDGCGWKFARSDELTRHYRKHTGHRPF	zinc-finger 2
LKLF	HCNWEGCGWKFARSDELTRHYRKHTGHRPF	
BTEB2	QCGV--CNFSFSRSDHLALHMKRH	
GKLF	QCQK--CDRAFSRSDHLALHMKRH	zinc-finger 3
LKLF	QCHL--CDRAFSRSDHLALHMKRH	

Figure 1. Sequence comparison of the zinc finger motifs among BTEB2, GKLF, and LFLF. The amino acid sequence is indicated by *single letter code*. Conserved two-cysteine, one-leucine, and two-histidine residues within the zinc finger motifs are *boxed*.

and paraffin embedded. Immunohistochemistry using anti-BTEB2 antibody was carried out by using the Vectastain Elite ABC kit (Vector Laboratories).

RESULTS

We attempted to isolate the DNA-binding protein that recognizes the *cis*-acting regulatory element (we refer to it as *SE1*) by Southwestern screening of the cDNA expression library prepared from C2/2 cells, a smooth muscle cell line derived from rabbit aorta. Among the positive clones was BTEB2. We obtained 2280 bp cDNA, which contained a full length of the rabbit BTEB2 protein coding region. Analysis of the predicted open reading frame encoding 219 amino acids reveals three putative zinc fingers that are highly conserved among the members of a family of Krupple-like transcription factors to which GKLF, EKLF, and LKLF belong [16] (figure 1). This family of transcription factors has been implicated in the regulation of tissue-specific gene expression [17–19]. EKLF was conclusively demonstrated to represent a CACCC-binding protein that controls the β-globin gene in vivo because destruction of the EKLF gene resulted in a profound reduction in β-globin expression. LKLF and GKLF are preferentially expressed in the lung and gut, respectively.

We next determined whether BTEB2 activates transcription from the SMemb promoter. The full-length BTEB2 cDNA under the control of the cytomegalovirus (CMV) promoter was cotransfected into COS-7 cells with a series of 5′-deletion constructs of rabbit SMemb promoter (figure 2). Overexpression of BTEB2 resulted in a significant induction of Del-105 reporter gene expression (6.5 ± 0.4-fold). Deletion of the sequence to −89 and further deletion to −32 resulted in a marked decrease in BTEB2-induced transactivation of SMemb promoter (figure 3).

To determine the regulation of BTEB2 expression in the aorta, we analyzed the BTEB2 mRNA levels in developing rabbit aorta. The expression levels of the

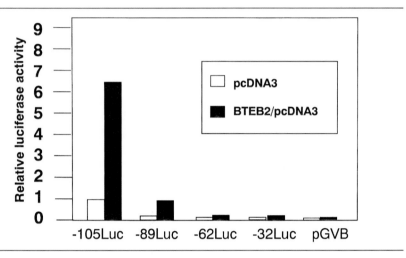

Figure 2. Activation of tissue factor and PAI-1 gene transcription by BTEB2. BTEB2 expression plasmid was cotransfected with indicated reporter genes. Promoters of tissue factor (TF) and PAI-1, but not of pGL3 (promoter-less control plasmid), were activated by BTEB2 expression vector.

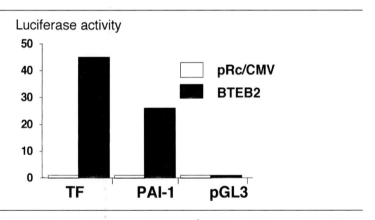

Figure 3. Effects of BTEB2 on SMemb promoter activity. The 5′-deletion analysis was carried out by using the constructs Del-105, Del-89, Del-62, and Del-32. COS7 cells were transfected with luciferase reporter constructs containing various lengths of the 5′-flanking region of the rabbit SMemb gene along with either empty vector (pcDNA3) or BTEB2 expression vector (BTEB2/pcDNA3). In the bar graph, results are shown as relative luciferase activities normalized with protein concentration of the cell lysate and are shown by the value relative to the activity of the Del-105 without BTEB2.

BTEB2 were more abundant in fetus and at 2 weeks of age compared to those in adult aorta, thus suggesting that BTEB2 expression is downregulated in the aorta during development. In addition, the immunohistochemistry indicated that the BTEB2 protein is markedly increased in neointima after balloon injury in rabbit aorta (data not shown).

BTEB2   Egr-1

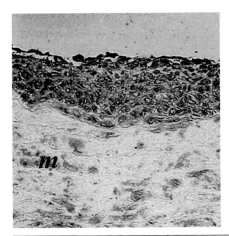 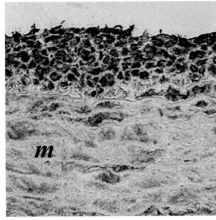

Figure 4. Expression of BTEB2 and Egr-1 after balloon injury. Rat aortic sections were stained with anti-BTEB2 or Egr-1. BTEB2 and Egr-1 were coexpressed strongly in neointimal layer (*i*) compared with medial layer (*m*) 2 weeks after balloon injury.

These data led us to hypothesize that BTEB2 plays a role in phenotypic modulation of vascular SMCs. To test this hypothesis, we cotransfected BTEB2 expression plasmid with a variety of reporter genes. As shown in figure 3, BTEB2 induced the promoter activity of tissue factor and plasminogen inhibitor-1 (PAI-1). Tissue factor and PAI-1 are known to play a key role in the development of atherosclerosis [3,4].

To determine the molecular mechanisms underlying this induction, we pursued our experiment to identify the regulatory mechanisms of BTEB2 expression. We have cloned the promoter region of the human BTEB2 gene and have identified *cis*-elements and *trans*-factors that govern the transcriptional expression of BTEB2 in vascular SMCs. Most notably, the BTEB2 promoter contains a consensus sequence of the Egr-1 binding site at −32, and gel shift assay demonstrates that this site is occupied by Egr-1. Incubation of the SMC nuclear extracts with anti-Egr-1 antibody clearly supershifted the complex. Transient transfection assays indicated that Egr-1 overexpression increased BTEB2 promoter activity, and deletion of the sequence attenuated this inducibility (data not shown). Immunohistochemistry of the balloon-injured rat aorta showed the expression of both Egr-1 and BTEB2 in the neointima (figure 4).

We reason that if Egr-1 regulates BTEB2 expression, the stimuli that can induce Egr-1 also induce BTEB2. Figure 4 shows that this is the case. Stimulation of serum-starved cultured vascular SMCs with PMA, the phorbol ester that activates protein kinase C, rapidly and transiently induced Egr-1 mRNA expression. We observed the concomitant increase in BTEB2 mRNA levels soon after PMA stimulation. Interestingly, induction of BTEB2 is sustained compared with that of Egr-1 (data not shown). These findings are intriguing because BTEB2 may play a role in regulating gene expression over the long term.

DISCUSSION

Our previous studies indicated that the SMemb gene in the arterial wall is almost exclusively expressed in proliferating vascular SMCs in neointima that developed in atherosclerosis and after balloon injury of rabbit aorta. Because SMemb is not a major isoform in normal aorta, these studies implicated SMemb as a molecular marker of neointimal SMCs [20]. In this study, we have cloned a cDNA encoding BTEB2, a member of zinc finger family of transcription factors, by using Southwestern screening methods, in which we employed a cis-acting regulatory element within the mouse SMemb gene as a hypridization probe. The major findings of this study are as follows: (1) BTEB2 can activate SMemb promoter activity, as assessed by the transient transfection of the SMemb–luciferase reporter plasmid into C2/2 cells; and (2) BTEB2 also induces the promoter activity of tissue factor and PAI-1, whose expression is known to be activated in vascular disease. These results suggest that BTEB2 can distinguish two phenotypes, namely, the synthetic form and the contractile form, and thus plays an important role in the development of vascular disease.

Recently, an induced expression of Egr-1 has been implicated in the development of vascular disease because of its rapid but transient induction of Egr-1 in endothelial cells in response to vascular injury. In contrast to the transient expression of Egr-1 in endothelial cells, our immunohistochemical study indicated that Egr-1 immunoreactivity remains positive 2 weeks after injury in the neointima and declines thereafter. In view of the fact that BTEB2 can increase Egr-1 promoter activity and that BTEB2 immunoreactivity is clearly detected 2 weeks after injury, persistent expression of Egr-1 in vascular SMCs may at least partly be due to BTEB2.

Transcription factors whose expression is limited to or is preferential in smooth muscle tissues have been cloned [21]. The Gax gene is expressed to a high degree in vascular SMCs but not in intestine [22]. The mRNA population particular to either phenotype of SMCs is determined in part by its characteristic array of transcription factors. In analogy to EKLF, whose expression is restricted predominantly to the erythroid lineage and whose targeted disruption in vivo causes severe β-globin deficiency, BTEB2 may play a critical role in the cell growth and differentiation of SMCs. Clearly, the function of BTEB2 in the in vivo context in phenotypic change and/or terminal differentiation awaits further study.

ACKNOWLEDGMENTS

We gratefully acknowledge Yasuharu Sasaki for providing us with the cultured smooth muscle cell line, C2/2, and Yoshiaki Fujii-Kuriyama and Kazuhiro Sogawa for providing human BTEB2 expression vector and advice.

REFERENCES

1. Aikawa M, Kim HS, Kuro-o M, Manabe I, Watanabe M, Yamaguchi H, Yazaki Y, Nagai R. 1995. Phenotypic modulation of smooth muscle cells during progression of human atherosclerosis as determined by altered expression of myosin heavy chain isoforms. Ann N Y Acad Sci 748:578–585.
2. Owens GK. 1995. Regulation of differentiation of vascular smooth muscle cells. Physiol Rev 75:487–517.
3. Ross R. 1995. Cell biology of atherosclerosis. Annu Rev Physiol 57:791–804.
4. Dzau VJ, Gibbons GH, Cooke JP, Omoigui N. 1993. Vascular biology and medicine in the 1990s: scope, concepts, potentials, and perspectives. Circulation 87:705–719.
5. Frid MG, Shekhonin BV, Koteliansky VE, Glukhova MA. 1992. Phenotypic changes of human smooth muscle cells during development: late expression of heavy caldesmon and calponin. Dev Biol 153:185–193.
6. Joseph LL, Miano M, Cserjesi P, Olson EN. 1996. SM22a, a marker of adult smooth muscle, is expressed in multiple myogenic lineages during embryogenesis. Circ Res 78:188–195.
7. Nagai R, Kuro OM, Babij P, Periasamy M. 1989. Identification of two types of smooth muscle myosin heavy chain isoforms by cDNA cloning and immunoblot analysis. J Biol Chem 264: 9734–9737.
8. Kawamoto S, Adelstein RS. 1991. Chicken nonmuscle myosin heavy chains: differential expression of two mRNAs and evidence for two different polypeptides. J Cell Biol 112:915–924.
9. Simons M, Wang M, McBride OW, Kawamoto S, Yamakawa K, Gdula D, Adelstein RS, Weir L. 1991. Human nonmuscle myosin heavy chains are encoded by two genes located on different chromosomes. Circ Res 69:530–539.
10. Babij P, Periasamy M. 1989. Myosin heavy chain isoform diversity in smooth muscle is produced by differential RNA processing. J Mol Biol 210:673–679.
11. Miano JM, Cserjesi P, Ligon KL, Periasamy M, Olson EN. 1994. Smooth muscle myosin heavy chain exclusively marks the smooth muscle lineage during mouse embryogenesis. Circ Res 75:803–812.
12. Watanabe M, Sakomura Y, Kurabayashi M, Manabe I, Aikawa M, Kuro-o M, Suzuki T, Yazaki Y, Nagai R. 1996. Structure and characterization of the 5'-flanking region of the mouse smooth muscle myosin heavy chain (SM1/2) gene. Circ Res 78:978–989.
13. Kuro-o M, Nagai R, Tsuchimochi H, Katoh, H, Yazaki Y, Ohkubo A, Takaku F. 1989. Developmentally regulated expression of vascular smooth muscle myosin heavy chain isoforms. J Biol Chem 264:18272–18275.
14. Singh H, LeBowitz JH, Baldwin AS Jr, Sharp PA. 1988. Molecular cloning of an enhancer binding protein: isolation by screening of an expression library with a recognition site DNA. Cell 52:415–423.
15. Vinson CR, LaMarco KL, Johnson PF, Landschulz WH, McKnight SL. 1988. In situ detection of sequence-specific DNA binding activity specified by a recombinard bacteriophage.
16. Sogawa K, Imataka H, Yamasaki Y, Kusume H, Abe H, Fujii KY. 1993. cDNA cloning and transcriptional properties of a novel GC box-binding protein, BTEB2. Nucleic Acids Res 21:1527–1532.
17. Chen X, Bieker JJ. 1996. Erythroid kruppel-like factor (EKLF) contains a multifunctional transcriptional activation domain important for inter- and intramolecular interactions. EMBO J 15: 5888–5896.
18. Miller IJ, Bieker JJ. 1993. A novel, erythroid cell-specific murine transcription factor that binds to the CACCC element and is related to the Kruppel family of nuclear proteins. Mol Cell Biol 13: 2776–2786.
19. Shields JM, Christy RJ, Yang VW. 1996. Identification and characterization of a gene encoding a gut-enriched Kruppel-like factor expressed during growth arrest. J Biol Chem 271:20009–20017.
20. Aikawa M, Nalla Sivam P, Kuro-o M, Kimura K, Nakahara K, Takewaki S, Ueda M, Yamaguchi H, Yazaki Y, Periasamy M, Nagai R. 1993. Human smooth muscle myosin heavy chain isoform as molecular markers for vascular development and atherosclerosis. Circ Res 73:1000–1012.
21. Morrisey EE, Ip HS, Lu MM, Parmacek MS. 1996. GATA-6: a zinc finger transcription factor that is expressed in multiple cell lineages derived from lateral mesoderm. Dev Biol 177:309–322.
22. Skopicki HA, Lyons GE, Schatteman G, Smith RC, Andres V, Schirm S, Isner J, Walsh K. 1997. Embryonic expression of the Gax homeodomain protein in cardiac, smooth, and skeletal muscle. Circ Res 80:452–462.

B. CARDIAC FAILURE IN THE HYPERTROPHIED HEART

N. Takeda, M. Nagano and N.S. Dhalla
(eds). The Hypertrophied Heart. Copyright
© 2000. pp. 253–263. Kluwer Academic
Publishers. Boston. All rights reserved.

PROTEIN KINASE C ACTIVATION IN CARDIAC HYPERTROPHY AND FAILURE

YASUCHIKA TAKEISHI, THUNDER JALILI, and RICHARD A. WALSH

Department of Medicine, Case Western Reserve University, 11100 Euclid Avenue, Cleveland, OH 44106, USA

Summary. It is clear from studies using neonatal rat ventricular myocytes that mechanical deformation activates the $G\alpha q$-phospholipase C signaling pathway and recapitulates the fetal gene program, followed by an increase in protein synthesis. In adult guinea pig heart, stretch stimulates phosphatidylinositol hydrolysis and translocation of protein kinase C (PKC). Cardiac-specific overexpression of the $G\alpha q$ and $PKC\beta_2$ in transgenic mice demonstrate a gene-dose-dependent induction of cardiac hypertrophy and contractile depression. $PKC\beta_2$-mediated phosphorylation of cardiac troponin I may decrease myofilament responsiveness to calcium and thus cause cardiomyocyte dysfunction. Furthermore, in failed human hearts, the expression and activity of $PKC\alpha$ and $PKC\beta$ are elevated. These results suggest a critical role of phospholipase C–PKC signaling in cardiac hypertrophy and heart failure. Treatment of the $PKC\beta_2$ transgenic mouse with a highly selective inhibitor of the $PKC\beta$ largely prevents and/or reverses the phenotype. Thus, selective inhibition of the $PKC\beta$ isoform may provide a novel therapeutic strategy for the prevention and treatment of congestive heart failure.

INTRODUCTION

Myocardial hypertrophy is an adaptive response to hormonal and mechanical stimuli that increase cardiac work. Initially, the resultant increased work is compensatory to normalize wall stress and maintain normal cardiac function. If the stimulus for pathologic hypertrophy is sufficiently intense and prolonged, decompensated hypertrophy ensues and ultimately leads to congestive heart failure [1]. Decompensated hypertrophy is characterized by an increase in chamber wall stress despite an increase in cardiac mass and is associated with symptoms and signs of pulmonary and systemic congestion. The molecular mechanisms that are responsible for compensated and decompensated hypertrophy are being elucidated by a number of studies that employ conventional experimental animal models, genetically engineered mice, and clinical investigation. However, precise mechanisms accounting for the transition from compensated to decompensated hypertrophy have not yet been completely characterized [2].

Protein kinase C (PKC) has been implicated as the intracellular mediator of several neurotransmitters, growth factors, and tumor promoters through multiple signal transduction pathways [3]. Currently, at least 11 isoforms have been identified in vivo and perhaps have played different functional roles in cell signaling leading to alterations in cardiac contractility, hypertrophic response, and tolerance to myocardial ischemia. Recently, we have reported a series of studies that suggest that PKC plays a critical role in the development of cardiac hypertrophy and failure. Here, we review the pathophysiological implications of PKC activation in cardiac hypertrophy and failure.

SIGNAL TRANSDUCTION THROUGH G PROTEIN, PHOSPHOLIPASE C, AND PKC

G proteins act as coupling proteins that become activated upon receptor stimulation [4,5]. In its GDP-bound form, the protein forms an inactive heterotrimer composed of three subunits (α, β, and γ). Upon ligand binding, a conformational shift in the receptor is transmitted to the α-subunit, resulting in the release of GDP and its replacement by GTP (figure 1). Subsequently, the α- and $\beta\gamma$-subunits become dissociated and are released from the receptor. Both the α- and $\beta\gamma$-subunits can activate a number of target systems. Deactivation of Gα occurs when GTP is hydrolyzed to GDP, a process that is mediated by the intrinsic GTPase activity of Gα and GTPase activating protein called *regulators of G protein signaling* (RGS). Gα with bound GDP reassociates with the $\beta\gamma$-subunit, forming a heterotrimetric complex that is poised for reactivation by the next extracellular signal. G proteins are classified on the basis of their Gα subunits. There are three major subfamilies of Gα protein, namely, Gαs, Gαi, and Gαq, which couple to different sets of receptors. Angiotensin II, α_1-adrenergic, and endothelin-1 receptors are coupled with Gαq, and the binding of ligands to their cognate receptors subsequently activates phospholipase C (PLC) β.

Four types of PLCβ exist ($-\beta_1$, $-\beta_2$, $-\beta_3$, and $-\beta_4$), and PLCβ_1 is the major isoform expressed in the heart [6]. PLCβ_1 hydrolyzes the membrane lipid phosphatidyl inositol-4-5 bisphosphate, and two biologically active intracellular second messengers, diacyl glycerol (DAG) and inositol triphosphate (IP$_3$), are generated by this hydrolytic process. Diacyl glycerol activates the serine/threonine kinase, PKC, while IP$_3$ binds to its receptor on the endoplasmic reticulum and stimulates the release of calcium [7].

Currently, 11 PKC isoforms have been identified and can be classified into three groups: conventional (or classical) isoforms responsive to calcium (α, β_1, β_2, and γ), novel isoforms that lack the calcium binding site (δ, ϵ, η, and θ), and atypical isoforms that do not respond to phorbol esters (ζ, λ, and μ). It is generally assumed that the activation of distinct PKC isoforms results in the activation of different sets of downstream targets and modulates transcriptional factors, gene expression, ion channels, Na$^+$–H$^+$ exchangers, sarcoplasmic reticular proteins, and myofibrillar proteins [8,9].

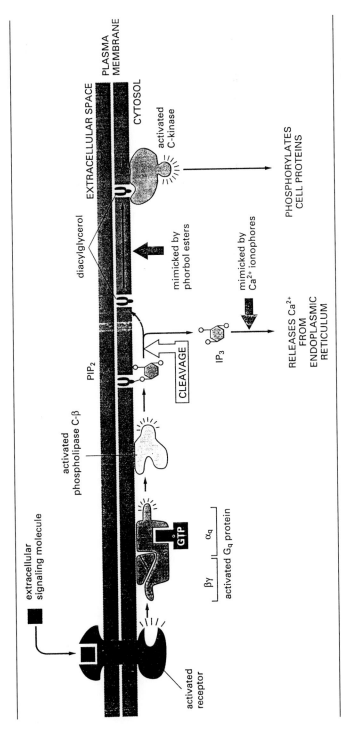

Figure 1. The G protein–phospholipase C signaling pathway. The activated receptor binds to a specific trimeric G protein (Gq), causing the α–subunit to dissociate and activate phospholipase Cβ, which cleaves phosphatidyl inositol biphosphate (PIP₂) to generate inositol triphosphate (IP₃) and diacylglycerol. Diacylglycerol activates PKC. PKC translocates from the cytosol to the inner face of the plasma membrane in the process of being activated. (Printed with permission from *Molecular Biology of the Cell*, figure 15-33.)

PHOSPHOLIPASE C–PKC SIGNALING IN CARDIAC HYPERTROPHY AND HEART FAILURE

Studies using neonatal cardiomyocytes

Dynamic or static stretch of the neonatal cardiomyocytes produces an increase in protein synthesis and resultant cardiac hypertrophy. This process may be mediated partly in the cardiomyocytes by stretch-activated sarcolemmal ion channels, $Na^+–H^+$ exchangers, tyrosine kinase-containing receptors, an extracellular matrix integrin-linked pathway, or G-protein-coupled receptors [10]. These mechanotransducers can then activate cytosolic signaling pathways that initiate gene transcription and translation of protein synthesis. In particular, it has been demonstrated that in the neonatal cardiomyocyte, mechanical deformation activates the $G\alpha q$-phospholipase C signaling pathway and reexpresses a number of genes, including atrial natriuretic factor (ANF), skeletal α-actin, and β-myosin heavy chain (MHC), followed by an increase in new protein synthesis [11,12]. Furthermore, it has been demonstrated that mechanical stretch induces secretion of angiotensin II from the cardiomyocyte, and secreted angiotensin II evokes cardiomyocyte hypertrophy [13,14]. Cardiomyocytes possess G-protein-coupled angiotensin II type-1 receptors that activate this pathway.

Phospholipase C signal transduction in the adult heart

However, the significance of this PLC pathway in response to pathophysiological stimuli in the adult heart has been poorly understood [10]. Since PKC isoform expression and responses to neurohormones are regulated differently during development [15], it was important to clarify this signaling pathway in the adult heart. Therefore, in isolated perfused adult guinea pig hearts, we characterized stretch-mediated phosphatidylinositol hydrolysis and PKC isoform translocation [16]. Balloon dilatation in the left ventricle with minimum diastolic pressure of 25 mmHg stimulated phosphatidylinositol hydrolysis with resultant translocation of the PKCε isoform. Perfusing the heart with angiotensin II and 4β-phorbol 12-myristate 13-acetate without stretch also translocated this isoform. Pretreatment of stretched heart with the specific angiotensin II type-1 receptor antagonist, losartan, abolished stretch-mediated accumulation of inositol phosphate and attenuated PKCε translocation. We demonstrated in that study that in the adult heart, mechanical stretch activates PLC, which results in phosphatidylinositol hydrolysis and PKC activation, in part by stimulation of the local renin–angiotensin system. However, the incomplete inhibition of PKC activation by angiotensin II type-1 receptor blockade suggests the presence of angiotensin II-independent processes for stretch-mediated signal transduction in matured myocardium.

Conventional animal models of heart failure

Hemodynamically loaded experimental animal models of hypertrophy and heart failure have been used in numerous studies. Depending on the degree or duration of loading, hemodynamic loads produce different types of heart conditions, from mild compensated hypertrophy to decompensated heart failure. In pressure-overloaded rat heart, Gu and Bishop have showed that PKCβ and ε isoforms are increased [17]. We also reported that the levels of PKCα and ε isoforms were increased during development of cardiac hypertrophy and failure induced by pressure overload in the guinea pig [18]. It is interesting to note that in failing rabbits hearts induced by both pressure overload and volume overload, expression of PKCα, β, γ, and ε are decreased [19]. These findings suggest that alterations in PKC isoform expression is likely to be species-specific in animal models of cardiac hypertrophy and failure induced by hemodynamic overload.

Studies using genetically engineered mice

The potential deleterious effects of activation of Gαq–PLC signal transduction has been suggested by a number of studies using cultured neonatal rat ventricular myocytes [11–14]. D'Angelo et al. transgenetically overexpressed the wild-type mouse Gαq protein in a postnatal cardiac-specific manner using the α-MHC promoter [20]. Transgenic cardiac-specific Gαq overexpression resulted in PKCε activation, cardiac hypertrophy, and recapitulation of fetal gene program in a gene-dose-dependent manner. It is noteworthy that in the presence of cardiac hypertrophy, extracellular-signal-regulated kinase (ERK) was not activated in the Gαq-overexpressing adult heart. Echocardiography and invasive hemodynamic study with a high-fidelity micromanometer demonstrated contractile depression associated with the cardiac hypertrophy. Higher level of Gαq expression resulted in overt congestive heart failure.

Inhibiting Gαq signaling may prevent cardiac hypertrophy in response to pressure overload. This finding is reported by Akhter et al. [21] in transgenic mice with cardiac-specific overexpression of a peptide fragment derived from the carboxy-terminus of Gαq that can effectively block Gαq receptor coupling. When pressure overload is surgically induced, the transgenic mice demonstrate significantly less ventricular hypertrophy than control animals. Incomplete attenuation of pressure overload-induced ventricular hypertrophy in mice with Gαq inhibitor overexpression suggests that other signaling pathways, perhaps tyrosine kinase mediated, play a role in the development of cardiac hypertrophy.

To examine the functional consequences of sustained activation of the PKCβ isoform, Wakasaki et al. generated transgenic mice with cardiac-specific overexpression of PKCβ$_2$ [22]. Postnatal cardiac-specific overexpression of the PKCβ$_2$ isoform in transgenic mice caused left ventricular hypertrophy, cardiomyocyte necrosis, and multifocal fibrosis and decreased in vivo left ventricular performance. The severity of phenotypes exhibited gene dose dependence. The expression of β-MHC, ANF, and c-fos were upregulated in hearts overexpressing PKCβ$_2$ (figure 2). This study represents the first successful in vivo overexpression of a PKC isoform in the cardiovascular system and demonstrates that sustained activation of PKC can produce cardiac hypertrophy and contractile depression.

Clinical investigation

To clarify the expression of PKC isoforms in failed human heart, explanted hearts of patients diagnosed with idiopathic dilated cardiomyopathy or ischemic car-

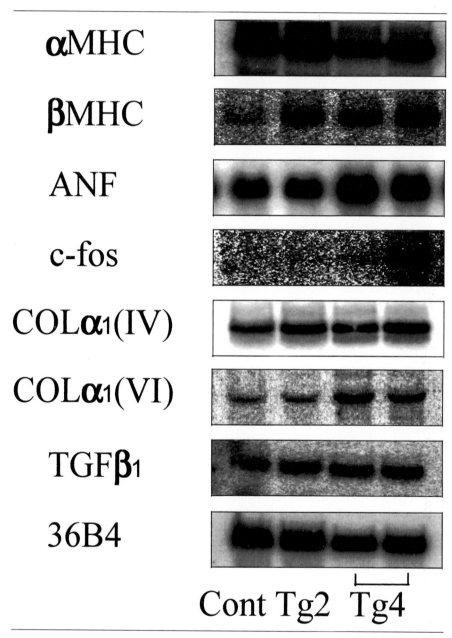

Figure 2. Expression of mRNAs in the $PKC\beta_2$ transgenic mouse heart. Northern blot analysis of total heart RNA from control (Cont) and transgenic mice (Tg2 and Tg4) at 8–12 weeks of age was performed. COL, Collagen. (Printed with permission from [22].)

diomyopathy were examined for PKC isoform content and compared with non-failed left ventricle from hearts rejected for transplant [23]. Expression of PKCα and β isoforms was elevated, but the PKCε isoform appeared to be unchanged or reduced in failed hearts. Total PKC activity and the contribution of the PKCβ isoform to total PKC activity were significantly increased in failed hearts. Immuno-histochemistry with antibody to PKCβ showed the intense staining in cardiomy-ocytes from failed hearts. To our knowledge, this is the first report on isoform-specific PKC activation in failed human heart.

FUNCTIONAL CONSEQUENCES OF PKC ACTIVATION

Cardiac hypertrophy

One of the consequences of PKC activation is the activation of transcription. This is, at least in part, mediated by the binding of the activator protein-1 (AP-1) complex to a consensus sequence [24]. AP-1 was subsequently identified as a heterodimer of the c-Jun and c-fos transcriptional factors.

NF-κB, a family of transcriptional activator proteins, triggers the transcription of early response genes. Phosphorylation by PKC appears to be an essential part of this pathway, both through the removal of NF-κB from the cytoplasmic inhibitory binding protein IκB-α and through augmentation of the transactivation potential of NF-κB itself [25].

The mitogen-activated protein kinases (MAPKs) are serine/threonine protein kinases and consisted of ERK, c-Jun NH_2-terminal protein kinase (JNK) and p38MAPK [26]. ERK is the first MAPK subfamily to be cloned and is activated by a variety of extracellular stimuli that produce proliferation or differentiation. In cardiomyocytes, PKC, but not the Src family or Ras, is critical for ERK activation [27]. A likely candidate through which PKC might activate ERK is Raf-1, a component of the Ras–Raf–MEK–ERK cascade. Mechanical stretch and angiotensin II activate Raf and ERK through PKC in neonatal cardiomyocytes [8]. Activation of ERK leads to the phosphorylation of transcriptional factors, such as c-Jun and Elk-1, and increases protein synthesis. When these outcomes are taken together, PKC isoform activation thereby initiates a phosphorylation cascade and may lead to changes in gene expression characteristics of the cardiac hypertrophic response.

Contractile function

PKC has been implicated in the modulation of cardiac contractile performance through phosphorylation of its substrate as well as in the control of cardiomyocyte hypertrophy [8,9]. In rat cardiomyocytes, Jideama et al. [28] have shown that PKCα and δ phosphorylate Ser-43/Ser-45 sites in troponin I and consequently reduce maximal activity of actomyosin MgATPase. PKCδ, but not PKCα, phosphorylates Ser-23/Ser-24, and reduces calcium sensitivity of MgATPase. In contrast, phospho-rylation of troponin T by PKCζ resulted in a slight increase of calcium sensitivity of MgATPase without affecting the maximal activity of MgATPase.

We reported that the percentage of shortening, rate of shortening, and rate of relengthening of cardiomyocytes were markedly reduced in PKCβ$_2$ overexpression mice compared to wild-type control mice, although the baseline level and amplitude of Ca^{2+} signals were similar [29]. These findings suggested a decreased myofilament responsiveness to Ca^{2+} in PKCβ$_2$ transgenic hearts. Therefore, the incorporation of [^{32}P] inorganic phosphate into cardiac myofibrillar and calcium cycling proteins was studied in Langendorff-perfused hearts. There was a significant increase in the degree of phosphorylation of troponin I in PKCβ$_2$-overexpressing transgenic mice. These findings indicate that in vivo PKCβ$_2$-mediated phosphorylation of troponin I may decrease myofilament Ca^{2-} responsiveness and thus cause cardiomyocyte dysfunction. Taken together, distinct PKC isoforms for phosphorylation of physiological substrates in the myocardium may produce differential functional consequences.

THERAPEUTIC IMPLICATIONS OF PKC INHIBITION

Angiotensin-converting enzyme (ACE) inhibitors have been widely used in human congestive heart failure of diverse etiology. These agents have been shown to improve symptoms, functional capacity, and survival of patients with heart failure compared to conventional diuretics and digoxin treatment. Therefore, we examined the effect of ACE inhibition on PKC isoform activation in our guinea pig model of decompensated hypertrophy produced by aortic banding [18]. Since the angiotensin II receptor is coupled with Gαq–phospholipase C, which activates PKC, we hypothesized that PKC activation by pressure overload could be blocked by ACE inhibition. Translocation of PKCα and ε isoforms was observed in banded animals, and this subcellular redistribution was attenuated by treatment with an ACE inhibitor, ramipril. This treatment was accompanied by prevention of downregulation of calcium cycling proteins, with a resultant improvement in cardiomyocyte calcium transient, isolated left ventricular function, and survival. These findings may represent a fundamental mechanism for the beneficial effects of this pharmacotherapy on cardiac function and survival in heart failure.

We reported that depressed intrinsic cardiomyocyte function of the PKCβ$_2$-overexpressing mouse improved and approached normal through a superfusion of a highly selective inhibitor of the PKCβ isoform (figure 3) [29]. The morphological and functional changes observed in the PKCβ$_2$ transgenic mouse were also prevented or reversed by chronic administration (8 weeks) of a PKCβ inhibitor (table 1) [22]. These results further support our proposal that depression of intrinsic cardiac function is in part related to excessive activation of the PKCβ isoform. The use of isoform-selective PKC inhibitors in a conventional animal model of cardiac failure will further elucidate the role of this signal transduction pathway in the progression from compensated hypertrophy to heart failure. Since PKC isoform activation appears to be involved in the structural and functional changes observed in human heart failure [23], selective inhibition of PKC isoforms may provide a novel therapeutic strategy for the prevention and treatment of this pathological process.

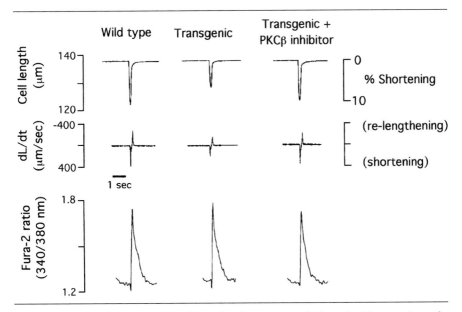

Figure 3. Representative analogue recordings of cardiomyocyte mechanics and calcium transients of cells isolated from a wild-type control mouse, a PKCβ₂ transgenic mouse, and a transgenic mouse treated with a PKCβ selective inhibitor. (Printed with permission from [29].)

Table 1. Echocardiographic measurements in transgenic mice and nontransgenic littermates with or without treatment of PKCβ inhibitor

	Nontreated		Treated With PKCβ inhibitor	
	Control ($n = 6$)	Transgenic ($n = 6$)	Control ($n = 6$)	Transgenic ($n = 6$)
LVEDD, mm	3.41 ± 0.29	2.91 ± 0.36[a]	3.30 ± 0.26	3.36 ± 0.26
LVESD, mm	1.76 ± 0.24	1.93 ± 0.34	1.77 ± 0.16	2.01 ± 0.17
%FS	48.4 ± 2.6	33.8 ± 7.5[a]	46.3 ± 4.3	40.0 ± 2.3[b]
IVS, mm	0.42 ± 0.03	0.61 ± 0.03[a]	0.42 ± 0.03	0.39 ± 0.03
PW, mm	0.39 ± 0.02	0.64 ± 0.05[a]	0.38 ± 0.05	0.38 ± 0.04
LV mass, mg	30.4 ± 4.3	40.5 ± 9.9[a]	28.8 ± 6.3	27.8 ± 5.3
Body weight, g	26.2 ± 3.3	25.4 ± 3.1	23.0 ± 2.2	23.7 ± 2.5
LV mass/body weight	1.17 ± 0.15	1.61 ± 0.38[a]	1.25 ± 0.26	1.18 ± 0.23
Heart rate, bpm	405 ± 54	363 ± 34	434 ± 44	372 ± 49

[a] $p < 0.05$ vs. nontreated control.
[b] $p < 0.05$ vs. treated control (ANOVA with Student–Newman–Keuls test).
LVEDD, left ventricular end-diastolic dimension; LVESD, left ventricular end-systolic dimension; IVS, interventricular septal wall thickness; PW posterior wall thickness; %FS, fractional shortening = (LVEDD − LVESD)/LVEDD × 100. (Printed with permission from [22].)

Taken together, our studies suggest that future studies of PKC signal transduction pathway in the heart may provide important insights into mechanisms for compensated and decompensated hypertrophy.

ACKNOWLEDGMENTS

These studies were supported in part by a Specialized Center of Research in Heart Failure grant (P50 HL52318) from the National Institutes of Health (R.A.W.). We thank Nancy A. Ball and Darryl L. Kirkpatrick for their excellent technical assistance with these studies.

REFERENCES

1. Wagoner LE, Walsh RA. 1996. The cellular pathophysiology of progression to heart failure. Curr Opin Cardiol 11:237–244.
2. Walsh RA, Dorn GW II. 1997. Growth and hypertrophy of the heart and blood vessels. In The Heart, 9th edi. Ed. JW Hurst, RC Schlant, CE Rackley, EH Sonnenblick, NK Wenger, 155–168. New York: McGraw-Hill.
3. Nishizuka Y. 1984. The role of protein kinase C in cell surface signal transduction and tumor promotion. Nature 308:693–697.
4. Neer EJ. 1995. Heterotrimetric G proteins: organizers of transmembrane signals. Cell 80:249–257.
5. Meij JT. 1996. Regulation of G protein function: implication for heart disease. Mol Cell Biochem 157:31–38.
6. Schnabel P, Gas H, Nohr T, Camps M, Bohm M. 1996. Identification and characterization of G protein–regulated phospholipase C in human myocardium. J Mol Cell Cardiol 28:2419–2427.
7. Nishizuka Y. 1992. Intracellular signaling by hydrolysis of phospholipids and activation of protein kinase C. Science 258:607–614.
8. Sugden PH, Bogoyevitch MA. 1995. Intracellular signaling through protein kinases in the heart. Cardiovasc Res 30:478–492.
9. Brodde OE, Michel MC, Zerkowski HR. 1995. Signal transduction mechanisms controlling cardiac contractility and their alterations in chronic heart failure. Cardiovasc Res 30:570–584.
10. Walsh RA. In press. The role of angiotensin II in stretch activated signal transduction of the normal, hypertrophied and failing adult heart. In Angiotensin II Blockade: Physiology and Clinical Implications. Ed. NS Dhalla, P Zahradka, IMC Dixon, and RE Beamish. Boston: Kluwer Academic Publishers.
11. Komuro I, Katoh Y, Kaida T, Shibazaki Y, Kurabayashi M, Takaku F, Yazaki Y. 1991. Mechanical loading stimulates cell hypertrophy and specific gene expression in cultured rat cardiac myocytes. J Biol Chem 266:1265–1268.
12. Sadoshima J, Jahn L, Takahashi T, Kulik TJ, Izumo S. 1992. Molecular characterization of the stretch-induced adaptation of cultured cardiac cells. J Biol Chem 267:10551–10560.
13. Sadoshima J, Xu Y, Slayter HS, Izumo S. 1993. Autocrine release of angiotensin II mediates stretch-induced hypertrophy of cardiac myocytes in vitro. Cell 75:977–984.
14. Yamazaki T, Komuro I, Kudoh S, Zou Y, Shiojima I, Mizuno T, Takano H, Hiroi Y, Ueki K, Tobe K, Kadowaki T, Nagai R, Yazaki Y. 1995. Angiotensin II partly mediates mechanical stretch-induced cardiac hypertrophy. Circ Res 77:258–265.
15. Rybin VO, Steinberg SF. 1994. Protein kinase C isoform expression and regulation in the developing rat heart. Circ Res 74:299–309.
16. Paul K, Ball NA, Dorn II GW, Walsh RA. 1997. Left ventricular stretch stimulates angiotensin II–mediated phosphatidylinositol hydrolysis and protein kinase C ε isoform translocation in adult guinea pig hearts. Circ Res 81:643–650.
17. Gu X, Bishop SP. 1994. Increased protein kinase C and isozyme redistribution in pressure-overloaded cardiac hypertrophy in the rat. Circ Res 75:926–931.
18. Takeishi Y, Bhagwat A, Ball NA, Kirkpatrick DL, Periasamy M, Walsh RA. 1999. Effect of angiotensin converting enzyme inhibition on protein kinase c and SR proteins in heart failure. Am J Physiol 276:H53–H62.

19. Rouet-Benzineb P, Mohammadi K, Perennec J, Poyard M, Bouanani NEH, Crozatier B. 1996. Protein kinase c isoform expression in normal and failing rabbit hearts. Circ Res 79:153–161.

20. D'Angelo DD, Sakata Y, Lorenz JN, Boivin GP, Walsh RA, Liggett SB, Dorn II GW. 1997. Transgenic Gαq overexpression induces cardiac contractile failure in mice. Proc Natl Acad Sci USA 94:8121–8126.

21. Akhter SA, Luttrell LM, Rockman HA, Iaccarino G, Lefkowitz RJ, Koch WJ. 1998. Targeting the receptor-Gq interface to inhibit in vivo pressure overload myocardial hypertrophy. Science 280:574–577.

22. Wakasaki H, Koya D, Schoen FJ, Hoit BD, Jirousek MR, Ways DK, Walsh RA, King GL. 1997. Targeted overexpression of protein kinase c β2 isoform in myocardium causes cardiomyopathy. Proc Natl Acad Sci USA 94:9320–9325.

23. Bowling N, Walsh RA, Song G, Estridge T, Sandusky GE, Fouts RL, Mintze K, Pickard T, Roden R, Bristow MR, Sabbah HN, Mizrahi JL, Gromo G, King GL, Vlahos CJ. 1999. Increased protein kinase C activity and expression of Ca^{2+}-sensitive isoforms in the failing human heart. Circulation 99:384–391.

24. Shubeita HE, Martinson EA, Van Bilsen M, Chien KR, Brown JH. 1992. Transcriptional activation of the cardiac myosin light chain 2 and atrial natriuretic factor genes by protein kinase C in neonatal rat ventricular myocytes. Proc Natl Acad Sci USA 89:1305–1309.

25. Schmitz ML, Dos Santos Silva MA, Baeuerle PA. 1995. Transactivation domain 2 (TA_2) of p65 NF-κB. Similarity of TA_1 and phosphorylation in intact cells. J Biol Chem 270:15576–15584.

26. Sugden PH, Clerk A. 1998. "Stress-responsive" mitogen-activated protein kinases (c-Jun N-terminal kinases and p38 mitogen-activated protein kinases) in the myocardium. Circ Res 83:345–352.

27. Zou Y, Komuro I, Yamazaki T, Aikawa R, Kudoh S, Shiojima I, Hiroi Y, Mizuno T, Yazaki Y. 1996. Protein kinase c, but not tyrosine kinase or Ras, plays a critical role in angiotensin II-induced activation of Raf-1 kinase and extracellular signal-regulated protein kinases in cardiac myocytes. J Biol Chem 271:33592–33597.

28. Jideama NM, Noland TA Jr, Raynor RL, Blobe GC, Fabbro D, Kazanietz MG, Blumberg PM, Hannun YA, Kuo JF. 1996. Phosphorylation specificities of protein kinase C isozymes for bovine cardiac troponin I and troponin T and sites within these proteins and regulation of myofilament properties. J Biol Chem 271:23277–23283.

29. Takeishi Y, Chu G, Kirkpatrick DL, Li Z, Wakasaki H, Kranias EG, King GL, Walsh RA. 1998. In vivo phosphorylation of cardiac troponin I by PKCβ2 decreases cardiomyocyte calcium responsiveness and contractility in transgenic mouse hearts. J Clin Invest 102:72–78.

N. Takeda, M. Nagano and N.S. Dhalla
(eds). The Hypertrophied Heart. Copyright
© 2000. pp. 265–278. Kluwer Academic
Publishers. Boston. All rights reserved.

ANGIOTENSIN II AND CONNECTIVE TISSUE HOMEOSTASIS

KARL T. WEBER

Division of Cardiovascular Diseases, University to Tennessee Health Science Center, Rm. 353 Dobbs Research Institute, 951 Court Avenue, Memphis, TN 38163, USA

Summary. Connective tissue homeostasis refers to self-regulated growth and structure of loose, dense, and specialized connective tissues. De novo generation and coinduction of signals that are either stimulatory or inhibitory to formation of these tissues provide for a reciprocal regulation of their composition. The octapeptide angiotensin (Ang) II is such a growth stimulator. Components involved in Ang II generation and its biologic activity, including angiotensin-converting enzyme (ACE) and Ang II receptors, are expressed by mesenchymal cells (e.g., fibroblasts, adipocytes) responsible for connective tissue turnover. ACE inhibition or AT$_1$ receptor antagonism each attenuate formation of these connective tissues. Endocrine properties of plasma Ang II involved in maintaining circulatory homeostasis can be broadened to encompass autocrine and paracrine effects of Ang II produced within connective tissues, where this peptide contributes to their homeostatic regulation of structure and composition.

INTRODUCTION

Angiotensin (Ang) II is widely recognized as an effector hormone of the circulating renin–angiotensin–aldosterone system. Its classic endocrine actions, brought about by receptor–ligand binding at classic cellular sites, are of paramount importance to circulatory homeostasis, which includes slat and water balance and vascular tonicity. An even broader portfolio of the physiologic relevance and pathophysiologic significance of Ang II in adult tissue has emerged in recent years based on a recognition of its de novo generation by a variety of cells, each possessing high-affinity membrane-bound receptors predominantly of the AT$_1$ receptor subtype. Autocrine/paracrine properties of locally generated Ang II regulate cell growth and behavior. Nowhere is this more obvious than in mesenchymal tissues that include loose, dense, and specialized connective tissues (e.g., extracellular matrix, adipose tissue, and bone and its marrow) and at sites of tissue repair. This chapter addresses several of the diverse actions of local Ang II in these tissues and in what is collectively referred to as *connective tissue homeostasis*.

CONNECTIVE TISSUE AND ITS HOMEOSTASIS

Normal connective tissue

Connective tissue is derived from mesenchyme, embryonic tissue formed by pluripotent mesodermal cells that differentiate along various cell lines to account for specific forms of connective tissue. Mesenchymal (or connective) tissue include specialized hematopoietic tissue, and loose and dense connective tissues distinguished according to their density of collagen fibers. Loose connective tissue is represented by the extracellular matrix of the heart, vasculature, and systemic organs and by adipose tissue. Dense connective tissue includes bone, dermis, tendons, and ligaments.

Extracellular matrix (ECM) includes not only structural proteins (collagens and elastin), of which fibrillar type I and type III collagens are dominant, but also an amorphous ground substance, composed principally of glycosaminoglycans and glycoproteins. The milieu of ECM microenvironment includes macrophages, fibroblasts, and endothelial cells, and various soluble, matrix- and cell membrane-bound molecules. Connective tissue is not inert. Its self-determination is based on an orchestrated balance between stimulators and inhibitors, operating in a paradigm of reciprocal regulation to govern cell behavior and ECM remodeling. Included here are metabolic functions intergal to fibrillar collagen turnover and the deposition and resorption of fat or bone.

Tissue homeostasis: the concept

Homeostasis is defined as a state of equilibrium that exists between different but interdependent elements or groups of elements in a living organism. This concept is often invoked when addressing the stability of an organism's internal environment, such as salt and water balance and factors intrinsic and extrinsic to kidneys, which serve to maintain constant the volume and composition of extracellular fluid. *Hormones*, or circulating signals, are generated at a site distant from their eventual activity in classic target cells. Their *endocrine* properties are expressed on target cells via specific receptors. It is now recognized that tissues can act independently of hormones to maintain their own circulatory homeostasis, through de novo generation of a variety of intrinsic substances that have *autocrine* and *paracrine* properties on constitutive cell populations. Organs express various substances that regulate the growth, specialized behavior, and survival of their constituent cell populations. Based on an emerging body of evidence derived from both in vivo and in vitro studies, the concept of connective tissue homeostasis emerges to describe an organ's self-regulation of extracellular matrix (ECM) structure and cellular composition—a self-determination of cell mobility, differentiation, replication, apoptosis, and the growth and regression of its structural protein scaffolding.

Connective tissue homeostasis

ECM homeostasis involves collagen synthesis and degradation. It also may depend on stromal cell differentiation, replication, and survival, each of which occurs within the dynamic microenvironment of the interstitial space containing a blood filtrate and soluble signals from ECM cells and parenchyma termed *tissue fluid*. The interstitial space is common to ventricles and atria [1]. It provides cardiac tissue with a dynamic microenvironment that includes self-aggregating macromolecules (e.g., TGF-β and matrix metalloproteinases and their respective inhibitors) involved in the regulation of cellular composition and matrix structure, or homeostasis.

Connective tissue homeostasis is based on fibroblasts having several requisite features [2]. First, fibroblasts must possess a genotype that permits de novo generation of signals and expression of their receptors that will control the destiny of ECM, including its growth and regression under normal or pathologic states [3]. A systemic reaction is not a requisite to the appearance of these signals. Local signals remain confined to their sites of production. Once formed, they do not promote a systemic response, an amplified version of their local effect, unless tissue injury is severe and the release of signals exceeds local inhibitors. Second, tissue-generated signals participate in a local system of reciprocal regulation, or negative feedback, where continuous and regulated production of stimulators and inhibitors resist change—checks and balances on cell behavior and ECM turnover. In most normal adult tissues, fibroblast growth and collagen turnover are modest, since stromal fibroblasts are quiescent, maintained in a Go state by growth inhibitors. Release from Go and progression into other phases of the cell cycle are related to the relative balance between a withdrawal of such suppressors and an excess production of growth stimulators. ACE and its catabolism of a growth suppressor, AcSDKP, may unleash cell proliferation at sites of repair while locally generated Ang II, via autocrine induction of macrophage-generated $TGF\beta_1$, serves to induce fibroblast differentiation into an active myofibroblast phenotype (expressing α-smooth muscle actin and vimentin) that regulates ECM formation. Simultaneous induction of nitric oxide and bradykinin by Ang II serves to inhibit tissue growth and induce a gene program that governs cell survival, thereby creating a self-limiting response to ECM formation that serves to minimize the possibility of unbridled fibrous tissue formation. This undoubtedly complex scenario is beginning to unfold, and further investigation will be necessary to elucidate it in detail.

ANGIOTENSIN II AND CONNECTIVE TISSUE HOMEOSTASIS

Angiotensin (Ang) II, an effector hormone of the circulating renin–angiotensin–aldosterone system (RAAS), has well-known endocrine properties expressed at cellular sites via stereospecific receptors that in adult tissues are predominantly of the AT_1 subtype [4,5]. These "classic" properties of plasma Ang II focus on *circulatory homeostasis*. In this connection, angiotensin-converting enzyme (ACE), an ectoenzyme bound to plasma membrane of endothelial cells, particularly of the pulmonary circulation, is well positioned and integral to the formation of circulating Ang II from inactive plasma Ang I substrate.

A broader perspective of Ang II is emerging as ongoing research uncovers an ever expanding arsenal to the physiologic relevance and pathophysiologic significance of this peptide, including its autocrine/paracrine actions I tissue, which can operate independent of its role as a plasma hormone. Several criteria must be fulfilled to substantiate de novo Ang II generation in any tissue and to qualify it as a local effector of cell behavior: (1) the presence of all components requisite to de novo Ang peptide generation, (2) target cell Ang II receptors and altered cell behavior in response to Ang II receptor binding; and (3), a direct or indirect regulation of a candidate gene(s) responsible for altered target cell behavior.

Connective tissue homeostasis is linked to fibroblast-derived Ang II, which in an autocrine manner regulates elaboration of $TGF\beta_1$, a fibrogenic cytokine responsible for connective tissue formation at normal and pathologic sites of collagen turnover. Spatial concordance exists between high-density ACE and Ang II receptor autoradiographic binding with fibroblast-like cells normally residing in heart valve leaflets or with the appearance of such fibroblast-like cells in response to injury (reviewed in [6]), including various tissues and diverse forms of injury: myocardial or renal infarction; pericardial inflammation; invasion of tissue by foreign body; or subcutaneous instillation of a chemical irritant. Additionally, these cells express $TGF\beta_1$ and type I collagen mRNA at each of these sites of repair. This indirect evidence linking Ang II production to fibroblasts involved in connective tissue formation is further supported by pharmacologic intervention. Through the use of ACE inhibition or AT_1 receptor antagonism, Ang II is linked to normal loose connective tissue homeostasis in utero and during neonatal growth and to fibrosis in adult rats at sites of injury. Additionally, components involved in Ang I and Ang II generation are present at transcription and translation levels in cultured fibroblast-like cells derived from either valve leaflets, scar tissue, or subcutaneous pouch tissue. AT_1 receptor binding in adult tissue promotes the expression of type I collagen mRNA. In this context, Ang II is a growth stimulator. AT_2 receptor binding inhibits growth to offset AT_1-mediated effects [7,8]. Thus, Ang II per se maintains a reciprocal regulation and stability to collagen turnover in normal adult tissues unless injury supervenes. Connective tissue fibroblast-like cells that appear at sites of repair express components requisite for de novo Ang peptide formation and Ang II receptors, integral to its biologic functions. Expression of angiotensinogen, an aspartyl protease (cathepsin D), and ACE is a function of differentiated fibroblast-like cells of connective tissue. De novo Ang II, however, does not operate independently of other factors involved in the reciprocal regulation of connective tissue. These include endothelins, aldosterone, and the $TGF\beta$ family of polypeptides, each of which functions as stimulators, and bradykinin, nitric oxide, and prostaglandins, which serve as inhibitors of collagen formation. ACE is integral to connective tissue homeostasis. It contributes to Ang II formation, which can influence the expression and secretion of these stimulators and inhibitors. Other substrates of ACE (in its dual capacity as a kininase II) include bradykinin, substance P, enkephalins, and a recently characterized tetrapeptide (N-acetyl-seryl-aspartyl-lysyl-proline). Referred to as AcSDKP, this peptide is a growth suppressor that maintains cells in their Go state [9,10]. It is present in plasma, circulating mononuclear cells and a variety of tissues, including bone marrow (vide infra). Given its metabolic profile, ACE is a physiologic regulator of inflammation, and as suggested previously, of connective tissue homeostasis [2].

Cardiovascular connective tissue

The heart's three-dimensional fibrillar collagen scaffolding maintains cardiac myocyte alignment throughout the cardiac cycle. Type I collagen imparts cardiac tissue with physical properties that include stiffness and resistance to deformation [11].

Formation of the heart's ECM begins in utero. Heart valve leaflet formation from endocardial cushions is linked to the expression of the TGFβ family of fibrogenic polypeptides [12,13]. Lamparter et al. [14] examined whether AT_1 or AT_2 receptor blockade would result in attenuation of collagen mRNA expression and fibrillar collagen accumulation and would alter $TGFβ_1$ mRNA expression in the developing fetal rat heart. Since Ang II receptor subtypes are developmentally regulated [15], pregnant rats received an antagonist of either AT_1 receptors (losartan) or AT_2 receptors (PD123319). Offspring were studied within 24 hours after birth and compared to fetuses of untreated age-matched controls. No birth defects or cardiac malformations were grossly evident in either treatment group. Birth weight was comparable in control and PD-treated animals but was reduced in losartan-treated newborn animals. Compared to untreated animals, type I collagen and $TGFβ_1$ mRNA expression in cardiac tissue were each equally reduced in response to losartan and PD123319 treatment, together with a significant decrease in total soluble cardiac collagen concentration confirmed by attenuated immunoreactivity of type I and type III collagen in whole heart extracts by Western blotting. The results of these pharmacologic interventions suggest that AT_1 and AT_2 receptors are each involved in the regulation of type I and type III collagen expression and structural protein expression during gestation. These effects appear to be mediated, at least in part, by attenuated cardiac $TGFβ_1$ levels. Functional and structural consequences of attenuated cardiac collagen formation in the fetus and newborn remains to be determined.

The collagen concentration of right and left ventricles in newborn rats is equivalent [16]. Collagen continues to accumulate in both ventricles and blood vessels for weeks after birth, despite a regression in right ventricular myocyte size that accompanies reduced right ventricular pressure work secondary to pulmonary vasodilatation. Despite normal differences in hemodynamic work loads between ventricles in young rats, the collagen concentration of the low-pressure right ventricle therefore is several times greater than that of its counterpart, the high-pressure left ventricle. Treatment of young rats with a nonpressor dose of an ACE inhibitor alters normal connective tissue formation. The collagen concentration of both ventricles, the aorta, and blood vessels is reduced (compared to untreated controls) in 10-week-old rats that had received enalapril for 6 weeks.

Heart valve leaflets and accompanying chordae tendineae represent an exteriorized segment of this scaffolding [17]. They offer a window of opportunity to study ECM homeostasis. High-density autoradiographic ACE binding is found in valve leaflets and adventitia of normal adult rat pulmonary artery, aorta, and intramyocardial coronary arteries (see figure 1A) [18–20]. High-density Ang II receptor binding is likewise present in heart valves and adventitia of the aorta and pulmonary artery (see figure 18B). Elsewhere in the heart, ACE and Ang II receptor binding densities are low (figure 1C and E). Fibroblast-like cells found in valve leaflets, also

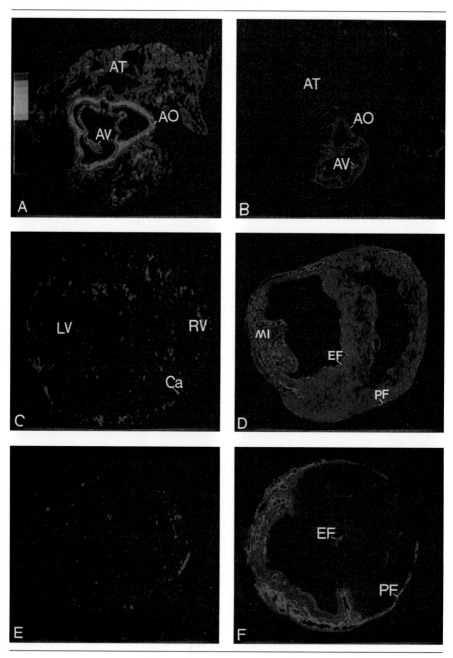

Figure 1. Autoradiographic ACE and Ang II receptor binding in the normal and infarcted rat heart. High binding density of ACE and Ang II receptors are seen in aortic valves (AV) and aorta (AO) of the normal rat heart (**A** and **B**, respectively). ACE and Ang II receptor binding is increased at the site of MI and at remote sites where endocardial (EF) and pericardial (PF) fibrosis appear (**D** and **F**) compared to normal heart with low ACE and Ang II receptor binding of right (RV) and left (LV) ventricles (**C** and **E**).

Examples of Angiotensin II and Connective Tissue Homeostasis

Connective Tissue Cells	Ang Components	Ang Receptors	Response
Myofibroblasts (valve leaflets, fibrous tissue)	Ao CathepsinD ACE	AT1	Synthesis of type I and III collagens
Adipocytes	Ao renin ACE	AT1>AT2	lipogenic enzymes and adipose mass
osteoblasts osteoclasts	?	AT1	bone formation and resorption
hematopoietic stem cells	?	AT1	erythropoiesis

Figure 2. Examples of angiotensin (Ang) II and connective tissue homeostasis. Ao, angiotensinogen; ACE, angiotensin-converting enzyme; AT1 and AT2, receptor subtypes. See text for discussion.

referred to as *myofibroblasts* or *valvular interstitial cells*, are a source of this binding. In culture, these cells express requisite components for Ang peptide generation, with Ang II regulating type I collagen synthesis of these cells via AT_1 receptor binding [21–24].

Adipose tissue

Loose connective tissue includes white and brown adipose tissue. Fat cells, or adipocytes, are scattered throughout cardiovascular connective tissue. Aggregates of predominantly adipocytes constitute adipose tissue that contain lobules of fat cells separated from each other by fibrous septa. Adipose tissue is richly perfused with vascular channels found in these septa.

Adipose tissue expresses components requisite to de novo Ang peptide generation and Ang II receptors (reviewed inn [25]). Adipocytes are a rich source of Ao, with its mRNA and secretion of protein a feature of white and brown adipocytes [26,27]. Specific renin activity is observed in brown adipose tissue without detection of renin mRNA by RT-PCR [28], suggesting either uptake of renal renin from the circulation or the presence of other proteases (e.g., cathepsins). ACE has been identified in rat and human adipose tissue [29,30]; however, its localization to adipocytes vs. stroma-vascular tissues remains controversial.

Unlike in the liver, Ao expression in adipose tissue is nutritionally regulated [31]. Ao mRNA and protein secretion are reduced within days of fasting and are reexpressed within days of refeeding—a reversible physiological response specific to this tissue without detectable changes in the liver and serum Ao concentrations. These responses in Ao to fasting and refeeding are each respectively associated with a respective fall and rise in blood pressure, implicating nutrition in adipose and circulatory homeostasis. Ao secretion is increased in a mouse model of obesity, and a theoretical model has been proposed wherein local Ao and Ang II generation in adipose tissue regulates its blood supply: less Ang II with vasodilatation during fasting to promote lipolysis and fatty acid efflux, while more Ang II during refeeding and local vasoconstriction promotes glucose metabolism [31]. It is further speculated that these responses could have pathological implications regarding hypotension of fasting and hypertension in obesity. Ao expression by 3T3/L1 cells, cloned from preadipocytes (an early developmental stage), is upregulated by insulin and downregulated by isoproterenol, a β-adrenergic receptor agonist [32].

Ang II increases lipogenesis of both cultured human adipocytes and 3T3/L1 cells. In the latter, this responses occurs via AT_2 receptor binding. Differences in developmental regulation of Ang II receptors notwithstanding, these observations further implicate paracrine properties of this locally derived peptide in adipose tissue homeostasis (adipocyte hypertrophy and metabolism) as expressed by autoregulation of adipocyte lipid synthesis and storage [33]. Ang II-induced differentiation of preadipocytes into adipocytes suggests that Ang II may also contribute to adipose tissue hyperplasia [34].

Ang II receptors of adipose tissue are regulated by age and fat mass. Adult rat adipose tissue, taken from epididymal, mesenteric, and retroperitoneal areas, and human tissue obtained from epigastric subcutaneous fat and peripheral omentum at the time of gastroplasty for morbid obesity have been examined and found to be predominantly of the AT_1 subtype [35]. Losartan, an AT_1 receptor antagonist, prevents adipose tissue hypertrophy in rats, independent of their nutritional status (35). Weight loss is reported to accompany chronic administration of an ACE inhibitor in hypertensive patients [36].

Hematopoietic tissue

Hematopoiesis

Stromal cells of bone marrow provide a microenvironment conducive to proliferation and differentiation of circulating blood cells. Stromal cells express angiotensinogen [37], whose function is uncertain but could contribute to hematopoiesis.

AcSDKP, a growth suppressor, prevents the recruitment of pluripotent hematopoietic stem cells and normal early progenitors into the S-phase of the cell cycle by maintaining them in the Go phase. AcSDKP is present in plasma, circulating mononuclear cells, and a variety of tissues, including bone marrow. The NH2-terminal domain of ACE is involved in the hydrolysis of AcSDKP; plasma and tissue ACE are likely involved in its catabolism [9]. ACE therefore is a physiologic regulator of AcSDKP, and its degradation of AcSDKP at sites of repair would permit cell proliferation. ACE expressed by mononuclear cells would foster the cell proliferation seen during early repair; myofibroblast and their expression of ACE could account for persistent cellular growth with later repair.

Erythrocytosis

Expression of AT$_1$ receptors by erythroid precursors appears when hematopoietic progenitor cells are maintained in culture together with erythropoietin. Ang II stimulation leads to proliferation of early erythroid progenitors, a response abolished by losartan [38]. The contribution of Ang II to the pathogenesis of renal transplant erythrocytosis remains uncertain, despite the clinical use of ACE inhibition to attenuate or even correct elevated hematocrit in this setting [38,40].

Leukocytes

Circulating granulocytes express and release angiotensinogen [37] and a serine protease (cathepsin G) that can generate Ang II from Ang I or directly from Ao [41–43]. Furthermore, activated monocytes express (mRNA, protein, and activity) ACE [44]. Ang II receptor binding sites have been reported in mononuclear leukocytes [45] and macrophages [46], although this finding is controversial and may also involve endocytosis [47,48]. As depicted in the schematic representation of tissue repair shown in figure 3, inflammatory cells are portrayed as providing an initial source of Ang II at sites of tissue injury, which promotes expression and release of TFGβ$_1$ from monocytes/macrophages in an autocrine/paracrine manner. This cytokine is considered integral to the differentiation of quiescent interstitial fibroblasts into their active myofibroblast phenotype [49]. Other potential effects of Ang II on macrophage functions have also been suggested [50,51].

Bone

Bone, a form of dense connective tissue, undergoes remodeling and thereby requires continuous regulation of osteoblast and osteoclast growth. As with hematopoiesis, the bone marrow microenvironment is integral to bone remodeling. Osteoblasts and osteoclasts are derived from hematopoietic stem cells, and Manolagas and Jilka (52) have suggested that hematopoiesis and genesis of osteoblasts and osteoclasts proceed along similar pathways and under identical regulatory controls. Osteoblast Ang II receptors have been identified, and this peptide is thought to influence osteoblast growth and bone formation [53,54]. ACE inhibitor-associated fetopathy, involving impaired calvarial bone formation, has been reported [55]. Ang II may also influence osteoclast-mediated bone resorption under circumstances that merit further investigation [56].

Fibrous tissue

Fibrous tissue is composed predominantly of type I and III collagens. It appears in response to or in the absence of myocyte necrosis (replacement and reactive forms of fibrosis, respectively). In vitro autoradiography identifies the heterogeneous densities of ACE and Ang II receptor binding that exists in the injured heart (reviewed in [6]). High-density binding is found at the infarct scar that forms following coronary artery ligation. Binding densities 4 weeks post-MI are shown in figure 1 and 1F. High-density ACE and Ang II receptor binding remains as late as 6 months post-

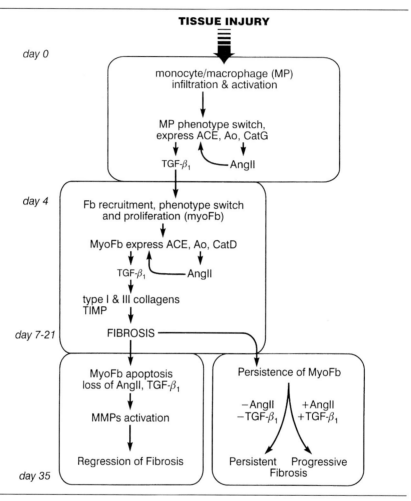

Figure 3. A paradigm of repair that follows tissue injury and that is based on an initial inflammatory cell response whose generation of Ang II is integral to the autocrine induction of TGFβ₁ that elicits differentiation of fibroblasts into myofibroblasts (myoFb). These latter cells are responsible for fibrous tissue formation based on their expression of type I and type III fibrillar collagens and inhibitors of matrix metalloproteinases (TIMP). The fate of myoFb determines whether there will be a regression, persistence, or progression to tissue fibrosis. (Reprinted with permission from Weber KT. 1997. Fibrosis, a common pathway to organ failure: angiotensin II and tissue repair. *Semin Nephrol* 17:467–491.)

MI. The expression of ACE and Ang II receptors is initially attributed to macrophages and the appearance of phenotypically transformed fibroblast-like cells that express alpha-smooth muscle actin (α-SMA) and are referred to as myofibroblasts (myoFb). Macrophages disappear from the site of repair by week 2 post-MI, while active myofibroblasts (α-SMA and vimentin positive) are persistent within the infarct scar, albeit at reduced numbers. Persistent activity is defined by myofibroblast expression of type I collagen and high-density binding for ACE and receptors for Ang II and TGFβ₁.

The rat MI model creates several other sites of tissue repair and subsequent fibrosis that are useful in the analysis of Ang II and connective tissue homeostasis (reviewed in [6]). Fibrosis in cardiac and noncardiac tissues involves a spatial and temporal coincidence between expression of ACE, Ang II receptors, TGFβ₁ and its receptors, type I collagen and α-SMA positive myofibroblasts. Fibrous tissue and its resident myofibroblasts generate Ang II de novo. This process has been demonstrated for valve leaflets, infarct scar tissue, pericardial fibrosis, and subcutaneous pouch tissue raised in response to croton oil. Additionally, pharmacologic intervention with either an AT_1 receptor antagonist or an ACE inhibitor attenuates expression of TGFβ₁, fibrous tissue formation, and tissue hydroxyproline concentration at these diverse sites, emphasizing an autocrine role for Ang II in regulating fibrogenesis and myofibroblast collagen turnover via AT_1 receptor binding.

CONCLUSIONS

Homeostasis is classically viewed as a state of equilibrium between different yet interdependent elements, such as salt and water balance. Homeostasis can also be applied to a tissue's autoregulation of its cellular composition and ECM: a self-determination of its cell alignment, differentiation, replication, hypertrophy, atrophy, and/or apoptosis, as well as growth or regression of ECM. De novo generation of stimulatory (e.g., Ang II) and inhibitory (e.g., NO) signals provides for a reciprocal regulation of ECM collagen turnover. All components involved in Ang II generation and activity, including ACE and Ang II receptors, are expressed by myofibroblasts responsible for fibrillar collagen synthesis at sites of active turnover such as valve leaflets and infarct scar. AT_1 receptor binding regulates myofibroblast expression of type I collagen in normal and pathologic states via autocrine induction of TGFβ₁. ACE inhibition or AT_1 receptor antagonism abrogates TGFβ₁ expression and retards normal connective tissue formation in utero, during early growth and development, and during fibrous tissue formation following injury. Classic concepts of homeostasis and endocrine properties of Ang II must each be broadened to recognize the autocrine and paracrine effects of Ang II that regulate ECM in normal and diseased tissues.

Man's ascent from prehistoric times involved adaptations to environmental stress. None has been more important than the ability to survive injury. Tissue injury, with blood loss and hypotension, invokes several homeostatic responses brought into play in sequential manner. Each is integral to survival. The first of these processes is circulatory homeostasis, which includes the need for coagulation and platelet aggregation at sites of bleeding; arteriolar vasoconstriction to preserve arterial pressure for a reduced intravascular volume; and renal resorption of salt and water to restore lost intravascular volume. Each of these responses is mediated, in part, by local Ang II and elevations in circulating Ang II that appear when renal perfusion is impaired and ischemic kidneys elaborate renin. Having compensated for the initial threat to survival, there follows a need to repair injured tissues. Healing is a property of all vascularized tissues. Through a biologic economy of action, mediators of circulatory homeostasis, such as Ang II, are likewise involved in connective tissue homeostasis that eventuates in tissue repair.

REFERENCES

1. Weber KT. 1991. Cardiac interstitium: extracellular space of the myocardium. In The Heart and Cardiovascular System, 2nd ed. Ed. HA Fozzard, E Haber, RB Jennings, AM Katz, and HE Morgan, 1465–1480. New York: Raven Press.
2. Weber KT, Swamynathan SK, Guntaka RV, Sun Y. 1999. Angiotensin II and extracellular matrix homeostasis. Int J Biochem Cell Biol 31:395–403.
3. Bayreuther K, Rodemann HP, Francz PI, Maier K. 1988. Differentiation of fibroblast stem cells. J Cell Sci Suppl 10:115–130.
4. Bottari SP, de Gasparo M, Steckelings UM, Levens NR. 1993. Angiotensin II receptor subtypes: characterization, signalling mechanisms, and possible physiological implications. Front Neuroendocrinol 14:123–171.
5. Timmermans PB, Wong PC, Chiu AT, Herblin WF, Benfield P, Carini DJ, Lee RJ, Wexler RR, Saye JA, Smith RD. 1993. Angiotensin II receptors and angiotensin II receptor antagonists. Pharmacol Rev 45:205–251.
6. Weber KT. 1997. Extracellular matrix remodeling in heart failure. A role for de novo angiotensin II generation. Circulation 96:4065–4082.
7. Stoll M, Steckelings UM, Paul M, Bottari SP, Metzger R, Unger T. 1995. The angiotensin AT2-receptor mediates inhibition of cell proliferation in coronary endothelial cells. J Clin Invest 95:651–657.
8. Nakajima M, Hutchinson HG, Fuginaga M, Hayashida W, Zhang L, Horiucki M, Pratt RE, Dzau VJ. 1995. The angiotensin II type 2 (AT2) antagonizes the growth effects of the AT1 receptor: gain-of-function study using gene transfer. Proc Natl Acad Sci USA 92:10663–10667.
9. Azizi M, Rousseau A, Ezan E, Guyene T-T, Michelet S, Grognet J-M, Lenfant M, Corvol P, Ménard J. 1996. Acute angiotensin-converting enzyme inhibition increases the plasma level of the natural stem cell regulatory N-acetyl-seryl-aspartyl-lysyl-proline. J Clin Invest 97:839–844.
10. Rousseau-Plasse A, Lenfant M, Potier P. 1996. Catabolism of the hemoregulatory peptide N-Acetyl-Ser-Asp-Lys-Pro: a new insight into the physiological role of the angiotensin-I-converting enzyme N-active site. Bioorg Med Chem 4:1113–1119.
11. Weber KT. 1989. Cardiac interstitium in health and disease: the fibrillar collagen network. J Am Coll Cardiol 13:1637–1652.
12. Nakajima Y, Mironov V, Yamagishi T, Nakamura H, Markwald RR. 1997. Expression of smooth muscle alpha-actin in mesenchymal cells during formation of avian endocardial cushion tissue: a role for transforming growth factor β3: Dev Dyn 209:296–309.
13. Potts JD, Dagle JM, Walder JA, Weeks DL, Runyan RB. 1991. Epithelial–mesenchymal transformation of embryonic cardiac endothelial cells is inhibited by a modified antisense oligodeoxynucleotide to transforming growth factor β3. Proc Natl Acad Sci USA 88:1516–1520.
14. Lamparter S, Sun Y, Weber KT. 1999. Angiotensin II receptor blockade during gestation attenuates collagen formation in the developing rat heart. Cardiovasc Res 43:165–172.
15. Grady EF, Sechi LA, Griffin CA, Schambelan M, Kalinyak JE. 1991. Expression of AT2 receptors in the developing rat fetus. J Clin Invest 88:921–933.
16. Caspari PG, Gibson K, Harris P. 1976. Changes in myocardial collagen in normal development and after β blockade. In Biochemistry and Pharmacology of Myocardial Hypertrophy, Hypoxia, and Infarction. Ed. P Harris, RJ Bing, and A Fleckenstein, 99–104. Baltimore: University Park Press. (Rona G, ed. Recent Advances in Studies on Cardiac Structure and Metabolism, vol. 7.)
17. Robinson TF, Geraci MA, Sonnenblick EH, Factor SM. 1988. Coiled perimysial fibers of papillary muscle in rat heart: morphology, distribution, and changes in configuration. Circ Res 63:577–592.
18. Sun Y, Diaz-Arias AA, Weber KT. 1994. Angiotensin-converting enzyme, bradykinin and angiotensin II receptor binding in rat skin, tendon and heart valves: an in vitro quantitative autoradiographic study. J Lab Clin Med 123:372–377.
19. Yamada H, Fabris B, Allen AM, Jackson B, Johnston CI, Mendelsohn FAO. 1991. Localization of angiotensin converting enzyme in rat heart. Circ Res 68:141–149.

20. Pinto JE, Viglione P, Saavedra JM. 1991. Autoradiographic localization and quantification of rat heart angiotensin converting enzyme. Am J Hypertens 4:321–326.
21. Katwa LC, Ratajska A, Cleutjens JPM, Sun Y, Zhou G, Lee SJ, Weber KT. 1995. Angiotensin converting enzyme and kininase-II-like activities in cultured valvular interstitial cells of the rat heart. Cardiovasc Res 29:57–64.
22. Katwa LC, Tyagi SC, Campbell SE, Lee SJ, Cicila GT, Weber KT. 1996. Valvular interstitial cells express angiotensinogen, cathepsin D, and generate angiotensin peptides. Int J Biochem Cell Biol 28:807–821.
23. Katwa LC, Campbell SE, Tyagi SC, Lee SJ, Cicila GT, Weber KT. 1997. Cultured myofibroblasts generate angiotensin peptides *de novo*. J Mol Cell Cardiol 29:1375–1386.
24. Katwa LC, Sun Y, Campbell SE, Tyagi SC, Dhalla AK, Kandala JC, Weber KT. 1998. Pouch tissue and angiotensin peptide generation. J Mol Cell Cardiol 30:1401–1413.
25. Zorad S, Fickova M, Zelezna B, Macho L, Kral JG. 1995. The role of angiotensin II and its receptors in regulation of adipose tissue metabolism and cellularity. Gen Physiol Biophys 14:383–391.
26. Cassis LA, Lynch KR, Peach MJ. 1998. Localization of angiotensinogen messenger RNA in rat aorta. Circ Res 62:1259–1262.
27. Campbell DJ, Habener JF. 1987. Cellular localization of angiotensinogen gene expression in brown adipose tissue and mesentery: quantification of messenger ribonucleic acid abundance using hybridization *in situ*. Endocrinology 121:1616–1626.
28. Shenoy U, Cassis L. 1997. Characterization of renin activity in brown adipose tissue. Am J Physiol 272:C989–C999.
29. Jonsson JR, Game PA, Head RJ, Frewin DB. 1994. The expression and localisation of the angiotensin-converting enzyme mRNA in human adipose tissue. Blood Press 3:72–75.
30. Crandall DL, Herzlinger HE, Saunders BD, Kral JG. 1994. Developmental aspects of the adipose tissue renin–angiotensin system: therapeutic implications. Drug Dev Res 32:117–125.
31. Frederich RC Jr, Kahn BB, Peach MJ, Flier JS. 1992. Tissue-specific nutritional regulation of angiotensinogen in adipose tissue. Hypertension 19:339–344.
32. Jones BH, Standridge MK, Taylor JW, Moustaïd N. 1997. Angiotensinogen gene expression in adipose tissue: analysis of obese models and hormonal and nutritional control. Am J Physiol 273:R236–R242.
33. Jones BH, Standridge MK, Moustaid N. 1997. Angiotensin II increases lipogenesis in 3T3-L1 and human adipose cells. Endocrinology 138:1512–1519.
34. Darimont C, Vassaux G, Ailhaud G, Negrel R. 1994. Differentiation of preadipose cells: paracrine role of prostacyclin upon stimulation of adipose cells by angiotensin-II. Endocrinology 135:2030–2036.
35. Crandall DL, Herzlinger HE, Saunders BD, Armellino DC, Kral JG. 1994. Distribution of angiotensin II receptors in rat and human adipocytes. J Lipid Res 35:1378–1385.
36. McGrath BP, Matthews PG, Louis W, Howes L, Whitworth JA, Kincaid-Smith PS, Fraser I, Scheinkestel C, MacDonald G, Rallings M. 1990. Double-blind study of dilevalol and captopril, both in combination with hydrochorothiazide, in patients with moderate to severe hypertension. J Cardiovasc Pharmacol 16:831–838.
37. Gomez RA, Norling LL, Wilfong N, Isakson P, Lynch KR, Hock R, Quesenberry P. 1993. Leukocytes synthesize angiotensinogen. Hypertension 21:470–475.
38. Mrug M, Stopka T, Julian BA, Prchal JF, Prchal JT. 1997. Angiotensin II stimulates proliferation of normal early erythroid progenitors. J Clin Invest 100:2310–2314.
39. Danovitch GM, Jamgotchian NJ, Eggena PH, Paul W, Barrett JD, Wilkinson A, Lee DBN. 1995. Angiotensin-converting enzyme inhibition in the treatment of renal transplant erythrocytosis. Clinical experience and observation of mechanism. Transplantation 60:132–137.
40. Julian BA, Gaston RS, Barker CV, Krystal G, Diethelm AG, Curtis JJ. 1994. Erythropoiesis after withdrawal of enalapril in post-transplant erythrocytosis. Kidney Int 46:1397–1403.
41. Wintroub BU, Klickstein LB, Watt KW. 1981. A human neutrophil-dependent pathway for generation of angiotensin II. Purification of the product and identification as angiotensin II. J Clin Invest 68:484–490.
42. Tonnesen MG, Klempner MS, Austen KF, Wintroub BU. 1982. Identification of a human neutrophil angiotensin II-generating protease as cathepsin G. J Clin Invest 69:25–30.
43. Klickstein LB, Kaempfer CE, Wintroub BU. 1982. The granulocyte–angiotensin system. Angiotensin I-converting activity of cathepsin G. J Biol Chem 257:15042–15046.
44. Friedland J, Setton C, Silverstein E. 1978. Induction of angiotensin converting enzyme in human myocytes in culture. Biochem Biophys Res Commun 83:843–849.

45. Shimada K, Yazaki Y. 1978. Binding sites for angiotensin II in human mononuclear leucocytes. J Biochem (Tokyo) 84:1013–1015.
46. Thomas DW, Hoffman MD. 1984. Identification of macrophage receptors for angiotensin: a potential role in antigen uptake for T lymphocyte responses? J Immunol 132:2807–2812.
47. Simon MR, Kamlay MT, Khan M, Melmon K. 1989. Angiotensin II binding to human mononuclear cells. Immunopharmocol Immunotoxicol 11:63–80.
48. Neyses L, Locher M, Wehling M, Pech H, Tenschert W, Vetter W. 1984. Angiotensin II binding to human mononuclear cells: receptor or free fluid endocytosis? Clin Sci 66:605–612.
49. Desmoulière A, Geinoz A, Gabbiani F, Gabbiani G. 1993. Transforming growth factor-β1 induces α-smooth muscle actin expression in granulation tissue myofibroblasts and in quiescent and growing cultured fibroblasts. J Cell Biol 122:103–111.
50. Fóris G, Dezsö B, Medgyesi GA, Füst G. 1983. Effect of angiotensin II on macrophage functions. Immunology 48:529–535.
51. Nairn R, Spengler ML, Hoffman MD, Solvay MJ, Thomas DW. 1984. Macrophage processing of peptide antigens: identification of an antigen complex. J Immunol 133:3225–3234.
52. Manolagas SC, Jilka RL. 1992. Cytokines, hematopoiesis, osteoclastogenesis, and estrogens. Calcif Tissue Int 50:199–202.
53. Hiruma Y, Inoue A, Hirose S, Hagiwara H. 1997. Angiotensin II stimulates the proliferation of osteoblast-rich populations of cells from rat calvariae. Biochem Biophys Res Commun 230:176–178.
54. Lamparter S, Kling L, Schrader M, Ziegler R, Pfeilschifter J. 1998. Effects of angiotensin II on bone cells in vitro. J Cell Physiol 175:89–98.
55. Barr M Jr, Cohen MM Jr. 1991. ACE inhibitor fetopathy and hypocalvaria: the kidney–skull connection. Teratology 44:485–495.
56. Hatton R, Stimpel M, Chambers TJ. 1997. Angiotensin II is generated from angiotensin I by bone cells and stimulates osteoclastic bone resorption in vitro. J Endocrinol 152:5–10.

N. Takeda, M. Nagano and N.S. Dhalla
(eds). The Hypertrophied Heart. Copyright
© 2000. pp. 279–302. Kluwer Academic
Publishers. Boston. All rights reserved.

BENEFICIAL EFFECTS OF ANGIOTENSIN BLOCKADE IN HEART FAILURE DUE TO MYOCARDIAL INFARCTION

NARANJAN S. DHALLA and XIAOBING GUO

Institute of Cardiovascular Sciences, St. Boniface General Hospital Research Centre, 351 Tache Avenue, and Department of Physiology, Faculty of Medicine, University of Manitoba, Winnipeg, Canada R2H 2A6

Summary. Although congestive heart failure is commonly associated with cardiac hypertrophy and/or cardiac dilation, the exact mechanisms for this complex syndrome are not clear. Furthermore, very little is known about the factors associated with the transition of cardiac hypertrophy to heart failure. Since the activation of both peripheral and tissue renin–angiotensin systems (RAS) is considered to be involved in the genesis of cardiac hypertrophy, we believe that the increased activity of RAS for a prolonged period constitutes one of the important factors in the development of congestive heart failure. Thus angiotensin blockade in animals or patients with congestive heart failure has been shown to exert beneficial effects in terms of preventing clinical signs, improving heart function, and reducing mortality. In this regard, it is pointed out that the blockade of RAS can be achieved either by using different types of angiotensin-converting enzyme (ACE) inhibitors or by angiotensin receptor blockers. Because of the role of the sarcoplasmic reticulum (SR) in the regulation of intracellular Ca^{2+} and the evidence that the occurrence of Ca^{2+}-handling abnormalities in cardiomyocytes plays a critical role in heart dysfunction, it is becoming clear that remodeling of the SR membrane with respect to changes in some of the Ca^{2+}-regulation proteins such as Ca^{2+}-pump ATPase, Ca^{2+}-release channels, and phospholamban is intimately associated with congestive heart failure. Some studies have now shown that the SR functional defects in congestive heart failure can be partially prevented by treatment with ACE inhibitors or inhibitors of the angiotensin receptors. Further, investigations with respect to the cardiac SR gene expression and protein contents in the failing hearts with or without RAS blockade are required to show whether ACE inhibitors and angiotensin receptor blockers prevent SR defects by affecting the cardiac gene expression in congestive heart failure.

INTRODUCTION

Congestive heart failure (CHF) represents an enormous clinical problem and is a symptomatic syndrome in which cardiac output is inadequate to meet the metabolic needs of the human body [1]. In the past several decades, two characteristic epidemiologic changes have been observed in the field of CHF. First, the incidence and prevalence of CHF and the resulting morbidity and mortality have dramatically increased, whereas the mortality and morbidity from most other cardiovascular diseases have decreased greatly. In the United States of America alone, there are 400,000 new cases of CHF each year, and more than 4.7 million people are suffering from this condition. In fact, CHF has become a major social and economic burden; the overall cost of managing CHF is estimated to be about $15 billion. Furthermore, the 5-year survival rate of CHF is as low as 25% in men and 38% in woman [2,3]. Second, the etiologies of CHF have significantly shifted from hypertension and valvular heart disease to coronary artery disease and diabetes [3]. Although etiologies of CHF include ischemia and myocardial infarction (MI), sustained hemodynamic pressure (hypertension), or volume overload and cardiomyopathies (myocarditis, dilated or hypertrophic cardiomyopathy) [4], the most frequent cause of heart failure in developed countries is ischemic heart disease [3]. This chapter is therefore focused on discussion of the pathophysiology and therapy of congestive heart failure subsequent to MI.

HEART FAILURE FOLLOWING MI

After MI, the cardiac pump failure due to the loss of contractile tissue evokes a series of responses that act to maintain systemic perfusion [2]. The structural remodeling of the left ventricle after MI is a time-dependent process that involves complex alterations in ventricular architecture, including both the infarcted necrotic heart and noninfarcted viable myocardium. Increased systolic and diastolic wall stress due to inefficient emptying of the left ventricle induces structural alterations in response to the enlarged cardiac volume [5,6]. Although contractile dysfunction may occur acutely in MI, heart failure usually arises more gradually and incrementally following the progressive left ventricular (LV) dilatation and remodeling of the viable myocardium. An acute MI, particularly with large and transmural infarct, can produce alterations in the topography of both the infarcted and noninfarcted areas of the ventricle [5,7]. Within hours of MI, necrosis, edema, and inflammation are localized to the infarcted area and are followed by a long-term period of fibroblast proliferation and collagen deposition. This process is referred to as *scar formation*, which is completed within weeks to months depending on species; for rats, the period of scar healing is about 3 weeks [2,5]. At the same time, the infarct expansion or thinning of the area of infarction occurs, and this process results in LV dilatation [2,5,6,8,9]; it is likely to be associated with complications such as the development of CHF, aneurysm formation, and myocardial rupture [5].

As a compensation to maintain the stroke volume after the loss of contractile tissue, ventricular enlargement and hypertrophy of the viable myocytes takes place. MI initiates time-dependent secondary changes in the noninfarcted tissue [5,6,8–10]. While the sarcomere from the enlarged human heart may be normal in length, the volume increase of the impaired ventricle may be due to a rearrangement of the myofibrils across the wall (myocyte slippage or a decrease in the number of cells), rather than a simple stretching of sarcomeres [2,5]. Whenever a precarious balance is exceeded, the increased cavity volume with insufficient compensatory hypertrophy and the resulting loading conditions further promote cardiac enlargement and dysfunction [2,5]. These changes after MI are regarded as the acute phase of ventricular remodeling, whereas the chronic phase occurs when the stimulus to volume enlargement still exists but the healing process of scar is complete [2].

It is well known that the remodeling process following MI is considerably more complex than that in any other models of pure hemodynamic overload. The process of remodeling is targeted to the heart as an organ and includes all cell types present in the heart: myocytes, interstitial cells, and fibroblasts in particular, and the vascular endothelium and the immune cells in some cases [11]. In the MI model, hemodynamic factors (increased LV volume, increased systolic and diastolic wall stresses), necrotic factors, inflammation factors, and myocardial ischemia exist and mix together [12]. The growth of vessel around the infarcted area normalizes the coronary vasodilatory capacity in 35 days [13]. In addition, the activation of the sympathetic nervous system and renin–angiotensin system (RAS) causes an enhancement in loading conditions in the failing ventricle and may accelerate the progression of CHF. Not only does the release of neurohormones in CHF exacerbate the hemodynamic abnormalities but also the continuous release of neurohormones initiates a series of self-reinforcing events that lead to LV dysfunction and CHF [14]. It was reported that high concentrations of neurohormones, such as atrial natriuretic peptide (ANP) and brain natriuretic peptide (BNP) in plasma, may affect both the LV dilatation and systolic dysfunction and play an important role in remodeling of the LV [15]. In addition, coronary artery occlusion promotes the accumulation of collagen, which decreases myocardial contractile strength, increases cardiac stiffness, and initiates the expansion of the infarcted tissue [16].

Under clinical conditions, the acute and long-term changes in ventricular remodeling after MI are the essential processes affecting ventricular function and survival. In addition to the initial insult during MI, the ventricular remodeling also has an important impact on the ultimate outcome after MI, and thus its therapy is important [5,17]. It is also considered that remodeling encompasses the transition from hypertrophy to CHF [18]; when the cardiac dilatation and geometry reach the critical point of heart weight [11], the LV remodeling itself may contribute to progression of CHF [4]. In terms of cellular alterations during the development of CHF, cardiac myocytes and the fibroblasts play a key role in remodeling where cardiomyocytes constitute the majority (76%) of the heart [11] and are more important. At the end-stage of heart failure in patients, remodeling of LV myocardium after MI is commonly associated with interstitial fibrosis in the noninfarcted hypertrophic myocardium, which is remote from the scar area [19].

MI RAT MODEL OF HEART FAILURE

The analysis of CHF relies on the use of appropriate and complementary experimental model systems; however, no animal model has all the salient pathophysiological features desired to mimic the clinical human conditions. Nonetheless, the post-MI rat is most frequently used as an experimentally induced model of CHF [18,20–22]. The procedure for the rat model of MI with coronary artery ligation has improved gradually and has been applied extensively to study CHF with respect to morphological features, metabolic and mechanical adaptations, and therapeutic evaluations [1,2,22–34]. It is now well accepted that left coronary artery ligation induces sustained and severe MI in rats, since the necrotic myocardium becomes completely replaced by scar tissue within 3 to 4 weeks [24] and cardiac failure begins to occur by 4 weeks after the induction of myocardial infarction [1,35,36]. CHF can be confirmed by hypertrophy of the viable myocardium, congested lungs, and hemodynamic alterations, including reduction of mean arterial blood pressure (MAP), left ventricular systolic pressure (LVSP), and left ventricular positive and negative dP/dt, in addition to a rise in left ventricular end–diastolic pressure (LVEDP). The defect in cardiac contractile function and loss of responsiveness to sympathetic stimulus, which are the hallmarks of failing human myocardium, are also observed in the MI rats. Rats with small infarcts have systolic dysfunction with reduced contractility and peak pressures, and those with large infarcts also have diastolic dysfunction with increased filling pressure. In some cases, the presence of ascites has also been reported [1,2,20,23,24,26,36–39]. The depression of LV function depends on the size of scar formation; the scar size of 30–40% [24] or greater [1,23] of the left ventricle has been reported to induce CHF. In the MI rat model, a large Q-wave (>1mV) is considered to have developed acute myocardial infarction, which is followed by heart failure [36]. Only animals with large Q waves in leads I, aVL, and V_5 were utilized by some investigators, and those with LVEDP less than 16mmHg were excluded from the infarcted groups [12].

In the MI model of CHF, not only does the left ventricle lose a part of its contractile mass but also the remaining myocardium develops hypertrophy; this viable tissue has been used to study the structural, functional, and morphological characteristics of surviving myocardium subsequent to MI [40]. The LV volume increased progressively as a time-dependent process that was related to the extent of histological damage. Although the predominant metabolic changes in the viable myocardium occur early during the thinning and expansion of the infarct, both dilation and eccentric hypertrophy of the viable myocardium also commence early and continue long after the MI healing [5]. The failing myocardium due to MI develops a lengthwise hypertrophy with series replication of sarcomeres, whereas the additional sarcomeric proteins assemble in parallel in the pressure-overload model [41]; the surviving myocardium is altered, leading to the development of CHF [41,42]. There is quantitatively a similar degree of cardiac myocyte hypertrophy, a 31% increase in cell volume compared to most models of pressure overload [12]. A depression in the mechanical function in cardiomyocytes isolated from the failing myocardium 6 weeks after MI has been reported [41], and the same phenomenon was observed in the skinned cardiac fibers as well [43]. However, some investigators have reported normal contractile function of cardiomyocytes from the infarcted failing rat heart [44]. In the MI rat, the collagen concentration appears to double in the viable free wall of the LV but increases by 27% in the noninfarcted septum [2]. Several therapeutic interventions have been tested in the MI rat model. Recombinant human growth hormone (GH) produced a 13% increase in the ejection fraction (EF) and a 50% increase in cardiac index, while there were no signs of additional hypertrophy [32]. However, GH replacement failed to improve LV function in hypophysectomized rats after MI [45]. Long-term administration of coenzyme Q_{10} was found to increase the cardiac output (CO) and stroke volume slightly but did not affect the survival rate [46]. The main disadvantage of the MI rat model is the high mortality—40–50% in the first 48 hours [24,25]; however, this experimental model has been shown to be quite reproducible.

There are several related animal models of CHF or cardiac hypertrophy that have been reported to exhibit ventricular remodeling. For example, MI in the dog has been shown to result in elevated LVEDP and decreased stroke volume [47]. Rabbits after MI were used to evaluate changes in the sarcoplasmic reticulum (SR) and sarcolemma (SL) function due to heart failure [48]. Animals with chronic diabetes induced by streptozotocin exhibited significantly depressed contractile force generation, SR Ca^{2+}-transport, and Ca^{2+}-stimulated ATPase activities; these alterations were reversed by insulin therapy but not by thyroid hormone [49]. Depressed Ca^{2+} mobilization and positive inotropic responses were also observed in this model of contractile dysfunction [50,51]. Heart failure due to aortic stenosis or pressure overload in guinea pigs [52,53], felines [54], ferrets [55], and rats [56,57] is induced by banding the descending thoracic aorta. Pressure overload in the rats is commonly induced by suprarenal abdominal aortic coarctation; these rats exhibit increased systolic LV pressure and LV hypertrophy [58,59], as well as reduced mRNA levels for SR Ca^{2+}-regulating proteins [29,60]. The genetically hypertensive rats belong to the pressure-overload model [61]. The volume overload in rats is induced by aortocaval shunt and the cardiac hypertrophy thus induced is considered to produce compensatory LV function [62]. Tachycardia in pigs and dogs has also been shown to result in CHF. The L-type Ca^{2+}-channel and SR Ca^{2+}-pump densities were reduced in the failing pig heart; these changes were recovered by a combination therapy with the ACE inhibitor benazeprilat and the angiotensin II (Ang II) type I receptor (AT_1) blocker valsartan; neither the ACE inhibitor nor the AT_1 receptor blocker alone had such effects [63]. In the tachycardia-induced CHF in dogs, it was shown that both the activity and protein level of SR Ca^{2+}-pump ATPase were reduced [64,65]. Cardiomyopathic Syrian hamsters have also been widely used for the study of both hypertrophic (BIO 14.6) [66] and dilated (BIO 5.58) [67,68] cardiomyopathy.

ROLE OF Ca^{2+} IN HEART FUNCTION

The LV function alterations in CHF may be due to changes in Ca^{2+}-handling, sarcomerogenesis, β-adrenergic signaling, and cytoskeleton [4]. However, cardiac muscle contraction and relaxation are mainly regulated by the intracellular concentration of free Ca^{2+} ($[Ca^{2+}]_i$), which is controlled by the SR Ca^{2+}-release and Ca^{2+}-uptake processes. The SR is a tubular network of membranes that participates in cardiac contraction and relaxation by raising and lowering the cytoplasmic levels of Ca^{2+} [69,70]. Most interventions that affect the strength of cardiac muscle contraction appear to exert this effect by altering $[Ca^{2+}]_i$ and/or the sensitivity of the contractile apparatus to Ca^{2+} [1,70–75]. Cardiac muscle contraction begins with Ca^{2+} influx through SL Ca^{2+} channels and ends with Ca^{2+} uptake by SR [1,36,73]. Abnormal-

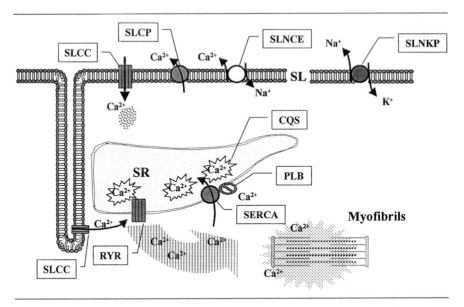

Figure 1. Calcium-induced calcium release in cardiomyocyte. SL, sarcolemma; SR, sarcoplasmic reticulum; RYR, ryanodine receptor; SERCA, sarcoplasmic reticulum Ca^{2+} pump; PLB, phospholamban; CQS, casequestrin; SLCC, sarcolemma Ca^{2+} channel; SLCP, sarcolemma Ca^{2+} pump; SLNKP, sarcolemma Na^+-K^+ pump; SLNCE, sarcolemma Na^+-Ca^{2+} exchanger.

ities in the intracellular Ca^{2+} handling are considered to represent the basis of depressed contractility in CHF [1,75]. Alterations in myocyte function are ascribed to changes at three sites in the excitation–contraction coupling (E-C coupling): the SL L-type calcium channel opening, Ca^{2+} release from the SR, and the reaction of myofilaments to Ca^{2+} [1,41,73] (figure 1).

The resting $[Ca^{2+}]_i$ is low (<200 nmol/L), whereas the extracellular Ca^{2+} concentration ($[Ca^{2+}]_o$) is high (1 mmol/L), and thus there is more than a 5000-fold gradient across the SL membrane. Various cation channels and transport proteins are involved in maintaining the low level of $[Ca^{2+}]_i$, and these include the SL Ca^{2+} pump and the Na^+-Ca^{2+} exchanger as well as the ryanodine receptor (RYR) and Ca^{2+}-pump ATPase (SERCA) [1,73]. The E-C coupling is a complex process in cardiomyocytes that is initiated by membrane electric activity. Extracellular Ca^{2+} enters the cardiomyocyte via specific SL Ca^{2+} channels (voltage-gated, L-type Ca^{2+} channel), and triggers Ca^{2+} release from the SR via the RYR. This process is called *Ca^{2+} induced Ca^{2+} release* (CICR) [73,75–77]. A "restricted space" where Ca^{2+} entry via SL is coupled to RYR and is adjacent to the junctional SR seems to play an important role in the process of E-C coupling [78]. The increased cardiac contractility in the hypertrophied heart of the spontaneously hypertensive rat was not associated with any changes in the SL L-type Ca^{2+} current in the SL or the SR Ca^{2+}-regulating proteins, and thus alterations in the microdomain between L-type

Ca^{2+}-channels and RYR were suggested to explain this observation [79]. While some Ca^{2+} may enter the cell via the reverse of Na^+–Ca^{2+} exchanger under certain conditions, Ca^{2+} released from the SR is considered to increase the $[Ca^{2+}]_i$ and result in a series of chemical events (cross-bridge formation) that initiate cell shortening and/or the generation of force. In this process of myofilament activation, most of the Ca^{2+} that causes contraction comes from the SR [73,78]; however, both endothelin and β-adrenergic agonists have also been shown to increase actomyosin ATPase activity directly [80]. In the last step of E-C coupling, Ca^{2+} interacts with troponin C, the regulatory complex of the contractile apparatus, to initiate the contraction [1].

The magnitude of contraction in different experimental models of heart failure is directly dependent upon the $[Ca^{2+}]_i$ in cardiomyocytes [1,27,73,74,79]. In failing hearts due to MI in rats, the diastolic $[Ca^{2+}]_i$ was increased and the systolic peak $[Ca^{2+}]_i$ was decreased while the contractile force development and relaxation of heart were reduced [27,81,82]. The time course of SR release function in the rabbit model was tested by the caffeine-induced contracture, and it was observed that both Ca^{2+} release and Ca^{2+} uptake were increased at 8 weeks but were normal at 15 weeks after MI [83]. It should be pointed out that not only the cardiac SR function is altered during CHF after MI but also the skeletal muscle SR is affected. There is significant reduction in skeletal muscle twitch and tetanic forces in addition to significant elevations in the rates of tension increase and decrease in the infarcted animals [84]. Accordingly, it has been concluded that both the cardiac and skeletal muscle SR functions are altered following MI.

SR Ca^{2+}-REGULATING PROTEINS AND THEIR FUNCTION

Due to its ability to take up and release free Ca^{2+}, SR is considered to play a key role in the process of E-C coupling for the regulation of intracellular Ca^{2+} in the heart on a beat-to-beat basis [1,36,73]. The regulation of Ca^{2+} by the SR is carried out by the Ca^{2+}-regulating proteins such as RYR, SERCA, PLB, and calsequestrin (CQS), which control the Ca^{2+} release, uptake, and storage activities. The RYR is located on the junctional SR and triggers the contraction of cardiac myocytes by releasing Ca^{2+} from the lumen of the SR into the cytoplasm. The RYR isolated from the heart and brain is a large protein of 4969 amino acids with Mr of 564,711 dalton, and its gene is located on chromosome 1 [85]. When exposed to micromolar concentrations of Ca^{2+}, the RYR is opened and thus releases Ca^{2+} from the SR into the cytoplasm of the cell [67,85–88]. The RYR has a high affinity to the alkaloid ryanodine. It has two important pharmacologic characteristics. First at low concentrations (<10 μmol/L) of ryanodine, the Ca^{2+}-release channel is opened in a state of a low–conductance configuration, secondly high concentrations of ryanodine completely block this channel [89,90]. Therefore, low concentrations of ryanodine are used to test the extent and speed of Ca^{2+} release from the SR [90]. It was also found that the Ca^{2+} release induced by inositol 1,4,5-triphosphate (IP_3) was reduced in the pressure-overloaded hypertrophied heart [56]. However, the amount of Ca^{2+} released by the SR depends on the size of Ca^{2+} load in the SR and on the size and duration of the initial Ca^{2+} trigger from the L-type Ca^{2+}-channel in the SL [91].

The SR Ca^{2+}-stimulated ATPase (SERCA) is localized in the cardiac longitudinal SR and works as a pump in which ATP is hydrolyzed for the transport of Ca^{2+} [29]. SERCA is a 100 kDa protein and is a major protein in the SR membrane [1]. SERCA is distributed all over the tubular SR [1,92], and its activity is dependent upon both Ca^{2+} and Mg^{2+}. There are three highly homologous genes in the SERCA pump family: SERCA1 (SERCA1a and SERCA1b) is restricted to the fast-twitch striated muscle and has a relatively high Ca^{2+} affinity [93], whereas SERCA2 and SERCA3 are expressed most abundantly in the myocardium, large and small intestine, thymus, and cerebellum [94,95]. Two isoforms of SERCA2 (SERCA2a and SERCA2b) [96] differ in their C-terminal sequences as a result of the alternative splicing [97]; SERCA2a in cardiomyocytes plays a key role for Ca^{2+} uptake into the SR, while SERCA2b is expressed in a variety of smooth muscle and nonmuscle tissues [95,98,99]. Two functional copies of the SERCA2 gene are required to maintain normal levels of SERCA2 mRNA, protein, and Ca^{2+}-sequestering activity [97]. However, it was found that SERCA1a can substitute for SERCA2a functionally and can be regulated by endogenous PLB in the heart in the transgenic mouse model [100]. Both ATP and potassium are known to regulate the function of SERCA2 [92,101].

Not only the rate and extent of cardiac relaxation but also the rate and amplitude of contraction are controlled by SERCA2. In the failing human heart, the beat duration was found to be longer than that in the normal heart, but this difference of contraction disappeared upon treatment of the normal heart with the SERCA inhibitor thapsigargin. The alteration of contraction in CHF was suggested to be due to decreased SR Ca^{2+} uptake [102] because the contraction is regulated by the amount of Ca^{2+} in the SR as well as by the Ca^{2+} gradient between the SR and the cytosol [75]. The overexpression of cardiac SERCA [103,104] in mouse was found to be associated with an increased maximum velocity of Ca^{2+} uptake (V_{max}) as well as an increased rate of contraction ($+dP/dt$) and rate of relaxation ($-dP/dt$). These results demonstrate that the enhancement in SERCA pump level can increase the cardiac contractile function by increasing the SR Ca^{2+} transport activity [103].

Phospholamban (PLB) is a phosphoprotein (25 kDa) that modulates the function of SERCA [105]. There is only one kind of PLB existing in the cardiac muscle and slow-twitch skeletal muscle [67]. In its unphosphorylated form, PLB binds to SERCA and prevents the transport of Ca^{2+} into the SR lumen. Phosphorylation of PLB by cAMP-dependent protein kinase (PKA) and protein kinase C (PKC) blocks the interaction between PLB and SERCA and thus increases the rate of Ca^{2+} uptake into the SR. Calmodulin, another Ca^{2+}-binding protein, is involved in the phosphorylation of PLB and plays a role in Ca^{2+} transport [1,75,106]. Calsequestrin (CQS) is a Ca^{2+}-binding protein in the SR with a molecular weight of 53 kDa [1]. It is confined to regions in the SR that store and release Ca^{2+} and is closely associated with the t-tubules and the nonjunctional SR [91]. In the cardiac SR, there is another Ca^{2+}-binding protein, calreticulin [67], whose function still remains to be defined clearly.

SR ALTERATIONS AND CHANGES IN GENE EXPRESSION IN CHF

The intracellular Ca^{2+} transients and cardiac contractions were markedly prolonged in the failing human heart [107,108]. Ca^{2+} homeostasis was disturbed in the failing human ventricular myocytes, and this was reflected by smaller and more slowly decaying Ca^{2+} transients. Ca^{2+} release from the SR was decreased, while the Ca^{2+} influx via the reverse mode of the Na^+–Ca^{2+} exchanger was increased [109]. It was identified that both the density and kinetics of L-type Ca^{2+} current were not significantly different in the post-MI remodeled rat myocytes compared with control [110]. On the basis of several such studies, it was concluded that the SR changes occur in human heart with CHF [111] (table 1).

The $[Ca^{2+}]_i$ was reduced due to a decrease in Ca^{2+} release from the SR in the infarcted rat heart [112,113]. By using the skinned fibers, it was shown that the amount of Ca^{2+} released from the SR was decreased upon stimulation with caffeine in CHF following MI in rats. Total RYR density (B_{max}) was reduced after 8 weeks of MI, while the receptor affinity (K_d) did not change. In addition, it was found that the decreased Ca^{2+} release in the failing heart was due to the downregulation of the SR Ca^{2+}-release channel [36,43]. In contrast, it has been reported that the density of RYR in cardiomyocytes from the MI rat heart is increased or unchanged [12]. Nonetheless, it was evident that Ca^{2+} sequestration by SERCA was impaired in the failing human myocardium [33,75] as well as in the MI rats [112–114]. It has been determined that the SERCA protein concentration was decreased and the ratio of SERCA to PLB or CQS was reduced in the human failing heart [115]; however, some investigators have reported that the SERCA concentration did not change in the failing heart [116]. A depression in the SERCA activity in CHF can be seen to result in the inability of myocardium to relax fully. For example, the protein level and the activity of SERCA begin to decrease in rats 4 weeks after MI; by 8 weeks, these drop to about 79% and 35% of control values, respectively [29]. On the other hand, in heterozygous mice with a null mutation in SERCA2, both the SERCA2a protein level and the rate of SR Ca^{2+} uptake were reduced by 35% on the appearance of CHF [97]. In the cardiomyocytes isolated from the nonin-

Table 1. Alterations in the cardiac SR Ca^{2+}-regulation protein contents in patients with heart failure

First authors [references]	Tissue source	RYR	SERCA2a	PLB	CQS
Movsesian [147]	CHF heart before transplantation	ND	—	—	—
Schwinger [116]	CHF heart before transplantation	ND	—	—	—
Hasenfuss [74, 148]	CHF heart of dilated and ischemic cardiomyopathy	ND	↓	↓	—
Linck [149]	CHF heart before transplantation	ND	↓	↓	ND
Meyer [15]	CHF heart of dilated cardiomyopathy	—	↓	—	—

ND, not detected; —, no change; ↓, decrease; RYR, ryanodine receptors; SERCA2a, sarcoplasmic reticular Ca^{2+}-pump; PLB, phospholamban; CQS, calsequestrin.

Table 2. Alterations in cardiac SR Ca^{2+}-regulation protein contents in animal models of heart failure

First author [references]	Tissue source	RYR	SERCA2a	PLB	CQS
Hisamatsu [62]	Rats after 12 weeks of aortocaval shunt	↓	↓	ND	ND
Yue [12]	Isolated myocytes of rats 6 weeks after MI	ND	—	—	ND
Qi [60]	8 weeks after abdominal aortic coarctation	ND	—	ND	ND
	16 weeks after abdominal aortic coarctation	ND	↓	ND	ND
Kiss [53]	Guinea pig after 8 weeks of aorta banding	ND	↓	↓	ND
Liu [150]	8 weeks after abdominal aorta banding in rats	ND	↓	ND	ND
O'Rourke [65]	Rapid pacing dogs	ND	↓	↓	ND
Periasamy [97]	Heterozygous mice with null mutation SERCA	ND	↓	ND	ND
Takeishi [140]	Aortic-banded guinea pigs	ND	↓	↓	ND

All abbreviations are the same as in table 1.

farcted region of the rat left ventricle 6 weeks after MI, the peak L-type Ca^{2+} current was not significantly changed, but peak Ca^{2+}-transients recorded by Fura-2 were decreased by 19% [41]. It was also found that when the SERCA in the infarcted heart was inhibited by thapsigargin ($1\,\mu M$), no further change of relaxation time was evident. These observations indicated that the function of SERCA2a was greatly downregulated in CHF [41].

The depressed SERCA activity in SR membranes from the viable left ventricle 16 weeks after MI was seen at different Ca^{2+}, K^+, and ATP concentrations; however, no alterations in the affinities of the enzyme for Ca^{2+} and ATP were observed. In addition, the SR phosphorylation (^{32}P incorporation) was reduced in the presence of Ca^{2+}–calmodulin or cAMP-dependent protein kinase (PKA) [40]. Other investigators showed a decrease in Ca^{2+}-pump ATPase activity in rats after MI [117]. These results reveal that the function of SERCA2a is decreased in rats after MI, and this may cause alterations of myocyte contraction in the hearts failing due to MI. On the other hand, despite a comparable degree of cellular hypertrophy and more severe hemodynamic decompensation, the expression of SERCA and PLB were not changed in MI-induced heart failure [12] or in some clinical studies [116]. CQS, unlike PLB, was unchanged during the development of CHF following MI (tables 1 and 2).

There is an immediate induction of the fetal/embryonic transcriptional gene program in the heart following MI in rats, which may precede myocyte hypertrophy and persist longer than in the pressure-overloaded hearts [12]. Abnormalities in SR Ca^{2+} transport in the CHF have been suggested to be due to changes in gene

Table 3. Alterations in cardiac mRNA levels for SR Ca^{2+}-regulation proteins in congestive heart failure

First author [references]	Tissue source	RYR	SERCA2a	PLB	CQS
Mercadier [151]	CHF heart before cardiac transplantation	ND	↓	ND	ND
Linck [149]	CHF heart before transplantation	ND	—	—	ND
Schwinger [116]	CHF heart before transplantation	ND	↓	—	ND
Arai [154]	CHF before cardiac transplantation	↓	↓	↓	—
Feldman [152]	Endomyocardial biopsies of human CHF heart	ND	ND	↓	ND
Feldman [153]	Failing LV of rats 20 weeks after aortic banding	ND	↓	—	ND
Yue [12]	Isolated myocytes of rats 6 weeks after MI	ND	—	—	ND
Iijima [117]	LV of rats 4 weeks after MI	—	↓	—	—
Qi [60]	8 weeks after abdominal aortic coarctation	ND	↓	ND	ND
	16 weeks after abdominal aortic coarctation	ND	↓↓	ND	ND
Periasamy [97]	Heterozygous mice with null mutation SERCA	ND	↓	ND	ND
Liu [150]	8 weeks after abdominal aorta banding in rats	ND	↓	ND	ND

All abbreviations are the same as in table 1.

expression for the SERCA protein in different models of heart failure [1]. The SERCA2 gene is expressed in high amounts in the heart and encodes the mRNA for two different isoforms [99]. The cardiac SERCA2 mRNA level drops significantly by 20% and 35% at 4 weeks and 16 weeks, respectively, after MI in rats. The alterations in mRNA and SERCA protein expression were comparable, while the SERCA activity was greatly reduced (table 3). These results demonstrate that changes in SERCA may be due to alterations at both the gene transcriptional level and the posttranscriptional level (mRNA stability) [29]. On the other hand, when the mRNA level of the cardiac SERCA was reduced by 45% in heterozygous mice with a null mutation of SERCA, the protein level and Ca^{2+}-uptake velocity were reduced markedly [97].

PRESENCE OF RAS IN THE CARDIOVASCULAR SYSTEM

RAS is one of the major systems regulating the cardiovascular function and includes different components. Angiotensinogen, a 452 amino acid globular glycoprotein of 55–56 kDa, is the precursor of Ang II. It is mainly localized in the pericentral zone of the liver lobules. The plasma is the major reservoir of angiotensinogen, and thus it is the major determinant of RAS activity [118]. Renin, a glycoproteolytic single-chain aspartyl protease of 37–40 kDa, is highly specific for its substrate, angiotensinogen, and is generated in the juxtaglomerular cells of the afferent arterioles of the kidney. The renin mRNA is found in almost all organs of the body, but its level in the heart is rather low. Renin cleaves a leucine–valine bond in the N-terminal region of angiotensinogen for the generation of angiotensin I (Ang I) [118,119]. Ang I is composed of 10 amino acids and does not have any significant effect of its own; however, it is converted by angiotensin-converting enzyme (ACE) to Ang II. ACE, a dipeptidyl carboxypeptidase, is a member of the family of zinc metal-lopeptidases, derived from the lung and other organs in the body. ACE is predom-inately attached to endothelial cells [2], and in addition to converting Ang I to Ang II, it inactivates a well-known vasodilator, bradykinin. Ang II plays the major role and shows almost all the effects of RAS when it combines with its receptors. An alternative pathway for Ang II production in the human heart is via chymase (a chymotrypsin-like proteinase), which is not affected by ACE inhibition [2]. Ang II receptor heterogeneity has been defined primarily by the use of nonpeptides to show that there are two distinct types of ACE receptors. Ang II type 1 (AT_1) recep-tor is composed of 359 amino acids with AT_{1A} and AT_{1B} subtypes [120]. It medi-ates most of the physiologic and pathophysiologic effects of Ang II, involves the translocation of protein kinase C (PKC) from the cytosol to the membranes, and is blocked by the specific AT_1 receptor antagonist, losartan [2,121]. The Ang II type 2 (AT_2) is present in the heart during fetal development and is blocked by PD123177. Although in adult ventricular myocytes, the AT_1 receptor subtype plays a major role [2], it was found that an inhibition of AT_2 receptor by PD123319 could amplify the immediate LV growth response to Ang II, with enhanced PKC translo-cation to membranes and reduced LV cGMP content [122].

Ang II receptors are widely distributed throughout the heart, and each receptor subtype accounts for about 50% of the specific binding by losartan or PD123177. The density of Ang II receptors is high in the atrioventricular node [123]. In the human atria, the ratio of $AT_2 : AT_1$ receptors is about 2 : 1, but in rats, the ratio is about 69% : 31%. However, most of the Ang II effects are mediated by the AT_1 recep-tor only [121]. The stimulation of AT_1 receptors activates phospholipase C (PLC) to produce phosphatidylinositol 4,5-bisphosphate, then forming diacylglycerol (DAG) and IP_3, which induces the SR Ca^{2+} release and increases the contractility [72,124]. On the other hand, DAG activates PKC and thus stimulates cardiac growth [125]. Ang II was observed to increase the $[Ca^{2+}]_i$ in rat cardiomyocytes, as mea-sured by Fura-2 AM fluorescence spectroscopy; this increase is dependent on the concentration of Ang II (0.01 to 10 µM) [124]. In the cardiac fibroblasts, Ang II decreased the activity of metalloproteinase I, which is the key enzyme for intersti-tial collagen degradation [11].

The existence of tissue RAS in the heart was identified by showing the presence of mRNA for angiotensinogen, ACE, and prorenin in cardiomyocytes [2]. It should be mentioned that Ang II has multiple effects on the heart and periphery, acting directly or indirectly on myocytes for the regulation of growth, vascular resistance, and contractility. The effects of Ang II are mediated via its receptors, which are located on ventricular and smooth muscle cells and are linked to guanine nucleotide-binding proteins (G proteins) that control the generation of various downstream second messenger pathways [2]. Mechanical stretch has been shown to initiate the release of Ang II, which acts as an initial mediator of the hypertrophic response in cardiac myocytes [126].

ROLE OF RAS IN MI AND CHF

The reduction of renal blood flow is detected by sensory receptors in the renal arterioles, and this initiates the release of renin from the kidney during the development of CHF. The formation of Ang II attenuates the baroreceptor sensitivity, and in fact the patients with CHF exhibit an excessive activation of the RAS at rest or during exercise [14]. In the pacing rabbits, elevated levels of plasma Ang II and decreased formation of nitric oxide were shown to be necessary for sustained increases in sympathetic nerve activity [127]. In the rat model of MI, the angiotensinogen mRNA levels were significantly elevated in the noninfarcted portion of the left ventricle at 5 days after infarction, and showed a significant correlation with infarct size and increased LVEDP. However, such alterations disappeared at 25 days after MI [128]. In this experimental model of MI, an increased expression of c-myc and c-jun was demonstrated in the viable myocytes of RV and LV 2 to 3 days after MI while the myocyte volume increased [2]. On the other hand, the Ang II receptors, mainly located on the nonmyocytes and fibroblasts [121], were found elevated in rats after MI; the AT_{1A} mRNA level was increased, while the AT_{1B} mRNA did not change [117]. The cardiac ACE activity was increased markedly in the infarcted area and moderately in the viable hypertrophied myocardium without any alteration of the affinity to the inhibitors [129]. Upregulation of ACE mRNA has been shown in experimentally induced pressure overload and in postinfarction heart failure [2]. In the CHF rats after MI, the ventricular myocytes were found to possess the AT_1 receptor subtype exclusively, whereas the Ang II-stimulated phosphoinositol turnover was enhanced 3.7-fold and 2.5-fold in the LV and RV myocytes, respectively [130]. It should be pointed out that RAS is involved in pathologic myocardial fibrosis because Ang II was reported to increase the collagen synthesis and inhibit the collagenase activity in cultured adult cardiac fibroblasts [2]. From this evidence, pharmacological interference with the RAS may be considered to be of potential physiological and clinical importance for remodeling of the infarcted left ventricle. In fact, inhibition of the RAS has become the therapeutic strategy to be used in clinical practice. The inhibition of the RAS can be achieved either by reduction of Ang II by using ACE inhibitors or by blockade of the Ang II receptors [131].

MODIFICATION OF CHF BY ACE INHIBITORS

The therapy of CHF with ACE inhibitors can be instituted at early stages of CHF [132], but these agents have also been shown to exert a marked beneficial effect even when therapy was initiated at late stages of CHF [133]. However, the mechanisms of action, time frame for the beneficial effects, and duration of therapy with

Table 4. Major clinical trials of enalapril for the treatment of congestive heart failure

Clinical trial [references]	Patients	Time	Dose	Effects
CONSENSUS I [155]	CHF not responsive to conventional therapies	—	—	Reduced mortality in the elderly CHF population
CONSENSUS-II [156]	6090 post-MI	24 hours–80 days	—	No improvement of survival in first 180 days after MI
VheFT II [157]	Mild to moderate CHF	2 years	20 mg/day	Improved survival; no great improvement of EF
SOLVD [158,159]	Asymptomatic and mild CHF	—	10 mg b.i.d.	Improved clinical symptoms
SOLVD [158]	—	—	11.2 mg/day	Reduced mortality and recurrence of MI

CHF, congestive heart failure; CONSENSUS, Cooperative New Scandinavian Enalapril Survival Study; EF, ejection fraction; MI, myocardial infarction; SOLVD, Studies of Left Ventricular Dysfunction; VHeFTII, Veteran's Administration Cooperative Vasodilator Heart Failure Trial II.

Table 5. Major animal experiments for enalapril in the treatment of MI and/or CHF

First author [reference]	Model	Duration	Dose	Effects
Sanbe [139]	MI rat	2nd–12th weeks	10 mg/kg/day	MAP ↓, LVEDP ↓, CO ↑ Metabolism ↑
Sanbe [28]	MI rat	2nd–12th weeks	10 mg/kg/day	CO ↑ β_1-adrenergic receptor density ↑
Schieffer [160]	MI rat	2nd–7th weeks	0.5 mg/kg/day	Coronary vascular resistance ↓ Interstitial fibrosis ↓

↑, increased; ↓, decreased; MI, myocardial infarction; CHF, congestive heart failure; MAP, mean arterial pressure; LVEDP, left ventricular end diastolic pressure; CO, cardiac output.

ACE inhibitors are still unknown [6]. It is pointed out that ACE inhibitors are considered to act via a decrease in the production of Ang II, which in turn results in an improvement of cardiac function and clinical outcome [134]. In CHF after MI, ACE inhibitors have been demonstrated to improve heart function and increase survival rate in rats and in humans; the clinical and hemodynamic benefits of ACE inhibitors in CHF in terms of improving exercise tolerance have now been well accepted [135,136]. Clinical trials of ACE inhibitors, such as enalapril (ENP), show reductions in morbidity and mortality of patients with CHF or after MI (table 4) [136,137]. In the infarcted rats, ACE inhibitors reduced ventricular volume and produced more favorable ventricular performance. ACE inhibitors not only reduced the LV filling pressure and ventricular distension but also reduced LV dilatation (table 5) without reducing the infarct size [43]. Irrespective of early versus delayed ACE inhibition in rats after MI, the LVSP, LVEDP, and central venous pressures were reduced; LV weight, LV cavity size, and LV collagen density were also decreased [133]. In clinical studies, long-term therapy with ACE inhibitors can favorably alter the loading conditions on the left ventricle and reduce the progressive ventricular enlargement; this attenuation of the ventricular enlargement was associated with a prolongation in survival [2,5,6,15,17,26,136].

ACE inhibitors are considered to affect heart failure by a combination of neurohormonal, hemodynamic, LV structural remodeling, and other effects [136]. First, ACE inhibitors directly decreased the circulating and tissue effects of Ang II by reducing its production. ACE inhibitors may suppress the sympathetic-mediated ventricular dilation caused by increased cardiac work load or direct trophic effects on the myocardium [2,6,136]. These drugs may also diminish the level of plasma aldosterone and prevent secondary sodium and volume retention [2,6,136]. The circulatory catecholamines are reduced, while the degradation of bradykinin is diminished by ACE inhibitors [2,136]. However, ACE inhibitors do not completely inhibit the production of Ang II, which can also be produced through the non-ACE pathway [125]. Secondly, these drugs can induce venodilation and arteriolar dilation, resulting in improved stroke volume and reduced atrial and ventricular diastolic volume without chronotropic stimulation [2,6,136]. In the patient treated with captopril, ischemia-related events were reduced during the first 3 to 12 months after MI, but there was a rebound phenomenon after the withdrawal of ACE inhibitor treatment. Such benefits are sustained with continued therapy in CHF; however, withdrawal can result in exacerbation of disease [138]. Thirdly, ACE inhibitors can decrease transmural wall stress, compensatory dilatation, and compensatory increase of end-diastolic and end-systolic volume. In addition, ACE inhibitors directly or indirectly alter the LV remodeling process and improve coronary flow distribution in both surface and transmural areas [2,6,136]. On a long-term basis (6 to 8 weeks), treatment with ACE inhibitors also reduces the abnormal accumulation of myocardial collagen in MI rats [2].

Several studies have been carried out for ACE inhibitor therapeutic effects (table 5). Long-term therapy with ENP in MI rats was observed to decrease MAP and LVEDP. ENP also prevents the reduction in cardiac output (CO) and stroke volume indices, in addition to reducing mitochondrial oxygen consumption by viable left and right ventricles. The underlying mechanism of therapy is attributable to recovery or preservation of the mitochondrial function, reduction in preload, and attenuation of the decrease of β_1-adrenergic receptor density [139]. In the pressure-overloaded rats with aortic–banding, ACE inhibitor therapy with ramipril improved the LV function and prevented the downregulation of Ca^{2+}-cycling protein expression, while the PKC levels were also attenuated [140]. It was found that the depression in the aortic flow, CO, and RYR density in SR [43] was attenuated after treatment of the infarcted rats with trandolapril. The major side effects of ACE inhibitors are cough, renal dysfunction, and first-dose hypotension, which are due to ACE inhibitor-induced bradykinin formation, but there are still some patients who have poor LV function despite the ACE inhibitor treatment [134].

MODIFICATION OF CHF BY ANG II RECEPTOR ANTAGONIST

An orally active antagonist, losartan (LOS), of the angiotensin receptors was first introduced into clinical practice at the beginning of this decade. LOS is a nonpeptide AT_1 subtype Ang II receptor antagonist without any agonistic actions [20,121]. Ang II receptor antagonists can directly block the action of Ang II by suppressing the receptors. LOS not only has been utilized as a tool to investigate the role of Ang II in CHF but also has been introduced as a new CHF therapy. The blockade of RAS by LOS was more specific than that by ACE inhibitors and was reported to show different effects [141]. LOS is devoid of the side effects caused by ACE inhibitors, especially those due to an increase in the level of bradykinin [125]. LOS alone improves the symptoms in CHF after MI or other diseases [142]. A comparison of the efficacy, tolerability, and effect on mortality of long-term Ang II receptor blockade and ENP is given in table 6 [143]. Furthermore, in the CHF patients who were severely symptomatic even during treatment with optimal doses (maximally recommended or tolerated) of ACE inhibitors, LOS was reported to enhance exercise capacity and to alleviate clinical symptoms [144]. In normal rat myocytes, LOS was shown to block the increase of $[Ca^{2+}]_i$ and cell beating stimulated by Ang II [124]. It was demonstrated that LOS either alone or combined with ENP could limit cardiac hypertrophy in MI rats; however, LOS did not have marked effects on nonmyocyte cellular proliferation [145]. Furthermore, there is some controversial data that LOS (10 mg/kg/day) did not exert marked beneficial effects on cardiac function in MI rats [131] and did not improve the cardiac output in pacing dogs [146]. Nonetheless, there is an ample body of evidence to show the beneficial effects of LOS and other AT_1 receptor antagonists in different types of heart failure.

Table 6. Major animal experiments for LOS treatment of MI and/or CHF

First author [reference]	Animal model	Method	Dose	Effects
Regitz–Zagrosek [142]	Human of CHF	Oral	5–150 mg once	MAP ↓, PCWP ↓, cardiac index ↑
	Human of CHF	Oral	5–15 mg/day for 12 weeks	MAP ↓, PCWP ↓
Raya [161]	MI rats	Oral	40 mg/kg/day	MAP −, LVEDP ↓
Smits [141]	MI rats	Oral	15 mg/kg/day	CO − Left ventricular hypertrophy ↓
Murakami [146]	Pacing dog	Venous	1.1 mol/kg	No effects on cardiac output
Liu [150]	Pressure-overload rat	Oral	20 mg/kg/day for 8 weeks	SERCA2 ⇈
Schieffer [160]	MI rat	2nd–7th weeks	3 mg/kg/day	Coronary vascular resistance ↓ Interstitial fibrosis ↓

⇈, partial increase compared to decrease in the sham-operated animal; PCWP, pulmonary capillary wedge pressure. All other abbreviations are the same as in table 5.

ACKNOWLEDGMENTS

The research work reported here from our laboratory was supported by a grant from the Medical Research Council of Canada (MRC Group in Experimental Cardiology). NSD holds MRC/Rx & D Chair in Cardiovascular Research supported by Merck Frosst of Canada.

REFERENCES

1. Dhalla NS, Afzal N, Beamish RE, Naimark B, Takeda N, Nagano M. 1993. Pathophysiology of cardiac dysfunction in congestive heart failure. Can J Cardiol 9:873–887.
2. Pfeffer JM, Fischer TA, Pfeffer MA. 1995. Angiotensin-converting enzyme inhibition and ventricular remodeling after myocardial infarction. Annu Rev Physiol 57:805–826.
3. Massie BM, Shah NB. 1997. Evolving trends in the epidemiologic factors of heart failure: rationale for preventive strategies and comprehensive disease management. Am Heart J 133:703–712.
4. Kurrelmeyer K, Kalra D, Bozkurt B, Wang F, Dibbs Z, Seta Y, Baumgarten G, Engle D, Sivasubramanian N, Mann DL. 1998. Cardiac remodeling as a consequence and cause of progressive heart failure. Clin Cardiol 21:114–119.
5. Pfeffer MA, Braunwald E. 1990. Ventricular remodeling after myocardial infarction. Experimental observations and clinical implications. Circulation 81:1161–1172.
6. Nelson KM, Yeager BF. 1996. What is the role of angiotensin-converting enzyme inhibitors in congestive heart failure and after myocardial infarction? Ann Pharmacother 30:986–993.
7. Anversa P, Sonnenblick EH. 1990. Ischemic cardiomyopathy: pathophysiologic mechanisms. Prog Cardiovasc Dis 33:49–70.
8. Roberts CS, Maclean D, Maroko P, Kloner RA. 1984. Early and late remodeling of the left ventricle after acute myocardial infarction. Am J Cardiol 54:407–410.
9. Erlebacher JA. 1985. Ventricular remodeling in myocardial infarction—the rat and the human [letter]. Am J Cardiol 56:910.
10. Sharpe N. 1992. Ventricular remodeling following myocardial infarction. Am J Cardiol 70:20C–26C.
11. Maisch B. 1996. Ventricular remodeling. Cardiology 87:2–10.
12. Yue P, Long CS, Austin R, Chang KC, Simpson PC, Massie BM. 1998. Post-infarction heart failure in the rat is associated with distinct alterations in cardiac myocyte molecular phenotype. J Mol Cell Cardiol 30:1615–1630.
13. Nelissen-Vrancken HJ, Debets JJ, Snoeckx LH, Daemen MJ, Smits JF. 1996. Time-related normalization of maximal coronary flow in isolated perfused hearts of rats with myocardial infarction. Circulation 93:349–355.
14. Packer M. 1988. Neurohormonal interactions and adaptations in congestive heart failure. Circulation 77:721–730.
15. Sigurdsson A, Swedberg K. 1996. The role of neurohormonal activation in chronic heart failure and postmyocardial infarction. Am Heart J 132:229–234.
16. Whittaker P. 1997. Collagen and ventricular remodeling after acute myocardial infarction: concepts and hypotheses. Basic Res Cardiol 92:79–81.
17. Rumberger JA. 1994. Ventricular dilatation and remodeling after myocardial infarction. Mayo Clin Proc 69:664–674.
18. Chien KR, Grace AA, Hunter JJ. 1999. Molecular and cellular biology of cardiac hypertrophy and failure. In Molecular Basis of Cardiovascular Disease—A Companion to Braunwald's Heart Disease. Ed. KR Chien, JL Breslow, JM Leiden, RD Rosenberg, and CE Seidman, 211–250. Philadelphia: WB Saunders.
19. Marijianowski MM, Teeling P, Becker AE. 1997. Remodeling after myocardial infarction in humans is not associated with interstitial fibrosis of noninfarcted myocardium [see comments]. J Am Coll Cardiol 30:76–82.
20. Sweet CS, Rucinska EJ. 1994. Losartan in heart failure: preclinical experiences and initial clinical outcomes. Eur Heart J 15:139–144.
21. Hasenfuss G. 1998. Alterations of calcium-regulatory proteins in heart failure. Cardiovasc Res 37:279–289.
22. Doggrell SA, Brown L. 1998. Rat models of hypertension, cardiac hypertrophy and failure. Cardiovasc Res 39:89–105.

23. Pfeffer MA, Pfeffer JM, Fishbein MC, Fletcher PJ, Spadaro J, Kloner RA, Braunwald E. 1979. Myocardial infarct size and ventricular function in rats. Circ Res 44:503–512.
24. Pfeffer JM, Pfeffer MA, Fletcher PJ, Braunwald E. 1984. Ventricular performance in rats with myocardial infarction and failure. Am J Med 76:99–103.
25. Anversa P, Beghi C, Kikkawa Y, Olivetti G. 1986. Myocardial infarction in rats. Infarct size, myocyte hypertrophy, and capillary growth. Circ Res 58:26–37.
26. Pfeffer JM. 1991. Progressive ventricular dilation in experimental myocardial infarction and its attenuation by angiotensin-converting enzyme inhibition. Am J Cardiol 68:17D–25D.
27. Capasso JM, Li P, Anversa P. 1993. Cytosolic calcium transients in myocytes isolated from rats with ischemic heart failure. Am J Physiol 265:H1953–H1964.
28. Sanbe A, Takeo S. 1995. Long-term treatment with angiotensin I-converting enzyme inhibitors attenuates the loss of cardiac beta-adrenoceptor responses in rats with chronic heart failure. Circulation 92:2666–2675.
29. Zarain-Herzberg A, Afzal N, Elimban V, Dhalla NS. 1996. Decreased expression of cardiac sarcoplasmic reticulum $Ca^{(2+)}$-pump ATPase in congestive heart failure due to myocardial infarction. Mol Cell Biochem 163/164:285–290.
30. Ye J, Yang L, Sethi R, Copps J, Ramjiawan B, Summers R, Deslauriers R. 1997. A new technique of coronary artery ligation: experimental myocardial infarction in rats in vivo with reduced mortality. Mol Cell Biochem 176:227–233.
31. Liu YH, Yang XP, Nass O, Sabbah HN, Peterson E, Carretero OA. 1997. Chronic heart failure induced by coronary artery ligation in Lewis inbred rats. Am J Physiol 272:H722–H227.
32. Isgaard J, Kujacic V, Jennische E, Holmang A, Sun XY, Hedner T, Hjalmarson A, Bengtsson BA. 1997. Growth hormone improves cardiac function in rats with experimental myocardial infarction. Eur J Clin Invest 27:517–525.
33. Hasenfuss G. 1998. Animal models of human cardiovascular disease, heart failure and hypertrophy. Cardiovasc Res 39:60–76.
34. Tajima M, Weinberg EO, Bartunek J, Jin H, Yang R, Paoni NF, Lorell BH. 1999. Treatment with growth hormone enhances contractile reserve and intracellular calcium transients in myocytes from rats with postinfarction heart failure. Circulation 99:127–134.
35. DeFelice A, Frering R, Horan P. 1989. Time course of hemodynamic changes in rats with healed severe myocardial infarction. Am J Physiol 257:H289–H296.
36. Yamaguchi F, Sanbe A, Takeo S. 1997. Cardiac sarcoplasmic reticular function in rats with chronic heart failure following myocardial infarction. J Mol Cell Cardiol 29:753–763.
37. Liu X, Shao Q, Dhalla NS. 1995. Myosin light chain phosphorylation in cardiac hypertrophy and failure due to myocardial infarction. J Mol Cell Cardiol 27:2613–2621.
38. Ganguly PK, Dhalla KS, Shao Q, Beamish RE, Dhalla NS. 1997. Differential changes in sympathetic activity in left and right ventricles in congestive heart failure after myocardial infarction. Am Heart J 133:340–345.
39. Sethi R, Elimban V, Chapman D, Dixon IM, Dhalla NS. 1998. Differential alterations in left and right ventricular G- proteins in congestive heart failure due to myocardial infarction. J Mol Cell Cardiol 30:2153–2163.
40. Afzal N, Dhalla NS. 1996. Sarcoplasmic reticular Ca^{2+} pump ATPase activity in congestive heart failure due to myocardial infarction. Can J Cardiol 12:1065–1073.
41. Holt E, Tonnessen T, Lunde PK, Semb SO, Wasserstrom JA, Sejersted OM, Christensen G. 1998. Mechanisms of cardiomyocyte dysfunction in heart failure following myocardial infarction in rats. J Mol Cell Cardiol 30:1581–1593.
42. Parmley WW. 1985. Pathophysiology of congestive heart failure. Am J Cardiol 55:9A–14A.
43. Yamaguchi F, Sanbe A, Takeo S. 1998. Effects of long-term treatment with trandolapril on sarcoplasmic reticulum function of cardiac muscle in rats with chronic heart failure following myocardial infarction. Br J Pharmacol 123:326–334.
44. Anand IS, Liu D, Chugh SS, Prahash AJ, Gupta S, John R, Popescu F, Chandrashekhar Y. 1997. Isolated myocyte contractile function is normal in postinfarct remodeled rat heart with systolic dysfunction. Circulation 96:3974–3984.
45. Shen YT, Wiedmann RT, Lynch JJ, Grossman W, Johnson RG. 1996. GH replacement fails to improve ventricular function in hypophysectomized rats with myocardial infarction. Am J Physiol 271:H1721–H1727.
46. Sanbe A, Tanonaka K, Niwano Y, Takeo S. 1994. Improvement of cardiac function and myocardial energy metabolism of rats with chronic heart failure by long-term coenzyme Q10 treatment. J Pharmacol Exp Ther 269:51–56.

47. Kumar R, Hood WB Jr, Abelmann WH. 1971. Hemodynamic spectrum of left ventricular failure in experimental myocardial infarction. Am Heart J 82:713–714.

48. Litwin SE, Bridge JH. 1997. Enhanced Na$^{(+)}$–Ca^{2+} exchange in the infarcted heart. Implications for excitation–contraction coupling. Circ Res 81:1083–1093.

49. Ganguly PK, Pierce GN, Dhalla KS, Dhalla NS. 1983. Defective sarcoplasmic reticular calcium transport in diabetic cardiomyopathy. Am J Physiol 244:E528–E535.

50. Xu YJ, Botsford MW, Panagia V, Dhalla NS. 1996. Responses of heart function and intracellular free Ca^{2+} to phosphatidic acid in chronic diabetes. Can J Cardiol 12:1092–1098.

51. Dhalla NS, Liu X, Panagia V, Takeda N. 1998. Subcellular remodeling and heart dysfunction in chronic diabetes [editorial]. Cardiovasc Res 40:239–247.

52. Ming Z, Nordin C, Siri F, Aronson RS. 1994. Reduced calcium current density in single myocytes isolated from hypertrophied failing guinea pig hearts. J Mol Cell Cardiol 26:1133–1143.

53. Kiss E, Ball NA, Kranias EG, Walsh RA. 1995. Differential changes in cardiac phospholamban and sarcoplasmic reticular Ca$^{(2+)}$–ATPase protein levels. Effects on Ca^{2+} transport and mechanics in compensated pressure-overload hypertrophy and congestive heart failure. Circ Res 77:759–764.

54. Bailey BA, Dipla K, Li S, Houser SR. 1997. Cellular basis of contractile derangements of hypertrophied feline ventricular myocytes. J Mol Cell Cardiol 29:1823–1835.

55. Wang J, Flemal K, Qiu Z, Ablin L, Grossman W, Morgan JP. 1994. Ca^{2+} handling and myofibrillar Ca^{2+} sensitivity in ferret cardiac myocytes with pressure-overload hypertrophy. Am J Physiol 267: H918–H9124.

56. Furukawa N, Bassett AL, Furukawa T, Myerburg RJ, Kimura S. 1991. Hypertrophy alters effect of Ins(1,4,5)P3 on Ca^{2+} release in skinned rat heart muscle. Am J Physiol 260:H612–H618.

57. Rupp H, Elimban V, Dhalla NS. 1998. Differential influence of fasting and BM13.907 treatment on growth and phenotype of pressure overloaded rat heart. Mol Cell Biochem 188:209–215.

58. Ohkusa T, Hisamatsu Y, Yano M, Kobayashi S, Tatsuno H, Saiki Y, Kohno M, Matsuzaki M. 1997. Altered cardiac mechanism and sarcoplasmic reticulum function in pressure overload-induced cardiac hypertrophy in rats. J Mol Cell Cardiol 29:45–54.

59. Delbridge LM, Satoh H, Yuan W, Bassani JW, Qi M, Ginsburg KS, Samarel AM, Bers DM. 1997. Cardiac myocyte volume, Ca^{2+} fluxes, and sarcoplasmic reticulum loading in pressure-overload hypertrophy. Am J Physiol 272:H2425–2435.

60. Qi M, Shannon TR, Euler DE, Bers DM, Samarel AM. 1997. Downregulation of sarcoplasmic reticulum Ca$^{(2+)}$-ATPase during progression of left ventricular hypertrophy. Am J Physiol 272: H2416–H2424.

61. Gomez AM, Valdivia HH, Cheng H, Lederer MR, Santana LF, Cannell MB, McCune SA, Altschuld RA, Lederer WJ. 1997. Defective excitation–contraction coupling in experimental cardiac hypertrophy and heart failure. Science 276:800–806.

62. Hisamatsu Y, Ohkusa T, Kihara Y, Inoko M, Ueyama T, Yano M, Sasayama S, Matsuzaki M. 1997. Early changes in the functions of cardiac sarcoplasmic reticulum in volume-overloaded cardiac hypertrophy in rats. J Mol Cell Cardiol 29:1097–1109.

63. Spinale FG, Mukherjee R, Iannini JP, Whitebread S, Hebbar L, Clair MJ, Melton DM, Cox MH, Thomas PB, de Gasparo M. 1997. Modulation of the renin–angiotensin pathway through enzyme inhibition and specific receptor blockade in pacing-induced heart failure: II. Effects on myocyte contractile processes. Circulation 96:2397–2406.

64. O'Rourke B, Kass DA, Tomaselli GF, Kaab S, Tunin R, Marban E. 1999. Mechanisms of altered excitation–contraction coupling in canine tachycardia-induced heart failure, I: experimental studies. Circ Res 84:562–570.

65. Winslow RL, Rice J, Jafri S, Marban E, O'Rourke B. 1999. Mechanisms of altered excitation–contraction coupling in canine tachycardia-induced heart failure, II: model studies. Circ Res 84:571–586.

66. Gertz EW. 1972. Cardiomyopathic Syrian hamster: a possible model of human disease. Prog Exp Tumor Res 16:242–260.

67. Arai M, Matsui H, Periasamy M. 1994. Sarcoplasmic reticulum gene expression in cardiac hypertrophy and heart failure. Circ Res 74:555–564.

68. Sapp JL, Howlett SE. 1994. Density of ryanodine receptors is increased in sarcoplasmic reticulum from prehypertrophic cardiomyopathic hamster heart. J Mol Cell Cardiol 26:325–334.

69. Dhalla NS, Ziegelhoffer A, Harrow JA. 1977. Regulatory role of membrane systems in heart function. Can J Physiol Pharmacol 55:1211–1234.

70. Dhalla NS, Das PK, Sharma GP. 1978. Subcellular basis of cardiac contractile failure. J Mol Cell Cardiol 10:363–385.

71. Dhalla NS, Pierce GN, Panagia V, Singal PK, Beamish RE. 1982. Calcium movements in relation to heart function. Basic Res Cardiol 77:117–139.
72. Morgan JP, Perreault CL, Morgan KG. 1991. The cellular basis of contraction and relaxation in cardiac and vascular smooth muscle. Am Heart J 1991. 121:961–968.
73. Barry WH, Bridge JH. 1993. Intracellular calcium homeostasis in cardiac myocytes. Circulation 87:1806–1815.
74. Hasenfuss G, Meyer M, Schillinger W, Preuss M, Pieske B, Just H. 1997. Calcium handling proteins in the failing human heart. Basic Res Cardiol 92:87–93.
75. Movsesian MA, Schwinger RH. 1998. Calcium sequestration by the sarcoplasmic reticulum in heart failure. Cardiovasc Res 37:352–359.
76. Fabiato A. 1983. Calcium-induced release of calcium from the cardiac sarcoplasmic reticulum. Am J Physiol 245:C1–C14.
77. Fabiato A. 1985. Simulated calcium current can both cause calcium loading in and trigger calcium release from the sarcoplasmic reticulum of a skinned canine cardiac Purkinje cell. J Gen Physiol 85:291–320.
78. Balke CW, Shorofsky SR. 1998. Alterations in calcium handling in cardiac hypertrophy and heart failure. Cardiovasc Res 37:290–299.
79. Shorofsky SR, Aggarwal R, Corretti M, Baffa JM, Strum JM, Al-Seikhan BA, Kobayashi YM, Jones LR, Wier WG, Balke CW. 1999. Cellular mechanisms of altered contractility in the hypertrophied heart: big hearts, big sparks. Circ Res 84:424–434.
80. Winegrad S. 1997. Endothelial cell regulation of contractility of the heart. Annu Rev Physiol 59:505–525.
81. Cheung JY, Musch TI, Misawa H, Semanchick A, Elensky M, Yelamarty RV, Moore RL. 1994. Impaired cardiac function in rats with healed myocardial infarction: cellular vs. myocardial mechanisms. Am J Physiol 266:C29–C36.
82. Li P, Park C, Micheletti R, Li B, Cheng W, Sonnenblick EH, Anversa P, Bianchi G. 1995. Myocyte performance during evolution of myocardial infarction in rats: effects of propionyl-L-carnitine. Am J Physiol 268:H1702–H1713.
83. Denvir MA, MacFarlane NG, Cobbe SM, Miller DJ. 1998. Sarcoplasmic reticulum Ca^{2+} loading in rabbits 8 and 15 weeks after coronary artery ligation. Pflugers Arch-Eur J Physiol 436:436–442.
84. Williams JH, Ward CW. 1998. Changes in skeletal muscle sarcoplasmic reticulum function and force production following myocardial infarction in rats. Exp Physiol 83:85–94.
85. Otsu K, Willard HF, Khanna VK, Zorzato F, Green NM, MacLennan DH. 1990. Molecular cloning of cDNA encoding the Ca^{2+} release channel (ryanodine receptor) of rabbit cardiac muscle sarcoplasmic reticulum. J Biol Chem 265:13472–13483.
86. Rousseau E, Smith JS, Meissner G. 1987. Ryanodine modifies conductance and gating behavior of single Ca^{2+} release channel. Am J Physiol 253:C364–C368.
87. Lai FA, Erickson HP, Rousseau E, Liu QY, Meissner G. 1988. Purification and reconstitution of the calcium release channel from skeletal muscle. Nature 331:315–319.
88. Anderson K, Lai FA, Liu QY, Rousseau E, Erickson HP, Meissner G. 1989. Structural and functional characterization of the purified cardiac ryanodine receptor-Ca^{2+} release channel complex. J Biol Chem 264:1329–1335.
89. Meissner G. 1986. Ryanodine activation and inhibition of the Ca^{2+} release channel of sarcoplasmic reticulum. J Biol Chem 261:6300–6306.
90. McPherson PS, Campbell KP. 1993. The ryanodine receptor/Ca^{2+} release channel. J Biol Chem 268:13765–13768.
91. Phillips RM, Narayan P, Gomez AM, Dilly K, Jones LR, Lederer WJ, Altschuld RA. 1998. Sarcoplasmic reticulum in heart failure: central player or bystander? Cardiovasc Res 37:346–351.
92. Jorgensen AO, Shen AC, Daly P, MacLennan DH. 1982. Localization of Ca^{2+} + Mg^{2+}-ATPase of the sarcoplasmic reticulum in adult rat papillary muscle. J Cell Biol 93:883–892.
93. Cantilina T, Sagara Y, Inesi G, Jones LR. 1993. Comparative studies of cardiac and skeletal sarcoplasmic reticulum ATPases. Effect of a phospholamban antibody on enzyme activation by Ca^{2+}. J Biol Chem 268:17018–17025.
94. Burk SE, Lytton J, MacLennan DH, Shull GE. 1989. cDNA cloning, functional expression, and mRNA tissue distribution of a third organellar Ca^{2+} pump. J Biol Chem 264:18561–18568.
95. Wu KD, Lee WS, Wey J, Bungard D, Lytton J. 1995. Localization and quantification of endoplasmic reticulum $Ca^{(2+)}$-ATPase isoform transcripts. Am J Physiol 269:C775–C784.
96. Zarain-Herzberg A, MacLennan DH, Periasamy M. 1990. Characterization of rabbit cardiac sarco(endo)plasmic reticulum $Ca^{2(+)}$-ATPase gene. J Biol Chem 265:4670–4677.

97. Periasamy M, Reed TD, Liu LH, Ji Y, Loukianov E, Paul RJ, Nieman ML, Riddle T, Duffy JJ, Doetschman T, Lorenz JN, Shull GE. 1999. Impaired cardiac performance in heterozygous mice with a null mutation in the sarco(endo)plasmic reticulum Ca^{2+}–ATPase isoform 2 (SERCA2) gene. J Biol Chem 274:2556–2562.

98. Verboomen H, Wuytack F, De Smedt H, Himpens B, Casteels R. 1992. Functional difference between SERCA2a and SERCA2b Ca^{2+} pumps and their modulation by phospholamban. Biochem J 286:591–595.

99. Zarain-Herzberg A, Rupp H, Elimban V, Dhalla NS. 1996. Modification of sarcoplasmic reticulum gene expression in pressure overload cardiac hypertrophy by etomoxir. FASEB J 10:1303–1309.

100. Ji Y, Loukianov E, Loukianova T, Jones LR, Periasamy M. 1999. SERCA1a can functionally substitute for SERCA2a in the heart. Am J Physiol 276:H89–H97.

101. Jones LR, Besch HR Jr, Watanabe AM. 1978. Regulation of the calcium pump of cardiac sarcoplasmic reticulum. Interactive roles of potassium and ATP on the phosphoprotein intermediate of the (K^+, Ca^{2+})–ATPase. J Biol Chem 253:1643–1653.

102. Davia K, Davies CH, Harding SE. 1997. Effects of inhibition of sarcoplasmic reticulum calcium uptake on contraction in myocytes isolated from failing human ventricle. Cardiovasc Res 33:88–97.

103. Baker DL, Hashimoto K, Grupp IL, Ji Y, Reed T, Loukianov E, Grupp G, Bhagwhat A, Hoit B, Walsh R, Marban E, Periasamy M. 1998. Targeted overexpression of the sarcoplasmic reticulum Ca^{2+}–ATPase increases cardiac contractility in transgenic mouse hearts. Circ Res 83:1205–1214.

104. Meyer M, Dillmann WH. 1998. Sarcoplasmic reticulum $Ca^{(2+)}$–ATPase overexpression by adenovirus mediated gene transfer and in transgenic mice. Cardiovasc Res 37:360–366.

105. Tada M, Kirchberger MA, Katz AM. 1975. Phosphorylation of a 22,000-dalton component of the cardiac sarcoplasmic reticulum by adenosine $3':5'$-monophosphate-dependent protein kinase. J Biol Chem 250:2640–2647.

106. Kirchberger MA, Antonetz T. 1982. Calmodulin-mediated regulation of calcium transport and $(Ca^{2+} + Mg^{2+})$- activated ATPase activity in isolated cardiac sarcoplasmic reticulum. J Biol Chem 257:5685–5691.

107. Gwathmey JK, Copelas L, MacKinnon R, Schoen FJ, Feldman MD, Grossman W, Morgan JP. 1987. Abnormal intracellular calcium handling in myocardium from patients with end-stage heart failure. Circ Res 61:70–76.

108. Morgan JP, Erny RE, Allen PD, Grossman W, Gwathmey JK. 1990. Abnormal intracellular calcium handling, a major cause of systolic and diastolic dysfunction in ventricular myocardium from patients with heart failure. Circulation 81:III21–III32.

109. Dipla K, Mattiello JA, Margulies KB, Jeevanandam V, Houser SR. 1999. The sarcoplasmic reticulum and the Na^+/Ca^{2+} exchanger both contribute to the Ca^{2+} transient of failing human ventricular myocytes. Circ Res 84:435–444.

110. Qin D, Zhang ZH, Caref EB, Boutjdir M, Jain P, El-Sherif N. 1996. Cellular and ionic basis of arrhythmias in postinfarction remodeled ventricular myocardium. Circ Res 79:461–473.

111. Limas CJ, Olivari MT, Goldenberg IF, Levine TB, Benditt DG, Simon A. 1987. Calcium uptake by cardiac sarcoplasmic reticulum in human dilated cardiomyopathy. Cardiovasc Res 21:601–605.

112. Zhang XQ, Moore RL, Tenhave T, Cheung JY. 1995. $[Ca^{2+}]i$ transients in hypertensive and postinfarction myocytes. Am J Physiol 269:C632–C640.

113. Zhang XQ, Tillotson DL, Moore RL, Zelis R, Cheung JY. 1996. Na^+/Ca^{2+} exchange currents and SR Ca^{2+} contents in postinfarction myocytes. Am J Physiol 271:C1800–C1807.

114. Zhang XQ, Moore RL, Tillotson DL, Cheung JY. 1995. Calcium currents in postinfarction rat cardiac myocytes. Am J Physiol 269:C1464–C1473.

115. Meyer M, Schillinger W, Pieske B, Holubarsch C, Heilmann C, Posival H, Kuwajima G, Mikoshiba K, Just H, Hasenfuss G. 1995. Alterations of sarcoplasmic reticulum proteins in failing human dilated cardiomyopathy. Circulation 92:778–784.

116. Schwinger RH, Bohm M, Schmidt U, Karczewski P, Bavendiek U, Flesch M, Krause EG, Erdmann E. 1995. Unchanged protein levels of SERCA II and phospholamban but reduced Ca^{2+} uptake and $Ca^{(2+)}$-ATPase activity of cardiac sarcoplasmic reticulum from dilated cardiomyopathy patients compared with patients with nonfailing hearts. Circulation 92:3220–3228.

117. Iijima K, Geshi E, Nomizo A, Arata Y, Katagiri T. 1998. Alterations in sarcoplasmic reticulum and angiotensin II type 1 receptor gene expression after myocardial infarction in rats. Jpn Circ J 62:449–454.

118. Griendling KK, Murphy TJ, Alexander RW. 1993. Molecular biology of the renin–angiotensin system. Circulation 87:1816–1828.

119. Dzau VJ, Burt DW, Pratt RE. 1988. Molecular biology of the renin–angiotensin system. Am J Physiol 255:F563–F573.
120. Furuta H, Guo DF, Inagami T. 1992. Molecular cloning and sequencing of the gene encoding human angiotensin II type 1 receptor. Biochem Biophys Res Commun 183:8–13.
121. Timmermans PB, Smith RD. 1994. Angiotensin II receptor subtypes: selective antagonists and functional correlates. Eur Heart J 15(Suppl D):79–87.
122. Bartunek J, Weinberg EO, Tajima M, Rohrbach S, Lorell BH. 1999. Angiotensin II type 2 receptor blockade amplifies the early signals of cardiac growth response to angiotensin II in hypertrophied hearts. Circulation 99:22–25.
123. Sechi LA, Griffin CA, Grady EF, Kalinyak JE, Schambelan M. 1992. Characterization of angiotensin II receptor subtypes in rat heart. Circ Res 71:1482–1489.
124. Shao Q, Saward L, Zahradka P, Dhalla NS. 1998. Ca²⁺ mobilization in adult rat cardiomyocytes by angiotensin type 1 and 2 receptors. Biochem Pharmacol 55:1413–1418.
125. Shao Q, Panagia V, Beamish RE, Dhalla NS. 1998. Role of renin–angiotensin system in cardiac hypertrophy and failure. In Angiotensin II Receptor Blockade: Physiological and Clinical Implications Ed. NS Dhalla, P Zahradka, I Dixon, and RE Beamish, 283–310. Boston: Kluwer Academic.
126. Sadoshima J, Xu Y, Slayter HS, Izumo S. 1993. Autocrine release of angiotensin II mediates stretch-induced hypertrophy of cardiac myocytes in vitro. Cell 75:977–984.
127. Liu JL, Zucker IH. 1999. Regulation of sympathetic nerve activity in heart failure: a role for nitric oxide and angiotensin II. Circ Res 84:417–423.
128. Lindpaintner K, Lu W, Neidermajer N, Schieffer B, Just H, Ganten D, Drexler H. 1993. Selective activation of cardiac angiotensinogen gene expression in post-infarction ventricular remodeling in the rat. J Mol Cell Cardiol 25:133–143.
129. Kohzuki M, Kanazawa M, Yoshida K, Kamimoto M, Wu XM, Jiang ZL, Yasujima M, Abe K, Johnston CI, Sato T. 1996. Cardiac angiotensin converting enzyme and endothelin receptor in rats with chronic myocardial infarction. Jpn Circ J 60:972–980.
130. Meggs LG, Coupet J, Huang H, Cheng W, Li P, Capasso JM, Homcy CJ, Anversa P. 1993. Regulation of angiotensin II receptors on ventricular myocytes after myocardial infarction in rats. Circ Res 72:1149–1162.
131. Zhu YC, Zhu YZ, Gohlke P, Stauss HM, Unger T. 1997. Effects of angiotensin-converting enzyme inhibition and angiotensin II AT1 receptor antagonism on cardiac parameters in left ventricular hypertrophy. Am J Cardiol 80:110A–117A.
132. Anthonio RL, van Veldhuisen DJ, van Gilst WH. 1998. Left ventricular dilatation after myocardial infarction: ACE inhibitors, beta-blockers, or both? J Cardiovasc Pharmacol 32:S1–S8.
133. Mulder P, Devaux B, Richard V, Henry JP, Wimart MC, Thibout E, Mace B, Thuillez C. 1997. Early versus delayed angiotensin-converting enzyme inhibition in experimental chronic heart failure. Effects on survival, hemodynamics, and cardiovascular remodeling. Circulation 95:1314–1319.
134. Pitt B. 1995. Importance of angiotensin-converting enzyme inhibitors in myocardial infarction and congestive heart failure: implications for clinical practice. Cardiology 86:41–45.
135. Cody RJ. Comparing angiotensin-converting enzyme inhibitor trial results in patients with acute myocardial infarction. Arch Intern Med 154:2029–2036.
136. Cody RJ. 1995. ACE inhibitors: myocardial infarction and congestive heart failure. Am Fam Physician 52:1801–1806.
137. Colucci WS. 1997. Molecular and cellular mechanisms of myocardial failure. Am J Cardiol 80:15L–25L.
138. van den Heuvel AF, van Gilst WH, van Veldhuisen DJ, de Vries RJ, Dunselman PH, Kingma JH. 1997. The Captopril and Thrombolysis Study (CATS) Investigators. Long-term anti-ischemic effects of angiotensin-converting enzyme inhibition in patients after myocardial infarction. J Am Coll Cardiol 30:400–405.
139. Sanbe A, Tanonaka K, Kobayasi R, Takeo S. 1995. Effects of long-term therapy with ACE inhibitors, captopril, enalapril and trandolapril, on myocardial energy metabolism in rats with heart failure following myocardial infarction. J Mol Cell Cardiol 27:2209–2222.
140. Takeishi Y, Bhagwat A, Ball NA, Kirkpatrick DL, Periasamy M, Walsh RA. 1999. Effect of angiotensin-converting enzyme inhibition on protein kinase C and SR proteins in heart failure. Am J Physiol 276:H53–H62.
141. Smits JF, van Krimpen C, Schoemaker RG, Cleutjens JP, Daemen MJ. 1992. Angiotensin II receptor blockade after myocardial infarction in rats: effects on hemodynamics, myocardial DNA synthesis, and interstitial collagen content. J Cardiovasc Pharmacol 20:772–778.

142. Regitz-Zagrosek V, Neuss M, Fleck E. 1995. Effects of angiotensin receptor antagonists in heart failure: clinical and experimental aspects. Eur Heart J 16:86–91.
143. Dickstein K, Chang P, Willenheimer R, Haunso S, Remes J, Hall C, Kjekshus J. 1995. Comparison of the effects of losartan and enalapril on clinical status and exercise performance in patients with moderate or severe chronic heart failure. J Am Coll Cardiol 26:438–445.
144. Hamroff G, Katz SD, Mancini D, Blaufarb I, Bijou R, Patel R, Jondeau G, Olivari MT, Thomas S, Le Jemtel TH. 1999. Addition of angiotensin II receptor blockade to maximal angiotensin-converting enzyme inhibition improves exercise capacity in patients with severe congestive heart failure. Circulation 99:990–992.
145. Taylor K, Patten RD, Smith JJ, Aronovitz MJ, Wight J, Salomon RN, Konstam MA. 1998. Divergent effects of angiotensin-converting enzyme inhibition and angiotensin II-receptor antagonism on myocardial cellular proliferation and collagen deposition after myocardial infarction in rats. J Cardiovasc Pharmacol 31:654–660.
146. Murakami M, Suzuki H, Naitoh M, Matsumoto A, Kageyama Y, Tsujimoto G, Saruta T. 1995. Blockade of the renin–angiotensin system in heart failure in conscious dogs. J Hypertens 13:1405–1412.
147. Movsesian MA, Karimi M, Green K, Jones LR. 1994. $Ca^{2(+)}$-transporting ATPase, phospholamban, and calsequestrin levels in nonfailing and failing human myocardium. Circulation 90:653–657.
148. Hasenfuss G, Reinecke H, Studer R, Meyer M, Pieske B, Holtz J, Holubarsch C, Posival H, Just H, Drexler H. 1994. Relation between myocardial function and expression of sarcoplasmic reticulum $Ca^{2(+)}$-ATPase in failing and nonfailing human myocardium. Circ Res 75:434–442.
149. Linck B, Boknik P, Eschenhagen T, Muller FU, Neumann J, Nose M, Jones LR, Schmitz W, Scholz H. 1996. Messenger RNA expression and immunological quantification of phospholamban and SR-$Ca^{2(+)}$-ATPase in failing and nonfailing human hearts. Cardiovasc Res 31:625–632.
150. Liu X, Sentex E, Golfman L, Takeda S, Osada M, Dhalla NS. 1999. Modification of cardiac subcellular remodeling due to pressure overload by captopril and losartan. Clin Exp Hypertens 21:145–156.
151. Mercadier JJ, Lompre AM, Duc P, Boheler KR, Fraysse JB, Wisnewsky C, Allen PD, Komajda M, Schwartz K. 1990. Altered sarcoplasmic reticulum $Ca^{2(+)}$-ATPase gene expression in the human ventricle during end-stage heart failure. J Clin Invest 85:305–309.
152. Feldman AM, Ray PE, Silan CM, Mercer JA, Minobe W, Bristow MR. 1991. Selective gene expression in failing human heart. Quantification of steady-state levels of messenger RNA in endomyocardial biopsies using the polymerase chain reaction. Circulation 83:1866–1872.
153. Feldman AM, Weinberg EO, Ray PE, Lorell BH. 1993. Selective changes in cardiac gene expression during compensated hypertrophy and the transition to cardiac decompensation in rats with chronic aortic banding. Circ Res 73:184–192.
154. Arai M, Alpert NR, MacLennan DH, Barton P, Periasamy M. 1993. Alterations in sarcoplasmic reticulum gene expression in human heart failure. A possible mechanism for alterations in systolic and diastolic properties of the failing myocardium. Circ Res 72:463–469.
155. The CONSENSUS Trial Study Group. 1987. Effects of enalapril on mortality in severe congestive heart failure. Results of the Cooperative North Scandinavian Enalapril Survival Study (CONSENSUS). N Engl J Med 316:1429–1435.
156. Swedberg K, Held P, Kjekshus J, Rasmussen K, Ryden L, Wedel H. 1992. Effects of the early administration of enalapril on mortality in patients with acute myocardial infarction. Results of the Cooperative New Scandinavian Enalapril Survival Study II (CONSENSUS II). N Engl J Med 327:678–684.
157. Cohn JN, Johnson G, Ziesche S, Cobb F, Francis G, Tristani F, Smith R, Dunkman WB, Loeb H, Wong M. 1991. A comparison of enalapril with hydralazine-isosorbide dinitrate in the treatment of chronic congestive heart failure. N Engl J Med 325:303–310.
158. The SOLVD Investigators. 1992. Effect of enalapril on mortality and the development of heart failure in asymptomatic patients with reduced left ventricular ejection fractions. [published erratum appears in N Engl J Med 327: 1768]. N Engl J Med 327:685–691.
159. The SOLVD Investigators. 1991. Effect of enalapril on survival in patients with reduced left ventricular ejection fractions and congestive heart failure. N Engl J Med 325:293–302.
160. Schieffer B, Wirger A, Meybrunn M, Seitz S, Holtz J, Riede UN, Drexler H. 1994. Comparative effects of chronic angiotensin-converting enzyme inhibition and angiotensin II type 1 receptor blockade on cardiac remodeling after myocardial infarction in the rat. Circulation 89:2273–2282.
161. Raya TE, Fonken SJ, Lee RW, Daugherty S, Goldman S, Wong PC, Timmermans PB, Morkin E. 1991. Hemodynamic effects of direct angiotensin II blockade compared to converting enzyme inhibition in rat model of heart failure. Am J Hypertens 4:334S–340S.

162. Richard S, Leclercq F, Lemaire S, Piot C, Nargeot J. 1998. Ca^{2+} currents in compensated hypertrophy and heart failure. Cardiovasc Res 37:300–311.
163. Wagner GS, Freye CJ, Palmeri ST, Roark SF, Stack NC, Ideker RE, Harrell FE Jr, Selvester RH. 1982. Evaluation of a QRS scoring system for estimating myocardial infarct size. I. Specificity and observer agreement. Circulation 65:342–347.
164. Chomczynski P, Sacchi N. 1987. Single-step method of RNA isolation by acid guanidinium thiocyanate-phenol-chloroform extraction. Anal Biochem 162:156–159.
165. Dixon IM, Hata T, Dhalla NS. 1992. Sarcolemmal calcium transport in congestive heart failure due to myocardial infarction in rats. Am J Physiol 262:H1387–H1394.
166. Ross J Jr. 1999. Growth hormone, cardiomyocyte contractile reserve, and heart failure. Circulation 99:15–17.
167. Shao, Q. 1999. Captopril treatment improves the sarcoplasmic reticular Ca^{2+} transport in heart failure due to myocardial infarction. J Mol Cell Cardiol 31:1663–1672.

N. Takeda, M. Nagano and N.S. Dhalla
(eds). The Hypertrophied Heart. Copyright
© 2000. pp. 303–320. Kluwer Academic
Publishers. Boston. All rights reserved.

ACTIVATED TGFβ SIGNALING IN THE HEART AFTER MYOCARDIAL INFARCTION

JIANMING HAO, TRACY SCAMMELL-LA FLEUR, and IAN M.C. DIXON

Laboratory of Molecular Cardiology, Institute of Cardiovascular Sciences, St. Boniface General Hospital Research Centre, Faculty of Medicine, University of Manitoba, 351 Tache Avenue, Winnipeg, Manitoba, Canada R2H 2A6

Summary. We have previously shown that myofibroblasts of the healed 8 week infarct scar overexpress transduction proteins that may be linked to elevated deposition of extracellular matrix components in this tissue. Other work suggests that $TGF\beta_1$ may be involved in cardiac fibrosis and myocyte hypertrophy. The significance of the altered TGFβ signaling in heart failure in the chronic phase of post-myocardial infarction (MI), particularly in the ongoing remodeling of the infarct scar, remains unexplored. Patterns of cardiac $TGF\beta_1$ and Smad 2, 3, and 4 protein expression were investigated 8 weeks after MI and were compared to relative collagen deposition in border tissues (containing remnant myocytes) and the infarct scar (nonmyocytes dominated by myofibroblasts). Both $TGF\beta_1$ mRNA abundance (Northern analysis) and protein levels (ELISA) were significantly increased in the infarct scar versus control values, and this trend was positively correlated to increased collagen type I expression in this tissues. Cardiac Smad 2, 3, and 4 proteins were significantly increased in border and scar tissues versus control values. Immunofluorescent studies indicated that Smad proteins were proximally localized to cellular nuclei in the infarct scar. TβRI (53 kDa) protein expression was significantly reduced in the scar, while the 75 kDa and 110 kDa isoforms of TβRII were unchanged and significantly increased respectively, in the infarct scar. These results indicate that TGFβ/Smad signaling may be involved in the remodeling of the infarct scar after the completion of wound healing per se, via ongoing stimulation of matrix deposition.

INTRODUCTION

Myocardial infarction (MI) is one of the major causes of heart failure [1]. After a large MI, ventricular chamber dilatation and sphericalization is attended by cardiac hypertrophy and fibrosis as well as wound healing in the scar, and these events are associated with the onset of heart failure [1–3]. TGFβ has been implicated in many fibrotic disorders, including glomerulonephritis, cirrhosis, lung fibrosis, and vascular restenosis [4]. As yet there is only limited information regarding the role of TGFβ in cardiac fibrosis and hypertrophy [5,6]. Increased expression of $TGF\beta_1$ mRNA and protein have been shown in myocardium bordering the infarct region 2 days after MI [7], suggesting a role in the cardiac wound-healing response. Recently, a major advance in our understanding of TGFβ signaling has been the identification of Smad proteins as downstream effectors of TGFβ. These proteins translocate to nuclei and initiate gene transcription in response to TGFβ binding to type II (TβRII) and subsequent dimerization with type I (TβRI) receptor [8,9]; however, the relationship between cardiac Smad protein activation and chronic cardiac remodeling of infarct scar or remnant tissue after MI is unknown.

TGFβ₁ is known to be expressed in the heart [10], and it has been shown that both cardiac myocytes and fibroblasts may release TGFβ₁ [11–14]. Similarly, TGFβ receptors are localized in both cardiac myocytes and nonmyocytes [15], and TGFβ₁ is known to alter myocardial gene expression in cultured neonatal cardiac myocytes [5]. Furthermore, TGFβ₁ is a powerful initiator for the production of fibrillar collagens and other major ECM components in a variety of cell types [16]. In cultured cardiac fibroblasts, TGFβ₁ has been shown to stimulate collagen deposition and to augment the synthesis of fibronectin and proteoglycans [17–20]. Thus the effects of TGFβ₁ on cardiac cells in vitro mimic changes that characteristically transpire during the development of cardiac fibrosis, hypertrophy, and failure.

It is possible that increased Smad signaling in cardiac cells may be linked to the development of cardiac hypertrophy and fibrosis of surviving myocardium and in the chronic remodeling of infarct scar tissue in post-MI hearts. Cardiac myofibroblasts are abundant at the site of cardiac tissue repair, are known to synthesize fibrillar collagens, and are major players in formation of infarct scar structure in the post-MI heart [21]. The healed infarct scar is specifically organized to confer anisotropic mechanical properties and to deform in a manner similar to noninfarcted myocardium, and thus may help to preserve ventricular function [22]. Thus inappropriate ongoing remodeling of the infarct scar by myofibroblast cells residing in that tissue is a possible mechanism for progressive loss of cardiac function after large MI. The present study was conducted to examine the relationships among expression patterns and cellular localization of TGFβ, Smad 2, 3, and 4, and fibrillar collagens in the infarct scar and border, as well as noninfarcted remnant tissues from animals in moderate heart failure due to MI (8 weeks post-MI). For the purpose of comparison, TβRI (ALK-5) and TβRII protein expression and localization in remnant left ventricle remote to the infarct scar, border, and infarct scar tissues of failing hearts were examined.

MATERIALS AND METHODS

Experimental model

All experimental protocols for animal studies were approved by the Animal Care Committee of the University of Manitoba, Canada, following guidelines established by the Medical Research Council of Canada. MI was produced in male Sprague–Dawley rats (weighing 200–250 g) by ligation of the left coronary artery, as described previously [23,24]. The mortality of all animals operated upon in this fashion was about 45% within 48 hours. Surviving rats from sham-operated and MI groups were sacrified at 8 weeks post-MI. Subsequently, cardiac tissues from different regions, including noninfarcted, viable, scar, and border tissues, were used for the following assays: (1) quantification of TGFβ$_1$; (2) detection of collagen type I and TGFβ$_1$ mRNA abundance; (3) localization and quantification of TβRI and TβRII protein; and (4) localization as well as quantification of Smad proteins.

Hemodynamic measurements

Left ventricular function of 8 week post-MI and age-matched sham-operated control groups were measured as described previously [23,25]. Briefly, rats were anesthetized by intraperitoneal injection of a ketamine:xylazine mixture (100 mg/kg: 10 mg/kg). A micromanometer-tipped catheter (2-0) (Millar SPR-249) was inserted into the right carotid artery. The catheter was advanced into the aorta to determine MAP, and then further advanced to the LV chamber to record LV systolic pressure (LVSP), LV end-diastolic pressure (LVEDP), the maximum rate of isovolumic pressure development ($+dP/dt_{max}$), and the maximum rate of isovolumic pressures decay ($-dP/dt_{max}$). Hemodynamic data was computed instantaneously and displayed using a computer data acquisition workstation (Biopac, Harvard Apparatus Canada).

Infarct size

After heart function recordings, the left ventricle was fixed by immersion in 10% formalin and embedded in paraffin. Six transverse slices were cut from the apex to the base, and serial sections (5 μm) were cut and mounted. The percentage of infarcted left ventricle was estimated at 8 weeks after coronary ligation by planimetric techniques as described previously [26]. Animals with large infarcts (>40% of the LV free wall) were used in this study.

Determination of cardiac total collagen

Samples from different groups were ground into powder in liquid nitrogen. Then 100 mg (wet weight) cardiac tissue was dried to constant weight. Tissue samples were digested in 6 M HCl (0.12 mL/mg dry weight) for 16 hours at 105°C. Hydroxyproline was measured as a marker for estimation of cardiac collagens according to the method of Chiariello et al. [27]. Collagen concentration was calculated by multiplying hydroxyproline levels by a factor of 7.46, assuming that interstitial collagen contains an average of 13.4% hydroxyproline [27]. The data were expressed as μg collagen per mg dry tissue.

ELISA assay for cardiac TGFβ$_1$

After excision, the heart was perfused with 5 mL cold PBS to flush out the remaining blood in the vascular lumen in myocardium in order to eliminate contamination by TGFβ$_1$ from blood sources. Approximately 0.5 g heart tissue was homogenized in 4 mL cold acid–ethanol (93% ethanol, 2% HCl, 85 μg/mL PMSF, and 5 μg/mL pepstatin A). Three samples were pooled in the case of border and scar tissues. After overnight extraction at 4°C by gentle rocking, extracts were subjected to centrifugation at $10,000 \times g$ for 10 minutes. The resulting supernatants were dialyzed extensively (3×100 volume) against 4 mM HCl at 4°C, using a 3500 MW-cutoff Spectrapore dialysis membrane and subjected to ELISA assay for $TGF\beta_1$ as previously described [28] with the exception that the captive agent was soluble $T\beta RII$ instead of anti-$TGF\beta_1$ antibody.

Immunofluorescent localization of $TGF\beta_1$ as well as Smad 2, 3, and 4, $T\beta RI$ (ALK-5), and $T\beta RII$

For these studies, a total of nine rats were used, including four sham-operated animals and five MI rats. LV tissue from sham and viable left ventricle remote to the infarct as well as border and scar tissues from MI rats were immersed in OCT compound (Miles Inc., Elkhart, IN, USA). Serial cryostat sections (7 μm) of ventricular tissue were mounted on gelatin coated slides. A minimum of six sections from different regions from hearts of each group were processed. Indirect immunofluorescence was performed as described in detail previously [26]. Tissue sections were fixed in 4% paraformaldehyde for 15 minutes. Polyclonal antibodies against active $TGF\beta_1$ as well as Smad 2, 3, and 4, $T\beta RI$, and $T\beta RII$ were diluted 1:50–1:100 with 1% BSA in PBS and applied as the primary antibodies. After incubation overnight at 4°C, the sections were washed with PBS and incubated with biotinylated, anti-goat (or rabbit) IgG secondary antibody and subsequently incubated with FITC-labeled streptavidin for 90 minutes. Staining of cellular nuclei in frozen sections of hearts was carried out using Hoechst dye 33342 at a final concentration of 10 μg/mL. The tissue sections were examined under a Nikon Labophot microscope equipped with epifluorescence optics and appropriate filters. The results were recorded by photography on Kodak TMAX 400 black and white film.

Western blot analysis of Smad 2, 3, 4 as well as $T\beta RI$ and $T\beta RII$

Western blot analysis was carried out as described previously [24,29]. For total cardiac Smad protein assays, tissues were homogenized with homogenization buffer containing 0.1% Triton X-100. This homogenate was sonicated for 5×5 seconds to disrupt nuclear membranes. The samples were allowed to lyse for 15 minutes on ice. After centrifugation at $10,000 \times g$ for 20 minutes at 4°C, the supernatant was retained for determination of Smad proteins. Total protein concentration of all samples was measured using the bicinchoninic acid (BCA) method [30]. Primary antibodies were diluted in TBS-T (Smad 2, 3, and 4 at 1:500 and $T\beta RI$, $T\beta RII$ at 1:250). The specific bands of target proteins were visualized by enhanced chemiluminescence (ECL) or by ECL Plus according to the manufacturer's instructions (Amersham Life Science Inc. Arlington Heights, IL, USA), and these bands were quantified using a CCD camera imaging densitometer (Bio-Rad, model GS 670).

RNA extraction and Northern blot analysis of cardiac $TGF\beta_1$ and type I fibrillar collagen mRNAs

Total RNA was isolated from noninfarcted left ventricles, viable, border, and scar tissues of infarcted left ventricle, 8 weeks after operation by the method of Chomczynski and Sacchi [31] as described previously [24,32]. A total of 12 animals were included in this assay. The cDNA fragments used in this study were human TGFβ₁, collagen type I, decorin, and glyceraldehyde-3-phosphate dehydrogenase (GAPDH). Northern bands were quantified by densitometry (Bio-Rad, GS 670), and these target mRNA signals were normalized to GAPDH signal to account for differences in loading and/or transfer of mRNA.

Reagents

Primary antibodies against Smad 2, 3, and 4 as well as TβRI, TβRII, and HRP-labeled anti-goat secondary antibody were from Santa Cruz Biotechnology, Inc. (Santa Cruz, CA, USA). Soluble TβRII, anti-TGFβ₁ antibody and recombinant human TGFβ₁ were obtained from R & D Systems (Minneapolis, MN, USA). Primary antibody against active TGFβ₁ was purchased from Promega Corporation (Madison, WI, USA). Complementary DNA probes for TGFβ₁, collagen type I, and GAPDH were obtained from the American Type Culture Collection (Rockville, MD, USA).

Statistical analysis

All values are expressed as mean ± SEM. One-way analysis of variance (ANOVA) followed by the Student–Newman–Keuls method was used for comparing the differences among multiple groups (SigmaStat). Significant differences among groups were defined by a probability of less than 0.05.

RESULTS

General observations: cardiac hypertrophy, total cardiac collagen concentration, and heart failure

Experimental animals in this study were characterized by the presence of large myocardial infarction (MI: $43 \pm 4\%$ of the total LV circumference), with an average total infarct scar weight of $0.26 \pm 0.03\,g$, which is comparable to values reported earlier [26]. Hearts of experimental animals were characterized by significant cardiac hypertrophy as reflected by an increase in the weight of the viable LV tissue and also by the increased ratio of LV weight to body weight (BW) in experimental animals compared to control values (table 1). The incidence and magnitude of LV hypertrophy noted in this study was comparable to our previous findings [23,24], as was the averaged transmural scar weight (one measure of the extent of MI) from experimental animals. Values for cardiac collagen in surviving myocardium remote to infarct ($48.6 \pm 4.3\,\mu g/mg$ dry wt) and border + scar tissues ($128.5 \pm 12.1\,\mu g/mg$ dry wt) were both significantly higher versus the control value ($21.9 \pm 2.7\,\mu g/mg$ dry wt) (figure 1A). The presence of heart failure, as reflected by an increase in left ventricular end-diastolic pressure (LVEDP), a decrease in the maximum rate of isovolumic pressure development or decay ($\pm dP/dt_{max}$) relative to their controls, and congested lung, has been characterized in this model (at the 8 week post-MI time point) from our previous studies [23,24].

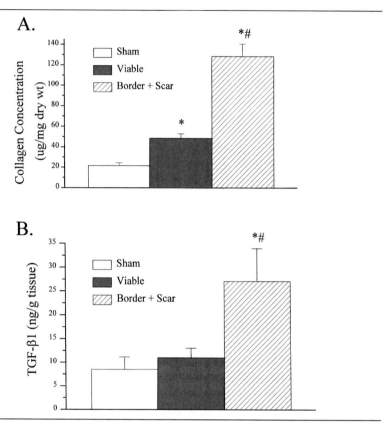

Figure 1. Total collagen concentration (**A**) and total cardiac transforming growth factor-β_1 (TGFβ_1) protein concentration (**B**) in 8 week sham-operated control hearts, viable tissue remote to the site of the infarct as well as border and scar tissues from hearts 8 weeks after the induction of myocardial infarction (MI). Total TGFβ_1 in cardiac samples was detected using ELISA. The data depicted are the mean ± SEM of five experiments. *, $p < 0.05$; #, $p < 0.05$ versus sham-operated control values and viable tissue values, respectively.

Alteration of total cardiac TGFβ_1

Quantitative assessment of total cardiac TGFβ_1 protein concentration in control and viable LV tissues as well as border + scar tissues of 8 week post-MI rats was carried out using ELISA. The results indicated that TGFβ_1 was increased by approximately 2.4-fold in border and scar tissues compared to that from control animals (figure 1B). There was no significant alteration of TGFβ_1 in samples from viable left ventricle versus control values.

Alteration of cardiac TGFβ_1 and collagen type I mRNA abundance

We addressed steady-state mRNA abundance of cardiac TGFβ_1 and collagen type I in tissues taken from various left ventricular regions of rats 8 weeks post-MI. Figure

Table 1. General and hemodynamic characteristics of sham and experimental rats 8 weeks after induction of myocardial infarction (MI)

Parameters	Sham-operated control	Myocardial infarction (MI)
BW, g	517 ± 9	478 ± 10
LVW, g	0.90 ± 0.02	1.01 ± 0.03★
LV/BW, mg/g	1.75 ± 0.03	2.09 ± 0.05★
Lung wet/dry wt ratio	3.45 ± 0.22	4.89 ± 0.23★
LVEDP, mmHg	3.6 ± 0.7	13.8 ± 1.6★
LVSP, mmHg	134 ± 9	118 ± 13
+dP/dt$_{max}$, mmHg/s	5612 ± 234	4422 ± 206★
−dP/dt$_{max}$, mmHg/s	5478 ± 229	3933 ± 243★

Experimental animals (MI) were characterized by large left ventricular myocardial infarction (43 ± 4% of the total LV circumference); sham-operated animals were noninfarcted age-matched controls; BW, body weight; LVW, left ventricular weight; LVEDP, LV end-diastolic pressure; LVSP, LV systolic pressure; +dP/dt$_{max}$, the maximum rate of isovolumic pressure development; −dP/dt$_{max}$, the maximum rate of isovolumic pressure decay. The data depicted is the mean ± SEM of 8–10 experiments. ★P < 0.05 *vs* sham-operated animals.

2 shows a representative Northern blot with autoradiographic bands specific for TGFβ$_1$, collagen type I, and GAPDH mRNAs from LV samples of sham, viable, and border + scar tissues. Estimation of the target gene mRNA abundance was calculated by the ratio of target gene to GAPDH signal. The ratios for TGFβ$_1$ and collagen type I were significantly increased in the border and scar regions versus values from viable tissue and control (histograms in figure 2).

Localization of active TGFβ$_1$ in cardiac tissue sections

Active TGFβ$_1$ was localized using immunofluorescent staining of frozen serial sections of control (sham-operated) left ventricle from age-matched rats, remnant (viable) LV tissue remote to the site of infarction, and border + scar tissue samples (figure 3). Active TGFβ$_1$ protein was localized mainly to the interstitial space in these sections. Compared to sham-operated control samples, viable tissues exhibited a relatively bright pattern of staining in the interstitial spaces, suggesting the presence of high levels of TGFβ$_1$. Intense staining of active TGFβ$_1$ protein was noted in the border + scar tissue in post-MI hearts as compared with that of sham hearts.

Quantification and localization of cardiac Smad 2, 3, and 4

Western analysis was used to determine cardiac Smad 2, 3, and 4 protein concentrations from 8 week sham-operated control hearts and different regions of postinfarct myocardium. Quantitative densitometry scanning of specific cardiac Smad 2 (55 kDa), Smad 3 (45 kDa), and Smad 4 (62 kDa) bands revealed that the concentrations of these proteins were significantly increased in border and scar tissues (lanes 7–9) when compared to control values (lanes 1–3; figure 4A). Furthermore, total Smad 2 and Smad 3 proteins were increased in the viable LV samples (lanes 4–6) from experimental animals versus controls. Immunofluorescence staining patterns of Smad 2, Smad 3, and Smad 4 are shown in sections of remnant (viable) LV tissue

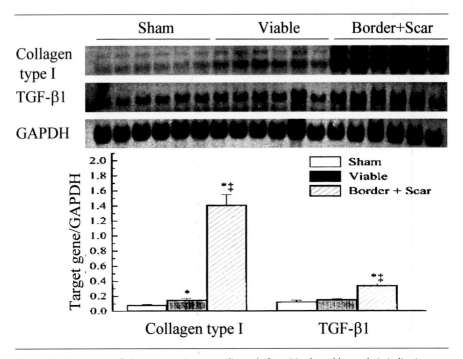

Figure 2. (Upper panel) A representative autoradiograph from Northern blot analysis indicating transforming growth factor-β_1 (TGFβ_1), collagen type I, and glyceraldehyde-3-phosphate dehydrogenase (GAPDH)-specific autoradiographic bands in sham-operated control and viable samples as well as border + scar tissues from rat hearts 8 weeks after induction of myocardial infarction. **(Bottom panel)** Data quantification (via CCD scanning densitometry) indicating target gene/GAPDH band intensity ratio in sham and viable as well as border + scar tissues. The data depicted are the mean ± SEM of six experiments. *, $p < 0.05$; ‡, $p < 0.05$ versus sham-operated controls and viable sample values, respectively.

remote to the infarct (figure 5A) and of the infarct scar (figure 5B) from 8 week post-MI rat heart. Double-staining of cellular nuclei in sections of infarct scar demonstrate the relative cellularity present in this tissue (figure 5Bii, iv, vi). We observed that in the remnant post-MI tissue sections, cardiac Smad 2, 3, and 4 proteins are localized mainly in the perivascular space (figure 5A). We observed marked localization of Smad 2, Smad 3, and Smad 4 proteins proximal to the nuclei of non-myocyte cells from sections of the infarct scar.

Quantification and localization of TβRI (ALK-5) and TβRII

Western blot analysis revealed that both TβRI and TβRII are detectable in the membrane fraction but not in the cytosolic fraction. Figure 6A (upper band) provides a representative blot illustrating the presence of a characteristic 53 kDa band for TβRI. It shows that there is a dramatic decrease of TβRI in the border and scar tissues. Figure 6A (bottom band) illustrates the bands specific for TβRII at 75 and 110 kDa

Sham   Viable   Border+Scar

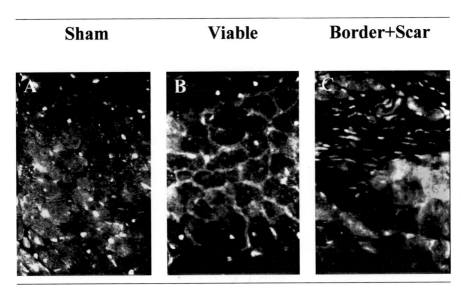

Figure 3. Immunofluorescent staining of active transforming growth factor-β1 (TGFβ₁) in frozen tissue sections of sham-operated control hearts (**A**), remnant heart remote to the site of infarct (**B**), and border + scar tissues (**C**) from 8 week post-MI rat hearts. Active TGFβ₁ protein appears as brightly stained material in all sections; these proteins appear to be localized in the interstitial spaces between myocytes in sham and viable sections. Magnification, ×400.

[33]. In contrast to TβRI, the major isoform of TβRII (75 kDa) was modestly decreased, but the 110 kDa isoform was markedly increased in the border + scar region. Figure 6B indicates relatively even loading of samples by amido black 10B staining of the same Western blot membrane. TGFβ₁ receptors and their distribution in 8 week experimental and age-matched control tissues were localized using immunofluorescent techniques. In a representative photomicrograph (figure 7), the staining pattern of immunoreactive TβRI (ALK-5) and TβRII appears as bright staining in and surrounding cardiac myocytes, as well as in the interstial space. Myocytes in the border region (lower portions of figure 7C and 7F) contain brightly stained material, which was taken to represent TβRI and TβRII immunostaining, respectively. Notably the infarct scar (present in the upper portions of figure 7C) is by the appearance of very little TβRI immunoreactive material. In contrast to the results addressing TβRI, stronger staining of TβRII was present in the scar and border region compared with sham and viable tissues.

DISCUSSION

Loss of normal left ventricular systolic pressure (LVSP), elevated LVEDP, decreased time to peak pressure development and decay ($\pm dP/dt_{max}$), and the presence of pulmonary congestion were confirmed in 8 week experimental animals. Although these findings were taken to reflect significant disruption of normal cardiac function, these

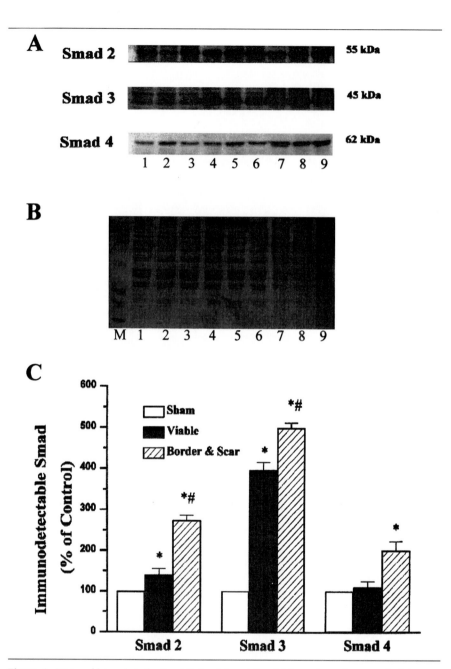

Figure 4. Western blot analysis for Smad 2, Smad 3, and Smad 4 in sections of age-matched sham-operated control hearts (lanes 1–3), as well as in viable tissues (lanes 4–6) and border + scar tissues (lanes 7–9) from experimental rat hearts 8 weeks post-MI. (**A**) A series of representative Western blot autoradiographs indicating the 55 kDa, 45 kDa, and 62 kDa bands specific for Smad 2, 3, and 4, respectively. Similar results were obtained in three experiments. (**B**) The Coomassie blue staining of the PVDF membrane, indicating the relative loading of total cardiac proteins for each sample. (**C**) Histograms for the quantified data of Smad protein expression (quantified by densitometric scanning), depicted as the mean ± SEM of three different experiments. *, $p < 0.05$; #, $p < 0.05$ versus values from sham-operated control and viable sample values, respectively.

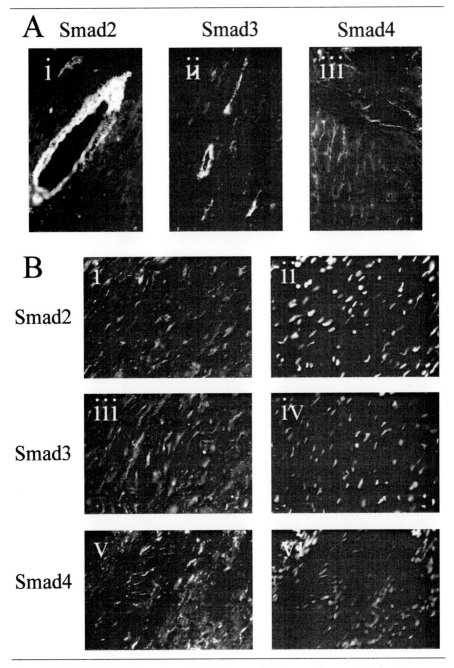

Figure 5. Smad localization in sections of viable tissue and infarct scar from post-MI heart. Immunofluorescent staining of Smad proteins in viable remnant tissue remote to the site of infarct (**A**) as well as infarct scar tissues (**B**) from rat hearts 8 weeks after the induction of MI. (**A**) Immunoreactive Smad 2 (Ai), Smad 3 (Aii), and Smad 4 (Aiii) proteins in the viable tissue localized to the perivascular space. (**B**) In the infarct scar, immunofluorescent staining for Smad 2 (Bi), Smad 3 (Biii), and Smad 4 (Bv) is shown on the left; sections Bii, Biv, and Bvi depict nuclei (Hoechst 33342) from the identical fields to the immediate left, respectively. Magnification, ×400.

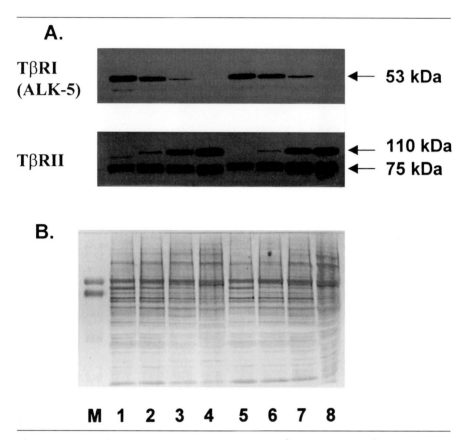

Figure 6. Western blot analysis of transforming growth factor-β receptor type I (TβRI, ALK-5) and transforming growth factor-β receptor type II (TβRII) protein concentration in sham-operated control, viable, border, and infarct scar tissues from 8 week experimental animals. (**A**) Representative Western blot showing specific bands of TβRI (ALK-5, 53 kDa) and TβRII (75 kDa and 110 kDa). Lanes 1 and 5 are samples from sham LV, lanes 2 and 6 are viable LV, lanes 3 and 7 are border tissue, and lanes 4 and 8 represent samples taken from infarct scar. (**B**) Amido black staining of the PVDF membrane, indicating the relative loading of total cardiac proteins for each sample.

animals did not display overt dyspnea, cyanosis, or marked lethargy and thus were considered to be in "moderate heart failure," as previously demonstrated [23,24]. This classification is based on our observations of the development of post-MI heart failure in rats with relatively large MI (≥40% LV free wall) and provides an arbitrary classification system to facilitate the comparison of differently timed experimental groups [23,24]. The incidence of cardiac hypertrophy in 8 week post-MI rat hearts, as indicated by increased LV weight and the ratio of LV weight to body weight, was also apparent when compared to noninfarcted controls. Significantly elevated deposition of cardiac collagens in the viable remnant tissue (cardiac fibrosis) and scar tissues (in chronic phase healing of the infarct scar) in post-MI hearts was

Sham	**Viable**	**Border + Scar**

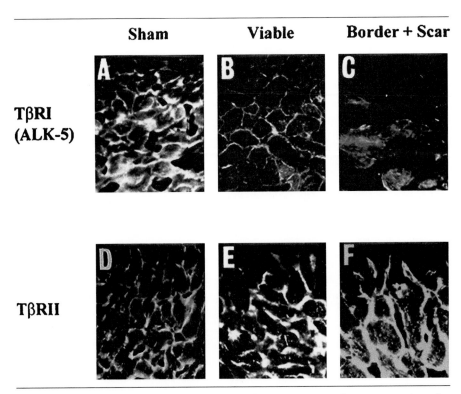

TβRI
(ALK-5)

TβRII

Figure 7. Immunofluorescent staining specific for TGFβ receptor type I (TβRI, ALK-5) and TGFβ receptor type II (TβRII) in sham hearts (**A, D**), viable myocardial sections (**B, E**), and border + scar (**C, F**) tissues, respectively, from rat hearts 8 weeks after MI. Immunoreactive TβRI and TβRII proteins appear as brightly stained material. Magnification, ×400.

confirmed in this investigation and was similar to the patterns of fibrosis observed in our previous studies [24,34]. Since the mechanical properties of the infarct scar are critical for cardiac function after MI [29], any alteration in the structure of the scar may influence cardiac function. Thus we chose to examine this stage of MI-associated heart failure to provide insights into the events associated with ongoing wound healing in various regions of the infarcted heart, including the infarct itself.

TGFβ contributes to an array of biological functions, including regulation of ECM production, wound repair, and growth inhibition [16,35]. These phenomena are mediated through transmembrane TGFβ receptors (TβRI and TβRII) that display serine/threonine kinase activity [9]. In experimental LV hypertrophy, the selective increase in expression of TGFβ$_1$ versus either TGFβ$_2$ or TGFβ$_3$ subtypes suggests that the former subtype is important in the pathogenesis of cardiac disease associated with hypertrophy [36]. TGFβ receptor activation occurs upon the binding of TGFβ to TβRII, which then recruits and phosphorylates TβRI [37]. It is now clear that phosphorylated Smad 2 (or Smad 3) proteins mediate TGFβ$_1$ signal transduction via binding of both Smad 4 [9,38,39] and FAST-1, a eukaryotic nuclear transcription factor [40]. The C-terminal region of FAST-1 protein binds specifically to Smad 2 [41], and the heterotrimeric complex is required for initiation of $TGF\beta_1$-mediated gene transcription. The phosphorylated TβRI is activated and phosphorylates cytosolic Smad 2 or possibly Smad 3 [8,9]. Phosphorylated Smad 2 (and/or Smad 3) then form(s) a heterotrimeric complex with Smad 4, and this complex accumulates in the nucleus, leading to the activation of target gene expression [9,38,39].

Interstitial fibrosis and attendant decreases in compliance of the surviving myocardium are believed to contribute to the occurrence of cardiac dysfunction [42], and it has become clear that the scar size is a reliable marker for the development of heart failure post-MI [43]. Although gross morphological examination of experimental hearts has indicated that scar formation is completed 3 weeks after MI [44], more detailed investigation suggests that the scar is not quiescent even 8 weeks after MI [24]. As opposed to interstitial fibrosis of remnant heart, normal fibrosis in the healing of the infarct scar may help to preserve ventricular function [22]. Although TGFβ stimulates ECM production, which is involved in the development of heart failure in post-MI heart [6], alteration of downstream Smad proteins in this pathology is unknown. The present study represents a first step in this regard, and our results support the hypothesis that elevated expression of $TGF\beta_1$ (both mRNA and protein) is positively correlated to the increased cardiac Smad protein expression, chronic phase healing of the infarct scar, and overt fibrosis of the viable remnant myocardium. Thus it may be possible that activation of Smads 2, 3, and 4 expression in post-MI heart is contributory to the ongoing scar remodeling. Although the precise significance of the predominance of Smad proteins in the cellular nuclei within the infarct scar is unclear, these proteins may participate in the stimulation of expression of matrix genes, i.e., fibrillar collagens. We suggest that by this mechanism, scar structure is chronically influenced in heart failure after MI. It is likely that balanced chronic infarct remodeling and marginal compensation of cardiac function is not maintained in the presence of large MI, since the functioning of experimental hearts rapidly deteriorates to overt decompensation by 16 weeks [23]. In the infarct scar, myofibroblasts (fibroblasts distinguished by their expression of α-actin and contractile ability) have been shown to be the predominant cell type in post-MI scar tissue in rat heart [21,29] and are likely candidate cells for the bulk of Smad protein expression in this tissue [45,46]. Furthermore, myofibroblasts may persist in infarct scar in post-MI patients for many years [45].

Since Smad 2 and Smad 3 may mediate growth inhibition by $TGF\beta_1$ [38,47,48], increased Smad protein expression may play a crucial role in the regulation of cardiac myofibroblast proliferation and collagen remodeling in post-MI hearts. It has been reported that angiotensin II (AII) concentration and AT_1 receptor density in myofibroblasts are significantly increased in the scar tissue post-MI [49–51]. Since AII has been implicated in the stimulation of cardiac fibroblast proliferation [52–54], the net proliferation of myofibroblasts may depend upon a balance between TGFβ signaling and other trophic factors, i.e., AII, during post-MI wound healing.

The significance of differential regulation of TβRII (increased) and TβRI (decreased) receptors in border and infarct scar is not easily explained by the current model of TGFβ receptor signaling. Since TβRI may act as a downstream component of TβRII [37,55,56], reduced expression of either receptor subtype may simply confer a loss of $TGF\beta_1$ responsiveness in target cells. On the other hand, recent evidence supports the view that the antiproliferative and fibrotic effects of $TGF\beta_1$ may be modulated independently in smooth muscle cells by selective changes in the TβRI/TβRII ratio [57]. Massague has speculated that the type II receptor may confer signal independently of the type I receptor by phosphorylating as yet unknown substrates [56]. The downregulation of TβRI may be due to the reciprocal regulation by stimulation of high concentrations of $TGF\beta_1$ in the scar and border tissues, and this view is supported by the demonstration that preexposure of osteoblasts to $TGF\beta_1$ is associated with decreased receptor density [58]. Conversely, TGFβ-mediated upregulation of TβRII receptors in vascular smooth muscle cells has been observed [59], and this autostimulatory mechanism may partially explain the expression in remnant border and infarct scar tissues in post-MI hearts.

In conclusion, increased Smad protein expression as well as increased $TGF\beta_1$ expression in infarct scar tissue in the chronic phase of post-MI hearts is positively correlated to elevated deposition of cardiac collagens. We suggest that overexpression of Smad proteins is involved in ongoing extracellular matrix remodeling of the infarct scar and in viable remnant regions is post-MI hearts by cardiac myofibroblasts, and that these changes are involved in the progression of heart failure. It follows that blockade of TGFβ signaling may inhibit $TGF\beta_1$-mediated fibrosis in post-MI heart. Thus the direct regulation of cardiac Smad protein expression and activation may represent a novel therapeutic approach for modulating fibrotic events in post-MI hearts.

ACKNOWLEDGMENTS

This study was supported by funding from the Medical Research Council of Canada (IMCD). I.M.C.D is a scholar of the Medical Research Council of Canada/PMAC health program with funding provided by Astra Pharma, Inc (Canada), J.H. is a recipient of a University of Manitoba Graduate Student Fellowship.

REFERENCES

1. Pfeffer JM, Fischer TA, Pfeffer MA. 1995. Angiotensin-converting enzyme inhibition and ventricular remodeling after myocardial infarction. Annu Rev Physiol 57:805–826.
2. Pfeffer MA, Braunwale E. 1990. Ventricular remodeling after myocardial infarction. Experimental observations and clinical implications. Circulation 81:1161–1172.
3. Weber KT, Sun Y, Katwa LC. 1996. Wound healing following myocardial infarction. Clin Cardiol 19:447–455.
4. Border WA, Noble NA. 1994. Transforming growth factor beta in tissue fibrosis. N Engl J Med 331:1286–1292.
5. Brand T, Schneider MD. 1995. The TGF beta superfamily in myocardium: ligands, receptors, transduction, and function. J Mol Cell Cardiol 27:5–18.
6. Eghbali M, Sigel A. 1995. Role of transforming growth factor beta-1 in the remodeling of collagen matrix in the heart. In Heart Hypertrophy and Failure. Ed. NS Dhalla, GN Pierce, V Panagia, and RE Beamish, 287–297. Boston: Kluwer Academic Publishers.

7. Thompson NL, Bazoberry F, Speir EH, Casscells W, Ferrans VJ, Flanders KC, Kondaiah P, Geiser AG, Sporn MB. 1988. Transforming growth factor beta-1 in acute myocardial infarction in rats. Growth Factors 1:91–99.

8. Macias Silva M, Abdollah S, Hoodless PA, Pirone R, Attisano L, Wrana JL. 1996. MADR2 is a substrate of the TGFbeta receptor and its phosphorylation is required for nuclear accumulation and signaling. Cell 87:1215–1224.

9. Massague J, Hata A, Liu F. 1997. Tgf-beta signalling through the Smad pathway. Trends Cell Biol 7:187–192.

10. Engelmann GL, Boehm KD, Birchenall Roberts MC, Ruscetti FW. 1992. Transforming growth factor-beta 1 in heart development. Mech Dev 38:85–97.

11. Eghbali M. 1989. Cellular origin and distribution of transforming growth factor-beta in the normal rat myocardium. Cell Tissue Res 256:553–558.

12. Lee AA, Dillmann WH, McCulloch AD, Villarreal FJ. 1995. Angiotensin II stimulates the autocrine production of transforming growth factor-beta 1 in adult rat cardiac fibroblasts. J Mol Cell Cardiol 27:2347–2357.

13. Flanders KC, Winokur TS, Holder MG, Sporn MS. 1993. Hyperthermia induces expression of transforming growth factor-betas in rat cardiac cells in vitro and in vivo. J Clin Invest 92:404–410.

14. Takahashi N, Calderone A, Izzo NJ Jr, Maki TM, Marsh JD, Colucci WS. 1994. Hypertrophic stimuli induce transforming growth factor-beta 1 expression in rat ventricular myocytes. J Clin Invest 94:1470–1476.

15. Engelmann GL, Grutkoski PS. 1994. Coordinate TGF-beta receptor gene expression during rat heart development. Cell Mol Biol Res 40:93–104.

16. Massague J. 1990. The transforming growth factor-beta family. Annu Rev Cell Biol 6:597–641.

17. Heimer R, Bashey RI, Kyle J, Jimenez SA. 1995. TGF-beta modulates the synthesis of proteoglycans by myocardial fibroblasts in culture. J Mol Cell Cardiol 27:2191–2198.

18. Chua CC, Chua BH, Zhao ZY, Krebs C, Diglio C, Perrin E. 1991. Effect of growth factors on collagen metabolism in cultured human heart fibroblasts. Connect Tissue Res 26:271–281.

19. Villarreal FJ, Lee AA, Dillmann WH, Giordano FJ. 1996. Adenovirus-mediated overexpression of human transforming growth factor-beta 1 in rat cardiac fibroblasts, myocytes and smooth muscle cells. J Mol Cell Cardiol 28:735–742.

20. Eghbali M, Tomek R, Sukhatme VP, Woods C, Bhambi B. 1991. Differential effects of transforming growth factor-beta 1 and phorbol myristate acetate on cardiac fibroblasts. Regulation of fibrillar collagen mRNAs and expression of early transcription factors. Circ Res 69:483–490.

21. Vracko R, Thorning D. 1991. Contractile cells in rat myocardial scar tissue. Lab Invest 65:214–227.

22. Holmes JW, Nunez JA, Covell JW. 1997. Functional implications of myocardial scar structure. Am J Physiol 272:H2123–H2130.

23. Dixon IMC, Lee SL, Dhalla NS. 1990. Nitrendipine binding in congestive heart failure due to myocardial infarction. Circ Res 66:782–788.

24. Ju H, Zhao S, Tappia PS, Panagia V, Dixon IMC. 1998. Expression of Gqalpha and PLC-beta in scar and border tissue in heart failure due to myocardial infarction. Circulation 97:892–899.

25. Dixon IMC, Hata T, Dhalla NS. 1992. Sarcolemmal calcium transport in congestive heart failure due to myocardial infarction in rats. Am J Physiol 262:H1387–H1394.

26. Ju H, Zhao S, Davinder SJ, Dixon IM. 1997. Effect of AT1 receptor blockade on cardiac collagen remodeling after myocardial infarction. Cardiovasc Res 35:223–232.

27. Chiariello M, Ambrosio G, Cappelli Bigazzi M, Perrone Filardi P, Brigante F, Sifola C. 1986. A biochemical method for the quantitation of myocardial scarring after experimental coronary artery occlusion. J Mol Cell Cardiol 18:283–290.

28. Junaid A, Rosenberg ME, Hostetter TH. 1997. Interaction of angiotensin II and TGF-beta 1 in the rat remnant kidney [published erratum appears in J Am Soc Nephrol 1998;9(1):154]. J Am Soc Nephrol 8:1732–1738.

29. Peterson D, Ju H, Panagia M, Chapman D, Dixon IMC. In press. Expression of Gia2 and Gsa in myofibroblasts localized to the infarct scar in heart failure due to myocardial infarction. Cardiovasc Res.

30. Smith PK, Krohn RI, Hermanson GT, Mallia AK, Gartner FH, Provenzano MD, Fujimoto EK, Goeke NM, Olson BJ, Klenk DC. 1985. Measurement of protein using bicinchoninic acid. Anal Biochem 150:76–85.

31. Chomczynski P, Sacchi N. 1987. Single-step method of RNA isolation by acid guanidinium thiocyanate-phenol-chloroform extraction. Anal Biochem 162:156–159.

32. Ju H, Scammel La Fleur T, Dixon IMC. 1996. Altered mRNA abundance of calcium transport genes in cardiac myocytes induced by angiotensin II. J Mol Cell Cardiol 28:1119–1128.

33. Hall FL, Benya PD, Padilla SR, Carbonaro Hall D, Williams R, Buckley S, Warburton D. 1996. Transforming growth factor-beta type-II receptor signalling: intrinsic/associated casein kinase activity, receptor interactions and functional effects of blocking antibodies. Biochem J 316:303–310.

34. Pelouch V, Dixon IM, Sethi R, Dhalla NS. 1993. Alteration of collagenous protein profile in congestive heart failure secondary to myocardial infarction. Mol Cell Biochem 129:121–131.

35. Roberts AB, Sporn MB. 1990. The transforming growth factor-betas. In Peptide Growth Factors and Their Receptors I. Ed. MB Sporn, AB Roberts, 420–472. New York: Springer-Verlag.

36. Li JM, Brooks G. 1997. Differential protein expression and subcellular distribution of TGF beta1, beta2 and beta3 in cardiomyocytes during pressure overload-induced hypertrophy. J Mol Cell Cardiol 29:2213–2224.

37. Wrana JL, Attisano L, Wieser R, Ventura F, Massague J. 1994. Mechanim of activation of the TGF-beta receptor. Nature 370:341–347.

38. Zhang Y, Feng X, We R, Derynck R. 1996. Receptor-associated Mad homologues synergize as effectors of the TGF-beta response. Nature 383:168–172.

39. Lagna G, Hata A, Hemmati Brivanlou A, Massague J. 1996. Partnership between DPC4 and SMAD proteins in TGF-beta signalling pathways. Nature 383:832–836.

40. Chen X, Weisberg E, Fridmacher V, Watanabe M, Naco G, Whitman M. 1997. Smad4 and FAST-1 in the assembly of activin-responsive factor. Nature 389:85–89.

41. Liu F, Pouponnot C, Massague J. 1997. Dual role of the Smad4/DPC4 tumor suppressor in TGFbeta-inducible transcriptional complexes. Genes Dev 11:3157–3167.

42. Weber KT. 1989. Cardiac interstitium in health and disease: the fibrillar collagen network. J Am Coll Cardiol 13:1637–1652.

43. Chareonthaitawee P, Christian TF, Hirose K, Gibbons RJ, Rumberger JA. 1995. Relation of initial infarct size to extent of left ventricular remodeling in the year after acute myocardial infarction. J Am Coll Cardiol 25:567–573.

44. Fishbein MC, Maclean D, Maroko PR. 1978. Experimental myocardial infarction in the rat: qualitative and quantitative changes during pathologic evolution. Am J Pathol 90:57–70.

45. Willems IE, Havenith MG, De Mey JG, Daemen MJ. 1994. The alpha-smooth muscle actin-positive cells in healing human myocardial scars. Am J Pathol 145:868–875.

46. Cleutjens JP, Verluyten MJ, Smits JF, Daemen MJ. 1995. Collagen remodeling after myocardial infarction in the rat heart. Am J Pathol 147:325–338.

47. Mucsi I, Goldberg HJ. 1997. Dominant-negative SMAD-3 interferes with transcriptional activation by multiple agonists. Biochem Biophys Res Commun 232:517–521.

48. Liu X, Sun Y, Constantinescu SN, Karam E, Weinberg RA, Lodish HF. 1997. Transforming growth factor beta-induced phosphorylation of Smad3 is required for growth inhibition and transcriptional induction in epithelial cells. Proc Natl Acad Sci USA 94:10669–10674.

49. Yamagishi H, Kim S, Nishikimi T, Takeuchi K, Takeda T. 1993. Contribution of cardiac renin–angiotensin system to ventricular remodelling in myocardial-infarcted rats. J Mol Cell Cardiol 25:1369–1380.

50. Lefroy DC, Wharton J, Crake T, Knock GA, Rutherford RA, Suzuki T, Morgan K, Polak JM, Poole-Wilson PA. 1996. Regional changes in angiotensin II receptor density after experimental myocardial infarction. J Mol Cell Cardiol 28:429–440.

51. Sun Y, Weber KT. 1996. Cells expressing angiotensin II receptors in fibrous tissue of rat heart. Cardiovasc Res 31:518–525.

52. Brilla CG, Zhou G, Matsubara L, Weber KT. 1994. Collagen metabolism in cultured adult rat cardiac fibroblasts: response to angiotensin II and aldosterone. J Mol Cell Cardiol 26:809–820.

53. Crabos M, Roth M, Hahn AW, Erne P. 1994. Characterization of angiotensin II receptors in cultured adult rat cardiac fibroblasts. Coupling to signaling systems and gene expression. J Clin Invest 93:2372–2378.

54. Sadoshima J, Izumo S. 1993. Molecular characterization of angiotensin II-induced hypertrophy of cardiac myocytes and hyperplasia of cardiac fibroblasts. Critical role of the AT1 receptor subtype. Circ Res 73:413–423.

55. Miyazono K. 1997. TGF-beta receptors and signal transduction. Int J Hematol 65:97–104.

56. Massague J. 1998. TGF-beta signal transduction. Annu Rev Biochem 67:753–91:753–791.

57. McCaffrey TA, Consigli S, Du B, Falcone DJ, Sanborn TA, Spokojny AM, Bush HLJ. 1995. Decreased type II/type I TGF-beta receptor ratio in cells derived from human atherosclerotic lesions. Conver-

sion from an antiproliferative to profibrotic response to TGF-beta1. J Clin Invest 96:2667–2675.

58. Centrella M, Ji C, Casinghino S, McCarthy TL. 1996. Rapid flux in transforming growth factor-beta receptors on bone cells. J Biol Chem 271:18616–18622.

59. Ward MR, Agrotis A, Jennings G, Bobik A. 1998. Vascular types I and II transforming growth factor-beta receptor expression: differential dependency on tyrosine kinases during induction by TGF-beta. FEBS Lett 422:197–200.

N. Takeda, M. Nagano and N.S. Dhalla
(eds). The Hypertrophied Heart. Copyright
© 2000. pp. 321–331. Kluwer Academic
Publishers. Boston. All rights reserved.

gp130-DEPENDENT SIGNALING PATHWAYS: RECENT ADVANCES AND IMPLICATIONS FOR CARDIOVASCULAR DISEASE

KEIKO YAMAUCHI-TAKIHARA, KEITA KUNISADA, YASUSHI FUJIO, HIDEMASA OH, EIROH TONE, AND TADAMITSU KISHIMOTO

Department of Molecular Medicine III, Osaka University Graduate School of Medicine, 2-2, Yamadaoka, Suita, Osaka 565-0871, Japan

Summary. Interleukin (IL)-6-related cytokines share gp130 as the signal-transducing protein. Cardiac myocytes produce various kinds of cytokines, including IL-6 and cardiotrophin-1. Activation of gp130 transduces hypertrophic and cytoprotective signals via JAK/STAT, MAP kinase, and PI3 kinase pathways. Besides various well-established mechanisms by which cardiac growth and myocardial remodeling are regulated, gp130 signaling may be a newly discovered mechanism that regulates these events in association with cytoprotective effects.

INTRODUCTION

Role of cytokines in cardiovascular disease

Cytokines are recognized as essential mediators of normal and pathological immune responses. It is also accepted that cytokines are involved in the cascade of events that lead to the wide range of inflammatory responses to exogenous and endogenous pathogens. The importance of cytokines in the cardiovascular system has been mainly studied from the perspective of hemodynamic effects, such as global myocardial dysfunction observed in septic shock, cardiac allograft rejection, and ischemic heart disease. Recent studies have indicated the additional importance of cytokines in the pathogenesis of myocarditis [1] and myocardial infarction [2]. Evidence of cytokine production by cardiac myocytes [3] has also contributed to the discovery of novel functions of cytokines in the regulation of cardiovascular disease.

Mechanisms inducing cardiac hypertrophy

Cardiac hypertrophy is induced by various stimuli, such as pressure or volume overload. Under these conditions, this hypertrophic response is assumed to be an important compensation to maintain mechanical function. Well-known stimuli of cardiac myocyte hypertrophy are mechanical stretch and various factors utilizing G protein-coupled receptors, including norepinephrine (NE) [4], endothelin-1 (ET-1) [5], and angiotensin II [6]. Recently, a novel interleukin (IL)-6 related cytokine, cardiotrophin-1 (CT-1), was cloned and characterized as a cardiac myocyte hypertrophy-inducing factor [7]. gp130 has been identified as a signal transducing protein of IL-6 related cytokines [8] (IL-6, IL-11, leukemia inhibitory factor [LIF], oncostatin M, ciliary neurotrophic factor [CNTF], and CT-1) and is widely expressed in various organs, including the heart. Double transgenic mice overexpressing IL-6 and the IL-6 receptor (which constitutively activate gp130) demonstrate myocardial hypertrophy at 20 weeks of age [9].

Signal transduction through gp130

IL-6 stimulation induces homodimerization of gp130, whereas stimulation by CT-1 and LIF leads to the formation of heterodimers composed of gp130 and LIF receptors [10]. Although gp130 possesses no tyrosine kinase domain, ligand-induced homo- or hetero-dimerization leads to activation of associated tyrosine kinases. Three members of the Janus kinase (JAK) family, namely, JAK1, JAK2, and Tyk2, are known to be associated with gp130 prior to stimulation and to be activated when gp130 is stimulated. Phosphorylated JAKs in turn phosphorylate a latent cytoplasmic transcription factor, STAT3, allowing it to bind to a responsive element of the target genes [8]. Moreover, the Ras/mitogen-activated protein kinase (MAPK) cascade is also activated, an event that is postulated to occur as the result of the interaction of an as yet unidentified adapter molecule with tyrosine-phosphorylated gp130.

Thus, gp130-mediated signaling appears to involve two distinct pathways, one Ras dependent and the other STAT dependent. In cardiac myocytes, the MAPK pathway is activated by many factors, such as NE, ET-1, and mechanical loading, and is thought to be an important pathway for the induction of hypertrophy [11].

Phosphatidylinositol 3 kinase (PI3K) is known to be activated by cytokine stimulation through different types of receptors to transduce intracellular responses. Several growth factor receptors, cytokine receptors, and G protein-coupled receptors are able to stimulate PI3K activity [12,13]. Furthermore, recent studies have revealed that PI3K plays an important role in the activation of p70 S6 kinase and the prevention of apoptosis [14].

We report here that the JAK/STAT, MAPK, and PI3K pathways are activated in association with the activation of gp130 and transduce hypertrophic and antiapoptotic signals in cardiac myocytes.

ACTIVATION OF gp130 TRANSDUCES HYPERTROPHIC SIGNALS IN CARDIAC MYOCYTES

Activation of gp130 transduces hypertrophic signals

Studies on the hypertrophic effects of gp130-dependent signaling have been conducted by using cultured neonatal rat cardiac myocytes. As shown in figure 1, LIF stimulation increases the size and induces the expression of c-fos, β-myosin heavy chain, and atrial naturiuretic peptide (ANP) mRNAs and stimulates [³H] leucine

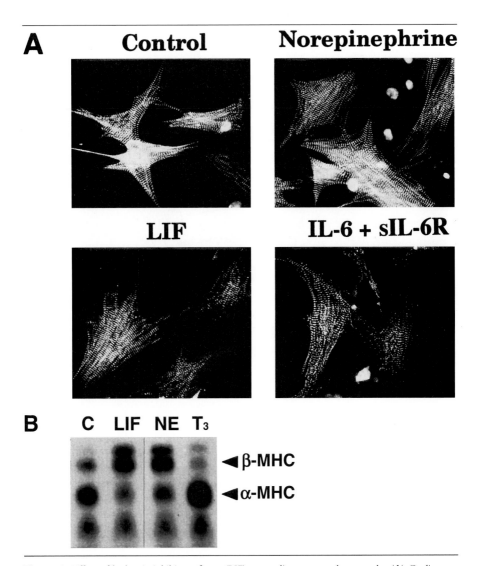

Figure 1. Effect of leukemia inhibitory factor (LIF) on cardiac myocyte hypertrophy. (**A**) Cardiac myocyte hypertrophy induced by norepinephrine, LIF, or a combination of IL-6 and soluble IL-6 receptor (sIL-6R). Cultured neonatal rat cardiac myocytes were plated on a glass coverslip coated with fibronectin, stimulated for 36 hours, and stained with antisarcomeric α-actinin antibody. (**B**) Myosin heavy chain (MHC) mRNA analysis by nuclease S1 protection assay. Increased expression of β-MHC mRNA is observed in neonatal rat cardiac myocytes stimulated with LIF (1×10^3 U/mL) or norepinephrine (NE; 2 μM), whereas α-MHC mRNA expression is augmented after thyroxine (T3; 0.02 μg/mL) stimulation.

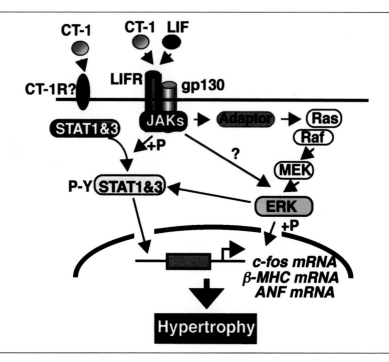

Figure 2. The signal transduction of gp130-dependent cardiac myocyte hypertrophy.

incorporation in cardiac myocytes [15]. To evaluate the molecular mechanisms involved in LIF–induced cardiac myocyte hypertrophy, the activation of the gp130-dependent signaling pathway was examined in cardiac myocytes. LIF stimulation rapidly tyrosine phosphorylates gp130 and subsequently activates both JAK1 and JAK2 within a few minutes, followed within 5 minutes by tyrosine phosphorylation of STAT3 in cardiac myocytes. LIF also activates MAPK in a characteristic way; i.e., the magnitude of activation is half of and the duration is shorter than that of NE-induced MAPK activation. This distinct kinetic pattern of MAPK activation observed after gp130 activation might be associated with a different physiological function in the gp130-dependent signaling pathway.

To summarize, the JAK/STAT and MAPK pathways are located downstream of gp130 in the cardiac myocyte and are rapidly activated by LIF both in vivo and in vitro [16] (figure 2).

Role of STAT3 in gp130-mediated cardiac myocyte hypertrophy

Studies focusing on the significance of STAT3 in inducing cardiac myocyte hypertrophy were pursued by using an adenovirus vector to overexpress wild-type STAT3 (WT) or dominant negative-type STAT3 (DN). Although STAT3 phosphorylation was not observed in WT before LIF stimulation, augmented

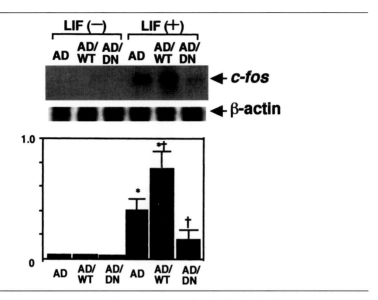

Figure 3. *c-fos* mRNA expression in cardiac myocytes stimulated with LIF. Cardiac myocytes were transfected with WT or DN and cultured for 2 days. They were starved for 6 hours and incubated for 30 minutes with LIF (1×10^3 U/mL). The lower panel presents the results from four independent experiments expressed as a relative intensity normalized to the expression level of β-actin mRNA. AD, adenovirus control vector *, $p < 0.05$ vs. LIF (−); †, $p < 0.05$ vs. AD.

phosphorylation was observed after the stimulation. In contrast, phosphorylation of STAT3 was not detected in DN, either with or without LIF stimulation. Pretreatment with PD98059, a MAPK kinase inhibitor, did not affect the level of tyrosine phosphorylation of STAT3 in cardiac myocytes. These results indicate that the activation of the JAK/STAT pathway, especially the STAT3-dependent pathway, is enhanced in STAT3-transfected but is not fully activated in DN-transfected cardiac myocytes after LIF stimulation, and that it is independent of the status of MAPK activation [17]. As shown in figure 3, *c-fos* and ANP mRNA expressions were significantly enhanced in WT and almost completely inhibited in DN after LIF stimulation. Although the expression of these mRNAs was reduced after PD98059 treatment, there were substantial differences in expression level between WT and DN [17].

To summarize, the induction of cardiac myocyte hypertrophy and of *c-fos* and ANP mRNA expressions by LIF was amplified by STAT3 overexpression, whereas it was attenuated under conditions that inhibited STAT3 signaling. Furthermore, when MAPK activation was inhibited, gene expression and protein synthesis were significantly suppressed even in the cells that overexpressed STAT3. This outcome could be explained by the cross-talk between JAK/STAT and MAPK cascades, both of which were necessary for maximal transcriptional upexpression.

Role of PI3K in gp130 mediated cardiac myocyte hypertrophy

The next studies focused on the role of PI3K in LIF-induced hypertrophic signals. Following the activation of gp130, a substantial increase in PI3K activity was observed in cardiac myocytes, with a rapid increase at 10 minutes and a decline at 60 minutes. In addition, JAK1 was found to bind to PI3K and LIF stimulation to increase the PI3K activity in JAK1 immunoprecipitates. A specific PI3K inhibitor, wortmannin, completely inhibited the LIF-induced activation of p70 S6 kinase and protein synthesis and partially inhibited MAPK activation in cardiac myocytes (figure 4). Therefore, the maximal stimulation of the protein kinase cascade by LIF requires the activation of PI3K, which may thus be an important mediator in LIF-induced transduction of hypertrophic signals [18].

ACTIVATION OF gp130 TRANSDUCES CYTOPROTECTIVE SIGNALS IN CARDIAC MYOCYTES

Cytoprotective function of IL-6-related cytokines

Cardiac myocyte survival is of central importance in the maintenance of cardiac function, as well as in the development of a variety of cardiac diseases. Adult cardiac myocytes are terminally differentiated and have lost their proliferative capacity. As a result, cardiac myocyte survival is critical for the maintenance of normal cardiac function. Although a wide variety of survival factors have been identified for neural cells and several other terminally differentiated cell types, relatively little is known about the specific growth factors or cytokines that are required for the maintenance of cardiac myocyte survival.

Two members of the IL-6 family of cytokines, CNTF and LIF, have been shown to play an important role in maintaining the viability of motoneurons in long-term culture [19,20]. Recent studies have further demonstrated that CT-1 is highly expressed in embryonic limb buds and has a protective effect on axotomy-induced degeneration in neural cells [21]. These results suggest that CT-1 can be expected to participate in normal motoneuron development and in the protection of human degenerative motoneuron disease. Therefore, the ligands that activate gp130 may play an important physiological role in regulating survival of terminally differentiated cell types.

In terms of a molecular basis of the cytoprotective effects of IL-6-related cytokines, IL-6 prevented the apoptosis induced by IL-6 depletion with the upregulation of bcl-xL in an IL-6-dependent myeloma cell line [22]. Bcl-x was identified as a bcl-2-related gene that functions as a regulator of apoptotic cell death. Bcl-x has two isoforms, namely, bcl-xL, a preventive isoform against apoptosis; and bcl-xS, a promotive isoform.

LIF induces bcl-xL in cardiac myocytes for an antiapoptotic effect

A recent study has provided direct evidence that one of the mechanisms by which LIF can promote the survival of cardiac myocytes is via activation leading to inhibition of the apoptotic signaling pathway. This study deployed an in vitro assay

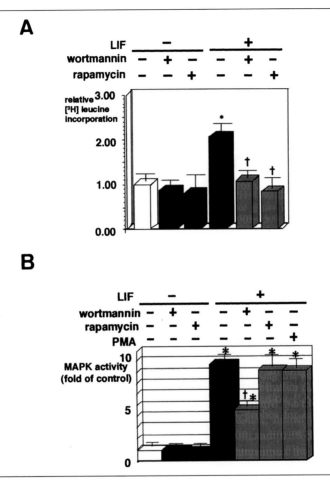

Figure 4. Association of PI3K activation in LIF-induced cardiac myocyte hypertrophy. (**A**) Increased protein synthesis induced by LIF is inhibited by wortmannin and rapamycin. Cultured cardiac myocytes were incubated in serum-free medium for 24 hours. Protein synthesis was measured by [³H] leucine incorporation 24 hours after LIF stimulation in the presence or absence of the indicated inhibitors. The results are standardized to the value obtained from LIF (−) (lane 1). ★, $p < 0.05$ vs. LIF (−) (lane 1); †, $p < 0.05$ vs. LIF (+) (lane 4). (**B**) LIF-induced MAPK activation is inhibited by wortmannin but not by rapamycin. The cell lysates were assayed for MAPK activity using BIOTRACK MAPK kit. Data are standardized to the value obtained from LIF (−) (lane 1). ★, $p < 0.05$ vs. LIF (−) (lane 1); †, $p < 0.05$ vs. LIF (+) (line 4).

system whereby cardiac myocytes entered the apoptotic signaling pathway after the deprivation of serum. LIF significantly improved cardiac myocyte survival and was associated with increased expression of bcl-x mRNA but not of bcl-2 mRNA. The isoform induced by LIF was identified as bcl-xL by Western blotting and RT-PCR using specific primers. The antisense oligonucleotide against bcl-x

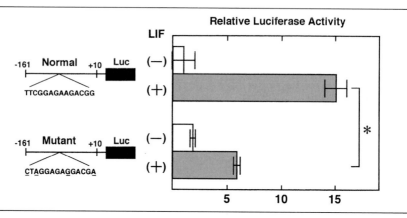

Figure 5. Effect of disruption of the GAS motif in the promoter activity of the *bcl-x* gene. Normal (TTCGGAGAAGACGG) or mutant (CTAGGAGAGGACGA) promoter-luciferase construct was transfected into cardiac myocytes and luciferase assay was performed. The transfected cells were stimulated with (gray bars) or without (open bars) $1 \times 10^3 \, \text{U/mL}$ LIF for 24 hours. The luciferase activity was normalized by β-galactosidase activity. *, $p < 0.05$.

mRNA inhibited the protective effect of LIF in conjunction with a reduction in bcl-xL protein [23].

Studies focusing on the LIF-induced transcriptional regulation of the bcl-x gene were pursued using the bcl-x promoter-luciferase reporter gene and electrophoretic mobility shift assays. Figure 5 shows the LIF-responsive *cis*-element located from −161 to +10 of the promoter region of the bcl-x gene, which contains a GAS motif, TTCGGAGAA, at position −41. This motif bound to STAT1, not to STAT3, and site-directed mutagenesis revealed that this motif was essential for LIF-responsive promoter activity [23]. There findings, taken together, indicate that LIF induces bcl-x mRNA via the STAT1 binding *cis*-element in cardiac myocytes, resulting in cyto-protective effects.

LIF activates Akt via PI3K in cardiac myocytes

The Akt encodes a serine threonine protein kinase that is activated by several growth factor-generated signals that are transduced via PI3K. Activation of Akt is known to deliver a survival signal that inhibits the apoptosis induced by growth factor with-drawal in neural cells and fibroblasts [24,25]. In addition, activation of Akt ultimately leads to inhibition of caspase activity and protection from apoptotic cell death. Bad is a distant member of the bcl-2 family that promotes cell death. The active but not the inactive forms of Akt were found to phosphorylate Bad and thus to act as an antiapototic. A recent study has further demonstrated that IL-3-induced Bad phos-phorylation is inhibited by PI3K-specific inhibitors [26].

To confirm the essential role of the PI3K cascade in the gp130-mediated sur-vival function, Akt activation was examined in LIF-stimulated cardiac myocytes. As

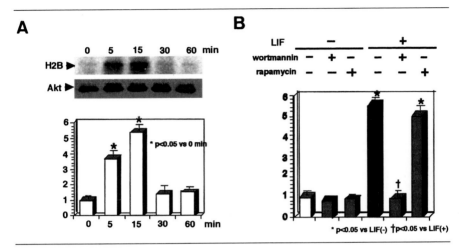

Figure 6. LIF-induced activation of Akt in cardiac myocytes. (**A**) Time course of Akt activation in cultured neonatal rat cardiac myocytes after LIF stimulation. Cardiac myocytes were incubated in serum-free medium for 24 hours and treated with 1×10^3 U/mL LIF for the time indicated. Cell lysates were immunoprecipitated with anti-Akt antibody preconjugated with protein G-sepharose, and the kinase activity was determined using $[\gamma^{-32}P]$ ATP and Crosstide as a substrate (lower panel). (**B**) LIF-induced Akt activation is sensitive to wortmannin, not to rapamycin.

shown in figure 6, LIF induced a rapid activation of Akt at 5 minutes, and the kinase activity reached a maximum at 15 minutes. Furthermore, LIF-induced Akt activation was completely inhibited by wortmannin but not by rapamycin [18]. Thus, LIF regulation of Akt employs PI3K but not p70 S6 kinase in cardiac myocytes. This is the first time that Akt was shown to be activated as a consequence of increased PI3K activity in cardiac myocytes. Although the activation of gp130 transduces cytoprotective signals through STAT1, as described above, PI3K is thus also recognized as crucial for gp130-mediated cell survival.

CONCLUSIONS

In conclusion, the JAK/STAT, MAPK, and PI3K pathways are all necessary for full activation of gp130-mediated hypertrophic and cytoprotective signals in cardiac myocytes. As discussed earlier, investigations of signaling pathways through gp130 in cardiac myocytes should uncover novel mechanisms of cardiac myocyte growth and survival. Although recent investigations have addressed the participation of cytokines in various cardiovascular diseases, we have but a limited understanding of their underlying functions and mechanisms. Our investigations of the hypertrophic and cytoprotective functions of IL-6-related cytokines are expected to provide new insights into the pathophysiological significance of cytokines in various myocardial diseases. Clarification of the regulation of these cascades in normal and diseased human hearts may well lead to a novel therapeutic approach to myocardial diseases.

ACKNOWLEDGMENTS

This study was supported by a grant-in-aid for general scientific research from the Ministry of Education, Science and Culture of Japan and research grants from the Ministry of Health and Welfare of Japan and the Study Group of Molecular Cardiology. The authors wish to thank Ms. M. Katayama for excellent secretarial assistance.

REFERENCES

1. Shioi T, Matsumori A, Sasayama S. 1996. Persistent expression of cytokine in the chronic stage of viral myocarditis in mice. Circulation 94:2930–2937.
2. Ono K, Matsumori A, Shioi T, Furukawa Y, Sasayama S. 1998. Cytokine gene expression after myocardial infarction in rat hearts. Circulation 98:149–156.
3. Yamauchi-Takihara K, Ihara Y, Ogata A, Yoshizaki K, Azuma J, Kishimoto T. 1995. Hypoxic stress induces cardiac myocyte-derived interleukin-6. Circulation 91:1520–1526.
4. Simpson P, McGrath A, Savion S. 1982. Myocyte hypertrophy in neonatal rat heart cultures and its regulation by serum and catecholamines. Circ Res 51:787–801.
5. Ito H, Hirata Y, Adachi S, Tanaka M, Tsujino M, Koike A, Nogami A, Marumo F, Hiroe M. 1993. Endothelin-1 is an autocrine/paracrine factor in the mechanism of angiotensin II-induced hypertrophy in cultured rat cardiomyocytes. J Clin Invest 98:398–403.
6. Sadoshima J, Xu Y, Slayter HS, Izumo S. 1993. Autocrine release of angiotensin II mediates stretch-induced hypertrophy of cardiac myocyte in vitro. Cell 95:997–984.
7. Pennica D, King KL, Shaw KJ, Luis E, Rullamas J, Luoh SM, Darbonne WC, Knutzon DS, Yen R, Chien KR, Baker JB, Wood WI. 1995. Expression cloning of cardiotrophin 1, a cytokine that induces cardiac myocyte hypertrophy. Proc Natl Acad Sci USA 92:1142–1146.
8. Kishimoto T, Taga T, Akira S. 1994. Cytokine signal transduction. Cell 76:253–262.
9. Hirota H, Yoshida K, Kishimoto T, Taga T. 1995. Continuous activation of gp130, a signal tansducing receptor component for IL-6-related cytokines, causes myocardial hypertrophy in mice. Proc Natl Acad Sci USA 92:4862–4866.
10. Pennica D, Shaw KJ, Swanson TA, Moore MW, Shelton DL, Zioncheck KA, Rosenthal A, Taga T, Paoni NF, Wood WI. 1995. Cardiotrophin-1. Biological activities and binding to the leukemia inhibitory factor receptor/gp130 signaling complex. J Biol Chem 270:10915–10922.
11. Yamazaki T, Tobe K, Hoh E, Maemura K, Kaida T, Komuro I, Tamemoto H, Kadowaki T, Nagai R, Yazaki Y. 1993. Mechanical loading activates mitogen-activated protein kinase and S6 peptide kinase in cultured rat cardiac myocytes. J Biol Chem 268:12069–12076.
12. Shubeita HE, McDonough PM, Harris AN, Knowlton KU, Glembotski CC, Brown JH, Chien KR. 1990. Endothelin induction of inositol phospholipid hydrolysis, sarcomere assembly, and cardiac gene expression in ventricular myocytes. A paracrine mechanism for myocardial cell hypertrophy. J Biol Chem 265:20555–20562.
13. Saward L, Zahradka P. 1997. Angiotensin II activates phosphatidylinositol 3-kinase in vascular smooth muscle cells. Circ Res 81:249–257.
14. Yao R, Cooper GM. 1995. Requirement for phosphatidylinositol-3 kinase in the prevention of apoptosis by nerve growth factor. Science 267:2003–2006.
15. Matsui H, Fujio Y, Kunisada K, Hirota H, Yamauchi-Takihara K. 1996. Leukemia inhibitory factor induces a hypertrophic response mediated by gp130 in murine cardiac myocytes. Res Commun Mol Pathol Pharmacol 93:149–162.
16. Kunisada K, Hirota H, Fujio Y, Matsui H, Tani Y, Yamauchi-Takihara K, Kishimoto T. 1996. Activation of JAK-STAT and MAP kinases by leukemia inhibitory factor through gp130 in cardiac myocytes. Circulation 94:2626–2632.
17. Kunisada K, Tone E, Fujio Y, Matsui H, Yamauchi-Takihara K, Kishimoto T. 1998. Activation of gp130 transduces hypertrophic signals via STAT3 in cardiac myocytes. Circulation 98:346–352.
18. Oh H, Fujio Y, Kunisada K, Hirota H, Matsui H, Kishimoto T, Yamauchi-Takihara K. 1998. Activation of phosphatidylinositol 3-kinase through gp130 induces protein kinase B and p70 S6 kinase phosphorylation in cardiac myocytes. J Biol Chem 273:9703–9710.
19. Oppenheim RW, Prevette D, Yin QW, Collins F, MacDonald J. 1991. Control of embryonic motoneuron survival in vivo by ciliary neurotrophic factor. Science 251:1616–1618.

20. Martinou JC, Martinou I, Kato A. 1992. Cholinergic differentiation factor (CDF/LIF) promotes survival of isolated rat embryonic motoneurons in vitro. Neuron 8:737–744.
21. Pennica D, Arce V, Swanson TA, Vejsada R, Pollock RA, Armanini M, Dudley K, Phillips HS, Rosenthal A, Kato AC, Henderson CE. 1996. Cardiotrophin-1, a cytokine present in embryonic muscle, support long term survival of spinal motoneurons. Neuron 17:63–74.
22. Schwarze MMK, Hawley RG. 1995. Prevention of myeloma cell apoptosis by ectopic bcl-2 expression or interleukin 6-mediated up-regulation of bcl-xL. Cancer Res 55:2262–2265.
23. Fujio Y, Kunisada K, Hirota H, Yamauchi-Takihara K, Kishimoto T. 1997. Leukemia inhibitory factor up-regulates bcl-x gene expression via STAT1 binding *cis*-element in cardiac myocytes. J Clin Invest 99:2898–2905.
24. Dudek H, Datta SR, Franke TF, Birnbaum MJ, Yao R, Cooper GM, Segal RA, Kaplan DR, Greenberg ME. 1997. Regulation of neuronal survival by the serine-threonine protein kinase Akt. Science 275:661–664.
25. Kulik G, Klippel A, Weber MJ. 1997. Antiapoptotic signalling by the insulin-like growth factor I receptor, phosphatidylinositol 3-kinase, and Akt. Mol Cell Biol 17:1795–1606.
26. Peso L, Gonzalez-Garcia M, Page C, Herrera R, Nunez G. 1997. Interleukin-3-induced phosphorylation of BAD through the protein kinase Akt. Science 278:687–689.

N. Takeda, M. Nagano and N.S. Dhalla
(eds). The Hypertrophied Heart. Copyright
© 2000. pp. 333–343. Kluwer Academic
Publishers. Boston. All rights reserved.

MOLECULAR GENETIC ASPECTS OF HYPERTROPHIC CARDIOMYOPATHY IN THE ORIENTAL

AKINORI KIMURA

Department of Molecular Pathogenesis, Division of Adult Diseases, and Etiology and Pathogenesis Research Unit, Medical Research Institute, Tokyo Medical and Dental University, Kandasurugadai 2-3-10, Chiyoda-ku, Tokyo 101-0062, Japan

Summary. To decipher the molecular etiologies of hypertrophic cardiomyopathy in Orientals, we have investigated mutations in the known disease genes in a large panel of Japanese and Korean patients including both familial and sporadic cases. Our analysis has revealed that about half of the familial cases and part of the sporadic cases could be attributed to mutations in the genes for cardiac sarcomere proteins. The clinical phenotypes of these mutations varied from one to another mutation, but there was a tendency of phenotypes to poor prognosis associated with which gene was mutated. In this report, the clinical implications of the mutational analysis will be discussed.

INTRODUCTION

Hypertrophic cardiomyopathy (HCM) is characterized by ventricular hypertrophy and reduced compliance of ventricles accompanied by disarray of myocytes and myofibrils in the absence of known causes of cardiac hypertrophy such as hypertention and metabolic diseases [1]. The etiology of HCM had been unknown because there were no HCM-specific biochemical or pathological changes. However, recent molecular genetic analyses based on linkage studies [2–6] and subsequent candidate gene approaches [7–11] have deciphered in part the molecular etiologies of HCM.

It is now well recognized that mutations in genes for components of the cardiac sarcomere, i.e., cardiac beta-myosin heavy chain (*MYH7*) [2,7], cardiac troponin T (*TNNT2*) [3,8], alpha-tropomyosin (*TPM1*) [4,8], cardiac myosin binding protein-C (*MYBPC3*) [5,9], ventricular myosin essential light chain (*MYL3*) [10], ventricular myosin regulatory light chain (*MYL2*) [10], and cardiac troponin I (*TNNI3*) [11] cause HCM (for a recent review, see [12]). Since the first discovery of an *MYH7* mutation in a large HCM family [7], molecular genetic analyses of HCM have been concerned with the identification of mutations in these genes, and genotype–

phenotype correlations have been reported for mutations in *MYH7* [13–15], *TNNT2* [16–18], *TPM1* [19–20], *MYBPC3* [21,22], *MYL3* [10], *MYL2* [10,23], and *TNNI3* [11]. The molecular basis of cardiac hypertrophy due to mutations in cardiac sarcomere components has also been investigated by in vitro [24–29] and in vivo [30–32] approaches, suggesting that cardiac hypertrophy in HCM is a compensation for reduced or impaired contractility of cardiac myocytes.

We have also investigated mutations in these HCM genes in Japanese and Korean HCM patients [12,33–45]. It is, however, still unclear which proportion of HCM patients has a mutation in these cardiac sarcomere components. This report will summarize our current data on the systematic mutational analyses of Oriental HCM patients and the clinical implications of these findings.

SUBJECTS AND METHODS

A total of 294 patients with HCM were analyzed for mutations in the seven known HCM genes by using single-stranded DNA confirmation polymorphism (SSCP) and sequencing methods, as described previously [11,12,33–45]. Among these patients, 184 have an apparent family history of HCM (familiar HCM, FHCM), and the others either have no family history or their family histories were unknown (sporadic HCM, SHCM). All the patients were genetically unrelated to each other. Family members and unrelated healthy individuals were also analyzed to investigate whether a detected sequence variation was a disease-causing mutation cosegregated with HCM in the family or a polymorphism not related to HCM. Blood samples were obtained from each subject after informed consent was obtained in the hospitals of clinical researchers in Japan and Korea, as noted in the acknowledgments.

RESULTS AND DISCUSSION

Identified mutations of cardiac sarcomere components

A total of 69 different sequence variations leading to changes in cardiac sarcomere proteins, i.e., amino acid substitutions, partial deletions, or truncations, were identified in the patients. Among these, 58 variations found in 118 patients were considered to be disease-related mutations because (1) the same variation was not found in more than 500 normal chromosomes (i.e., in more than 250 healthy controls), (2) the variation was found at the evolutionary conserved amino acid residue in sarcomere isoforms among various spicies, and/or (3) the variation was cosegregated with disease in corresponding multiplex families of FHCM. In the cases of SHCM, familial segregation of each sequence variation was not tested. However, when the variation was not found in the healthy controls, and when the variation was also found in other FHCM patients, was a de novo mutation, or led to gross structural changes such as splicing or nonsense mutations, the variation was considered to be a disease-related mutation. The disease-related mutations are shown in table 1.

In contrast, 11 other variations leading to amino acid replacements were considered to be polymorphisms or non-disease-related variations because they were also found in unrelated healthy individuals and/or they were not cosegreated with the

Table 1. HCM gene mutations found in Oriental patients with HCM

Gene	Exon	Codon	Change	Nature	Ethnic origin	Reference
MYH7	3	36	Ala26Val	missense	Jpn	37
MYH7	3	59	Val59Ile	missense	Jpn	37
MYH7	5	143	Arg143Gln	missense	Jpn	36
MYH7	5	143	Arg143Trp	missense	Jpn	37
MYH7	8	214	Gly214Asp	missense	Jpn	this study
MYH7	14	453	Arg453Cys	missense	Jpn	36
MYH7	15	498	Gln498Glu	missense	Jpn	43
MYH7	15	527	Pro527Ser	missense	Jpn	this study
MYH7	16	587	Asp587Val	missense	Jpn	37
MYH7	16	602	Asn602Ser	missense	Jpn	37
MYH7	16	615	Lys615Asn	missense	Jpn	33
MYH7	16	624	Tyr624Asn	missense	Jpn	42
MYH7	19	691	His691Pro	missense	Jpn	43
MYH7	19	716	Gly716Arg	missense	Kor	44
MYH7	20	731	Pro731Leu	missense	Jpn	38
MYH7	20	736	Ile736Met	missense	Jpn	37
MYH7	20	741	Gly741Arg	missense	Jpn	37
MYH7	20	741	Gly741Trp	missense	Jpn	37
MYH7	20	742	Ala742Val	missense	Jpn	this study
MYH7	21	778	Asp778Gly	missense	Jpn	34
MYH7	21	797	Ala797Pro	missense	Jpn	36
MYH7	22	843	Ala843Val	missense	Jpn	this study
MYH7	22	870	Arg870Cys	missense	Jpn, Kor	41
MYH7	22	870	Arg870His	missense	Jpn	38
MYH7	22	870	Arg870Trp	missense	Jpn	this study
MYH7	23	926	Leu926Pro	missense	Jpn	43
MYH7	23	935	Glu935Lys	missense	Jpn	35
TNNT2	9	92	Arg92Trp	missense	Jpn	43
TNNT2	9	92	Arg92Gln	missense	Jpn	this study
TNNT2	9	94	Arg94Leu	missense	Jpn	43
TNNT2	9	110	Phe110Ile	missense	Jpn	43
TNNT2	10	130	Arg130Cys	missense	Jpn	43
TNNT2	10	134	Arg134Trp	missense	Kor	this study
TNNT2	11	160	Glu160 del3	1 aa deletion	Jpn	43
TNNT2	11	163	Glu163Lys	missense	Jpn	43
TPM1	3	102	Ala102Asp	missense	Jpn	36
MYBPC3	3	129	Glu129ter	termination	Jpn	this study
MYBPC3	6	258	Glu258Arg	missense	Jpn	41
MYBPC3	13	386	Glu386ter	termination	Jpn	this study
MYBPC3	17	495	Arg495Gln	missense	Jpn	this study
MYBPC3	18	552–7	552–7 del18	6 aa deletion	Jpn	this study
MYBPC3	18	589	Arg589Cys	missense	Jpn	this study
MYBPC3	18	593	Ser593 del1	frameshift	Jpn	11
MYBPC3	18	597	Arg597Gln	missense	Jpn	this study
MYBPC3	24	773	Asp773 ins1	frameshift	Jpn	this study
MYBPC3	27	945	Arg945 del2	frameshift	Jpn, Kor	11
MYBPC3	27	969	Gln969ter	termination	Jpn	this study
MYBPC3	IVS27	at +1	g to a	splicing	Jpn, Kor	11
MYBPC3	30	1105	Ala1105 ins2	frameshift	Kor	this study
MYBPC3	33	1238	Leu1238Pro	missense	Kor	this study
MYL3	3	57	Ala57Gly	missense	Jpn, Kor	41
MYL2	4	57	Arg57Gln	missense	Jpn	41
TNNI3	7	145	Arg145Gln	missense	Jpn	11
TNNI3	7	145	Arg145Gly	missense	Kor	11
TNNI3	7	162	Arg162Trp	missense	Jpn	11
TNNI3	7	183	Lys183 del3	1 aa deletion	Jpn	11
TNNI3	8	203	Gly203Ser	missense	Jpn	11
TNNI3	8	206	Lys206Glu	missense	Jpn	11

Table 2. HCM gene polymorphisms with amino acid change

HCM gene	Exon	Polymorphism		Reference
		Codon	Change	
MYH7	3	54	Arg54ter	38
TNNT2	14	253	Lys253Arg	8
MYBPC3	2	95	Ile95Leu	this study
MYBPC3	4	160	Arg160Trp	this study
MYBPC3	6	236	Ser236Gly	this study
MYBPC3	17	507	Gly507Arg	this study
MYBPC3	28	998	Gln998Glu	this study
MYBPC3	29	1046	Thr1046Met	this study
TNNI3	5	58	Lys58Asn	11
TNNI3	5	74	Arg74Ser	11
TNNI3	5	79	Arg79Cys	11

disease in multiplex families. These non-disease-related variations or polymorphisms are listed in table 2.

In addition, we have identified many other sequence variations in the patients (data not shown). However, these were not leading to structural change of sarcomere proteins, i.e., synonymous substitutions in exons or base substitutions in introns not affecting the splicing consensus sequences, and were also found in unrelated healthy controls, indicating that they were polymorphisms. Some examples of these polymorphisms were reported previously for the *TNNI3* gene [11].

Disease phenotype of the sarcomere mutations

The phenotypes of mutations—e.g., the extent and localization of cardiac hypertrophy, transmission to dilated phase, and disease-related sudden death—in the Oriental HCM patients and their family members varied from one to another mutation. The phenotypes also varied among the mutation-prone individuals in the same family. However, there was a tendency of disease-related phenotypes to poor prognosis depending on which gene was mutated, as shown in table 3. These tendencies were deduced from the analysis of each mutation-prone individual, especially those with mutations in *MYH7*, *TNNT2*, *MYBPC3*, and *TNNI3* genes, because in these cases a considerable number of mutation-prone individuals could be analyzed. As for mutation in the *TPM1*, *MYL2*, and *MYL3* genes, only one mutation in each gene was found in the Orientals, indicating that the phenotype in table 3 reflected the phenotypic expression of the mutant allele itself rather than the mutated gene.

The extent of cardiac hypertrophy, in general, is less in association with *TNNT2* mutations than in association with *MYH7* and *MYBPC3* mutations [40,45]. It was found that the carriers of *MYBPC3* mutations developed cardiac hypertrophy later than those of *MYH7* mutations [45], suggesting that the *MYBPC3* mutations were associated with late-onset HCM, as has been reported in Caucasian patients [22]. It

Table 3. Clinical phenotypes of HCM gene mutations in the Oriental HCM families

HCM gene	No. of mutations	No. of analyzed families	IVS thickness (mm)	Transmission to dHCM	Sudden death
MYH7	27	54	21 ± 7	variable (from 50s)	variable
TNNT2	8	20	16 ± 5	relatively frequent (from 40s)	variable
TPM1	1	1	13 ± 2	none	rare
MYBPC3	14	32	19 ± 7	rare (only 2 cases, from 60s)	rare
MYL3	1	2	12 ± 2	non	non
MYL2	1	2	15 ± 6	variable (from 40s)	rare
TNNI3	6	7	15 ± 2	none	rare

also was observed that the development of dilated-phase HCM (dHCM) was more frequently and occurred earlier in patients with TNNT2 mutations than in the others, except that the carriers of the Phe110Ile mutation in the TNNT2 gene rarely developed dHCM [40], as was reported by Anan et al. [46]. The TNNI3 mutation was more frequently found in the patients who had cardiac hypertrophy in the apex or apical-sided septum (apical hypertrophy or AHCM) than in patients with typical HCM [11].

An interesting finding was that the extent of cardiac hypertrophy was not correlated with the risk of disease-related death, because the TNNT2 mutations were strongly associated with the risk but showed relatively mild cardiac hypertrophy [40]. Another interesting finding was that some MYH7 mutations were related to a poor survival prognosis, while other MYH7 mutations were not. Examples of cumulative survival of mutation-prone individuals and obligatory carriers are shown in figure 1. The Asp778Gly mutation found in six different Japanese multiplex families [34,38] and the Arg716Gly mutation found in a Korean FHCM family [44] showed quite a poor prognosis, whereas the Arg870His [38], Arg870Cys, and Arg143Gln mutations found in 4, 3, and 2 unrelated families, respectively, did not (figure 1).

It has been speculated from similar analyses in Caucasian FHCM families that the MYH7 mutations leading to the charge alteration, especially those replacing the Arg residue, were associated with poor prognosis [14,15]. However, this hypothesis was not the case for the Arg870Cys and Arg143Gln mutations found in the Orientals. Mapping of these MYH7 mutations, as well as the MYH7 mutations in the literature for which cumulative survival curves have been reported [13–15], onto a structural model of human MYH7 protein deduced from the crystallography of chicken skeletal myosin heavy chain [47] suggested that the MYH7 mutations in three functionally important domains of myosin heavy chain—i.e., ATP-binding domain, actin-interacting domain, and essential light chain-interacting domain—were associated with poor survival prognosis [41], especially when they lead to the change alterations. In contrast, the MYH7 mutations that were mapped to the other domains, especially those mapped onto the head–rod junctional part of myosin, were associated with favorable survival prognosis, even when they change the charge of the myosin heavy chain.

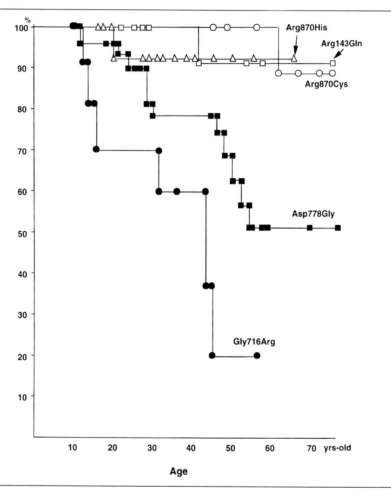

Figure 1. Cumulative survival curves of the Oriental patients and their family members who have myosin heavy chain gene mutations. The curves refer to individuals in whom each myosin heavy chain mutation was associated with hypertrophic cardiomyopathy.

Frequency of sarcomere mutations in Oriental HCM

Our systematic analysis of mutations in the seven known HCM genes has revealed that a substantial portion of patients have the sarcomere mutations. The frequency of sarcomere mutations in the unrelated familial cases (FHCM, probands of multiplex families) was about 47% and that in the unrelated sporadic cases (SHCM) was about 14%, as shown in table 4.

The method employed in the screening of mutations in all protein-coding exons and adjacent introns was based on the SSCP analysis, by which about 90% of sequence variations could be detected. It was, then, speculated that only about half

Table 4. Frequency of HCM gene
mutations in Oriental HCM patients

HCM gene	FHCM proband ($n = 184$)	SHCM ($n = 110$)
MYH7	17.93%	1.82%
TNNT2	10.87%	2.73%
TPM1	0.54%	0.00%
MYBPC3	12.50%	4.54%
MYL3	1.09%	1.82%
MYL2	1.09%	0.00%
TNNI3	2.72%	2.73%
Total	46.74%	13.64%

of Oriental FHCM could be attributable to mutations in these known HCM genes. This speculation in turn suggests that there may be still other disease genes responsible for HCM.

One example is a still unknown gene mapped onto chromosome 7q3 (*CMH6* locus), suggested from a linkage analysis in a multiplex family where many affected individuals were reported to have Wolff–Parkinson–White (WPW) syndrome [6]. In our study, however, there were five FHCM patients with WPW syndrome, and two of them had a mutation in the *MYBPC3* or *TNNI3* gene [11], demonstrating that not all HCM with WPW syndrome could be attributable to the *CMH6* locus. Our observation also suggests that WPW syndrome in the *CMH6*-linked HCM might be a coincidental event and not a characteristic clinical entity of HCM. Nevertheless, identifications of the responsible gene in the *CMH6* locus and the other unknown HCM genes will resolve the molecular basis of WPW syndrome found in 5–10% of HCM patients.

Another interesting finding was that we found sarcomere mutations in the sporadic cases. Because the sporadic cases in this study were defined as having no apparent family history, they should include bona fide familial cases having mutations of low penetrance. Indeed, several mutations found in the SHCM cases were also found in other unrelated FHCM cases, where the disease penetrance was found to be relatively low [11,45]. Another possibility is that some mutations may be de novo, as was reported previously for a *TNNI3* mutation [11]. Nevertheless, a lower frequency of sarcomere mutations in SHCM than in FHCM suggests that considerable portions of SHCM may not be inheritable disease but rather acquired disease.

In this respect, it is interesting to note that about 10% of HCM patients were reported to have antibodies against hepatitis C virus (HCV), suggesting that HCV infection may manifest the HCM phenotype [48]. Matsumori et al. reported that the HCV genome could be detected in some patients with HCM; more than half of them were sporadic cases and/or apical hypertrophy [49]. We also tested about 40 patients for anti-HCV antibodies and found that about 10% of them were positive, but none of them had a sarcomere mutation (data not shown). On the other hand, we analyzed for sarcomere mutations in 30 patients with apical hypertrophy, a clinical subtype of HCM with lower incidence of family history, and found mutations in only four cases, supporting the notion that a considerable portion of apical hypertrophy as well as sporadic HCM cases may be acquired disease or so-called *multifactorial disease*—disease defined as a consequence of interaction between many genetic polymorphisms and environmental factors.

ACKNOLEDGMENTS

I am grateful to the patients and their family members for generously providing blood samples for this study. I also thank Profs. H. Toshima, H. Yasuda, Y. Yazaki, S. Sasayama, T. Imaizumi, Y. Koga, M. Yokoyama, S. Kawamura, T. Izumi, R. Nagai, T. Toyo-oka, M. Matsuzaki, Y. Doi, and J.E. Park; Drs. H. Nishi, T. Sakamoto, A. Hiroe, A. Matsumori, F. Teranishi, K. Nakamura, H. Kitaoka, W.H. Lee, T.H. Hwang, and the other members of the Research Society of Idiopathic Cardiomyopathy, Japan, for their contributions in blood sampling and clinical investigations; and Drs. H. Harada, M. Satoh, M. Takahashi, T. Sasaoka, S. Hiroi, T. Nakamura, N. Ohbuchi, and T. Arimura for their contributions in the mutational analyses. This work was supported in part by research grants from the Ministry of Health and Welfare, Japan, from the Ministry of Education, Science, Sports and Culture, Japan, from the Japan Science Promotion Society, from the Culture, Japan, from the Japan Science Promotion Society, from the National Cardiovascular Research Center, from the Kato Memorial Foundation, from the Atsuko Ouchi Memorial Fund, and from the Uehara Memorial Foundation.

REFERENCES

1. Maron BJ, Bonow RO, Cannon RO 3d, Leon MB, Epstein SE. 1987. Hypertrophic cardiomyopathy: interrelations of clinical manifestations, pathophysiology, and therapy. N Engl J Med 316: 780–789.
2. Jarcho JA, McKenna W, Pare JAP, Solomon SD, Holcombe RF, Dickie S, Levi T, Danis-Keller H, Seidman JG, Seidman CE. 1989. Mapping a gene for familial hypertrophic cardiomyopathy to chromosome 14q1. N Engl J Med 321:1372–1378.
3. Watkins H, MacRae C, Thierfelder L, Chou YH, Frennaux M, McKenna W, Seidman JG, Seidman CE. 1993. A disease gene for familial hypertrophic cardiomyopathy maps to chromosome 1q3. Nature Genet 3:333–337.
4. Thierfelder L, MacRae C, Watkins H, Tomfohrde J, Williams M, McKenna W, Bohm K, Noeske G, Schlepper M, Bowcock A, Seidman CE, Seidman JG. 1993. A familial hypertrophic cardiomyopathy locus maps to chromosome 15q2. Proc Natl Acad Sci USA 90:6270–6274.
5. Carrier L, Hengstenberg C, Beckmann JS, Guicheney P, Dufour C, Bercovici J, Dausse E, Berebbi-Bertrand I, Wisnewsky C, Pulvenis D, Komajda M, Schwartz K. 1993. Mapping of a novel gene for familial hypertrophic cardiomyopathy to chromosome 11. Nature Genet 4:311–313.
6. MacRae CA, Ghaisas N, Kass S, Donnelly S, Basson CT, Watkins HC, Anan R, Thierfelder LH, McGarry K, Rowland E, McKenna WJ, Seidman JG, Seidman CE. 1995. Familial hypertrophic cardiomyopathy with Wolff–Parkinson–White syndrome maps to a locus on chromosome 7q3. J Clin Invest 96:1216–1220.
7. Geisterfer-Lowrance AAT, Kass S, Tanigawa G, Vosberg HP, McKenna W, Seidman CE, Seidman JG. 1990. A molecular basis for familial hypertrophic cardiomyopathy: a beta cardiac myosin heavy chain gene missense mutation. Cell 62:999–1006.
8. Thierfelder L, Watkins H, MacRae C, Lamas R, McKenna W, Vosberg HP, Siedman JG, Seidman CE. 1994. Alpha tropomyosin and cardiac troponin T mutation cause familial hypertrophic cardiomyopathy: a disease of the sarcomere. Cell 77:701–712.
9. Watkins H, Conner D, Thierfelder L, Jarcho JA, MacRae C, McKenna WJ, Maron BJ Seidman JG, Seidman CE. 1995. Mutations in the cardiac myosin binding protein-C gene on chromosome 11 cause familial hypertrophic cardiomyopathy. Nature Genet 11:434–437.

10. Poetter K, Jiang H, Hassenzadeh S, Master SR, Chang A, Dalakas MC, Rayment I, Sellers JR, Fananapazir L, Epstein ND. 1996. Mutations in either essential or regulatory light chains of myosins are associated with a rare myopathy in human heart and skeletal muscle. Nature Genet 13:63–69.

11. Kimura A, Harada H, Park JE, Nishi H, Satoh M, Takahashi M, Hiroi S, Sasaoka T, Ohbuchi N, Nakamura T, Koyanagi T, Hwang TH, Choo JA, Chung KS, Hasegawa A, Nagai R, Okazaki O, Nakamura H, Matsuzaki M, Sakamoto T, Toshima H, Koga Y, Imaizumi T, Sasazuki T. 1997. Mutations in the cardiac troponin I gene associated with hypertrophic caridomyopathy. Nature Genet 16:379–382.

12. Bonne G, carrier L, Richard B, Hainque B, Schwartz K. 1998. Familial hypertrophic cardiomyopathy: from mutations to functional defects. Circ Res 83:580–593.

13. Epstein ND, Cohn GM, Cyran F, Fananapazir L. 1992. Difference in clinical expression of hypertrophic cardiomyopathy associated with two distinct mutations in the beta-myosin heavy chain gene: a 9081Leu → Val mutation and a 403Arg → Gln mutation. Circulation 86:345–352.

14. Watkins H, Rosenzweig T, Hwang DS, Levi T, McKenna W, Seidman CE, Seidman JG. 1992. Characteristic and prognostic implications of myosin missense mutations in familial hypertrophic cardiomyopathy. N Engl J Med 326:1106–1114.

15. Anan R, Greve G, Thierfelder L, Watkins H, McKenna WJ, Solomon S, Vecchio C, Shono H, Nakao S, Tanaka H, Seidman JG, Seidman CE. 1994. Prognostic implications of novel beta myosin heavy chain gene mutations that cause familial hypertrophic cardiomyopathy. J Clin Invest 93:280–285.

16. Watkins H, McKenna W, Thierfelder L, Spirito P, Matsumori A, Maravec CS, Seidman JG, Seidman CE. 1995. Mutations in the genes for cardiac troponin T and alpha-tropomyosin in hypertrophic cardiomyopathy. N Engl J Med 332:1058–1064.

17. Moolman JC, Corfield VA, Posen B, Ngumbela K, Seidman C, Brink PA, Watkins H. 1997. Sudden death due to troponin T mutations. J Am Coll Cardiol 29:549–555.

18. Nakajima-Taniguchi C, Matsui H, Fujio Y, Nagata S, Kishimoto T, Yamauchi-Takihara K. 1997. Novel missense mutation in cardiac troponin T gene found in Japanese patient with hypertrophic cardiomyopathy. J Mol Cell Cardiol 29:839–843.

19. Yamauchi-Takihara K, Nakajima-Taniguchi C, Matsui H, Fujia Y, Kunisada K, Nagata S, Kishimoto T. 1996. Clinical implications of hypertrophic cardiomyopathy associated with mutations in the alpha-tropomyosin gene. Heart 76:63–65.

20. Coviello DA, Maron BJM, Spirito P, Watkins H, Vosberg HP, Thierfelder L, Schoen FJ, Seidman JG, Seidman CE. 1997. Clinical features of hypertrophic cardiomyopathy caused by mutation of a "hot spot" in the alpha-tropomyosin gene. J Am Coll Cardiol 29:635–640.

21. Carrier L, Bonne G, Bahrend E, Yu B, Richard P, Niel F, Hainque B, Cruaud C, Gary F, Labeit S, Bouhour JB, Dubourg O, Desnos M, Hagege AA, Trent RJ, Komajda M, Fiszman M, Schwartz K. 1997. Organization and sequences of human cardiac myosin binding protein C gene (MYBPC3) and identification of mutations predicted to produce truncated proteins in familial hypertrophic cardiomyopathy. Circ Res 80:427–439.

22. Niiumura H, Bachinski LL. Sangwatanaroj S, Watkins H, Chudley AE, McKenna W, Kristinsson A, Roberts R, Sole M, Maron BJ, Seidman JG, Seidman CE. 1998. Mutations in the gene for cardiac myosin-binding protein C and late-onset familial hypertrophic cardiomyopathy. N Engl J Med 338:1248–1257.

23. Flavigny J, Richard P, Isnard R, Carrier L, Charron P, Bonne G, Forissier JF, Desnos M, Dubourg O, Komajda M, Schwartz K, Hainque B. 1998. Identification of two novel mutations in the ventricular regulatory light chain gene (MYL2) associated with familial and classical forms of hypertrophic cardiomyopathy. J Mol Med 76:208–214.

24. Lankford EB, Epstein ND, Fananapazir L, Sweeney HL. 1995. Abnormal contractile properties of muscle fibers expressing beta-myosin heavy chain gene mutations in patients with hypertrophic cardiomyopathy. J Clin Invest 95:1409–1414.

25. Cuda G, Fananapazir L, Epstein ND, Sellers JR. 1997. The in vitro motility activity of beta-cardiac myosin depends on the nature of the myosin heavy chain mutation in hypertrophic cardiomyopathy. J Muscle Res Cell Motif 18:275–283.

26. Watkins H, Seidman CE, Seidman JG, Feng HS, Sweeney HL. 1996. Expression and functional assesement of a truncated cardiac troponin T that causes hypertrophic cardiomyopathy. J Clin Invest 98:2456–2461.

27. Marian AH, Zhao G, Seta Y, Roberts R, Yu QT. 1997. Expression of a mutant (Arg92Gln) human cardiac troponin T, known to cause hypertrophic cardiomyopathy, impairs adult cardiac myocyte contractility. Circ Res 81:76–85.

28. Bottinelli R, Coviello DA, Redwood CS, Pellegrino MA, Maron BJ, Spirito P, Watkins H, Reggiani C. 1998. A mutant tropomyosin that causes hypertrophic cardiomyopathy is expressed in vivo and associated with an increased calcium sensitivity. Circ Res 82:106–115.

29. Bing W, Redwood CS, Purcell IF, Esposito G, Watkins H, Marston SB. 1997. Effects of two hypertrophic cardiomyopathy mutations in alpha-tropomyosin, Asp175Asn and Glu180Gly, on Ca2+ regulation of thin filament motility. Biochem Biophys Res Commun 236:760–764.

30. Geisterfe-Lowrance AAT, Christe M, Conner DA, Ingwall JS, Schoen FJ, Seidman CE, Seidman JG. 1996. A mouse model of familial hypertrophic cardiomyopathy. Science 272:731–734.

31. Vikstrom KL, Factor SM, Leinwald LA. 1996. Mice expressing mutant myosin heavy chains are a model for familial hypertrophic cardiomyopathy. Mol Med 2:556–567.

32. Tardiff JC, Factor SM, Tompkins BD, Hewett TE, Palmer BM, Moore RL, Schwartz S, Robbins J, Leinwand LA. 1998. A truncated cardiac troponin T molecule in transgenic mice suggests multiple cellular mechanisms for familial hypertrophic cardiomyopathy. J Clin Invest 101:2800–2811.

33. Nishi H, Kimura A, Harada H, Toshima H. Sasazuki T. 1992. Novel missense mutation in cardiac beta-myosin heavy chain gene found in a Japanese patient with hypertrophic cardiomyopahty. Biochem Biophys Res Commun 188:379–387.

34. Harada H, Kimura A, Nishi H, Sasazuki T, Toshima H. 1993. A missense mutation of cardiac beta-myosin heavy chain gene linked to familial hypertrophic cardiomyopathy in affected Japanese families. Biochem Biophys Res Commun 194:791–798.

35. Nishi H, Kimura A, Harada H, Adachi K, Koga Y, Sasazuki T, Toshima H. 1994. Possible gene dose effect of a mutant cardiac beta-myosin heavy chain gene on the clinical expression of hypertrophic cardiomyopathy. Biochem Biophys Res Commun 200:549–556.

36. Kimura A, Harada H, Nishi H, Yasunaga S, Koyanagi T, Koga Y, Imaizumi T, Toshima H, Sasazuki T. 1995. Genetic approaches to identification of a novel responsible gene for familial hypertrophic cardiomyopathy. In Cardiac Development and Gene Regualtion. Ed. Y. Yazaki, 127–144. Tokyo: Excerpta Medica.

37. Kimura A, Nishi H, Harada H, Noguchi M, Ashizawa N, Koga Y, Yano K, Yazaki Y, Kitabatake A, Toshima H, Sasazuki T. 1995. Genetic analysis of hypertrophic cardiomyopathy in Japan. In Developmental Mechanisms of Heart Disease. Ed. EB Clark, RR Markwald, and A Takao, 113–120. New York: Futura Press.

38. Nishi H, Kimura A, Harada H, Matsuyama K, Koga Y, Sasazuki T, Toshima H. 1995. A myosin missense mutation, not a null allele, causes hypertrophic cardiomyopathy. Circulation 91:2911–2915.

39. Kato M, Takazawa K, Kimura A, Ruegg JC, Amano K, Wang Y, Sakaki Y, Toyo-oka T. 1995. Altered actin binding with myosin mutation in hypertrophic cardiomyopathy and sudden death. Lancet 345:1247.

40. Koga Y, Toshima H, Kimura A, Harada H, Koyanagi T, Nishi H, Nakata M, Imaizumi T. 1996. Clinical manifestations of hypertrophic cardiomyopathy with mutations in the cardiac beta-myosin heavy chain and cardiac troponin T genes. J Cardiac Failure 2:S97–S103.

41. Kimura A, Harada H, Nishi H, Koyanagi T, Yasunaga S, Date Y, Nakata M, Imaizumi T, Sasazuki T, Koga Y, Toshima H. 1996. Mutations in seven different genes cause hypertrophic cardiomyopathy in Japanese patients. In An Approach to Diseases. Ed. Y. Niho, 142–151. Fukuoka: Kyushu University Press.

42. Ohsuzu F, Katsushika S, Akanuma M, Nakamura H, Harada H, Satoh M, Hiroi S, Kimura A. 1997. Hypertrophic obstructive cardiomyopathy due to a novel T-to-A transition at codon 624 in the beta-myosin heavy chain possibly related to the sudden death. Int J Cardiol 62:203–209.

43. Kimura A. 1997. Molecular genetics of hypertrophic cardiomyopathy in Japan. Intern Med 36:152–154.

44. Hwang TH, Lee WH, Kimura A, Satoh M, Nakamura T, Kim MK, Choi SK, Park JE. 1998. Early expression of a malignant phenotype of familial hypertrophic cardiomyopathy associated with a Gly716Arg myosin heavy cahin mutation in a Korean family. Am J Cardiol 82:1509–1513.

45. Doi YL, Kitaoka H, Hitomi N, Satoh M, Kimura A. 1999. Clinical expression in patients with hypertrophic cardiomyopathy caused by cardiac myosin-binding protein C gene mutation. Circulation 100:448–449.

46. Anan R, Shono H, Kisanuki A, Arima S, Nakao S, Tanaka H. 1998. Patients with familial hypertrophic cardiomyopathy caused by a Phe110Ile missense mutation in the cardiac troponin T gene have variable cardiac morphologies and a favorable prognosis. Circulation 98:391–397.

47. Rayment I, Rypniewski WR, Schmidt-Base K, Smith R, Tomchick DR, Benning MM, Winkelmann DA, Wesenberg G, Holden HM. 1993. Three-dimensional structure of myosin subfragment-1: a molecular motor. Science 261:50–58.

48. Matsumori A, Ohashi N, Hasegawa K, Sasayama S, Eto T, Fujisawa H, Imaizumi T, Izumi T, Kawamura K, Kawana M, Kimura A, Kitabatake A, Matsuzaki M, Nagai R, Tanaka H, Hiroe M, Hori M, Inoko H, Seko Y, Sekiguchi M, Shimotohno T, Sugishita Y, Takeda N, Takihara K, Tanaka M, Tokuhisa T, Toyooka T, Yokoyama H. 1998. Hepatitis C virus infection and heart disease: a multicenter study in Japan. Jpn Circ J 62:389–391.
49. Matsumori A, Matobe Y, Nishio R, Shioi T, Ono K, Sasayama S. 1996. Detection of hepatitis C cirus RNA from the heart of patients with hypertrophic cardiomyopathy. Biochem Biophys Res Commum 222:678–682.

N. Takeda, M. Nagano and N.S. Dhalla
(eds). The Hypertrophied Heart. Copyright
© 2000. pp. 345–353. Kluwer Academic
Publishers. Boston. All rights reserved.

HEPATITIS C VIRUS INFECTION IN HYPERTROPHIC OR DILATED CARDIOMYOPATHY

AKIRA MATSUMORI

Department of Cardiovascular Medicine, Kyoto University Graduate School of Medicine, 54 Kawaracho Shogoin, Sakyo-ku, Kyoto 606-8397, Japan

Summary. The myocardium may be the target of several types of viral infections. Enteroviruses, particularly coxsackievirus B, are believed to be the most common pathogens responsible for viral myocarditis, but the importance of hepatitis C virus (HCV) infection has been recently noted in patients with hypertrophic cardiomyopathy (HCM) or dilated cardiomyopathy (DCM). In a collaborative research project of the Committees of the Study of Idiopathic Cardiomyopathy, HCV antibody was found in 74 of 697 patients (10.6%) with HCM and in 42 of 663 patients (6.3%) with DCM; these prevalences were significantly higher than those found in volunteer blood donors in Japan. HCV antibody was detected in 650 of 11,967 patients (5.4%) seeking care in five academic hospitals. Various cardiac abnormalities were found, and arrhythmias were the most frequent. These observations suggest that HCV infection is an important cause of a variety of otherwise unexplained heart diseases.

INTRODUCTION

The myocardium is affected in a wide range of viral infections. In some cases, myocarditis may be the primary problem; in others, myocarditis may occur as part of the general disease. Myocarditis is thought to be most commonly caused by enteroviruses, particularly coxsackievirus B. However, in many cases when myocarditis has been assumed on clinical grounds, no definite evidence of viral origin is obtained, despite extensive laboratory investigation. The evidence often is only circumstantial, and direct conclusive proof of cardiac involvement is not available [1–3]. However, accumulating evidence links viral myocarditis with the eventual development of dilated cardiomyopathy [4–8].

Viral myocarditis presents differently. When myocardial necrosis occurs diffusely, congestive heart failure develops and, later, dilated cardiomyopathy. If myocardial lesions are localized, ventricular aneurysm occurs. When complicated with arrhythmia, myocarditis presents as arrhythmogenic right ventricular dysplasia [8,9]. When myocardial necrosis is localized to the subendocardial region, restrictive cardiomy-

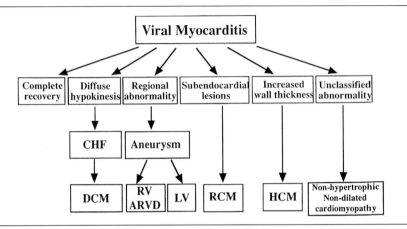

Figure 1. Natural history of viral myocarditis. When myocardial necrosis occurs diffusely, congestive heart failure develops and, later, dilated cardiomyopathy. If myocardial lesions are localized, ventricular aneurysm occurs. When complicated with arrhythmia, myocarditis presents as arrhythmogenic right ventricular dysplasia. When myocardial necrosis is localized to subendocardial regions, restrictive cardiomyopathy may develop. Although it has not been proved yet, hypertrophic cardiomyopathy may be a sequela of viral myocarditis. CHF, congestive heart failure; DCM, dilated cardiomyopathy; RV, right ventricle; ARVD, arrhythmogenic right ventricular dysplasia; LV, left ventricle; RCM, restrictive cardiomyopathy; HCM, hypertrophic cardiomyopathy. (Reproduced from [9], with permission.)

opathy may develop. It has not been proved yet that hypertrophic cardiomyopathy may be a sequela of viral myocarditis, but in fact asymmetrical septal hypertrophy is sometimes seen in patients with myocarditis [10] (figure 1).

The development of molecular biological techniques made possible the detection of viral nucleic acid in small endomyocardial tissue samples. This development has not only strengthened the pathogenetic link between myocarditis and dilated cardiomyopathy but has also provided some evidence that the presence of virus may have prognostic implications [11]. However, reported results have varied widely, probably due to the different detection procedures adopted by the various investigators. This discrepancy emphasizes the need for a detection assay that is reliable, sensitive, and specific. More recently, it has been shown that enterovirus is not a primary cause of dilated cardiomyopathy [12]. Baboonian et al. [13] reviewed the published literature as well as statistical analyses of the cumulative molecular data relating enteroviruses to dilated cardiomyopathy and compared these findings with the information available on the role of enteroviruses in acute myocarditis. Twelve papers reported studies of acute myocarditis, of which 11 found higher percentages of enteroviral RNA positivity in the diseased population, giving an overall odds ratio of 4.4. Seventeen papers reported studies in dilated cardiomyopathy, with 11 recording higher positivity rates in these patients. Cumulative analysis of these data suggests an overall odds ratio of 3.8. The causative role of enteroviruses in acute myocarditis, particularly in children, is supported by meta-analysis of the available literature. However, the data on dilated cardiomyopathy are only suggestive of an association, since a proportion of the studies are negative.

Martin et al. [14] reported that adenovirus was more prevalent (68%) than enterovirus in pediatric patients with acute myocarditis by PCR. Recently, an association of HIV infection with dilated cardiomyopathy has been reported, and the occurrence of dilated cardiomyopathy has been suggested to be related either to a direct action of HIV on the myocardial tissue or to an autoimmune process induced by HIV, possibly in association with other cardiotrophic viruses [15].

HEPATITIS C VIRUS AND DILATED CARDIOMYOPATHY

We evaluated patients with cardiomyopathy and myocarditis by PCR for the presence of RNA viruses such as enterovirus, cardiovirus, hepatitis A virus, human immunodeficiency viruses 1 and 2, human T-lymphocytic leukemia virus I, influenza A and B viruses, and reovirus. We also evaluated patients with cardiomyopathy and myocarditis for DNA viruses such as adenovirus, cytomegalovirus, Epstein–Barr virus, hepatitis B virus, human herpesvirus 6, varicella-zoster virus, and herpes simplex virus types 1 and 2. However, enterovirus RNA was detected in only one patient with dilated cardiomyopathy, and no other virus genomes were found [16]. On the contrary, we found hepatitis C virus (HCV) RNA in six patients with cardiomyopathy. Further studies have suggested the importance of hepatitis C virus infection in cardiomyopathy and myocarditis [16–20].

Over an 8-year period, we identified eight patients (15.1%) with dilated cardiomyopathy who had evidence of HCV infection on the basis of a positive immunoradiometric assay (table 1), whereas only one patient (2.5%) of those with ischemic heart disease was positive for the HCV antibody. The difference was statistically significant. None of the patients with HCV antibody in this study had known risk factors for HCV infection, such as a history of intravenous drug use, previous blood transfusions, acute hepatitis, or abnormal liver function. Mildly elevated levels of serum transaminase were found in four patients. The primary findings at presentation were congestive heart failure and cardiac arrhythmias (table 2). Of the eight patients with HCV antibodies, five patients had HCV RNA in the serum, and all five patients had type 1b HCV, HCV RNA was found in the hearts of five patients. Negative strands of HCV RNA were detected in the heart of three

Table 1. Incidence of antibodies against hepatitis C virus

	M/F	Age (mean ± SD)	Anti-hepatitis C virus antibody	
			Positive/N	Frequency (%)
Dilated cardiomyopathy	32/21	53.2 ± 16.5	8/53	15.1[a]
Hypertrophic cardiomyopathy	41/29	57.7 ± 9.6	11/70	15.7[a]
Ischemic heart disease	1/40	57.7 ± 8.2	1/40	2.5

[a] $p < 0.05$ vs. control, Fisher's exact test.

Table 2. Clinical profiles of patients with dilated cardiomyopathy with positive anti-hepatitis C virus antibody

	Case number							
	1	2	3	4	5	6	7	8
Age	57	22	61	66	61	17	62	49
Sex	F	M	M	F	F	F	F	M
NYHA	III	IV	II	III	III	III	II	III
Onset	CHF	CHF	VT	CHF	CHF	CHF	CHF	CHF
HR	70	75	56	103	102	99	68	60
CI	2.0	2.8	2.5	2.1	3.6	2.0	3.1	2.7
PCWP	15	13	8	27	6	24	8	5
LVEDP	13	18	18	27	4	32	12	12
LVEDVI	157	142	156	222	94	105	84	96
LVEF	25	25	26	24	37	26	35	45
AST (11–27 IU/L)	27	57	21	46	42	17	21	41
ALT (6–27 IU/L)	16	75	28	42	50	8	17	35
Outcome	Died of CHF	Died of CHF	Sudden death	CHF	Improved	CHF	CHF	CHF

CHF, congestive heart failure; VT, ventricular tachycardia; AST, aspartate aminotransferase; ALT, alanine aminotransferase.

Table 3. Clinical profiles of patients with dilated cardiomyopathy with positive anti-hepatitis C virus antibody

	Case number							
	1	2	3	4	5	6	7	8
Anti-HCV Ab	+	+	+	+	+	+	+	+
HCV RNA in serum	+	+	−	+	+	−	+	ND
Type	1b	1b	−	1b	1b	−	1b	ND
Titer	ND	1×10^3	−	2×10^3	8×10^2	−	1.2×10^3	ND
HCV RNA in the heart								
(+) strand	+	+[a]/−[b]	−	+	+	−	+	−
(−) strand	+	−	ND	+	−	−	+	−

[a] Biopsy specimen.
[b] Autopsy specimen.
ND, not done.

patients (table 3). Because negative RNA molecules are considered to be intermediates in the replication of the HCV genome [21], it was supposed that HCV replicates in myocardial tissues.

HEPATITIS C VIRUS AND HYPERTROPHIC CARDIOMYOPATHY

In our study, we found 11 of 70 (15.7%) patients with hypertrophic cardiomyopathy who were positive for HCV antibody (table 1). Of these 11 patients, five were men and six were women; their average age was 59.7 years (range 50–71 years). Three patients had a history of mild hypertension, and one had a family history of hypertrophic cardiomyopathy. Symptoms consisted of chest pain in two patients, exertional shortness of breath in four patients, and palpitation in two patients. Two patients had histories of chronic hepatitis, while the others had no known risk factors for HCV infection, such as a history of intravenous drug use or previous blood transfusions. Mildly elevated serum aminotransferases were measured in six patients. HCV RNA was found in the hearts of all six patients studied, and negative strands of HCV RNA were found in the hearts of two patients. As seen in the heart of patients with dilated cardiomyopathy, the detection of negative strands of HCV in the heart also suggests that the HCV replicates in the heart of patients with hypertrophic cardiomyopathy.

Of the 11 infected patients with hypertrophic cardiomyopathy, six patients had ace of spades-shaped deformities of the left ventricle, showing apical hypertrophy. Apical hypertrophic cardiomyopathy was originally described by Sakamoto [22] and Yamaguchi [23] as a morphologic variant of the disease in which hypertrophy is present predominantly in the apical region of the left ventricle. The present study suggests that HCV infection is an important cause of the apical and other forms of hypertrophic cardiomyopathy.

HEPATITIS C VIRUS INFECTION AND HEART DISEASES: A MULTICENTER STUDY IN JAPAN

As a collaborative research project of the Committees for the Study Idiopathic Cardiomyopathy, under the auspices of the Japanese Ministry of Health and Welfare, a questionnaire was submitted to 19 Japanese medical institutions in 1997, and was returned by 11 participants. The questionnaire inquired specifically about the prevalence of antibody against HCV in patients with dilated and hypertrophic cardiomyopathy. The prevalence of antibody was also measured among all patients seeking care in five academic hospitals. Clinical diagnosis and electrocardiographic and echocardiographic findings were detailed in patients with positive anti-HCV antibody. In addition, the prevalence of the antibody among Japanese volunteer blood donors in 1990 was obtained from the records of the Japan Red Cross Blood Center. The presence of HCV antibody was found in 74 of 697 patients (10.6%) with hypertrophic cardiomyopathy and in 42 of 663 patients (6.3%) with dilated cardiomyopathy (table 4). In contrast, the prevalence of positive HCV antibody among volunteer blood donors 50–59 years of age in November, 1990, was 2.4% (25 of 1039) [24]. Hypertrophic and dilated cardiomyopathies were both associated with significantly higher prevalences of positive antibodies than were measured among blood donors. In addition, positive HCV antibody was more prevalent in patients with hypertrophic cardiomyopathy than in those with dilated cardiomyopathy.

The clinical diagnoses in random patients with positive HCV antibody are listed in table 5. Among several cardiac abnormalities observed in these patients, arrhythmias were the most frequent. Electrocardiographic abnormalities were found in 130

Table 4. Incidence of antibodies against hepatitis C virus in
patients with dilated or hypertrophic cardiomyopathy—a multicenter study

		Anti-hepatitis C antibody	
	Mean age (yr)	Positive/Total (n)	Frequency (%)
Dilated cardiomyopathy	56.5	42/663	6.3[a]
Hypertrophic cardiomyopathy	57.7	74/697	10.6[a,b]
Controls (blood donors)	(50–59)	25/1039	2.4

[a] $p < 0.05$ vs. controls.
[b] $p < 0.01$ vs. dilated cardiomyopathy.

Table 5. Clinical diagnosis of patients
with positive HCV antibody ($n = 349$)

Clinical diagnosis	n	Frequency (%)
Arrhythmia	75	21.5
Hypertension	71	20.3
Myocardial infarction	57	16.3
Diabetes mellitus	50	14.3
Angina pectoris	45	12.9
Renal disease	41	11.7
Valvular heart disease	33	9.5
Congestive heart failure	28	8.0
Hypertrophic cardiomyopathy	23	6.6
Postvalvular replacement and/or CABG	22	6.3
Dilated cardiomyopathy	20	5.7
Cerebrovascular disease	7	2.0
Unclassified cardiomyopathy	2	0.6
Myocarditis	1	0.3

Reproduced from [19], with permission.

of 349 patients tested (62.8%), most often in the form of arrhythmias or conduction disturbances (table 6). Echocardiographic examination suggested that HCV infection was associated with left ventricular hypertrophy in over 50% of the patients, ventricular dilatation in 40%, and decreased left ventricular systolic function in 34% (table 7).

This survey found a high prevalence of HCV antibody in patients with hypertrophic and dilated cardiomyopathy, supporting previous results pointing to the importance of HCV infection in the pathogenesis of cardiomyopathies [16–20]. Interestingly, the prevalence of positive anti-HCV antibody was higher in hypertrophic than in dilated cardiomyopathy. The study also suggests that several cardiac abnormalities other than myopathic disorders—for example, arrhythmias—may result from HCV infection, and that HCV infection may be a risk factor for such conditions (hypertension, myocardial infarction, etc), although further study is necessary to confirm these associations.

Table 6. Electrocardiographic findings
in patients with positive HCV antibody

EKG	n/total	Frequency (%)
Normal	130/349	37.2
LVH	79/219	36.1
ST-T changes	56/219	25.6
Abnormal Q	22/219	10.0
Arrhythmia and conduction disturbance	102/219	46.6
RBBB	42/102	41.2
AV block	29/102	28.4
Af	22/102	21.6
VPC	11/102	10.8
LAD	7/102	6.9
SVT	3/102	2.9

Reproduced from [19], with permission.

Table 7. Echocardiographic findings
in patients with positive HCV antibody

	n/total	Frequency (%)
IVST > 10 mm	110/167	65.9
LVPWT > 10 mm	98/166	59.0
LVDd > 50 mm	113/281	40.2
LVEF < 50%	62/180	34.4
IVST/LVPWT ≧ 1.3	48/166	28.9

Reproduced from [19], with permission.

HCV causes persistent infection and progression to chronicity. The disease is often overlooked, since it may remain remarkably indolent for years, producing few signs and symptoms. These observations suggest that HCV infection is an important cause of various heart diseases of previously undetermined etiologies.

An increasing body of evidence suggests that, in addition to the well-known classic risk factors, some microbial infections may be associated with the development of atherosclerosis and myocardial infarction. Recently, high levels of antibodies against enterovirus-common antigen have been shown to be associated with myocardial infarction, and the study suggests that enterovirus infections increased the risk of myocardial infarction. However, further studies are needed to understand the possible clinical significance of this observation [25].

INTERFERON THERAPY FOR CARDIOMYOPATHIES ASSOCIATED WITH HEPATITIS C VIRUS INFECTION

Our results emphasize the need for studies to determine whether interferon therapy is effective in treating patients with myocarditis and cardiomyopathy who are infected with HCV. Further studies are under way in our institution.

REFERENCES

1. Kawai C, Matsumori A, Fujiwara H. 1987. Myocarditis and dilated cardiomyopathy. Annu Rev Med 38:221–239.
2. Abelmann WH, Lorell BH. 1989. The challenge of cardiomyopathy. J Am Coll Cardiol 13:1219–1239.
3. Olinde KD, O'Connell JB. 1994. Inflammatory heart disease: pathogenesis, clinical manifestations, and treatment of myocarditis. Annu Rev Med 45:481–490.
4. Caforio ALP, Stewart JT, McKenna WJ. 1990. Idiopathic dilated cardiomyopathy. Br Med J 300:890–891.
5. Johnson RA, Palacios I. 1982. Dilated cardiomyopathies of the adult (second of two parts). N Engl J Med 307:1119–1126.
6. Matsumori A, Kawai C. 1982. An experimental model for congestive heart failure after encephalomyocarditis virus myocarditis in mice. Circulation 65:1230–1235.
7. Matsumori A, Kawai C. 1982. An animal model of congestive (dilated) cardiomyopathy: dilatation and hypertrophy of the heart in the chronic stage in DBA/2 mice with myocarditis caused by encephalomyocarditis virus. Circulation 66:377–380.
8. Matsumori A. 1993. Animal models: pathological findings and therapeutic considerations. In Viral Infection of the Heart. Ed. JE Banatvala, 110–137. Kent: Edward Arnold.
9. Matsumori A. 1997. Molecular and immune mechanisms in the pathogenesis of cardiomyopathy. Jpn Circ J 61:275–291.
10. Kawano H, Kawai S, Nishijo T, Shirai T, Inagaki Y, Okada R. 1994. An autopsy case of hypertrophic cardiomyopathy with pathological findings suggesting chronic myocarditis. Jpn Heart J 35:95–105.
11. Why HJF, Meany BT, Richardson PJ, Olsen EGJ, Bowles NE, Cunningham L, Freeke CA, Archard LC. 1994. Clinical and prognostic significance of detection of enteroviral RNA in the myocardium of patients with myocarditis or dilated cardiomyopathy. Circulation 89:2582–2589.
12. Giacca M, Severini GM, Mestroni L, Salvi A, Lardieri G, Falaschi A, Camerini F. 1994. Low frequency of detection by nested polymerase chainreaction of enterovirus ribonucleic acid in endomyocardial tissue of patients with idiopathic dilated cardiomyopathy. J Am Coll Cardiol 24:1033–1040.
13. Baboonian C, Treasure T. 1998. Meta-analysis of the association of enteroviruses with human heart disease. Heart 78:539–543.
14. Martin AB, Webber S, Fricker FJ, Jaffe R, Demmler G, Kearny D, Zhang Y-H, Bodurtha J, Gelb B, Ni J, Bricker JT, Towbin JA. 1994. Acute myocarditis. Rapid diagnosis by PCR in children. Circulation 90:330–339.
15. Barbaro G, Di Lorenzo G, Grisorio B, Barbarini G. 1998. Incidence of dilated cardiomyopathy and detection of HIV in myocardial cells of IV-positive patients. Gruppo Italiano per lo Studio Cardiologico dei Pazienti Affetti da AIDS. N Engl J Med 339:1153–1155.
16. Matsumori A, Matoba Y, Sasayama S. 1995. Dilated cardiomyopathy associated with hepatitis C virus infection. Circulation 92:2519–2525.
17. Okabe M, Fukuda K, Arakawa K, Kikuchi M. 1997. Chronic variant of myocarditis associated with hepatitis C virus infection. Circulation 96:22–24.
18. Matsumori A, Matoba Y, Nishio R, Shioi T, Ono K, Sasayama S. 1996. Detection of hepatitis C virus RNA from the heart of patients with hypertrophic cardiomyopathy. Biochem Biophys Res Commun 222:678–682.
19. Matsumori A, Ohashi N, Hasegawa K, Sasayama S, Eto T, Imaizumi T, Izumi T, Kawamura K, Kawana M, Kimura A, Kitabatake A, Matsuzaki M, Nagai R, Tanaka H, Hiroe M, Hori M, Inoko H, Seko Y, Sekiguchi M, Shimotohno K, Sugishita Y, Takeda N, Takihara T, Tanaka M, Tokuhisa T, Toyo-oka T, Yokoyama M. 1998. Hepatitis C virus infection and heart diseases. A multicenter study in Japan. Jpn Circ J 62:389–391.
20. Matsumori A, Ohashi N, Sasayama S. 1998. Hepatitis C virus infection and hypertrophic cardiomyopathy. Ann Intern Med 129:749–750.
21. Aria KTN, Sallie R, Sangar D, Alexander GJM, Smith H, Byrne J, Portmann B, Eddleston ALWF, Williams R. 1993. Detection of genomic and intermediate replicative strands of hepatitis C virus in liver tissue by in situ hybridization. J Clin Invest 91:2226–2234.
22. Sakamoto T, Tei C, Murayama M, Ichiyasu H, Hada Y. 1976. Giant T-wave inversion as a manifestation of asymmetrical apical hypertrophy (AAH) of the left ventricle. Echocardiographic and ultrasonocardiotomographic study. Jpn Heart J 17:611–629.

23. Yamaguchi H, Ishimura T, Nishiyama S, Nagasaki F, Nakanishi S, Takatsu F, Nishijo T, Umeda T, Machii K. 1979. Hypertrophic nonobstructive cardiomyopathy with giant negative T waves (apical hypertrophy): ventriculographic and echocardiographic features in 30 patients. Am J Cardiol 44: 401–412.

24. Sugiyama Y, Mizui M, Moriya T, Tanaka J, Yoshizawa H. 1992. Epidemiology of HCV infection. Rinshoi 18:544–548 (in Japanese).

25. Roivainen M, Alfthan G, Jousilahti P, Kimpimäki M, Hovi T, Tuomilehto J. 1998. Enterovirus infections as a possible risk factor for myocardial infarction. Circulation 98:2534–2537.

N. Takeda, M. Nagano and N.S. Dhalla
(eds). The Hypertrophied Heart. Copyright
© 2000. pp. 355–362. Kluwer Academic
Publishers. Boston. All rights reserved.

ENHANCEMENT OF EARLY DIASTOLIC FILLING PROVOKED BY DOBUTAMINE INFUSION IN DILATED CARDIOMYOPATHY

SHINGO KUROKAWA, NAOKI TOKITA, MASAHIKO MORIGUCHI,
NAOTO FUKUDA, YOUJI MACHIDA, and TOHRU IZUMI

*Department of Internal Medicine and Cardiology, Kitasato University School of Medicine, 1-15-1, Kitasato,
Sagamihara 228-8555, Japan*

Summary. In considering whether to extend β-blocker therapy to dilated cardiomyopathy, we encountered a valuable case. A 40-year-old man with dilated cardiomyopathy developed heart failure with quite poor systolic function. After administration of β-blocker, his pump function improved. In echocardiographic monitoring before β-blocker therapy, only his early diastolic filling velocity was very responsive to dobutamine loading among functional parameters, including the systolic phase. This finding supports the hypothesis that the enhancement of left ventricular filling by dobutamine loading is a useful predictor in dilated cardiomyopathic patients of whether β-blocker will be effective or not.

During the last decade, β-blocker therapy adjunctive to fundamental drugs has been well developed and has dramatically contributed to improved outcomes for dilated cardiomyopathic patients. In considering whether to extend this therapy, we encountered an outstanding case. The patient responded well to β-blocker therapy. In echocardiographic monitoring before β-blocker therapy, his sensitivity to a β-agonist was very suggestive: although during dobutamine loading his systolic functional parameters could not be further augmented, his early diastolic filling velocity was exceptionally enhanced.

CASE REPORT

A 40-year-old man who was admitted to our hospital for heart failure was checked for underlying disease of chronic heart failure. He had been hospitalized elsewhere twice before this consultation because of congestive heart failure. His past history and family history were not unique. His cardiac function was NYHA III.

Physical examination on admission revealed the following: His blood pressure was 102/50 mmHg, with a regular pulse rate of 72 beats/min. On auscultation, a protodiastolic gallop was documented. Breath sounds were clear, and no peripheral

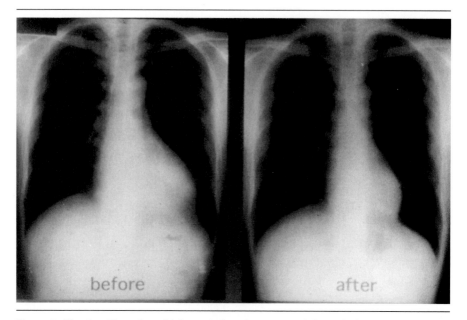

Figure 1. The chest X-ray showed left ventricular enlargement, and the cardiothoracic ratio was 68% on admission. There was no congestion in the lung field (left). Four months after β-blocker therapy, the size of left ventricle distinctly diminished, indicating a cardiothoracic ratio down to 44% (right).

edema was present. Routine hematological study showed normal counts and normal figures. The serum glutamic pyruvic transaminase was 60 IU/L (normal 30–40), serum creatine kinase was 130 IU/L, and C-reactive protein was negative. The plasma concentration of brain natriuretic peptide (BNP) was 220 pg/mL on admission, and this value was moderately higher than normal. Four months later after treatment with β-blocker (metoprolol 60 mg/day), the plasma concentration of BNP improved into the normal level: 9.1 pg/mL.

A chest X-ray showed left ventricular enlargement and the cardiothoracic ratio was 68% on admission (figure 1). Pulmonary congestion was not seen on admission. Four months after administration of β-blocker, the size of his left ventricle distinctly diminished, indicating a cardiothoracic ratio of 44% (figure 1). An electrocardiogram (ECG) on admission revealed sinus rhythm and poor R-wave progression in V1 to V4 leads. This abnormality in ECG remained even after treatment.

A transthoracic two-dimensional echocardiogram taken after fundamental therapy with digitalis glycosides and diuretics for 3 weeks showed diffuse severe hypokinesis at most portions of left ventricle. Severe hypokinesis of the interventricular septum and the left ventricular posterior wall at the papillary muscle level was documented in an M-mode echocardiogram, as shown in figure 2. The left ventricular diastolic and systolic dimension (LVDd and LVDs) were 60 mm and 56 mm, respectively. Fractional shortening of the left ventricle was calculated as 6%. Low-

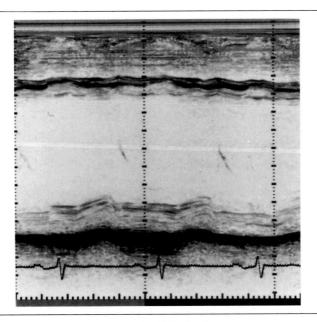

Figure 2. M-mode echocardiogram at rest before β-blocker therapy.

dose dobutamine stress echocardiography was performed to evaluate systolic and diastolic function, specifically, the concentration of dobutamine administered rose from 2.0 μg/kg/min to 8.0 μg/kg/min in increments every 3 minutes (figure 3). Early diastolic filling velocity, E/A ratio, and early diastolic inflow deceleration time were checked before loading. These were measured as 45.5 cm/sec, 0.98, and 87 msec, respectively (figure 4). At the last concentration of dobutamine loading (8.0 μg/kg/min), early diastolic filling velocity (79.5 cm/sec) became much higher than that observed before infusion (figure 5), which resulted in a higher E/A value (1.79). There were no significant changes among systolic parameters even in M-mode echocardiography, as shown in figure 3. After adjunctive treatment with β-blocker for four months, M-mode echocardiogram at the papillary muscle level revealed obvious wall motion improvement, with a decreased size of the left ventricle (LVDd, from 60 to 55 mm; LVDs, from 56 to 42 mm). Consequently, the fractional shortening of the left ventricle was increased up to 24% (figure 6). After β-blocker therapy, early diastolic filling velocity, E/A ratio, and early diastolic inflow deceleration time were 63.9 cm/sec, 1.09, and 170 msec at rest, respectively (figure 7).

Cardiac catheterization was performed before the use of the β-blocker. The coronary angiogram was normal, and the histopathologic features of the biopsy specimens were not specific, i.e., the size of cardiomyocytes varied from large to small, a decrease of myofibrils and a large amount of interstitial fibrosis were remarked, but neither inflammatory infiltrates nor cellular necrosis were seen.

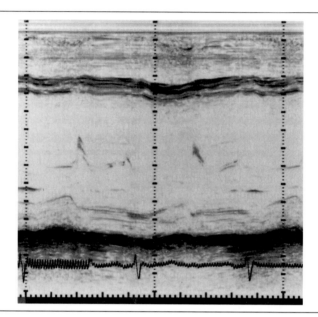

Figure 3. M-mode echocardiogram during dobutamine loading before β-blocker therapy. There was no improvement of the left ventricular wall motion.

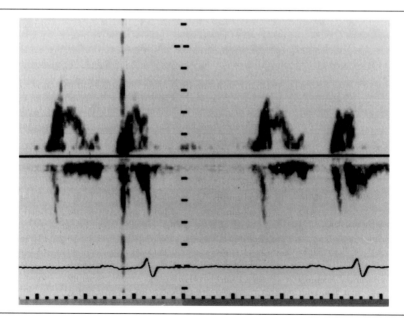

Figure 4. Diastolic inflow filling pattern at rest before β-blocker therapy.

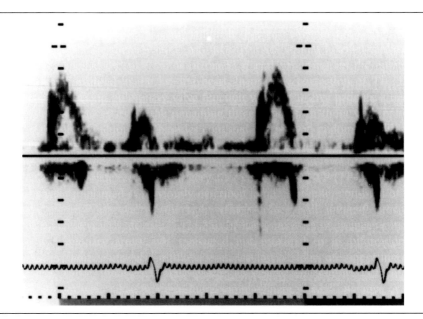

Figure 5. Diastolic inflow filling pattern during dobutamine loading before β-blocker therapy. Significant enhancement of the left ventricular filling velocity can be seen in early diastole.

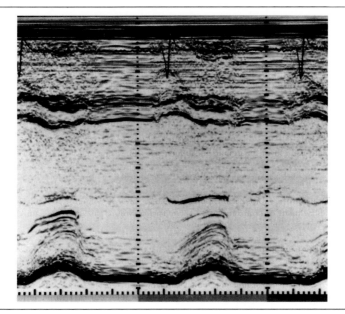

Figure 6. M-mode echocardiogram at the papillary muscle level after β-blocker therapy four months later. Obvious improvement of the wall motion can be seen in both the interventricular septum and left ventricular posterior wall.

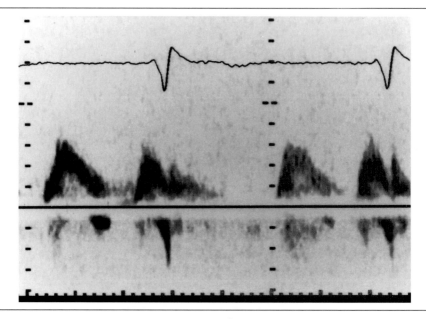

Figure 7. Diastolic inflow filling pattern at rest after β-blocker therapy.

DISCUSSION

Since Waagstein et al. [1] proposed the effect of chronic β-adrenergic receptor blocker in dilated cardiomyopathy, many studies [2–6] have been carried out until now. At present, β-blocker therapy has become an effective treatment for patients with dilated cardiomyopathy, including the serious stage of chronic heart failure. However, there still remain many clinical tasks to be resolved. The most difficult one is how to determine which patients are unable to tolerate β-blocker therapy before administration. To answer this question completely, it is necessary to study the clinical characteristics of good responders to β-blocker therapy. The literature has already emphasized that good responders to β-blocker have tachycardia, a high plasma concentration of catecholamines, interfascicular fibrosis in the biopsies, and amelioration of regional wall motion by dobutamine loading echocardiography [1,2,7–11], but these features are not universal and are not helpful for all dilated cardiomyopathic patients. Generally speaking, β-blockers have been shown to exert a beneficial effect on systolic function in patients with dilated cardiomyopathy, whereas less attention has been paid to the possible beneficial effects on diastolic function. A recent study [12] confirms a reduction in early diastolic filling after β-blocker therapy, with decreases of the E/A ratio and early diastolic inflow deceleration time. These phenomena may be explained by the displacement of filling from the early to the late diastolic phases. This understanding encourages a hypothesis that a decrease in the E/A ratio and an early diastolic inflow deceleration time are very sensitive indicators after β-blocker therapy, and that this tendency will therefore occur in good responders. Unfortunately, however, we cannot predict the effectiveness of such an observation before use of β-blocker therapy. We hypothesize that this change in left ventricular diastolic filling after the therapy elucidates the pharmacological effect of the β-blocker. In the present case, the early diastolic inflow deceleration time was prolonged. Therefore, by using Doppler-obtained left ventricular filling dynamics at rest, we could assess whether the amount of β-blocker was adequate or not. But we failed to predict the effectiveness of β-blocker before its administration.

The β-blocker inhibits specific receptor and blocks transmembrane signal transduction. Contraction and relaxation of the heart are regulated by cytoplasmic Ca^{2+} concentration, and this process is dependent on cyclic AMP. The β-stimulators cause an increase of the cyclic AMP concentration and cytoplasmic Ca^{2+} concentration through a Ca^{2+}-induced Ca^{2+} release mechanism and causes Ca^{2+} mobilization from the sarcoplasmic reticulum. The β-stimulators accelerate both contraction and relaxation of the heart. During dobutamine loading, an overall increase in left ventricular filling velocity occurs in normal subjects. A reduction in early diastolic filling in patients with coronary artery disease has already been reported [13]. The relaxation of the heart is considered as a process of Ca^{2+} reuptake into the sarcoplasmic reticulum. Therefore, the change of Doppler signals obtained during early diastolic filling after dobutamine loading seems reflect the potentiality of the reserved capacity concerning the Ca^{2+} reuptake into the sarcoplasmic reticulum.

It has been indicated that myocardial lesions in dilated cardiomyopathy progress uniformly. However, the abnormality of left ventricular wall motion is often nonuniform. This observation explains why myocardial damage in patients with dilated cardiomyopathy is not similar even when the pump function seems to be damaged to same level. Among the left ventricular segments presenting the same degree of wall motion abnormality at rest, the responses to dobutamine loading are quite different [10]. From our understanding, this nonuniform response has a tendency to be amplified in the diastolic property in comparison with the systolic one, probably because diastolic filling, which may reflect the capacity of Ca^{2+} reuptake into the sarcoplasmic reticulum, is easily stimulated by dobutamine. In the present case, the dobutamine had no effect on the systolic function; in contrast, the loading remarkably accelerated the early diastolic filling velocity. This finding can be interpreted to mean that the β-blocker contributes a beneficial effect to even dilated cardiomyopathic patients in the case of only enhancement of diastolic filling with no augmentation of systolic function by dobutamine loading.

In conclusion, we have given a case report of an outstanding responder to β-blocker therapy who had no beneficial effect on systolic function but who only had an increase of early diastolic filling by dobutamine loading before β-blocker administration. As a result of this experience, we would like to emphasize that when dilated cardiomyopathic patients respond positively to dobutamine loading during early diastole, the β-blocker will still be effective, even if they belong to the group of patients with quite poor systolic function.

ACKNOWLEDGMENTS

This study was supported by a grant from Mitsui Life Social Welfare Foundation of 1997.

REFERENCES

1. Waagstein F, Hjalmarson A, Varnauskas E, Wallentin I. 1975. Effect of chronic beta-adrenergic receptor blockade in congestive cardiomyopathy. Br Heart J 37:1022.
2. Anderson JL. 1988. Treatment of cardiac myopathies with beta blocker. What do we know, where do we go from here? Postgrad Med 29:104–112.
3. Waagstein F, Caidahl K, Wallentin I, Bergh CH, Hjalmarson A. 1989. Long-term β-blockade in dilated cardiomyopathy. Effect of short- and long-term metoprolol treatment followed by withdrawal and readministration of metoprolol. Circulation 80:551–563.
4. Yokota Y, Nomura H, Kawai H, Fukuzaki H. 1992. Effect of long-term β-blockade therapy in patients with dilated cardiomyopathy. Serial clinical and echocardiographic observation. Jpn Circ J 56:52–61.
5. Waagstein F, Bristow MR, Swedlberg K, Camerini F, Fowler MB, Silver MA, Gilbert EM, Johnson MR, Goss FG, Hjalmarson A. 1994. Beneficial effects of metoprolol in idiopathic dilated cardiomyopathy. Metoprolol in dilated cardiomyopathy (MDC) trial study group. Lancet 342:1441–1446.
6. Packer M, Bristow MR, Cohn JN, Colucci WS, Gibert EM, Shusterman NH. 1996. The effect of carvedilol on morbidity and mortality in patients with chronic heart failure. U.S. Carvediol heart failure study group. N Engl J Med 334(21):1349–1355.
7. Cohn J, Levine TB, Olivari MT, Lura D, Francis GS, Simon AB, Rector T. 1984. Plasma norepinephrine as a guide to prognosis in patients with chronic congestive heart failure. N Engl J Med 311:819–823.
8. Engelmeier RS, O'Connel IB, Walsh R, Rad N, Scanlon PJ, Gunnar RM. 1985. Improvement in symptoms and exercise tolerance by metoprolol in patients with dilated cardiomyopathy: a double-blind, randomized, placebo-controlled trial. Circulation 72:536–546.
9. Fowler MB, Bristow MR. 1985. Rationale for beta-adrenergic blocking drugs in cardiomyopathy. AM J Cardiol 55:120D–124D.
10. Nakanishi M, Yokota Y, Fukuzaki H. 1989. Regional wall motion abnormality and its relation to myocardial histopathological change and clinical prognosis in dilated cardiomyopathy. Usefulness of dobutamine loading echocardiography. Jpn Circ J 54:249–259.
11. Yamada T, Fukunami M, Ohmori M, Iwakura K, Kumagai K, Kondoh N, Minamino T, Tsujimura E, Nagareda T, Kotoh K, Hoki N. 1993. Which subgroup of patients with dilated cardiomyopathy would benefit from long-term beta-blocker therapy. J Am Coll Cardiol 21:628–633.
12. Andersson B, Caidahl K, Lenarda A, Warren S, Goss F, Waldenstom A, Persson S, Wallentin I, Hjalmarson A, Waagstein F. 1996. Changes in early and late diastolic filling patterns induced by long-term adrenergic β-blockade in patients with idiopathic cardiomyopathy. Circulation 94:673–682.
13. El-said EM, Roelandt JRTC, Fioretti PM, Mcneill AJ, Forster T, Boersma H, Linker DT. 1994. Abnormal left ventricular early diastolic filling during dobutamine stress Doppler echocardiography is a sensitive indicator of significant coronary artery disease. J Am Coll Cardiol 24:1618–1624.

N. Takeda, M. Nagano and N.S. Dhalla
(eds). The Hypertrophied Heart. Copyright
© 2000. pp. 363–374. Kluwer Academic
Publishers. Boston. All rights reserved.

DNA FRAGMENTATION IS A POSSIBLE MECHANISM FOR HEART FAILURE IN CARDIOMYOPATHY

YOSHIKI SAWA,[1] SATOSHI TAKETANI,[1] NAOMASA KAWAGUCHI,[2] KOJI KAGISAKI,[1] SHUNZO ONISHI,[2] and HIKARU MATSUDA[1]

[1] First Department of Surgery and [2] Applied Physiology, Osaka University Medical School, 2-2 Yamada-oka, Suita, Osaka, Japan

Summary. Involvement of DNA fragmentation in the mechanism for the transition to heart failure in cardiomyopathy was evaluated in six patients with end-stage dilated cardiomyopathy (DCM) and in cardiomyopathic Syrian hamsters (UM-X7.1(UM), $n = 30$). In the clinical study, patients with DCM showed low FS, DNA fragmentation in the nuclei of myocytes as detected by TUNEL staining, change of mitochondrial membrane protein as detected by 7A6 staining, and morphological change of nuclei as evaluated by electron microscopy. In the experimental study, UM showed a significantly higher percentage of DNA-damaged myocytes as evaluated by flowcytometric analysis, change of mitochondrial membrane protein as detected by 7A6 staining, and apoptotic body in terms of the ultrastructure. UM showed apparent histological damages in association with the significant deterioration of cardiac function as compared with the control (C, $n = 30$). These results demonstrated that DNA fragmentation in association with the change of mitochondrial protein related to the deterioration of cardiac function both in patients with end-stage DCM and in cardiomyopathic hamsters. Thus, DNA fragmentation following mitochondrial membrane change may relate to a mechanism for the transition to heart failure in cardiomyopathy.

INTRODUCTION

The myocardium in patients with dilated cardiomyopathy (DCM) is known to deteriorate progressively, leading the reduction of left ventricular contractility. However, the pathogenetic mechanisms responsible for the transition to cardiac dysfunction and heart failure in DCM are as yet not well understood. Patients with end-stage DCM underwent implantation of a left ventricular assist device (LVAD) to prolong their survival until cardiac transplantation. The implantable LVAD has been reported to provide excellent hemodynamic support [1–6] and to decrease neurohormonal hyperreactibility, probably due to improvement in hemodynamic status [2]. However, the LVAD appears to still have some limitations, and further investigation, including elucidation of the mechanisms of DCM, might be needed in order to obtain better clinical results. Apoptosis or DNA fragmentation is an endogenous cellular process by which an external signal activates a metabolic pathway that results in cell death. It is speculated that DNA fragmentation, suggesting apoptosis, may be involved in the pathogenesis of the transition to heart failure in cardiomyopathy. However, this mechanism has never been clarified. In this study, we describe morphological deterioration and DNA fragmentation in Syrian cardiomyopathic hamsters and in patients with end-stage DCM who underwent long-term LVAD support.

CLINICAL STUDY

Study subjects

This study was performed on six patients (age 51.8 ± 6.1 years old). All patients were diagnosed as having end-stage dilated cardiomyopathy. All patients were implanted with a Toyobo–NCVC LVAD (Toyobo, Tokyo, Japan). The Toyobo–NCVC LVAD is an extracorporeal pneumatic diaphragm device made of segmented poly-ether polyurethane and includes Bjork–Shiley inlet and outlet valves. The effective pump stroke volume is 70 mL. All the LVAD implantations were performed under cardiopulmonary bypass. The inflow cannula was placed in the left atrium, and the outflow cannula was approximated to the ascending aorta [7]. Four of these patients died of multiple organ failure within 3 months. One patient died of massive cere-bral hemorrhage at 154 days after implantation. One patient is alive on LVAD support at present.

Echocardiographic studies were obtained at three specific intervals: (1) before LVAD implantation, (2) in the operation room just before and after LVAD implan-tation, and (3) 30 days after LVAD implantation, when the patient was stable on LVAD support. Images were recorded with a Hewlett-Packard SONOS OR and SONOS 1500 (Hewlett-Packard, Andover, MA, USA). Acoustic quantification tech-niques also were used to determine the right ventricular fractional area of change by means of automatic boundary detection [8]. Transgastric or basal views were used to measure left ventricular diastolic diameters (LVDd) and systolic diameters (LVDs), and fractional shortening (FS) was calculated as

(LVDd − LVDs)/LVDd.

The specimens of the left ventricular myocardium were obtained by endomyocar-dial biopsy before the operation, at LVAD implantation, and at autopsy. Before the operation and at LVAD implantation, three pieces of the myocardium with a diam-eter of 2 to 3 mm were obtained from the inside of the left ventricle. Two of the specimens were then embedded in Tissue-Tek (Miles Inc., Elkhart, IN, USA) and placed in liquid nitrogen at −196°C, and one was fixed in 10% neutral formalde-hyde and embedded in paraffin. Eight serial sections were obtained from each spec-imen embedded in paraffin and were stained with hematoxylin and eosin for light microscopic examination. The myocardial cell diameter was determined from 100 measurements of cross-sectioned myocyte at the exact level of the nucleus and calculated with the aid of an image analysis system (SPICCA II, Olympus, Tokyo, Japan) and by using the method of Chalkley [9], Arai [10] and their coworkers. The percent of interstitial fibrosis (% fibrosis) was determined as the average of the ratios of the fibrosis area to the total area from the eight sections, and the fibrosis area was calculated with the use of an image analysis system (SPICCA II, Olympus, Tokyo, Japan).

For immunohistochemical staining of the mitochondria membrane protein 7A6 Ag (a 38 kDa protein localized to the mitochondria membrane) in the myocardium, an enzyme-labeled streptavidin technique was employed that uses sheep polyclonal antibody against a synthetic peptide sequence that is completely conserved in mouse 7A6 Ag (APO2.7, Immunotech, Marseille, France). Briefly, eight sections with a thickness of 4 μm were obtained with the use of Cryostat (HM500, Microme, Germany) from two frozen specimens, mounted on glass slides, immediately fixed in 95% methanol for 2 minutes, and then air dried. These sections were placed in methanolic hydrogen peroxide (0.3%) for 30 minutes. After rinsing for 5 minutes in phosphate-buffered saline (PBS), the sections were exposed to normal rabbit serum to minimize nonspecific binding. Four sections were incubated with the primary antibody (10 μg/mL), as shown above, overnight at 4°C. The sections were then washed three times for 5 minutes with PBS, incubated with the second antibody—the biotinylated rabbit anti-mouse immunoglobulin (Dako, Tokyo, Japan)—for 10 minutes at room temperature, rinsed, and then treated with peroxidase-labeled streptavidin (Dako). The peroxidase activity was visualized in 0.05 M Tris-HCl buffer and 0.01% hydrogen peroxide for 10 minutes at room temperature. The other four sections used as controls were stained without the primary antibody, as described above.

TUNEL staining was performed as follows: eight sections with a thickness of 4 μm were obtained with the use of Cryostat (HM500, Microme) from two frozen specimens, mounted on glass slides, immediately fixed in 95% methanol for 2 minutes, and then air dried. This procedure was used to label the photolysis-induced DNA stained breaks. The samples were processed by using the TdT Kit (ApopTag TM), kindly provided by Oncor Inc (Gaithersburg, MD, USA), as described elsewhere [11,12]. Incorporation of digoxygenin-conjugated dUTP (d-dUTP) into DNA, using this kit, is catalyzed by exogenous TdT; the incorporated d-dUTP is then detected with fluorescein-labeled digoxygenin antibodies [13]. In addition, we also tested the phycoerythrin (PE)-conjugated digoxygenin antibodies (Molecular Probe). DNA was counterstained with 5 μg/mL preputium iodide in the presence of 100 μg/mL DNase-free RNase (Sigma).

To evaluate the degree of expression of DNA fragmentation in the myocardium, 100 nuclei of the myocardial cells were examined randomly and %DNA fragmentation was defined as the number of nuclei in which DNA fragmentation was detected.

For purposes of comparison, normal values for quantitative angiographic and left ventricular function data were obtained form five normal subjects who had undergone catherization for atypical chest pain. Their mean age (± SD) was 44 ± 8 years.

Statistics

Data are expressed as means ± standard deviation (SD). Statistical evaluation was performed by using analysis of variance (ANOVA). Scheffe's test was used for individual comparisons between groups when a significant change was observed by ANOVA. Statistical significance was determined as a p-value less than 0.05.

Clinical results

Baseline and postoperative echocardiograms were available for six patients. In this group, left ventricular dimensions had markedly decreased in all patients (LVDd: 73 ± 14 mm vs. 52 ± 10 mm, $p < 0.01$, before LVAD implantation vs. 30 days after LVAD implantation; see table 1). Left ventricular fractional shortening also was markedly reduced in all patients (0.08 ± 0.03 mm vs. 0.14 ± 0.09 mm, $p < 0.01$; table 1). Intraoperative echocardiography confirmed that the aortic valve die not open during device function and that the left ventricle was unloaded.

The respective mean values for myocardial cell diameter and % fibrosis were 18.5 ± 5.4 μm (range 8 to 22 μm) and 18.5 ± 8.5% (range 12% to 20%) in the myocardium of patients with DCM who underwent cardiac catheterization before the operation (figure 1a; table 2). Both these values increased at LVAD implantation (myocardial cell diameter 22.2 ± 6.8 μm [range 15 to 30 μm]; % fibrosis 28.2 ± 5.5% [range 20% to 36%]; see figure 1b). Further, the increases were observed at autopsy (myocardial cell diameter 34.2 ± 12.8 μm [range 21 to 48 μm]; % fibrosis 40.2 ± 16.3% [range 24% to 56%]; see figure 1c).

These parameters were significantly higher than those for the five normal controls who underwent cardiac catheterization and myocardial biopsy because of suspected coronary artery disease (myocardial cell diameter 8 ± 4.2 μm [range 6 to 12 μm]; % fibrosis 4 ± 4.2% [range 2% to 8%]).

Table 1. LV function before and after LVAD

	Before LVAD implantation ($n = 6$)	30 days after LVAD implantation ($n = 6$)	
LVDd (mm)	73 ± 14	52 ± 10	$p < 0.01$
FS (mm)	0.08 ± 0.03	0.14 ± 0.09	$p < 0.01$

Table 2. Histological change in the serial specimens of the left ventricular myocardium before and after LVAD

	Before LVAD implantation ($n = 8$)	LVAD implantation ($n = 8$)	Autopsy ($n = 8$)	
CD (μm)	18.5 ± 5.4	22.2 ± 6.8	34.2 ± 12.8	$p < 0.01$
% Fb (%)	18.5 ± 8.5	28.2 ± 5.5	40.2 ± 16.3	$p < 0.01$
% TUNEL (%)	0	0.27 ± 0.15	3.1 ± 1.2	$p < 0.01$
APO2.7 positive	0/8	8/8	8/8	
TUNEL positive	0/8	4/8	8/8	

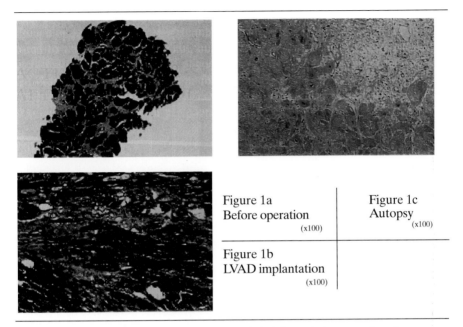

Figure 1a
Before operation
(x100)

Figure 1c
Autopsy
(x100)

Figure 1b
LVAD implantation
(x100)

Figure 1. Histological findings. The serial specimens of the left ventricular myocardium from a representative case are shown. All the samples were stained with hematoxylin and eosin. (**a**) Before LVAD implantation (×100); (**b**) at LVAD implantation (×100); (**c**) at autopsy (×100).

Mitochondria membrane protein was detected by mean of APO 2.7 in the myocardial cells of all patients both at LVAD implantation and at autopsy (figure 2b, 2c), but not before operation, and in none of the normal controls (figure 2a; table 2).

DNA fragmentation was detected by TUNEL in the nuclei of the myocardial cells of six patients at autopsy (% TUNEL positive 3.1 ± 1.2% [range 0.5% to 5.5%]; see figure 3c) and of four patients at LVAD implantation (% TUNEL positive 0.27 ± 0.25% [range 0.01% to 0.5%]), but not before operation, and in none of the normal controls (figure 3a; table 2).

EXPERIMENTAL STUDY

Materials and methods

In this study, cardiomyopathic Syrian hamster (UM-X7.1) and its normal control hamster were used. The UM-X7.1 (UM) group and the control hamster group were evaluated at the ages of 30 days, 60 days, 90 days, 120 days, and 180 days after birth. Both groups had 30 animals. The age-related changes of hypertrophy were evaluated in terms of cardiac weight–body weight ratio and morphological changes using hematoxylin eosin staining.

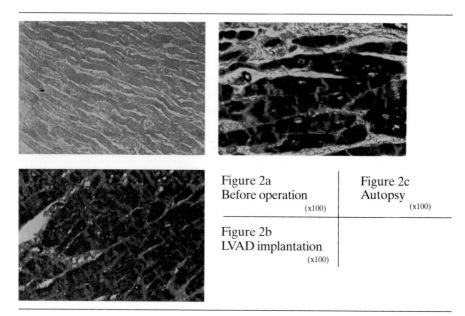

Figure 2a
Before operation
(x100)

Figure 2c
Autopsy
(x100)

Figure 2b
LVAD implantation
(x100)

Figure 2. Expression of mitochondria membrane protein. The serial specimens of the left ventricular myocardium were stained with APO2.7. These specimens were obtained from the same patient as in figure 1. (**a**) Before LVAD implantation (×100); (**b**) at LVAD implantation (×100); (**c**) at autopsy (×100).

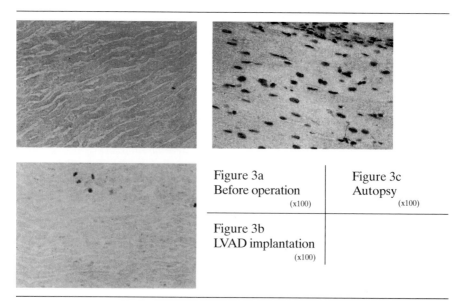

Figure 3a
Before operation
(x100)

Figure 3c
Autopsy
(x100)

Figure 3b
LVAD implantation
(x100)

Figure 3. Expression of TUNEL in the myocardium nuclei. The serial specimens of the left ventricular myocardium were stained by TUNEL. These specimens were obtained from the same patient as in figure 1. (**a**) Before LVAD implantation (×100); (**b**) at LVAD implantation (×100); (**c**) at autopsy (×100).

At age of 120 days after birth, the hearts were isolated and the left ventricular functions were evaluated using the Langendorff perfusion system in both the UM group and control group. DNA fragmentation was assessed by nick and labeling staining and electron microscopy in the tissues, as described above.

To evaluate the DNA damage in myocytes quantitatively, the hearts in both groups were excised and subjected to Langendorff perfusion with acalcemic Krebs–Henseleit buffer. After administration of an enzyme solution containing collagenase, cardiomyocytes were isolated using percoll gradient method and cultured in medium. Then DNA staining was performed as follows: cardiomyocytes were fixed with 70% ice-cold ethanol, then RNase was added. After 30 minutes incubation at 37°C, cells were stained with propidium iodide (PI). Then flow cytometric analyses were made using a FACScan analyzer. DNA analysis was performed as follows: only the viable cells were gated, and the percentage of DNA content less than 2C peak was counted as the DNA damaged cells.

Statistics

Data are expressed as means ± standard deviation (SD). Statistical evaluation was performed by using analysis of variance (ANOVA). Scheffe's test was used for individual comparisons between groups when a significant change was observed by ANOVA. Statistical significance was determined as a p-value less than 0.05.

Experimental results

At 90 days after birth, the UM group showed apparent hypertrophy and significant increase in the ratio of ventricular weight to body weight as compared with the same age group of control hamsters (table 3). The UM group showed apparent increase of fibrosis evaluated by Congo-red staining (figure 4), and its percentage increased significantly 120 days after birth in comparison with the control group.

At 60 days after birth, the UM group showed morphological changes in myocytes, such as myolysis, granulation, and calcification. These changes increased even at 120 days after birth (table 4).

At day 90 after birth, the UM group showed apoptosis in myocytes detected by nick end labeling (figure 5). Moreover, in the electron microscopic findings, apoptotic nuclear body was detected in the UM group (figure 5).

In terms of DNA analysis in isolated hamster myocytes, the UM group showed a significant higher percentage of DNA-damaged myocytes at day 90 after birth than the control group (figure 6).

DISCUSSION

In the clinical study, serial myocardial biopsies showed increases in myocardial cell diameter and intercellular fibrosis even under excellent hemodynamic support by LVAD. A change in mitochondrial membrane protein was detected during LVAD implantation. DNA fragmentation detected by TUNEL staining in the nuclei of myocytes was not detected before LVAD. The results of the experimental study using

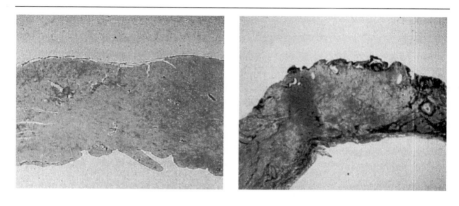

Control (120d)   UM-X7.1 (120d)

Figure 4. Histological finding. All the samples were stained with Congo-red staining. The UM group showed an apparent increase of fibrosis.

Table 3. Change in cardiac weight per body weight

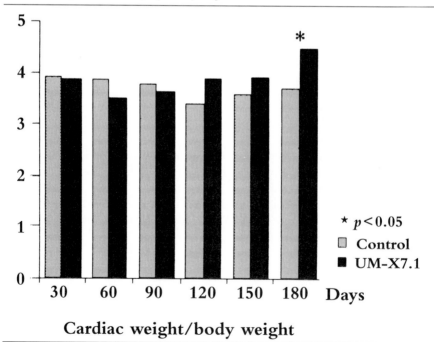

Cardiac weight/body weight

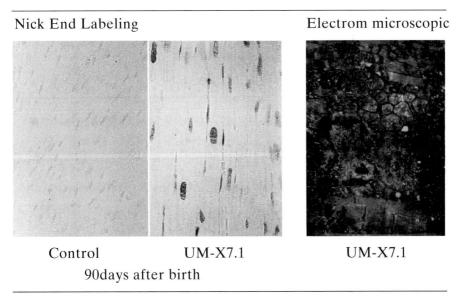

Nick End Labeling   Electrom microscopic

Control   UM-X7.1   UM-X7.1
90days after birth

Figure 5. Expression of TUNEL and electron microscopy in the myocardium nuclei.

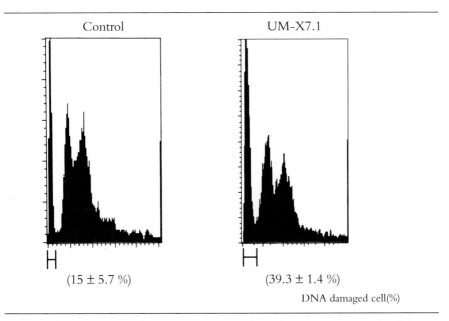

Control   UM-X7.1

(15 ± 5.7 %)   (39.3 ± 1.4 %)

DNA damaged cell(%)

Figure 6. Flow cytometric analysis. Percentage of DNA-damaged myocytes at day 90 after birth: UM group and control group.

Table 4. Histological change in UM group

Days	30	60	90	120	150	180
Myolysis	±	++	+	±	±	±
Granulation	–	+++	++	±	±	±
Calcification	–	++	++	++	±	±

cardiomyopathic Syrian hamster enhanced these clinical results. These results demonstrated that DNA fragmentation in association with the change of mitochondrial protein related to the deterioration of cardiac function both in patients with end-stage DCM and in cardiomyopathic hamsters. Thus, DNA fragmentation following mitochondrial membrane change may relate to a mechanism for the transition to heart failure in cardiomyopathy.

Myocyte cell loss and myocyte reactive hypertrophies are major components of ventricular remodeling in heart failure, and myocyte cell loss has been supposed to relate to apoptosis [14]. Apoptosis is physiologically important in the maturation of organ systems and the renewal of mature cells, as well as in senescence [15–17]. Terminally differentiated cells such as myocardial or neuronal cells are not believed to undergo apoptosis under natural conditions. Zhang et al. reported that cell sorting and DNA fragmentation experiments revealed that 7A6-positive cells, but not 7A6-negative cells, had apparent DNA fragments characteristic of cells undergoing apoptosis. By mean of immunoblotting, under reducing conditions, anti-7A6 detected a 38 kDa protein band in the cell lysate prepared from apoptotic cells. Immunoelectron microscopy showed 7A6 Ag to be localized to the membrane of mitochondria in apoptotic Jurkat cells [18]. Our results indicated that 7A6-positive cells were marked in myocytes in patients with end-stage DCM. These data confirm our hypothesis that mitochondrial change in association with apoptosis may be involved in the pathogenesis of human DCM.

DCM is characterized by dilatation of the left and/or right ventricle, resulting in ventricular dysfunction that is not associated with coronary artery disease, valvular disease, or congenital heart disease; however, the cause of DCM has not been clarified yet [1]. Patients with end-stage DCM show a decrease in left ventricular ejection fraction and may die of congestive heart failure unless they undergo cardiac transplantation, despite full medical treatment. Morphological cellular changes in chronic failure of the myocardium due to DCM have not been systematically described. Schaper et al. reported that the myocardium of DCM is characterized by an increase in interstitial fibrosis, degeneration of hypertrophied myocytes, irregular distribution of desmin in myocytes, and alterations of the cytoskeleton. These histological changes develop progressively and result in myocardial dysfunction and cardiac failure despite medical treatment [17]. Narula and Olivetti have reported that loss of myocytes due to apoptosis (irreversible change) occurs in patients with end-stage cardiomyopathy and may contribute to progressive myocardial hypertrophy and dysfunction [19,20]. Our data coincide with these reports and confirm that patients in the final stage of DCM show progression of apoptosis even under the unloading of LVAD.

This study showed that progressive deterioration of the myocardium is accompanied by increases in myocyte diameter and collagen volume fraction, despite improvement in hemodynamics as a result of LVAD support. The appearance of myocyte disalignment, granulation tissue, and degeneration is associated with DNA fragmentation in patients with DCM even during long-term LVAD support. These data suggest that left ventricular function may not be improved with the implantation of LVAD when DNA fragmentation has already occurred in the heart. Therefore, more fundamental strategies including gene therapy are needed to treat the irreversible damaged myocardium in DCM.

In summary, in patients with end-stage DCM and in cardiomyopathic hamsters, serial myocardial biopsies showed increases in myocardial cell diameter, intercellular fibrosis, and DNA fragmentation in association with changes of mitochondrial protein. These results demonstrated that DNA fragmentation in association with change of mitochondrial protein related to the deterioration of cardiac function both in patients with end-stage DCM and in cardiomyopathic hamster. Thus, DNA fragmentation following mitochondrial membrane change may relate to a mechanism for the transition to heart failure in cardiomyopathy.

REFERENCES

1. Report of the WHO/ISFC task on the definition and classification of cardiomyopathies. 1980. Br Heart J 44:672–673.
2. James KB, McCarthy PM, Jaalouk S, Bravo EL, Betkowski A, Thomas JD, Nakatani S, Fouad Tarazi FMTI. 1996. Plasma volume and its regulatory factors in congestive heart failure after implantation of long-term left ventricular assist devices. Circulation 93:1515–1519.
3. Scheinin SA, Capek P, Radovancevic B, Duncan JM, McAllister HA Jr, Frazier OH. 1992. The effect of prolonged left ventricular support on myocardial histopathology in patients with end-stage cardiomyopathy. ASIO J 38:M271–M274.
4. McCarthy PM, Nakatani S, Vargo R, Kottke Marchant K, Harasaki H, James KB, Savage RM, Thomas JD. 1995. Structural and left ventricular histologic changes after implantable LVAD insertion. Ann Thorac Surg 59:609–613.
5. Frazier OH, Benedict CR, Radovancevic B, Bick RJ, Capek P, Springer WE, Macris MP, Delgado R, Buja LM. 1996. Improved left ventricular function after chronic left ventricular unloading. Ann Thorac Surg 62:675–681.
6. Kormos RL, Murali S, Dew MA, Armitage JM, Hardesty RL, Borovetz HS, Griffith BP. 1994. Chronic mechanical circulatory support: rehabilitation, low morbidity, and superior survival. Ann Thorac Surg 57:51–57.
7. Takano H, Taenaka Y, Noda H, Kinoshita M, Yagura A, Tatsumi E, Sekii H, Sasaki E, Umezu M. 1989. Multi-institutional studies of the National Cardiovascular Center Ventricular Assist System: use in 92 patients. ASAIO Trans 35:541–544.
8. Vandenberg BF, Rath LS, Stuhlmuller P, Melton HE Jr, Skorton DJ. 1992. Estimation of left ventricular cavity area with an on-line, semiautomated echocardiographic edge detection system. Circulation 86:159–166.
9. Chalkley HW, Cornfield J, Park H. 1949. A method of estimating volume surface ration. Science 110:295–297.
10. Arai S, Machida A, Nakamura T. 1968. Myocardial structure and vascularization of hypertrophied hearts. Tohoku J Exp Med 95:35–54.
11. Gorczyca W, Gong J, Darzynkiewicz Z. 1993. Detection of DNA strand breaks in individual apoptotic cells by the in situ terminal deoxynucleotidyl transferase and nick translation assays. Cancer Res 53:1945–1951.

12. Li X, Traganos F, Melamed MR, Darzynkiewicz Z. 1995. Single-step procedure for labeling DNA strand breaks with fluorescein- or BODIPY-conjugated deoxynucleotides: detection of apoptosis and bromodeoxyuridine incorporation. Cytometry 20:172–180.
13. Afanas'ev VN, Korol' BA, Mantsygin YA, Nelipovich PA, Pechatnikov VA, Umansky SR. 1987. Flow cytometry biochemical analysis of DNA degradation characteristic of two types of cell death. FEBS Lett 194:347–350.
14. Kajstura J, Zhang X, Liu Y, Szoke E, Cheng W, Olivetti G, Hintze TH, Anversa P. 1995. The cellular basis of pacing-induced dilated cardiomyopathy. Circulation 92:2306–2317.
15. Wyllie AH. 1980. Glucocorticoid-induced thymocyte apoptosis is associated with endogenous endonuclease activation. Nature 284:555–556.
16. Gottlieb RA, Burleson KO, Kloner RA, Babior BM, Engler RL. 1994. Reperfusion injury induces apoptosis in rabbit cardiomyocytes. J Clin Invest 94:1621–1628.
17. Tanaka M, Ito H, Adachi S, et al. 1994. Hypoxia induces apoptosis with enhanced expression of Fas antigen messenger RNA in cultured neonatal rat cardiomyocyte. Circ Res 75:426–433.
18. Zhang C, Ao Z, Seth A, Schlossman SFA. 1996. Mitochondrial membrane protein defined by a novel monoclonal antibody is preferentially detected in apoptotic cells. J Immunol 157:3980–3987.
19. Narula J, Haider N, Virmani R, DiSalvo TG, Kolodgie FD, Hajjar RJ, Schmidt U, Semigran MJ, Dec GW, Khaw BA. 1996. Apoptosis in myocyte in end-stage heart failure. N Engl J Med 335:1182–1189.
20. Olivetti G, Abbi R, Quaini F, Kajstura J, Cheng W, Nitahara JA, Quaini E, Di Loreto C, Beltrami CA, Krajewski S, Reed JC, Anversa P. 1997. Apoptosis in the failing human heart. N Engl J Med 336:1131–1141.

N. Takeda, M. Nagano and N.S. Dhalla
(eds). The Hypertrophied Heart. Copyright
© 2000. pp. 375–382. Kluwer Academic
Publishers. Boston. All rights reserved.

THE DIFFERENCE IN PHOSPHORYLATION OF DESMIN AND MYOSIN LIGHT CHAIN 2 IN THE BIO14.6 CARDIOMYOPATHIC HEART

TAKUJI HAYAKAWA,[1] HIROAKI MINAMI,[1] SAIJI MASUKAWA,[1]
TADATO NAGANE,[1] KATSURO TAKEUCHI,[1] OSAMU YAHARA,[2]
and KENJIRO KIKUCHI[1]

[1] First Department of Internal Medicine, Asahikawa Medical College, Nishikagura 4-5-3-11, Asahikawa
078-8510, Japan; [2] Douhoku National Hospital, Asahikawa, Japan

Summary. Desmin is one of the intermediate filaments and is important to maintain cell integrity. To investigate the function and regulation of desmin in hypertrophic cardiomyopathic hearts, we determined the content of desmin and measured the change of phosphorylation of desmin and myosin light chain 2 (MLC2) in the Bio14.6 cardiomyopathic hamster at 23 weeks of age by two-dimensional electrophoresis. The content of desmin and phosphorylated desmin was increased significantly in Bio14.6 compared to that of controls. On the other hand, MLC2 was decreased. The decline of phosphorylated MLC2, which attenuates Ca^{2+} sensitivity, seems to be a significant mechanism of hypertrophic cardiomyopathy. Considering the fact that phosphorylation of desmin leads to a disassembly of desmin filament and that dephosphorylation induces formation of it, this result strongly suggested that accumulated phosphorylated desmin might relate to disruption of muscle architecture, weakness, and degeneration of cardiomyocytes.

INTRODUCTION

The intermediate filaments in cardiomyocytes are composed of desmin, a 55 kDa polypeptide that is encoded by a single copy gene. Phosphorylation and dephosphorylation of desmin is very crucial for the assembly–disassembly of intermediate filaments [1]. Phosphorylation leads to disassembly of desmin filaments, and dephosphorylation induces formation of desmin filaments. From clinical study, d'Amati found that the pattern of desmin filaments is altered in hypertrophic cardiomyopathy [2]. Schaper indicated that the amount of desmin was increased, with disorderly arrangement, in the myocardium of dilated cardiomyopathy [3]. Furthermore, Rappaport reported that phosphorylated desmin was accumulated in deltoid muscle of familial myopathy [4]. On the other hand, myosin light chain 2 (MLC2), which is a contractile protein, increases Ca^{2+} sensitivity when phosphorylated [5]. However, it is not well known how the regulation of desmin filament formation and MLC2 phosphorylation exists in the cardiomyopathic hearts. We investigated the level of desmin content and the change of phosphorylation of desmin and MLC2 in the Bio14.6 cardiomyopathic hamster hearts.

MATERIALS AND METHODS

Experimental animals

Six male F1b Syrian hamsters (F1b) and Bio14.6 cardiomyopathic hamsters (Bio14.6) were used at 23 weeks of age. The hamsters were anesthetized with a peritoneal injection of pentobarbital sodium (20 mg/kg). The left and right ventricles were weighed separately and stored at −80°C.

Determination of desmin content

The heart muscles were homogenized with 8M guanidine hydrochloride, followed by dialysis with 7M urea solution. This solution was centrifuged at 14,000 rpm for 15 minutes, and the supernatant was employed as the sample. After prerun, isoelectric focusing gel electrophoresis was done according to the method of Hirabayashi, using agarose in the first dimension [6]. First-dimension electrophoresis was carried out at 500 V (constant) for 16 hours. The prepared gels were removed and put on a plate gel for second-dimension electrophoresis. Electric equilibrium was obtained with agarose as a fixative to which SDS, glycerol, and 2-mercaptoethanol were added. The slab gel was composed in a similar way to that of Laemmli. After being submitted to the second electrophoresis for 6 hours, the slab gels were stained with 0.13% Coomassie Brilliant Blue R-250 (CBBR)/45% ethanol/9.2% acetic acid solution overnight and then destained by constantly stirring with 5% ethanol/7.5% acetic acid solution at 37°C. Each structural protein spot of cardiac muscle was identified according to the observation reported by Hirabayashi [6] and Murakami [7].

Determination of phosphorylated desmin

The heart muscles were homogenized with 8M urea solution. This solution was centrifuged at 3000 rpm for 15 minutes, and the supernatant was employed as a sample. The first-dimension electrophoresis was performed using the method of Hubbard [8]. Electrophoresis was carried out at 500 V for 15 hours and 800 V for 55 minutes. The second-dimension electrophoresis, staining, and destaining were done according to the same method of evaluating desmin content.

Determination of phosphorylated myosin light chain 2

The frozen heart muscles were powdered in liquid nitrogen, immediately homogenized in 10% TCA, and stirred for 15 minutes on ice. This solution was centrifuged at 5000 rpm for 10 minutes, and the supernatant was discarded. The precipitation was washed with ethanol/ether solution, then centrifuged at 3000 rpm for 10 minutes. The protein pellet was dissolved with 7M urea solution, then centrifuged at 3000 rpm for 10 minutes, and the supernatant was employed as the sample. First-dimension electrophoresis was performed according to the method of Morano [9]. The second-dimension electrophoresis, staining, and destaining were done according to the method of determinating desmin content described above.

Quantitation of CBBR-stained proteins

Each spot was cut out and weighed. Then 25% pyridine solution appropriate to its weight was added to it, according to the method of Murakami [7] and Fenner [10]. The CBBR that was bound to the protein was extracted by agitating the sample slowly overnight. Absorption was analyzed at 605 nm to measure the protein content and percentage of phosphorylation of desmin and MLC2.

Protein determination

The protein concentration of the heart muscles used as a specimen was determined by the modified Lowry method, using bovine serum albumin (BSA) as a standard.

Statistical analysis

Results are expressed as mean ± S.E. To test statistical significance, Student's t-test was used, and the difference was judged significant at $p < 0.05$.

RESULTS

Body weight and heart weight (table 1)

The body weight of Bio14.6 was decreased significantly compared to that of aged-matched F1b. The heart weight of Bio14.6 was increased significantly compared to that of controls. The ratio of body weight to heart weight of Bio14.6 was increased significantly compared to that of F1b. These data showed that the hearts of Bio14.6 at the age of 23 weeks were hypertrophied.

Determination of desmin content

Figure 1 shows a representative example of a two-dimensional electrophoretogram focused on desmin. The desmin spot of Bio14.6 was prominently enlarged compared with that of control. The desmin content of F1b hearts was 8.7 ± 4.4 pmol/mg

Table 1. A comparison of F1b and Bio14.6 at 23 weeks

23 weeks	F1b	Bio14.6
B.W. (g)	127.5 ± 8.4	130.0 ± 14.1[a]
H.W. (mg)	401.6 ± 15.6	486.5 ± 64.1[a]
LV.W. (mg)	282.9 ± 15.4	360.1 ± 48.5[a]
RV.W. (mg)	43.8 ± 11.2	95.0 ± 15.5[a]
H.W./B.W. (mg/g)	3.16 ± 0.12	3.80 ± 0.29[a]

[a] Significant difference ($p < 0.05$) in comparison with F1b.
Values are mean ± S.E. B.W., body weight; H.W., heart weight; LV.W., left ventricular weight; RV.W., right ventricular weight.

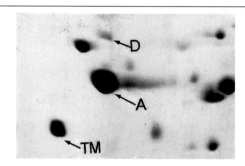

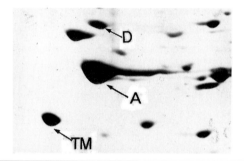

Figure 1. Two-dimensional electrophoretogram of left ventricular myocardium of F1b and Bio14.6 cardiomyopathic heart. D, desmin; A, actin; TM, Tropomyosin.

protein, while that of Bio14.6 was 15.6 ± 4.8 pmol/mg protein. The desmin of Bio14.6 cardiomyopathic hearts at the age of 23 weeks was increased significantly compared with that of controls.

Phosphorylated desmin

Figure 2 shows a two-dimensional electrophoretogram presenting phosphorylated and dephosphorylated desmin. Phosphorylated desmin of the F1b myocardium was 35.8 ± 4.2% and that of Bio14.6 was 50.3 ± 1.3%. Phosphorylated desmin of Bio14.6 was increased markedly compared to that of controls.

Phosphorylated MLC2

A two-dimensional electrophoretogram demonstrates phosphorylated and dephosphorylated MLC2 (figure 3). Phosphorylated MLC2 of the myocardium of F1b was 24.9 ± 6.0% and that of Bio14.6 was 17.8 ± 8.2%. Phosphorylated MLC2 of the myocardium of the Bio14.6 was decreased significantly compared to that of controls.

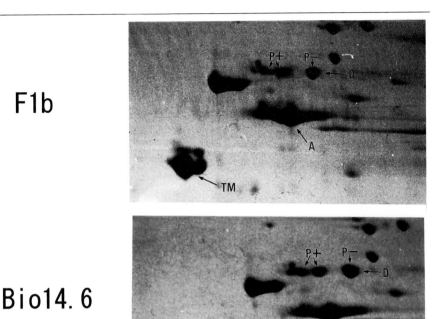

Figure 2. Two-dimensional electrophoretogram of phosphorylated and dephosphorylated desmin of F1b and Bio14.6 cardiomyopathic heart. P+, phosphrylated form; p−, dephosphorylated form.

DISCUSSION

Desmin is known to be a cytoskeletal element that forms an interlinking transverse scaffold around the myofibrils at the Z-disc level, with connections to the sarcolemma and to the nuclear membrane. The content of desmin varies considerably among the different muscle tissues. The myocardium contains much more desmin than skeletal muscles, probably because the intermediate lattice provides elasticity, limits cell distortion in cell that change shape over 60 times a minutes, and resists the intermittent severe tension. Immunoelectron microscopic study demonstrated an increased amount of desmin, oriented longitudinally either in the intermyofiblillar space linking Z bands or along digitations of the intercalated discs connecting neighboring desmosomes in the experimental hypertrophied rat heart [11]. In a previous study, we demonstrated the increase in desmin content of the hypertrophied right ventricle exposed to hypoxia [12] and of the noninfarcted hypertrophied left ventricle after myocardial infarction in rat [13]. Recent studies of desmin knockout mice demonstrated that, although such mice develop and reproduce normally,

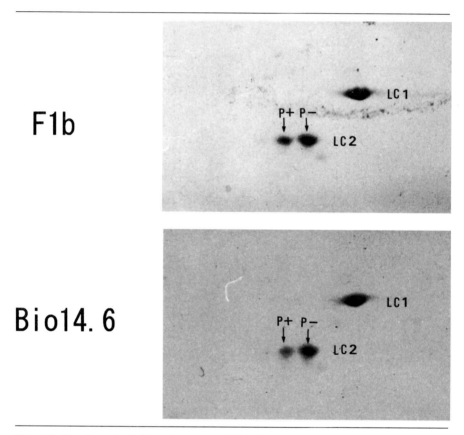

Figure 3. Two-dimensional electrophoretogram of phosphorylated and dephosphorylated myosin light chain 2 (MLC2) of F1b and Bio14.6 cardiomyopathic heart. P+, phosphorylated form; p–, dephosphorylated form; LC1, myosin light chain 1; LC2, myosin light chain 2.

cardiovascular lesions and skeletal myopathy were observed in growing and adult stages [14,15]. These results strengthen the notion that desmin filaments are required to maintain the integrity of the cardiomyocytes.

At present, no disease has been found to be directly related to lack of desmin in humans. However, severe myopathies have been described in which desmin filaments are disrupted, increased, and arranged in a disorderly way. In this study, we investigated the pathophysiological importance of desmin in hypertrophic cardiomyopathy using Bio14.6 cardiomyopathic hamster. First, we determined the amount of myocardial desmin using our modified two-dimensional electrophoresis and found that the desmin content was increased in the cardiomyopathic heart compared to that of controls. This result in animal models is compatible with the information gained in human specimens, namely, that desmin accumulates in hypertrophic cardiomyopathic hearts.

Concerning the formation of desmin filaments, Geisler [16] and Inagaki [1] reported that phosphorylation of desmin induced disassembly of desmin filaments and dephosphorylation of desmin led to formation of it. Rapaport reported the storage of phosphorylated desmin in the skeletal muscle biopsies of a familial myopathy [4]. On the other hand, our previous study demonstrated that dephosphorylated desmin was increased in noninfarcted areas of the hypertrophied left ventricle [13]. In our second examination, we analyzed the phosphorylated and dephosphorylated form of desmin in the cardiomyopathic hearts and found that the amount of phosphorylated desmin was increased compared to those of controls. This result indicates that the accumulation of phosphorylated desmin, which loses the ability to form intermediate filaments, may be one of the important reasons for disruption of muscle architecture, weakness, and degeneration of cardiomyocytes in hypertrophied cardiomyopathy.

Phosphorylation of MLC2 is known to play an important part in the modulation of force production in cardiac muscle. Phosphorylation of MLC2 increases Ca^{2+} sensitivity. Morano demonstrated the decline in phosphorylation of MLC2 in spontaneously hypertensive rats [17]. Liu found a decline in phosphorylated MLC2 in the left ventricle after experimental myocardial infarction [18] and indicated that depressed phosphorylation of MLC2 is related to impaired cardiac performance. Our result—that phosphorylated MLC2 was decreased in 23-week-old Bio14.6 hearts— suggests that the depression in phosphorylation of MLC2 had already begun even in the hypertrophied stage, not the heart failure stage, and that this was the significant mechanism leading to heart failure.

This study demonstrated different changes in two proteins: phosphorylated desmin was increased but phosphorylated MLC2 was decreased. In vitro, phosphorylation of desmin is reported to be dependent on the kinase activity of PKA, PKC, and cdc2 kinase [19]. On the other hand, MLC2 is phosphorylated by a Ca^{2+}–calmodulin-dependent myosin light chain kinase (MLCK), which requires both calcium and calmodulin for activation [6]. Dephosphorylation of MLC2 is catalyzed by a myosin light chain phosphatase [5]. Furthermore, recent studies inform us that PKC may play a role in the phosphorylation of MLC2. In considering why the phosphorylation of these two proteins moved in opposite directions, one explanation is that, although some kinase surely phosphorylates both proteins, phosphorylation of these two proteins is primarily done by different kinases, as indicated above. Mohammadi insists that PKC activity and expression declines in rabbit left ventricular hearts [20]. Similarly, the other possible explanation is the abnormality of signal transduction in the cardiomyopathic hypertrophied heart. Further investigation of signal transduction, focused especially on phosphorylation of these proteins, will lead to a greater understanding of the pathophysiological importance of intermediate filaments and contractile proteins in cardiomyopathic hearts.

REFERENCES

1. Inagaki M, Gonda Y, Matsuyama M, Nishizawa K, Nishi Y, Sato C. 1988. The role of phosphorylation on the assembly–disassembly of desmin. J Biol Chem 263:5970–5978.

2. Francalanci P, Gallo P, Bernucci P, Silver MD, d'Amati G. 1995. The pattern of desmin filaments in myocardial disarray. Hum Pathol 26:262–266.
3. Schaper J, Froede R, Hein S, Buck A, Hashizume H, Speiser B, Friedl A, Bleese N. 1990. Impairment of the myocardial ultrastructure and changes of the cytoskeleton in dilated cardiomyopathy. Circulation 83:504–514.
4. Rappaport L, Contard F, Samuel JL, Delcayre C, Marotte F, Tome F, Fardeau M. 1988. Storage of phosphorylated desmin in a familial myopathy. FEBS Lett 231:421–425.
5. Sweeney HL, Bowman BF, Stull JT. 1993. Myosin light chain phosphorylation in vertebrate striated muscle: regulation and function. Am J Physiol 264:C1085–C1095.
6. Hirabayashi T, Tamura R, Mitsui I, Watanabe Y. 1983. Investigation of actin in Tetrahymena cells. A comparison with skeletal muscle actin by a devised two-dimensional gel electrophoresis method. J Biochem 93:461–468.
7. Murakami U, Uchida K. 1985. Contents of myofibrillar proteins in cardiac, skeletal, and smooth muscle. J Biochem 98:187–197.
8. Hubbard BD, Lazarides E. 1979. Copurification of actin and desmin from chicken smooth muscle and their copolymerization in vitro to intermediate filaments. J Cell Biol 80:166–182.
9. Morano I, Arndt H, Gartner C, Ruegg JC. 1988. Skinned fibers of human atrium and ventricle: myosin isoenzymes and contractility. Circ Res 62:632–639.
10. Fenner C, Traut RR, Mason DT, Wikman-Coffelt J. 1975. Quantification of Coomassie Blue stained proteins in polyacrylamide gels based on analyses of eluted dye. Anal Biochem 63:595–602.
11. Watkins SC, Samuel JL, Marotte F, Bertier-Savalle B, Rappaport L. 1987. Microtubles and desmin filaments during onset of heart hypertrophy in rat: a double immunoelectron microscope study. Circ Res 60:327–336.
12. Minami H, Yahara O, Nagane T, Matsumoto H, Nakano H, Osanai S, Akiba Y, Takeda A, Hayakawa T, Yamashita H, Onodera S, Kikuchi K. 1994. Structural proteins in the hypertrophied right ventricle exposed to hypoxia. Analysis by two-dimensional electrophoresis. In The Adapted Heart. Ed. M Nagano, N Takeda, NS Dhalla, 161–171. New York: Raven Press.
13. Nagane T, Minami H, Yahara O, Masukawa S, Hayakawa T, Kikuchi K. 1996. Alteration in structural proteins in noninfarcted region during remodeling after myocardial infarction. Analysis by two-dimensional electrophoresis. Jpn J Electrophoresis 40:13–20.
14. Li Z, Colucci-Guyon E, Pincon-Raymond M, Mericskay M, Pournin S, Paulin D, Babinet C. 1996. Cardiovascular lesions and skeletal myopathy in mice lacking desmin. Dev Biol 175:362–366.
15. Milner DJ, Weitzer G, Tran D, Bradley A, Capetanaki Y. 1996. Disruption of muscle architecture and myocardial degeneration in mice lacking desmin. J Cell Biol 134:1255–1270.
16. Geisler N, Weber K. 1988. Phosphorylation of desmin in vitro inhibits formation of intermediate filaments; identification of three kinase A sites in the aminoterminal head domain. EMBO J 7:15–20.
17. Morano I, Monika L, Lengsfeld M, Ganten U, Ganten D, Ruegg JC. 1988. Chronic hypertension changes myosin isoenzyme pattern and decreases myosin phosphorylation in the rat heart. J Mol Cell Cardiol 20:875–886.
18. Liu X, Shao Q, Dhalla NS. 1995. Myosin light chain phosphorylation in cardiac hypertrophy and failure due to myocardial infarction. J Mol Cell Cardiol 27:2613–2621.
19. Kusubata M, Matsuoka Y, et al. 1993. Cdc2 kinase phosphorylation of desmin at three serine/threonine residues in the amino-terminal head domain. Biochem Biophysiol Res Commun 190(3):927–934.
20. Mohammadi K, Rouet-Benzineb P, Laplace M, Crozatier B. 1997. Protein kinase C activity and expression in rabbit left ventricular hypertrophy. J Mol Cell Cardiol 29:1687–1694.

N. Takeda, M. Nagano and N.S. Dhalla
(eds). The Hypertrophied Heart. Copyright
© 2000. pp. 383–392. Kluwer Academic
Publishers. Boston. All rights reserved.

CARDIAC REMODELING IN CARDIOMYOPATHIC HAMSTER HEARTS

HIDEAKI KAWAGUCHI

Department of Laboratory Medicine, Hokkaido University, School of Medicine, N-15, W-7, Kita-ku, Sapporo 060-8638, Japan

Summary. Recent reports have shown that angiotensin-converting enzyme inhibitors have a role in cardiac remodeling and have beneficial effects on congestive heart failure. But calcium antagonist therapy has been controversial in the treatment of congestive heart failure. The present study examined the effects of the calcium antagonist amlodipine on the morphological changes in the cardiac muscle cells and extracellular matrix and on progressive left ventricular dysfunction in cardiomyopathic hamsters. The effects of amlodipine were compared with enalapril.

Between the ages of 5 and 20 weeks, BIO53.58 hamsters (dilated model of cardiomyopathy) received orally either 20 mg/kg/day of enalapril or 10 mg/kg/day of amlodipine. During the study period, cardiac function of hamsters were assessed by echocardiography. At 20 weeks of age, each heart was fixed, and serial sections were stained.

At 20 weeks of age, the left ventricular percent fractional shortening (%FS) significantly improved in the enalapril group ($26.7 \pm 4.6\%$, $p < 0.05$) and in the amlodipine group ($35.2 \pm 5.0\%$, $p < 0.0001$) compared with the control group ($20.8 \pm 4.0\%$). The left ventricular diastolic dimension (LVDd) significantly decreased in the enalapril group (6.1 ± 0.4 mm, $p < 0.05$) and in the amlodipine group (5.5 ± 0.8 mm, $p < 0.001$) compared with the control group (6.8 ± 0.4 mm). The fibrous tissue volume tended to decrease, and the ratio of fibrous tissue to ventricular volume significantly decreased in the amlodipine group ($11.2 \pm 1.8\%$, $p < 0.05$) compared with the no-treatment group ($14.6 \pm 1.9\%$). At 20 weeks of treatment with amlodipine, the fibrous tissue volume significantly decreased (15.4 ± 2.8 mm^3, $p < 0.05$) compared with the control group (21.0 ± 2.4 mm^3).

Enalapril and amlodipine can prevent progressive remodeling and can reduce cardiac dysfunction in cardiomyopathic hamsters (BIO53.58). Enalapril is not as effective as amlodipine for prevention of cardiac remodeling in cardiomyopathic hamsters.

INTRODUCTION

The accumulation of fibrillar collagen in the cardiac interstitium is one of the major morphological features of left ventricular hypertrophy accompanied by genetic hypertension, acquired hypertension, and myocardial infarction. This morphological change is called *structural remodeling*, and it may account for the abnormal ventricular function that eventually leads to congestive heart failure. Several lines of evidence suggest that both circulating and tissue renin–angiotensin systems may be involved in the remodeling of the myocardium. Treatment with only a low dose of angiotensin-converting enzyme (ACE) inhibitor, without subsequent lowering of the blood pressure, causes a decrease in left ventricular hypertrophy [1]. Treatment with the ACE inhibitor lisinopril has been shown to reverse interstitial collagen accumulation in spontaneously hypertensive rats with established left ventricular hypertrophy [2]. These results suggest that angiotensin II acts as a growth factor for myocytes and other cells in the heart. Angiotensin II may affect ventricular remodeling by acting as a growth factor, as previously suggested, thus promoting myocyte hypertrophy [3]. Several clinical [4,5] and experimental [2,6] studies have demonstrated that ACE inhibitor suppresses cardiac fibrosis.

Protective effects of verapamil in cardiomyopathic Syrian hamsters have been reported [7–11]. But calcium antagonist therapy has been controversial in the treatment of congestive heart failure. The negative inotropic action and the vasorelaxing effect of the drug and its consequent reflex augmentation of beta-adrenergic activity are thought to lead to the deterioration of heart failure. A recent clinical trial demonstrated a beneficial effect of amlodipine on heart failure. There are several reports that the negative inotropic action of amlodipine is weak and that it does not augment beta-adrenergic activity. But the effect of amlodipine on cardiac remodeling is not clear. And it is expected that amlodipine exerts its beneficial effects by improving intracellular calcium handling in the failing heart.

We evaluated the calcium antagonist amlodipine for its effects on morphological changes in cardiac muscle cells and in the extracellular matrix, as well as on progressive left ventricular dysfunction, in an animal model of dilated cardiomyopathy comparing the effects of long-term treatments with the ACE inhibitor enalapril.

MATERIALS AND METHODS

Experimental animals

The BIO53.58 strain of cardiomyopathic golden Syrian hamsters develops abnormalities of the cardiac and skeletal muscles that are inherited as an autosomal recessive trait [12]. Between 4 and 20 weeks of age, BIO53.58 hamsters gradually develop cardiac dilation that is accompanied by diffuse cell death. This strain also has a significantly shorter life span and demonstrates reduced cardiac function at an earlier age than the hypertrophic cardiomyopathic hamster (BIO14.6 hamster) [13,14].

In contrast to the BIO14.6 hamster, BIO53.58 hamsters do not develop myolysis or hypertrophy before dilation [15]. Therefore, the BIO53.58 hamster provides a good model of cardiac dilation and congestive heart failure. Experiments were carried out using 50 male, dilated cardiomyopathic hamsters (BIO53.58) aged 5 weeks (BIO Breeders, Fitchburg, MA, USA). Male F1b hamsters ($n = 50$), a noncardiomyopathic F1 hybrid of BIO1.5 and BIO87.2 hamsters, were used as controls. BIO53.58 hamsters were randomly assigned to one of three groups, receiving either enalapril (20 mg/kg/day po, BANYU Pharmaceutical Co., Ltd.), amlodipine (10 mg/kg/day po, Pfizer Pharmaceutical Co., Ltd.), or no treatment. The study period was 15 weeks in the enalapril group and in the amlodipine groups.

During the study period, we performed transthoracic echocardiography on each hamster under urethane anesthesia (0.5 mg/g body weight intraperitoneal injection) with an ultrasound system (Hitachi EUB565A), using a 7.5 MHz sector scanner. We recorded M-Mode echocardiograms at the chorda level, measured the left ventricular diastolic dimension and left ventricular systolic dimension using the conventional "leading edge" method [16], and calculated percent fractional shortening (%FS) as the percent difference between the left ventricular diastolic (LVDd) and systolic (LVDs) dimensions:

$$\%FS = 100 \times (LVDd - LVDs)/LVDd.$$

Histological analysis

Hamsters from each group were also used for histological analysis. The ventricles and atria were excised from each heart, and the blood was carefully washed out with saline. Hearts were fixed with 10% formaldehyde, embedded in paraffin after dehydration through a graded alcohol series, and sectioned transversely using a microtome (Leitz Wetzlar: 33776) from the atria to the apex in 8 μm serial sections. The sections were stained with Gomori's aldehyde fuchsin using the Masson–Goldner method [17] and periodic acid shiff (PAS)-hematoxylin for light microscopy.

Cardiac tissue volumes were determined by a point counting method [18,19]. The sections were picked up at 400 μm intervals from serial sections and enlarged to 44× with a light microscope projector on a sheet of paper that had regular triangle lattice of points spaced 20 mm from the nearest neighbors. At such a magnification, each point is 0.45 mm apart in the sections and represents a hexagonal area of 0.45 mm × 0.45 mm × $\sqrt{3}/2$ mm^2. The numbers of points lying in the myocytes, nonmyocytes, calcified area, or fibrotic area projected on the paper were counted. The volume (V) was obtained from the sum of the points, the representative area (a) for one point and the sectional interval being

$$V(mm^3) = \sum(point \times a \times 0.4 \, mm)$$

The volume of ventricles (VV) was largely divided into the volume of myocytes (MV) and the other space (NMV):

$$VV(mm^3) = MV(mm^3) + NMV(mm^3)$$

In the present study, because the volume of nonmyocytes was negligibly small compared with the volume of fibrous tissue and calcified lesions, NMV was considered as the volume of fibrous tissue and calcified lesions. VV, MV, NMV, and the NMV to VV ratio (= NMV/VV × 100) were calculated.

Histometry

The section that had the largest diameter of the left ventricle was selected from the serial sections to measure myocyte breadth and to count nuclear density.

Short diameters of myocytes were measured using an eyepiece micrometer with a 1 μm scale at a magnification of 1000×. Lines that ran transversely on the left ventricular wall were selected from the anterior, lateral, posterior, and septal wall. The myocyte diameters were measured along each line from epicardium to endocardium. The mean value was used as a representative for each specimen.

Numbers of myocyte nuclei were counted in 16 randomly selected fields from the left ventricular myocyte space through an eyepiece with a 250 μm square micrometer at a magnification of 400× under the light microscope. The nuclei that seemed to be degenerated were not counted. Numbers of nuclei calculated per square millimeter were used as the density of viable myocytes.

DNA probes

Three cDNA probes were used for Northern blot analyses; a probe for cardiac ryanodine receptor mRNA, a 1348 bp Hind III fragment of pHRR105 (Recombinant Bluescript KS plasmid) [20] corresponding to nucleotides 5071–6418 of the rabbit cardiac RyR cDNA; a probe for phospholamban mRNA, a 159 bp fragment corresponding to nucleotides of coding region of BIO53.58 hamster phospholamban cDNA, which was cloned by our group as below; and a probe for glyceraldehyde-3-phosphate dehydrogenase mRNA, an Xba I/Hind III fragment of cDNA (#57091, American Type Culture Collection, Rockville, MD, USA). All cDNA probes were uniformly labeled with random primers using Klenow and α-P32dCTP to a specific activity of more than 105 cpm/mg.

The phospholamban cDNA probe was cloned from BIO53.58 hamster heart total RNA. Sense and antisense primers—PHL-185S (ATGGAAAAAGTCCAATACCT) and PHL-343A (TCACAGAAGCATCACAATGA), respectively—were designed based on the published sequence for the rat heart phospholamban [21] (numbers designating each oligonucleotide refer to the position in the published sequence). First-strand cDNA was synthesized using 1 μg of total BIO53.58 hamster heart RNA and 3 μg of random primer (BIBCO BRL Cat. No. 48190-011) with moloney murine leukemia reverse transcriptase at 37°C for 1 hour. Forty cycles of polymerase chain reaction with Taq DNA polymerase (GIBCO BRL Cat. No. 18038-018) were then performed on 5% of the products of first-strand cDNA synthesis with 2 μmol of each primer through use of the following parameters: 30 second denaturation at 94°C, 30 second annealing at 40°C for the first 3 cycles and thereafter at 45°C, and 30 second extension at 72°C. The polymerase chain reaction products were separated from primers on low-melt agalose gels, and a 159 bp cDNA product was excised, purified, and subcloned into pBluescript (Stratagene,

La Jolla, CA, USA). This cDNA clone was sequenced with Sanger method and is shown as follows:

ATGGAAAAAGTCCAATACCTCACTCGCTCTGCTATCAGGAGAGCCTCAA
TATTGAAATGCCTCAGCAAGCACGTCAAAATCTCCAGAATCTATTTAT
CAACTTCTGTCTCATCTTGATATGTCTCCTGCTGATCTGCATCATTGTGAT
GCTTCTGTGA.

Statistical analysis

Values are given as mean ± SD. Comparisons between two groups were performed with the unpaired Student's t-test or Mann–Whitney U-test when the t-test was inappropriate, and comparisons between three groups were performed with one-way factorial ANOVA. $p < 0.05$ was considered the limit of significance [21].

RESULTS

Cardiac function in cardiomyopathic hamster heart

The left ventricular diastolic dimension was significantly ($p < 0.05$) enlarged in cardiomyopathic hamsters (6.8 ± 0.4 mm) at 20 weeks of age as compared with age-matched F1b hamsters (4.9 ± 0.4 mm). The percent fractional shortening of the left ventricles of BIO53.58 hamsters was significantly decreased at 5 weeks of age (57.3 ± 7.9% vs. 66.5 ± 5.9%; $p < 0.05$) and decreased further at 20 weeks of age (20.8 ± 4.0% vs. 63.3 ± 5.8%; $p < 0.01$) as compared with age-matched F1b hamsters.

Treatment with amlodipine and enalapril

At 15 weeks of treatment, enalapril significantly reduced ventricular weight in both BIO53.58 and F1b hamsters (table 1), as compared with hamsters that received no treatment. But amlodipine did not significantly change either body weight or ventricular weight (table 1).

The left ventricular diastolic dimension decreased significantly in the enalapril group (6.1 ± 0.4 mm, $p < 0.05$) and in the amlodipine group (5.5 ± 0.8 mm, $p < 0.001$) compared with the no-treatment group (6.8 ± 0.4 mm).

Table 1. Alteration of body weight (g) and ventricular weight (mg)

Group	Drug	Body weight (g)	Ventricular weight (mg)
BIO 53.58	Enalapril	104.8 ± 7.4	277.8 ± 10.8[a]
	Amlodipine	105.6 ± 5.7	328.3 ± 50.4
	No treatment	106.5 ± 3.9	340.5 ± 35.3
F1b	Enalapril	118.3 ± 11.1	327.8 ± 29.6
	Amlodipine	166.0 ± 11.5	420.2 ± 20.9
	No treatment	165.2 ± 6.4	394.6 ± 21.0

[a] $p < 0.05$ compared with the no-treatment group.
Values are expressed as mean ± SD.

Left ventricular percent fractional shortening increased in the enalapril group (26.7 ± 4.6%, $p < 0.05$) and in the amlodipine group (35.2 ± 5.0%, $p < 0.0001$) compared with the no-treatment group (20.8 ± 4.0%).

The area of necrosis, fibrosis, and calcification were decreased in both the enalapril and amlodipine groups. The left ventricular wall remained thick in both the enalapril and amlodipine groups compared with the thinning ventricular wall of the no-treatment group.

Myocyte size was smaller and myocytes were more concentrated in both the enalapril and amlodipine groups than in the no-treatment group.

Total ventricular volume tended to increase in the enalapril group. As mentioned above, ventricular weight of the amlodipine group did not change, but ventricular volume tended to increase in this group.

Fibrous tissue volume tended to decrease and the ratio of fibrous tissue to ventricular volume significantly decreased in the amlodipine group (11.2 ± 1.8%, $p < 0.05$) compared with the no-treatment group (14.6 ± 1.9%). On the other hand, fibrous tissue volume tended to decrease in the enalapril group, but the change was not significant. At 20 weeks, it decreased significantly in the amlodipine group (15.4 ± 2.8 mm³, $p < 0.05$) compared with the no-treatment group (21.0 ± 2.4 mm³) (table 2).

The myocyte diameter tended to decrease and the density of myocytes significantly increased in the amlodipine group (557.50 ± 42.95/mm², $p < 0.001$) compared with no-treatment group (396.5 ± 24.15/mm²) (table 3). But enalapril could not improve myocyte breadth and cell density at 20 weeks (table 3).

Table 2. The volume of ventricles, myocytes, and fibrous tissue in the cardiomyopathic hamster

Drug	Ventricles (mm³)	Myocytes (mm³)	Fibrous tissue (mm³)
Enalapril	141.2 ± 4.1	123.9 ± 3.5	17.3 ± 0.4
Amlodipine	142.3 ± 13.0	126.9 ± 11.4	15.4 ± 2.8[a]
No treatment	142.9 ± 18.5	121.9 ± 17.8	21.0 ± 2.4

[a] $p < 0.05$ compared with the no-treatment group.
Values are expressed as mean ± SD.

Table 3. Cell diameter and cell number in cardiomyopathic hamster

Drug	Cell breadth (μm)	Cell number (/mm²)
Enalapril	11.6 ± 1.1	452.5 ± 5.0
Amlodipine	11.2 ± 0.6	557.5 ± 43.0[a]
No treatment	12.0 ± 0.4	396.5 ± 24.2

[a] $p < 0.001$ compared with the no-treatment group.
Cell diameter is the short diameter of the myocyte and cell number is the nuclear density of myocytes per square millimeter. Values are expressed as mean ± SD.

RNA expression in cardiomyopathic hamster heart

RNA from control and cardiomyopathic hamsters hybridizes to a cDNA probe specific for the cardiac ryanodine receptor and a cDNA probe specific for phospholamban. The cardiac ryanodine receptor mRNA levels are decreased in cardiomyopathic hamsters (0.54 ± 0.4, $p < 0.05$) compared with control hamsters (2.5 ± 1.7). But phospholamban mRNA levels did not change in cardiomyopathic hamsters. Amlodipine treatment did not modify the expressions of these two genes.

DISCUSSION

Amlodipine prevented cardiac dilation and improved cardiac systolic function in the 20-week-old cardiomyopathic hamsters. Histological studies showed that amlodipine suppressed cardiac fibrosis and preserved the volume of myocytes space by preventing myocyte cell death. The calcium overload of myocytes has been implicated in the etiology of cardiac abnormalities in this cardiomyopathic hamster. However, the cause of the calcium overload is still unknown. Our studies demonstrated the downregulation of ryanodine receptor mRNA levels in this animal model of cardiomyopathic hamster (BIO53.58). The ryanodine receptor mRNA levels of BIO53.58 were lower by 80% than those of control hamster (F1b). On the other hand, the phospholamban mRNA levels of BIO53.58 were not downregulated and equal to that of F1b. These two proteins, locating in the sarcoplasmic reticulum (SR) and related to calcium transport through the SR, are regulated in a differential way. The downregulation of Ca^{2+}-release proteins/ryanodine receptor could result in systolic dysfunction and could be a cause of abnormal calcium handling. Phospholamban, one of the modulators of Ca^{2+} uptake proteins/SR Ca^{2+}ATPase, could modify the diastolic function. Our results show that there is little regulatory effect of phospholamban on cardiac dysfunction through this gene expression. Ca^{2+} uptake proteins/SR Ca^{2+}–ATPase is more directly related to the diastolic function, and it is necessary whether the gene expression is altered or not in the cardiomyopathic hamster. Northern blot analysis demonstrated that amlodipine did not modify the SR gene expressions of ryanodine receptor and phospholamban. The ryanodine receptor mRNA levels remained downregulated and equal to that of the no-treatment group. The phospholamban mRNA levels remained normal and equal to that of no-treatment group. It is postulated that the improvement of cardiac function by amlodipine is due to afterload reduction, prevention of myocyte necrosis, and prevention of cardiac fibrosis. Similar hemodynamic effects of amlodipine are shared by other calcium antagonists. However, calcium antagonist therapy is controversial in the treatment of congestive heart failure. A recent randomized, double-blind study revealed that nifedipine, a calcium channel blocker, increased the severity of the symptoms of congestive heart failure patients [23]. Although nifedipine-mediated reduction in cardiac muscle force development in patients with normal left ventricular function is usually offset by the vasorelaxing effect of the drug and its consequent reflex augmentation of beta-adrenergic activity, this mechanism often fails in patients with congestive heart failure in whom baroreceptor sensitivity is known to be attenuated. In addition to this effect, nifedipine increases plasma renin activity and may lead to increased angiotensin II, which is a vasoconstrictor and causes retention of sodium and water. These effects are considered to contribute to the deterioration of congestive heart failure patients. Compared with other calcium antagonists, the negative inotropic action of amlodipine is weak [24]. Therefore, all the properties of amlodipine contribute not only to the improvement of myocardial tissue but also to the amelioration of cardiac systolic function. Amlodipine also increased cell viability. Densities of myocytes (NA) significantly increased and the volume (V) of myocyte space tended to increase in the amlodipine group. The number (N) of myocytes, being calculated as $N = NA \times V$ and thought to be proportional to the total number of myocytes in the whole ventricle, increased significantly in the amlodipine group compared with the no-treatment group. The breadth of each myocyte was smaller in the amlodipine group than in the no-treatment group, showing that amlodipine prevented myocyte cell growth by its direct effect on the cell or by reducing mechanical forces (e.g., stretch) acting on each myocyte. The increased weight of myocyte space seems to counterbalance the decreased weight of fibrotic space, and as a result, amlodipine did not reduce ventricular weight. It is postulated that amlodipine improved calcium handling, ameliorated calcium overload, and prevented calcium-mediated cell death. It seems that amlodipine ameliorated calcium overload by inhibiting Ca^{2+} influx through sarcolemmal voltage-dependent Ca^{2+} channels and not by modifying the gene expression of ryanodine receptor and phospholamban. However, sarcoplasmic reticulum Ca^{2+}–ATPase or sarcolemmal Na^{+}–Ca^{2+} exchange are also related to homeostasis of intracellular calcium handling. Therefore, we must next investigate whether the expression of these proteins could be altered by amlodipine.

Treatment for 15 weeks with enalapril improved carciac function and prevented cardiac dilation, but prevention of fibrosis was not significant. The 15-week treatment with ACE inhibitor may not have been long enough to change collagen metabolism, especially the degradation of collagen, even if angiotensin II-induced collagen synthesis was inhibited. In our preliminary experiments, enalapril treatment for 25 weeks significantly suppressed the fibrosis of ventricles in cardiomyopathic hamsters compared with the no-treatment group. The total amount of collagen increase in BIO53.58 hamsters correlated with the pathological progression of fibrosis. The increase of collagen gives ventricles stiffness and impairs the cardiac diastolic function. Furthermore, it is known that angiotensin II stimulates collagen synthesis in cultured cardiac fibroblasts [25]. A recent clinical study reported that ACE inhibitors caused regression of cardiac hypertrophy. In addition, the remarkable effectiveness of ACE inhibitor's in preventing heart failure and the mounting evidence for additional cardioprotective effects of drugs related to the renin–angiotensin system have promoted an intense interest in the cardiac tissue renin–angiotensin system and its role in both normal and diseased hearts. Therefore, the tissue renin–angiotensin system may be implicated in cardiac hypertrophy and other cardiac disorders in humans.

In the present study, enalapril tended to inhibit myocyte cell death and cell growth and significantly improved cardiac fibrosis in cardiomyopathic hamsters. However, enalapril did not show as dramatic an effect for prevention of cell death as amlodipine did. Our data demonstrated a mild increase in the volume of myocyte space and a significant decrease in fibrosis in the enalapril group. Enalapril decreased ventricular weight significantly compared with the no-treatment group. It seems that the decrease in ventricular weight is largely due to the reduction of fibrosis. Whereas amlodipine significantly inhibited cell death by ameliorating calcium overload of myocytes, the major effects of enalapril are thought to suppress fibrosis by inhibiting the production of angiotensin II. In the present study, the cardioprotective effect of enalapril was weaker than that of amlodipine. The reason may be that the dose of enalapril (20 mg/kg) was not strong enough to inhibit cardiac remodeling, or that cardiomyopathic hamsters (BIO53.58), whose etiology is presumed to be abnormal handling of calcium [12], are more sensitive to treatment with amlodipine than with enalapril. A recent clinical study demonstrated that ACE inhibitors improve cardiac function and suppress cardiac dilation in chronic heart failure [26]. Even in acute myocardial infarction, early treatment with ACE inhibitors improves cardiac remodeling. Our results support the clinical study, and have proved that ACE inhibitor suppresses the development of fibrosis in heart failure. However, our study suggests that the calcium antagonist amlodipine may be more effective than the angiotensin-converting enzyme enalapril in some type of heart failure whose main etiology is abnormal calcium handling.

Enalapril significantly suppressed fibrosis and improved cardiac function in the cardiomyopathic hamster. It seems that the longer period of treatment with enalapril is more effective for prevention of fibrosis. Amlodipine preserved myocyte viability by preventing cell death, suppressed fibrosis, and significantly improved cardiac function in the cardiomyopathic hamster.

These data suggest that the major effect of enalapril is the suppression of fibrosis and that the major effect of amlodipine is the prevention of calcium-mediated cell death. Amlodipine was more effective than enalapril in preventing cardiac remodeling in cardiomyopathic hamsters, BIO53.58.

ACKNOWLEDGMENTS

The author would like to thank Dr. Masashi Watanabe for contributing the experiments.

REFERENCES

1. Sen S, Bumpus FM. 1979. Collagen synthesis in development and reversal of cardiac hypertrophy in spontaneously hypertensive rats. Am J Cardiol 44:954–958.
2. Brilla CG, Janicki JS, Weber KT. 1991. Cardioreparative effects of lisinopril in rats with genetic hypertension and left ventricular hypertrophy. Circulation 83:1771–1779.
3. Baker KM, Aceto JF. 1990. Angiotensin—stimulation of protein synthesis and cell growth in chick heart cells. Am J Physiol 259:H610–H618.
4. Pfeffer MA, Lamas GA, Vaughan DE, Parisi AF, Braunwawald E. 1988. Effect of captopril on progressive ventricular dilatation after anterior myocardial infarction. N Engl J Med 319.

5. Sharpe N, Murphy J, Smith H, Hannan S. 1988. Treatment of patients with symptomless left ventricular dysfunction after myocardial infarction. Lancet (8580) 1:255–264.
6. Weber KT, Brilla CG. 1991. Pathological hypertrophy and cardiac interstitium: fibrosis and renin–angiotensin–aldosterone system. Circulation 83:1849–1865.
7. Jasmin G, Solymoss B. 1975. Prevention of hereditary cardiomyopathy in the hamster by verapamil and other agent. Proc Soc Exp Biol Med 149:193–198.
8. Yamashita T, Kobayashi A, Yamazaki N, Miura K, Shirasawa H. 1986. Effects of L-carnitine and Verapamil on myocardial carnitine concentration and histopathology of Syrian hamster BIO14.6. Cardiovasc Res 20:614–620.
9. Wrogemann K, Nylen EG. 1978. Mitochondrial calcium overloading in cardiomyopathic hamsters. J Moll Cell Cardiol 10:185–195.
10. Kobayashi A, Yamashita T, Kaneko M, Nishiyama T, Hayashi H, Yamazaki N. 1987. Effects of verapamil on experimental cardiomyopathy in the BIO14.6 Syrian hamster. J Am Coll Cardiol 10:1128–1134.
11. Factor SM, Cho S, Scheuer J, Sonnenblick EH, Ashwani M. 1988. Prevention of hereditary cardiomyopathy in the Syrian hamster with chronic verapamil therapy. J Am Coll Cardiol: 1599–1604.
12. Bajusz E. 1969. Hereditary cardiomyopathy: a new disease model. Am Heart J 77:686–696.
13. Homburger F, Baker JR, Nixon CW, Whitney R. 1962. Primary generalized polymyopathy and cardiac necrosis in an inbred line of Syrian hamsters. Med Exp 6:339–345.
14. Bajusz E, Baker JR, Nixon CW, and Homburger F. 1969. Spontaneous hereditary myocardial degeneration and congestive heart failure in a strain of Syrian hamsters. Ann NY Acad Sci: 105–129.
15. Strobeck JE, Factor SM, Bhan A, Sole M, Liew CC, Fein F, Sonnenblick EH. 1979. Hereditary and acquired cardiomyopathies in experimental animals: mechanical, biochemical, and structural features. Ann NY Acad Sci 317:59–88.
16. Crawford M, Grant D, O'Rourke R, Starling M, Groves BM. 1980. Accuracy and reproducibility of new M-mode echocardiographic recommendation for measuring left ventricular dimensions. Circulation 61:137–143.
17. Sano Y. 1976. Histological Techniques: theoretical and Applied. Tokyo: NANZANDO.
18. Abe K, Ito T. 1972. A new stereological method for determination of the size of spherical objects in electron microscopy: its application to small lymphocytes of the mouse thymus. Arch Histol Jpn 34:203–214.
19. Watanabe S, Abe K, Anbo Y, Katoh H. 1995. Changes in the mouse exocrine pancreas after pancreatic duct ligation: a qualitative and quantitative histological study. Arch Histol Cytol: 365–374.
20. Nakai J, Imagawa T, Hakamata Y, Shigekawa M, Takeshima H, Numa S. 1990. Primary structure and functional expression from cDNA of the cardiac ryanodine receptor/calcium release channel. FEBS Lett 271:169–177.
21. Moorman AFM, Vermeulen JLM, Koban MU, Schwartz K, Lamers WH, Boheler KR. 1995. Patterns of expression of sarcoplasmic reticulum Ca^{2+}-ATPase and phospholamban mRNA during rat heart development. Circ Res 76:616–625.
22. Wallenstein S, Zucker CL, Fleiss JL. 1980. Some statistical methods useful in circulation research. Circ Res 47:1–9.
23. Elkayam U, Amin J, Mehra A, Vasquez J, Weber L, Rahimtoola SH. 1990. A prospective, randamized, double-blind, crossover study to compare the efficacy and safety of chronic nifedipine therapy with that of isosorbide dinitrate and their combination in the treatment of chronic congestive heart failure. Circulation 82:1954–1961.
24. Nakaya H, Hattori Y, Nakao Y, Kanno M. 1988. Cardiac versus vascular effect of a new dihydropyridine derivative: CV-4093: in vitro comparison with other calcium antagonist. Eur J Pharmacol 146:35–43.
25. Sano H, Okamoto H, Kitabatake A, Lizuka K, Murakami T, Kawaguchi H. 1998. Increased mRNA expression of cardiac renin–angiotensin system and collagen synthesis in spontaneously hypertensive rats. Mol Cell Biochem 178:51–58.
26. The SOLVED Investigators. 1992. Effects of the angiotensin converting enzyme inhibitor enalapril on the long-term progression of left ventricular dysfunction in patients with heart failure. Circulation 86:431–438.

N. Takeda, M. Nagano and N.S. Dhalla
(eds). The Hypertrophied Heart. Copyright
© 2000. pp. 393–398. Kluwer Academic
Publishers. Boston. All rights reserved.

HUMAN MYOCARDIAL Na,K–ATPase IN REMODELING

KELD KJELDSEN

Department of Medicine B2142, The Heart Center, Rigshospitalet, University of Copenhagen, Blegdamsvej 9, DK-2100 Copenhagen, Denmark

Summary. Hypertrophy and dilatation are important parts of the architectural structure changes of the heart in remodeling. The sarcolemmal Na,K–ATPase is of importance for heart rhythm and contractility. By measurements of ^{3}H-ouabain binding in small biopsies, it has become possible to quantify the Na,K–ATPase with high accuracy and precision in the human heart. The normal human left ventricular myocardium has a Na,K–ATPase density of 728 pmol/g wet weight. In early stages of compensated myocardial hypertrophy, human myocardial Na,K–ATPase concentration tends to be increased. In later, decompensated stages of hypertrophy, the Na,K–ATPase density is reduced by as much as 56%. In heart failure associated with dilated cardiomyopathy, the Na,K–ATPase concentration is reduced by as much as 89%. A positive, linear correlation exists between the left ventricular ejection fraction and Na,K–ATPase concentration. Such major changes at the level of sarcolemmal ion homeostasis during remodeling may be expected to be of major general importance for the function of the myocardium. Furthermore, they may have bearing for digoxin therapy, pointing to a putative benefit of keeping such patients at low plasma-digoxin levels.

INTRODUCTION

Remodeling can be defined as all the architectural changes occurring in the heart during physiological development as well as in response to pathophysiological conditions. Thus, hypertrophy and dilatation are important aspects of myocardial remodeling. Over the last 10–15 years, it has been realized that complex alterations in left ventricular architecture develop concomitantly with clinical manifestations of heart failure [1]. Numerous processes are involved in these aspects of heart physiology and pathophysiology [2,3]. Remodeling as a consequence of pathophysiological stimuli may be adaptive in the early phase, but the enlarged cardiac volume inevitably results in accentuation of left ventricular dysfunction and becomes a marker for poor prognosis [4]. In this chapter, the importance of human myocardial Na,K–ATPase concentration is reviewed in relation to remodeling. The regulation of the quantity of Na,K–ATPase is of importance for myocardial membrane function and thus for heart rhythm and contraction.

METHODOLOGICAL CONSIDERATIONS

In the evaluation of myocardial protein expression, e.g., Na,K–ATPase quantity in remodeling, a potential problem is that many entities may change at the same time. Accordingly, the way that specific protein levels should be presented may be subject to discussion. Protein expression is often given relative to wet weight of tissue, since this value is generally easy to determine; furthermore, it can often be determined on the sample prior to use of the sample for a biochemical assay. This is of major importance in studies using precious human material such as small endomyocardial samples taken during heart catheterization. Myocardial water content may, of course, be subject to regulation during remodeling. Thus, water content may need to be determined at least in some representative tissue samples. It might also be considered relevant to relate protein expression to other parameters. Expressing a change in the content of a specific protein relative to overall protein content may give information as to whether regulation of a certain protein is selective or unselective compared to other proteins. Expressing a specific change relative to membrane markers or other proteins may also give such information. It may also be considered relevant to express protein content relative to DNA content—which may, from many points of views, be considered to be the "gold standard." If the mass of the heart can be estimated, then expressing the amount of a protein per total heart may also give valuable information. Thus, growth or shrinkage of the heart may cause an apparent down- or upregulation of protein concentration or density, even though the total amount of the protein in the entire heart is unchanged. In general, seen from a biochemical, physiological or pathophysiological point of view, it is clear that the most information will be obtained by giving a certain protein regulation relative to as many factors as possible. From the viewpoint of clinical research and practice, the relation of a protein to the simple wet weight parameter will often suffice. This has often been considered to be the case in studies of the regulation of human myocardial Na,K–ATPase concentration [5,6].

When putative quantitative changes are addressed in human myocardial Na,K–ATPase in remodeling, specific methodological problems must be taken into consideration. Thus, methods must be used that are applicable for quantitative evaluations. The major problem is the presence of large quantities of nonspecific ATPases in the myocardium. This situation is different from, e.g., the kidneys, where the major part of ATPase is Na,K–ATPase. In myocardial preparation, this situation necessitates purification procedures prior to traditional Na,K–ATPase activity measurements, and accordingly, membrane material is lost [7,8]. It has been calculated that the recovery of Na,K–ATPase in measurements of Na,K–ATPase activity in purified myocardial membranes may be as low as only a few percent of that in the original material. Furthermore, it cannot be ensured that the protein is recovered equally in the compared conditions. Thus, methods developed applying crude myocardial tissue homogenates or intact myocardial samples must be employed, e.g. enzyme activity measurements in crude homogenates or ^{3}H-ouabain binding in intact tissue samples. [5,6]. Furthermore, caution should be taken in the use of molecular biology techniques in the studies of quantitative aspects of Na,K–ATPase in the myocardium. Thus, when immunoblotting is applied at the protein level, the risk for affinity change of the protein for the antibody in the pathophysiological condition should be considered. Furthermore, in studies applying immunoblotting at the mRNA level, it cannot be ensured that the subsequent protein expression is not infringed upon by the pathophysiological condition per se. Thus, whereas studies on the various myocardial Na,K–ATPase isoforms as well as on the expression of the Na,K–ATPase at mRNA level might be of interest from a molecular biological point of view, this approach has added very little to the knowledge of the quantative regulation of Na,K–ATPase in the human myocardium during remodeling.

Finally, it should be noted that caution is due during the extrapolation of results of studies of one single transport protein to a clinical setting. Downregulation at the level of one transport protein might be counteracted by upregulation of another transport protein and vice versa, thus balancing out the effects. It may be anticipated that in the future, important new knowledge about ion homeostasis in myocardial remodeling may come from studies evaluating the regulatory interplay among myocardial ion transporters.

HUMAN MYOCARDIAL Na,K–ATPase REGULATION

In recent years, much effort has been applied to determine the quantity of Na,K–ATPase in the normal human myocardium. Probably the hitherto best reported value comes from studies in which the heart transplantation program allowed access to normal, vital, human myocardial tissue from explanted normal hearts that were not used for transplantation for various reasons. Such studies offered for the first time access to the ultimately normal, human myocardium. Thus, a value of $728 \pm 58\,pmol/g$ wet weight ($n = 5$) was obtained in the left ventricular myocardium [9].

Early studies on endomyocardial biopsies taken during heart catheterization indicated a tendency toward an increase in human myocardial Na,K–ATPase concentration in hypertrophy [10,11]. Later studies on human left myocardium obtained at autopsy showed a significant reduction of 25%. This reduction was obtained when groups of hearts with high and low left ventricular total weight, respectively, were compared [12]. Recently, a study of intact samples of left ventricular myocardial biopsies obtained during open aortic valve replacement surgery for severe aortic stenosis with ensuing myocardial hypertrophy showed a significant reduction of 56% in myocardial Na,K–ATPase concentration [13]. When these results are taken together with animal studies they suggest that an upregulation of Na,K–ATPase concentration may be anticipated in the early stages of myocardial hypertrophy. Furthermore, it seems at present to be without doubt that the quantity of human myocardial Na,K–ATPase is significantly reduced in severe myocardial hypertrophy. Indications are that myocardial Na,K–ATPase per hart is reduced, indicating that the observed downregulation is not merely the simple outcome of increased cardiac mass relative to membranes but represents a reduction in Na,K–ATPase per se. It might be hypothesized that the Na,K–ATPase concentration is upregulated in the early phases of hypertrophy, where protein synthesis is known to be increased, whereas the Na,K–ATPase concentration is downregulated when hypertrophy becomes decompensated and protein synthesis is reduced. Further elucidation of Na,K–ATPase regulation in human myocardial hypertrophy studies quantifying the Na,K–ATPase at various stages of hypertrophy seems, however, to be needed.

The effect of dilated heart disease on human myocardial Na,K–ATPase concentration has been studied in endomyocardial biopsies obtained during heart catheterization for diagnostic purposes. A total of 52 patients were investigated, and a downregulation of Na,K–ATPase concentration of around 40% was observed. It is of interest that a significant, positive, linear correlation between ejection fraction (EF) determined angiographically and myocardial Na,K–ATPase concentration was established. A maximum reduction in Na,K–ATPase concentration of 89% was obtained when EF was reduced to 20%. The possibility was excluded that down-regulation was the simple outcome of an increase in water content or of the content of collagen tissue; it was found to be selective relative to overall protein synthesis regulation [10,11]. Since a number of patients had been treated with digoxin, and since this treatment has been shown to cause a functional decrease in Na,K–ATPase of about 25% [9,14], part of the downregulation observed might be due to digitalization per se. When these findings are taken together, however, it seems without doubt that the reduction in Na,K–ATPase concentration in human myocardium with dilated heart disease is of the magnitude 25%. This finding is also consistent with a meta-analysis concluding that there is a consistent decrease of 26–32% in Na,K–ATPase concentration in the failing human heart [15]. Indications are that total myocardial Na,K–ATPase per heart increases in severe dilatation. However, the Na,K–ATPase synthesis seems unable to match the increasing cell size, resulting in a reduction in Na,K–ATPase density. A comparison of the Na,K–ATPase value obtained in explanted normal, vital human hearts [9] with that found in endomyocardial biopsies from a subgroup of patients with heart disease but preserved ejection fraction [10] shows that the downregulation of Na,K–ATPase concentration occurs before left ventricle ejection fraction decreases. This finding may indicate the pathophysiological importance of the Na,K–ATPase downregulation.

PERSPECTIVES

The observed changes in Na,K–ATPase concentration with remodeling are of importance for ion homeostasis [16] across the myocyte membrane and will thus have a bearing on the generation of arrhythmias as well as on changes in contractile capacity. Furthermore, since myocardial Na,K–ATPase is generally accepted as the receptor for the inotropic action of digoxin [17], the downregulation of Na,K–ATPase in heart failure may have a bearing on digoxin therapy, suggesting a putative benefit of keeping such patients at low plasma digoxin levels. It is of major interest that cell growth factors may stimulate Na,K–ATPase [18]. Here especially, the treatment with growth hormones of heart failure patients has, at least in initial evaluation, shown beneficial effects [19,20]. The application of mechanical left ventricular assist devices in the treatment of terminal heart failure may, in certain cases, result in recovery by reverse remodeling and an improvement in left ventricular ejection fraction. Unloading of the failing left ventricle by mechanical left ventricular device systems has now been shown in 19 weaned patients to be associated with a decrease in left ventricular end-diastolic diameter of 75% and an increase in left ventricular ejection fraction of 180% [21]. Hitherto, not much has been known about the possibility for spontaneous recovery in heart failure. However, it has been a well-known clinical experience that protracted bed rest might, in some cases, be beneficial. Thus, future experiments evaluating the effect of, e.g., growth factors on human myocardial Na,K–ATPase during remodeling, together with studies during reverse remodeling, seem promising.

ACKNOWLEDGMENTS

The studies were supported by The Danish Heart Foundation and The Villadsen Family Foundation.

REFERENCES

1. Cohn JN. 1996. Structural basis for heart failure. Ventricular remodeling and its pharmacologic inhibition. Circulation 91:2504–2507.
2. Maisch B. 1996. Ventricular remodeling. Cardiology 87(Suppl 1):2–10.
3. Francis GS. 1998. Changing the remodeling process in heart failure: basic mechanisms and laboratory results. Curr Opin Cardiol 13:156–161.
4. Katz AM. 1994. The cardiomyopathy of overload: an unnatural growth response in the hypertrophied heart. Ann Intern Med 121:362–371.
5. Nørgaard A. 1986. Quantification of the Na,K–ATPase pumps in mammalian skeletal muscle. Acta Pharmacol Toxicol 58(Suppl 1):1–34.
6. Schmidt TA. 1997. Human myocardial and skeletal muscular Na,K–ATPase in relation to digoxin treatment of heart failure. Dan Med Bull 44:499–521.
7. Jones LR, Besch HR. 1984. Isolation of canine cardiac sarcolemmal vesicles. Meth Pharmacol 5:1–12.
8. Hansen O, Clausen T. 1988. Quantitative determination of Na,K–ATPase and other sarcolemmal components in muscle cells. Am J Physiol 254:C1–C7.
9. Schmidt TA, Allen PD, Colluci WS, Marsh JD, Kjeldsen K. 1993. No adaption to digitalization as evaluated by digitalis receptor (Na,K–ATPase) quantification in explanted hearts from donors without heart disease and from digitalized patients in endstage heart failure. Am J Cardiol 70:110–114.
10. Nørgaard A, Bagger JP, Bjerregaard P, Baandrup U, Kjeldsen K, Thomsen PEB. 1988. Relation of left ventricular function and Na,K-pump concentration in suspected idiopathic dilated cardiomyopathy. Am J Cardiol 61:1312–1315.
11. Nøgaard A, Kjeldsen K. 1989. Human myocardial Na,K-pumps in relation to heart disease. J Appl Cardiol 4:239–245.
12. Ellingsen Ø, Holthe MR, Svindland A, Aksnes G, Sejersted OM, Ilebekk A. 1994. Na,K-pump concentration in hypertrophied human hearts. Eur Heart J 15:1184–1190.
13. Larsen JS, Schmidt TA, Bundgaard H, Kjeldsen K. 1997. Reduced concentration of myocardial Na,K–ATPase in human aortic valve disease as well as of Na,K– and Ca–ATPase in rodents with hypertrophy. Mol Cell Biochem 169:85–93.
14. Rasmussen HH, Okita GT, Hartz RS, ten-Eick RE. 1990. Inhibition of electrogenic Na-pumping in isolated atrial tissue from patients treated with digoxin. J Pharmacol Exp Ther 252:60–64.
15. Shamraj OI, Grupp IL, Grupp G, Melvin D, Gradoux N, Kremers W, Lingrel JB, De Pover A. 1993. Characterization of Na,K–ATPase, its isoforms, and the inotropic response to ouabain in isolated failing human hearts. Cardiovasc Res 27:2229–2237.
16. Skou JC. 1965. Enzymatic basis for active transport of Na and K across cell membrane. Physiol Rev 45:596–617.
17. Smith TW. 1988. Digitalis. Mechanisms of action and clinical use. N Engl J Med 318:358–365.
18. Clausen T. 1996. Long- and short-term regulation of the Na^+–K^+ pump in skeletal muscle. News Physiol Sci 11:24–30.

19. Fazio S, Sabatini D, Brunella C, Vigorito C, Giordano A, Guida R, Pardo F, Biondi B, Saccà L. 1996. A preliminary study of growth hormone in the treatment of dilated cardiomyopathy. N Engl J Med 334:809–814.
20. Dreifuss P, Anker SD, Coats AJS. 1998. Growth hormone in chronic heart failure. Circulation 97: 1650–1651.
21. Müller J, Hetzer R. 1998. Weaning from LVAD as the new "bridge to recovery"—Mechanical bed rest with the Novacor LVAD. Frontiers in heart failure treatment. 1:16–18.

N. Takeda, M. Nagano and N.S. Dhalla
(eds). The Hypertrophied Heart. Copyright
© 2000. pp. 399–407. Kluwer Academic
Publishers. Boston. All rights reserved.

NITRIC OXIDE SYNTHASE GENE TRANSFER INHIBITS PROTEIN SYNTHESIS OF RAT CARDIAC MYCOCYTES

UICHI IKEDA,[1] YOSHIKAZU MAEDA,[1] KEN-ICHI OYA,[1] MASAHISA
SHIMPO,[1] SHUICHI UENO,[1] MASASHI URABE,[2] AKIHIRO KUME,[2] JOHN
MONAHAN,[3] KEIYA OZAWA,[2] AND KAZUYUKI SHIMADA[1]

[1] Department of Cardiology and [2] Division of Genetic Therapeutics, Center for Molecular Medicine, Jichi Medical
School, Minamikawachi-machi, Tochigi 329-0498, Japan; [3] Avigen Inc., Alameda, CA, USA

Summary. We investigated whether nitric oxide (NO) synthase gene transfer could attenuate α-adrenergic agonist-induced growth of cardiac myocytes. First, we investigated the effects of exogenous NO and a cGMP analogue on protein synthesis of cultured neonatal rat cardiac myocytes. The NO donor, morpholinosydnonimine (SIN-1), and 8-bromo-cGMP caused concentration-dependent decreases in phenylephrine (Phe)-induced ^{3}H-leucine incorporation into myocytes. We then transferred endothelial NO synthase (eNOS) gene into cardiac myocytes using adeno-associated virus (AAV) vectors. eNOS gene transfer into cardiac myocytes induced 140 kDa eNOS protein expression and significantly increased cGMP contents of myocytes compared with control cells. eNOS gene transfer also inhibited ^{3}H-leucine incorporation into cardiac myocytes in response to Phe, which was significantly recovered in the presence of the NOS inhibitor N^G-monometyl-L-arginine acetate. These results indicate that authentic NO attenuates the effects of the α-adrenergic agonist-induced cardiac hypertrophy at least partially via cGMP production, suggesting that eNOS gene transfer using AAV vectors is promising for the gene therapy of cardiac hypertrophy.

INTRODUCTION

Nitric oxide (NO) is synthesized in various types of cells and appears to play important roles, including vascular tone [1,2], neurotransmission [3], and immunoregulation [4]. There are two classes of NO synthases (NOS), namely, constitutive and inducible [5]. The constitutive enzymes were initially identified in the brain (NOS I or nNOS) [6] and endothelial cells (NOS III or eNOS) [7–9]. These enzymes are regulated by reversible binding of calcium–calmodulin. The inducible NOS isoform (NOS II or iNOS) is typically expressed in cells only after exposure to cytokines and is calcium independent [10,11]. NO activates soluble guanylate cyclase, which increases intracellular guanosine 3′,5′-cyclic monophosphate (cGMP), thereby inducing vasorelaxation and inhibiting platelet aggregation [12–14]. Previous studies have demonstrated that NO inhibits proliferation of various kinds of cells such as vascular smooth muscle cells [15] and mesangial cells [16] in vitro. Chronic administration of L-arginine, a substrate of NOS, to spontaneously hypertensive rats (SHR) attenuated cardiac hypertrophy independently of blood pressure and increased myocardial content of cGMP and nitrate/nitrite [17], suggesting that NO also has a protective effect against cardiac hypertrophy. In this study, we investigated whether endogenously generated NO by eNOS gene transfer could inhibit hypertrophy in cultured neonatal rat cardiac myocytes induced by the α-adrenergic agonist phenirephrine (Phe).

MATERIALS AND METHODS

Cell culture

Cardiac myocytes were prepared from ventricles of 1-day-old Sprague–Dawley rats as described previously [18]. Briefly, after dissociation with 0.25% trypsin, cell suspensions were washed with DMEM supplemented with 10% fetal calf serum (FCS; CSL Limited) and centrifuged at $500 \times g$ for 10 minutes. The cell pellets were then resuspended in DMEM (GIBCO BRL) containing 10% FCS. For selective enrichment of cardiac myocytes, the dissociated cells were preplated for 1 hour, during which nonmyocytes readily attached to the bottom of the culture dishes. The resulting suspensions of myocytes were plated onto 24-well dishes at a density of 5×10^5 cells/well. Thymidine (0.6 mg/mL) was added during the first 72 hours to prevent proliferation of nonmyocytes. Using this method, we routinely obtained enriched cultures containing more than 95% myocytes, as assayed by immunofluorescence staining with an anti-myosin heavy chain antibody.

Leucine incorporation assay

Protein synthesis in cardiac myocytes was measured by leucine incorporation into the cells. The cardiac myocytes were incubated with Phe for 12 hours, followed by addition of ^{3}H-leucine (100 μCi/mL, Amersham) for another 6 hours. The cells were washed with PBS twice and then lysed with 1N NaOH and 0.1% sodium dodecyle sulfate (SDS). Radioactivity was measured by liquid scintillation counting.

Production of AAV–NOS

The full-length bovine eNOS, cDNA, a kind gift from D.G. Harrison (Emory University School of Medicine), was isolated from Bruescript SK+ vector (pBS-NOS) by restriction enzyme digest with *Sal I* (4096 bp). To generate p1.1c-NOS, this *Sal I*-digested fragment was ligated into the *Sal I* cloning site of the p1.1c expression plasmid (4050 bp). The p1.1c vectors were engineered by introducing cytomegalovirus immediate early promotor, human growth hormone 1st intron, and simian virus 40 polyadenylation signal into pUC 18 vectors. The p1.1c-NOS plasmids were digested with *BstB I* in order to delete human growth hormone 1st intron (269 bp) and then self-ligated to generate p1.1c-NOS (7877 bp). The resulting *Not I–Not I* expression cassette (5146 bp) was inserted between the inverted terminal repeats of a pUC-based plasmid containing both adeno-associated virus (AAV) inverted terminal repeats and AAV *rep* and *cap* genes outside the inverted terminal repeats (pWee1909-NOS; 12020 bp).

Immunoblot analysis of eNOS protein

Cell were rinsed with ice-cold PBS and resuspended into the lysis buffer (1% Nonidit P-40, 50 mmol/L Tris-HCl, pH 7.4 150 mmol/L NaCl, 220 U/mL aprotinine, 1 mmol/L PMSF). After incubation on ice for 30 minutes, cell extracts were centrifuged to remove cell debris. eNOS protein was immunoprecipitated from 1 mg of cell lysates with anti-bovine eNOS antibody (Affinity Bioreagents, Inc.) and protein A-Sepharose 4B beads (Sigma), and eluted into lysis buffer. The immune complexes were then separated through 7.5% polyacrylamide gel electrophoresis and blotted onto polyvinylidene difluoride membrane (Immunobin; Millipore). The membrane was incubated for 1 hour at room temperature in Tris-buffered saline with Tween 20 (TBST: 20 mmol/L Tris-HCl, pH 7.4, 150 mmol/L NaCl, 0.05% Tween 20) with 4% nonfat milk. The membrane was then incubated with anti-eNOS antibody (1:1000) overnight at 4°C in TBST. Specific binding of the antibody was visualized by the ECL detection system (Amersham) according to the manufacturer's instruction.

cGMP measurements

For determination of intracellular cGMP levels, 0.5 mmol/L IBMX, a cyclic nucleotide phosphodiesterase inhibitor, was added to each well 30 minutes before the addition of Phe to prevent breakdown of accumulated cGMP. After incubation with Phe for 1 hour, cells were immediately immersed in 0.2 mL of 0.1 N HCl to stop the reaction. Cells were then collected into glass tubes with a rubber policeman, boiled for 5 minutes, and then centrifuged at $2500g$ for 15 minutes at room temperature. The supernatants were decanted, and after 0.05 mL of 50 mmol/L sodium acetate was added to each tube, cells were kept at −70°C until assayed for cGMP contents. The pellets were dissolved in 0.2 mL of 1% SDS and kept at 4°C until assayed for protein. Intracellular cGMP contents were measured with a commercial enzyme immunoassay kit using the manufacturer's high-sensitivity acetylation protocol (Amersham International plc).

Statistical analysis

Values are expressed as means ± SE. Differences of values were assessed by one-factor ANOVA. A value of $p < 0.05$ was considered statistically significant.

RESULTS

Effects of NO donor and 8 Br-cGMP on protein synthesis

We used Phe to stimulate protein synthesis of cardiac myocytes. Addition of Phe increased leucine incorporation into cardiac myocytes in a dose-dependent manner

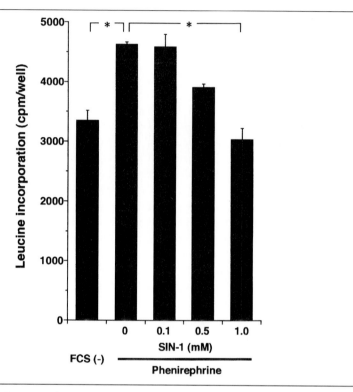

Figure 1. Effects of SIN-1 on ³H-leucine incorporation into cardiac myocytes. After cardiac myocytes were incubated with 10^{-6} mol/L phenirephrine and various concentrations of SIN-1 for 12 hours, ³H-leucine was added to the culture medium, and the cells were further incubated for 6 hours. ³H-leucine incorporation into cardiac myocytes treated with SIN-1 was significantly lower than that into control cells. Data are mean ± SE of four samples. $\star$, $p < 0.05$.

($10^{-8} \sim 10^{-6}$ mol/L). We first investigated whether exogenous NO could inhibit Phe-induced increase in protein synthesis of cardiac myocytes. Cardiac myocytes were incubated with 10^{-6} mol/L Phe and the NO donor morpholinosydnonimine (SIN-1) for 12 hours. As shown in figure 1, SIN-1 inhibited Phe-induced protein synthesis of cardiac myocytes in a dose-dependent manner, indicating the growth-inhibitory effects of exogenous NO on cardiac myocytes.

To investigate whether this inhibitory effect is mediated via formation of cGMP, a second messenger of NO, we next investigated the effect of a cGMP analogue, 8-bromo-cGMP, on protein synthesis in cardiac myocytes. We found that 8-bromo-cGMP did not influence leucine incorporation into unstimulated cardiac myocytes. On the other hand, 8-bromo-cGMP significantly supressed leucine incorporation into Phe-stimulated cardiac myocytes (figure 2). This result suggests that exogenous NO could suppress cardiac hypertrophy at least in part via a cGMP production.

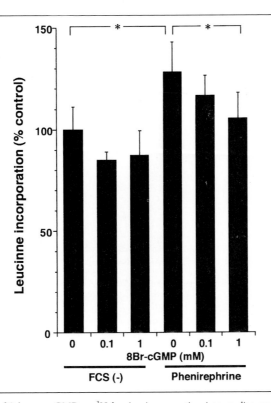

Figure 2. Effects of 8-bromo-cGMP on ^{3}H-leucine incorporation into cardiac myocytes. After cardiac myocytes were incubated with 10^{-6} mol/L phenirephrine and 8-bromo-cGMP for 12 hours, ^{3}H-leucine was added to the culture medium, and the cells were further incubated for 6 hours. ^{3}H-leucine incorporation into cardiac myocytes treated with 8-bromo-cGMP was significantly lower than that into control cells. Data are mean ± SE of four samples, *, $p < 0.05$.

eNOS gene transfer into cardiac myocytes

Previously, we have reported that AAV vectors could efficiently transduce cardiac myocytes [19]. The particle titer of AAV-NOS we have generated was $6.9 \pm 1.3 \times 10^{10}$ particles/mL (data not shown). We thus transduced cardiac myocytes with AAV-NOS (MOI: 1.0×10^4) to examine the effect of endogenously generated NO on protein synthesis in Phe-stimulated cardiac myocytes. Immunoblot analysis revealed that nontransduced cardiac myocytes did not express eNOS protein; however, eNOS-transduced cells expressed 140 kDa eNOS protein (data not shown).

We then measured cGMP contents in cardiac myocytes. cGMP levels in eNOS-transduced cardiac myocytes were significantly higher than those in nontransduced cells (166.7 ± 30.6 vs. 70.7 ± 28.7 fmol/well). This increase in cGMP was partially but significantly suppressed in the presence of the NOS inhibitor N^G-monometyl-L-arginine acetate (L-NMMA; 1 mmol/L, Research Biochemicals Inc.). These

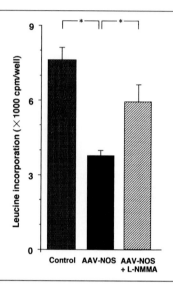

Figure 3. Effects of eNOS gene transfer on ^{3}H-leucine incorporation into cardiac myocytes. After cardiac myocytes were incubated with 10^{-6} mol/L phenylephrine for 12 hours, ^{3}H-leucine was added to the culture medium, and the cells, were further incubated for 6 hours. ^{3}H-leucine incorporation into cardiac myocytes transduced with AAV-NOS was significantly lower than that into the control myocytes. This inhibition was partially but significantly reduced in the presence of 1 mmol/L L-NMMA. Data are mean ± SE of four samples. $\star$, $p < 0.05$.

findings indicate that eNOS gene transfer into cardiac myocytes using AAV vectors resulted in functional eNOS expression and increased cGMP production.

Effects of eNOS gene transfer on protein synthesis

We next investigated the effect of eNOS gene transfer on Phe-induced leucine incorporation into cardiac myocytes. After a 24-hour incubation with or without (control) AAV-NOS (MOI: 1.0×10^4), cardiac myocytes were cultured with serum-free medium for 24 hours. Phe with or without 1 mmol/L L-NMMA was added to the culture medium, and leucine incorporation into the cells was measured as described in the Materials and Methods section. Leucine incorporation into cardiac myocytes was significantly increased by Phe, and this Phe-induced leucine incorporation was significantly inhibited by eNOS gene transfer, and was partially recovered in the presence of L-NMMA at any Phe concentrations (figure 3).

DISCUSSION

NO, a potent vasodilator produced by endothelial cells, is thought to be the endothelium-dependent relaxing factor (EDRF) that mediates vascular tone in response to acetylcholine, bradykinin, and substance P in various vascular beds [1,2]. Recently, eNOS-knockout mice were shown to be hypertensive [20]. Thus, NO has been implicated in the regulation of blood pressure and hypertension. On the other hand, cardiac hypertrophy is one of the compensatory mechanisms against high blood pressure. Previous studies have demonstrated that NO inhibits proliferation of various kinds of cells such as vascular smooth muscle cells [15] and mesangial cells [16]. Very recently, Kullo et al. [21] reported that gene transfer of ecNOS to porcine vascular smooth muscle cells resulted in the expression of a functional enzyme and inhibition of cellular proliferation in response to serum. On the other hand, NO might be implicated in the development of cardiac hypertrophy independent of blood pressure levels. Nava et al. [22] reported that the Ca^{2+}-dependent NOS activity was upregulated in cardiac endothelial cells of SHR. The high activity of cardiac Ca^{2+}-dependent NOS was related to increased arterial pressure of these animals. Nava et al. speculated that in the heart, endothelial cells respond with a higher production of NO as a compensatory mechanism against high blood pressure and its damaging effects on the heart. Matsuoka et al. [17] also demonstrated that chronic L-arginine administration to SHR attenuated cardiac hypertrophy independently of blood pressure and increased myocardial content of cGMP and nitrate/nitrite. In the present study, we demonstrated NO-donor, SIN-1-attunated protein synthesis of Phe-stimulated cardiac myocytes. We also found that 8-bromo-cGMP, a cGMP analogue, mimicked this effect, suggesting that the inhibitory effect of NO on protein synthesis might be mediated via cGMP production.

There are many gene transfer vehicles, including adenovirus, retrovirus, and liposome. Although adenoviral vectors have been shown to be able to transduce cells with high efficiency, gene expression is transient due to its episomal feature. In addition, adenoviral vectors may have some direct cytopathic effects and may induce immunological responses to transduced cells, because leaky expression of adenoviral genes cannot be completely eliminated. These features are limitations of this vector for clinical applications. Retroviral vector transduces cells less efficiently. Moreover, this vector cannot transduce nondividing cells. Adeno-associated virus (AAV) vectors are based on a nonpathogenic parvovirus. It is known that lung epithelial cells [23], neuronal cells [24], skeletal muscle cells [25,26], and cardiac myocytes [19] are efficiently transduced with AAV vectors, and transgene expression persists for long periods. These characteristics are advantages in the application of AAV vectors for chronic heart disease such as cardiac hypertrophy. Using this AAV vector, we demonstrated that eNOS gene transfer into cardiac myocytes resulted in functional eNOS protein expression and elevated cGMP contents. We further demonstrated here that eNOS gene transfer inhibited Phe-induced protein synthesis of cardiac myocytes. These results indicate that authentic NO attenuates the effects of the α-adrenergic agonist-induced cardiac hypertrophy at least partially via cGMP production, suggesting that eNOS gene transfer using AAV vectors is promising for the gene therapy of cardiac hypertrophy.

ACKNOWLEDGMENTS

This work was supported in part by grants from the Ministry of Health and Welfare of Japan, Grants-in-Aid for Scientific Research from the Ministry of Education, Science, Sports and Culture of Japan.

REFERENCES

1. Ignarro L. 1989. Biological actions and properties of endothelium-derived nitric oxide formed and released from artery and vein. Circ Res 65:1–21.
2. Furchgott RF, Zawadzki JV. 1980. The obligatory role of endothelial cells in the relaxation of arterial smooth muscle by acetylcholine. Nature 288:373–376.
3. Bredt DS, Snyder SH. 1989. Nitric oxide mediates glutamate-linked enhancement of cGMP levels in the cerebellum. Proc Natl Acad Sci USA 86:9030–9033.
4. Garthwaite J, Garthwaite G, Palmer RM, Moncada S. 1989. NMDA receptor activation induces nitric oxide synthesis from arginine in rat brain slices. Eur J Pharmacol 172:413–416.
5. Hibbs JJ, Taintor RR, Vavrin Z, Rachlin EM. 1988. Nitric oxide: a cytotoxic activated macrophage effector molecule. Biochem Biophys Res Commun 157:87–94.
6. Nathan C, Xie QW. 1994. Nitric oxide synthase; roles, tolls, and controls. Cell 78:915–918.
7. Lamas S, Marsden PA, Li GK, Tempst P, Michel T. 1992. Endothelial nitric oxide synthase: molecular cloning and characterization of a distinct constitutive enzyme isoform. Proc Natl Acad Sci USA 89:6348–6352.
8. Forstermann U, Closs EI, Pollock JS, Nakane M, Schwarz P, Gath I, Kleinert H. 1994. Nitric oxide synthase isozymes. Characterization, purification, molecular cloning, and functions. Hypertension 23:1121–1131.
9. Marsden PA, Heng HH, Scherer SW, Stewart RJ, Hall AV, Shi XM, Tsui LC, Schappert KT. 1993. Structure and chromosomal localization of the human constitutive endothelial nitric oxide synthase gene. J Biol Chem 268:17478–17488.
10. Stuehr DJ, Griffith OW. 1992. Mammalian nitric oxide synthases. Adv Enzymol Rel Areas Mol Biol 65:287–346.
11. Lowenstein CJ, Glatt CS, Bredt D, Snyder SH. 1992. Cloned and expressed macrophage nitric oxide synthase contrasts with the brain enzyme. Proc Natl Acad Sci USA 89:6711–6715.
12. Marin J, Sanchez FC. 1990. Role of endothelium-formed nitric oxide on vascular responses. Gen Pharmacol 21:575–587.
13. Radomski MW, Palmer RMJ, Moncada S. 1987. The role of nitric oxide and cGMP in platelet adhesion to vascular endothelium. Biochem Biophys Res Commun 148:1482–1489.
14. deGraaf JC, Banga JD, Moncada S, Palmer RMJ, deGroot PJ, Sixma JJ. 1992. Nitric oxide functions as an inhibitor of platelet adhesion under flow conditions. Circulation 85:2284–2290.
15. Garg UC, Hassid A. 1989. Nitric oxide-generating vasodilators and 8-bromo-cyclic guanosine monophosphate inhibit mitogenesis and proliferation of cultured rat vascular smooth muscle cells. J Clin Invest 83:1774–1777.
16. Garg UC, Hassid A. 1989. Inhibition of rat mesangial cell mitogenesis by nitric oxide-generating vasodilators. Am J Physiol 257:F60–F66.
17. Matsuoka H, Nakata M, Kohno K, Koga Y, Nomura G, Toshima H, Imaizumi T. 1996. Chronic L-arginine administration attenuates cardiac hypertrophy in spontaneously hypertensive rats. Hypertension 27:14–18.
18. Yamamoto K, Ikeda U, Seino Y, Tsuruya Y, Oguchi A, Okada K, Ishikawa S, Saito T, Kamitani K, Hara Y, Shimada K. 1993. Regulation of Na, K–ATPase gene expression by sodium ions in cultured neonatal rat cardiocytes. J Clin Invest 92:1889–1895.
19. Maeda Y, Ikeda U, Shimpo M, Ueno S, Ogasawara Y, Urabe M, Kume A, Takizawa T, Saito T, Colosi P, Kurtzman G, Shimada K, Ozawa K. 1998. Efficient gene transfer into cardiac myocytes using adeno-associated virus (AAV) vectors. J Mol Cell Cardiol 30:1341–1348.
20. Huang PL, Huang Z, Mashimo H, Bloch KD, Moskowitz MA, Bevan JA, Fishman MC. 1995. Hypertension in mice lacking the gene for endothelial nitric oxide synthase. Nature 377:239–242.
21. Kullo IJ, Mozes G, Schwartz RS, Gloviczki P, Crotty TB, Barber DA, Katusic ZS, O'Brien T. 1997. Adventitial gene transfer of recombinant endothelial nitric oxide synthase to rabbit carotid arteries alters vascular reactivity. Circulation 96:2254–2261.
22. Nava E, Noll G, Luscher TF. 1995. Increased activity of constitutive nitric oxide synthase in cardiac endothelium in spontaneous hypertension. Circulation 91:2310–2313.
23. Flotte TR, Afione SA, Conrad C, McGrath SA, Solow, R, Oka H, Zeitlin PL, Guggino WB, Carter BJ. 1993. Stable in vivo expression of the cystic fibrosis transmembrane conductance regulator with an adeno-associated virus vector. Proc Natl Acad Sci USA 90:10613–10617.
24. Kaplitt MG, Leone P, Samulski RJ, Xiao X, Pfaff DW, O'Malley KL, During MJ. 1994. Long-term gene expression and phenotypic correction using adeno-associated virus vectors in the mammalian brain. Nat Genet 8:148–154.

25. Kessler PD, Podsakoff GM, Chen X, McQuiston SA, Colosi PC, Matelis LA, Kurtzman GJ, Byrne BJ. 1996. Gene delivery to skeletal muscle results in sustained expression and systemic delivery of a therapeutic protein. Proc Natl Acad Sci USA 93:14082–14087.
26. Fisher KJ, Jooss K, Alston J, Yang Y, Haecker SE, High K, Pathak R, Raper SE, Wilson JM. 1997. Recombinant adeno-associated virus for muscle directed gene therapy. Nature Med 3:306–312.

N. Takeda, M. Nagano and N.S. Dhalla
(eds). The Hypertrophied Heart. Copyright
© 2000. pp. 409–421. Kluwer Academic
Publishers. Boston. All rights reserved.

HUMAN HEART FAILURE:
A MECHANISTIC ASSESSMENT OF ALTERED VENTRICULAR FUNCTION

NORMAN R. ALPERT and LOUIS A. MULIERI

Department of Molecular Physiology and Biophysics, University of Vermont College of Medicine, Burlington, Vermont 05405-0068, USA

Summary. Human heart failure is associated with high mortality and morbidity. From a functional viewpoint, the failing heart has low power (rate of doing work) and an inadequate cardiac output to meet the metabolic needs of the periphery. We use myothermal and mechanical techniques on specially prepared thin epicardial muscle strips from nonfailing (coronary bypass surgery) and failing (idiopathic dilated cardiomyopathy, NYHA IV) human hearts to assess the mechanistic basis for the depressed power and cardiac output. The isometric peak force, rate of force development, and rate of relaxation are reduced to 53%, 49%, and 54%, respectively, in the failing heart while the time to peak tension is increased by 15%. The total activity-related heat, initial heat, tension-dependent heat, tension-independent heat, and tension-independent heat rate were substantially and significantly reduced in the failing preparations. The ratio of total activity-related heat to initial heat is an index of the ability of mitochondria to resynthesize ATP from ADP and is found to be unchanged in the failing myocardium. The amount of calcium cycled per beat and the rate of calcium uptake can be calculated from the tension-independent heat. In the failing myocardium, both of these are reduced to 31% of nonfailing values. The average cross-bridge force time integral can be calculated from the fiber strip force-time integral divided by the number of cross-bridge cycles per half sarcomere per twitch. The latter is obtained from the tension-dependent heat. The average cross-bridge force-time integral is increased by 41% in the failing heart. The depression in isometric force correlates with the decrease in calcium cycled per beat. This in itself contributes to the reduced ventricular performance. Added to that, there is a blunting of the force–frequency relationship and a decrease in the velocity of unloaded shortening. These fundamental changes at the molecular level result in a decrease in power output of the ventricle and ultimately lead to the serious morbid and mortal consequences found in congestive heart failure.

INTRODUCTION

The failing heart is incapable of pumping a sufficient amount of blood to meet the metabolic needs of the organism. Despite heroic efforts for early diagnosis and treat-

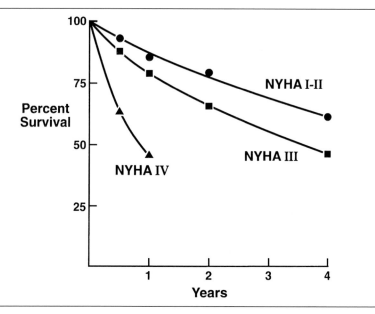

Figure 1. The relationship between percent survival and NYHA classification as a function of years after diagnosis. (Redrawn from the FIRST [2] and SOLVD [3] studies.)

ment of this disease, ventricular failure remains a serious public health problem, affecting about three persons per thousand per year [1]. Persons with heart failure are at substantial risk for morbid and mortal events. The mortality risk is best illustrated by comparing percent survival at given times following diagnosis for different degrees of failure based on the simple clinical assessment provided by the NYHA categories[1] I–IV (figure 1). There is also a relationship between survivability and ejection fraction, with survivability being 75.7%, 67.8%, and 49.9% for ejection fractions 30–40%, 20–30%, and less than 20%, respectively [4]. The relationship of functional performance as well as clinical assessment with mortality suggests that there is a severe deficit in ventricular function associated with heart failure. This chapter is directed at uncovering the molecular alterations in the failing ventricular muscle that account for the functional impairment. Strips of human ventricular muscle from failing (F) and nonfailing (NF) hearts are used for a myothermal-mechanical assessment of heart muscle mechanics with the view of pinpointing the nature of the changes in the contractile and excitation contraction coupling systems that cause the depressed function.

METHODS AND RESULTS

Patient population and epicardial strip preparation

Subepicaridal strips from nonfailing hearts (NF) were obtained immediately after cardioplegic arrest from patients undergoing coronary artery bypass surgery where the ejection fraction was greater than 60%; strips of failing hearts (F) from patients with idiopathic dilated cardiomyopathy (NYHA Class IV, ejection fraction $13 \pm 1\%$) were obtained immediately following transplantation. Both the NF and F strips were placed in a Krebs butanedione monoxime (30 mmoles/l BDM) protection solution prior to final thin-strip dissection for myothermal and mechanical measurements [5].[2] Following the surgical excision of the tissue from the epicardial surface of the heart, the rough strip was placed in oxygenated protective solution for 1 hour to ensure recovery from the trauma of biopsy at the time of surgery. Thin strips, consisting of parallel running fibers, were sculpted from the original biopsy material so that the final preparation was 0.2–0.3 mm in diameter [5]. The BDM protective solution was washed out and all subsequent measurements were made, following incubation, in oxygenated (95% O_2/5% CO_2) Krebs–Ringer.

Myothermal and mechanical measurements

The myothermal and mechanical measurements were made at 37°C. The apparatus and protocol for carrying out mechanical and myothermal measurements on thin strips of heart tissue have been described in detail elsewhere [6]. The mechanical measurements (peak force, time to peak tension, $\pm dP/dt$) were made in each muscle strip at the optimum of the tension–length relationship [7,8]. The cross-sectional area of the strip was obtained from the ratio of the length at L_{max} (3–4 mm) to the blotted weight (0.2–0.6 mg). The steady-state force–frequency relation was obtained following 5 minutes of stimulation at each frequency from 0.2 Hz and increasing in 0.2 Hz increments.

The sculpted thin muscle strip is placed on the centrally located measuring junctions of the thermopile, with the bottom end of the strip fixed to a stationary supporting hook and the upper end of the strip attached to the force transducer. The strip is mounted on the thermopile so that the flat portion of the muscle is apposed to the measuring junctions. After mounting, the muscle and thermopile system are incubated in normal Krebs–Ringer solution for 90 minutes to completely wash out the BDM–Ringer protective solution. The washout solution is then drained and replaced with fresh oxygenated Ringer (95% O_2/5% CO_2), and the muscle is stimulated while being stretched in small increments (0.05 mm). The strip is stimulated end-to-end by means of 25-μm platinum-wire stimulating electrodes threaded into the 4-0 noncapillary braided silk ligatures used to tie the muscle to the force transducer and the stationary hook. After complete equilibration, the chamber is drained of all solutions and the measurements of force and heat are made.

Thermodynamic considerations

For the purpose of this analysis, the heart muscle strip can be considered to be a thermodynamic closed system. Under these circumstances, the total enthalpy change ($-\Delta H$) is equal to the heat liberated (q) and the work done (w) (see Eq. 1). Under isometric conditions where no external work is done, the enthalpy change ($-\Delta H$) is equal to the heat liberated (q) (see Eq. 2). The changes in enthalpy can be attributed to the changes in enthalpy of all the reactions coupled to the contraction–relaxation cycle (see Eq. 3), where n_i is the number of moles involved in the ith reaction and $-\Delta H_i$ is the change in enthalpy per mole for the ith reaction. Eqs. 1, 2, and 3 are statements of the first law of thermodynamics. The change in free energy $(-\Delta G)$ is the driving force for the relationships described. The free energy change $(-\Delta G)$ is related to the enthalpy change $(-\Delta H)$ by the second law of thermodynamics (see Eq. 4), where $T\Delta S$ is the entropy change.

$$-\Delta H = q + w \tag{1}$$

$$-\Delta H = q \tag{2}$$

$$-\Delta H = \Sigma_o^i n_i, X \times (-\Delta H_i) \tag{3}$$

$$-\Delta H = -\Delta G + T\Delta S \tag{4}$$

In muscle contraction and relaxation, the terminal phosphate bond of ATP is the primary source of energy (see Eq. 5). The hydrolysis of ATP with the production of ADP is very tightly coupled to the resynthesis of ATP from the ADP by the creatine phospho-transferease reaction (see Eq. 6). The equilibrium constant of 20 for the resynthesis of ATP assures that in the inherently slow contraction of cardiac muscle there is a virtually instantaneous resynthesis of the hydrolyzed ATP (Eq. 6). The enthalpy change for the hydrolysis of the key phosphate bond is 34 kJ/mole or 56 pnJ/molecule (56×10^{-21} J/molecule = $(34 \times 10^3$ J/mole)$/6.022 \times 10^{23}$ molecules/mole) [9].

$$ATP \rightarrow ADP + Pi \tag{5}$$

$$CrP + ADP \rightarrow ATP + Cr \tag{6}$$

Analysis of myothermal data

The cardiac muscle strip, in contact with the heat measuring junctions of the thermopile and stretched to the optimum length (L_{max}), liberates heat at a steady rate. The resting heat (RH) is associated with the maintenance of the internal environment of the muscle, with about 70% associated with maintenance of the ionic milieu and 30% related to protein synthesis [10]. When the muscle is stimulated to contract isometrically, the total activity-related heat (T_A) is liberated in two phases. There is an initial rapid heat liberation (I) associated with the mechanics of contraction and relaxation and a secondary slower heat liberation, reflecting recovery processes, that occurs at a mono-exponentially decreasing rate (R) (Eq. 7) (figure 2). Because R is liberated at a mono-exponentially decreasing rate, it is readily extrapolated to zero time; subtracting R from T_A thus provides the initial heat (I) (Eq. 8). The initial heat is a reflection of calcium cycling (TIH, tension-independent heat) and cross-bridge cycling (TDH, tension-dependent heat) (Eq. 9). The initial heat is partitioned

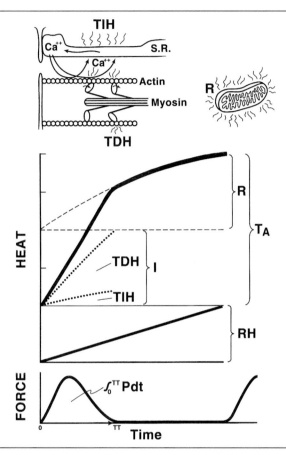

Figure 2. A drawing of a typical record of resting and total activity-related heat production in the isometrically contracting heart muscle strip. The following abbreviations are used: RH, resting heat; T_A, total activity-related heat; R, recovery heat; I, initial heat; TDH, tension-dependent heat; TIH, tension-independent heat; and $\int Pdt$, FTI, force–time integral. For the contribution to heat production of mitochondria, calcium cycling, and cross-bridge cycling, see figure 1. R is associated with the mitochondrial resynthesis of ATP from the ADP produced during the contraction and relaxation cycle. TDH is associated with the obligatory hydrolysis of a high-energy phosphate bond during the cross-bridge cycle. TIH is heat liberated during the removal of Ca^{2+} from the cytosol by the sarcoplasmic reticulum and sarcolemma.

into its components by incubating the strip in a low concentration of BDM–Krebs (2–5 mMolar), which decreases or eliminates the tension-dependent heat (TDH), leaving the tension–independent heat (TIH) [11]. The TIH can be used to calculate the amount of calcium released into the cytosol per beat and the rate of calcium uptake (where K is 0.75 and takes into account the difference in energy requirements between the sarcolemma and the sarcoplasmic reticulum for the removal of Ca^{2+}; the $CrP:Ca^{2+}$ coupling ratio is 2) (Eq. 10). The cross-bridge force–time integral (FTI_{XBr}) is equal to the muscle force–time integral (FTI_{muscle}) divided by the number of cross-bridge cycles that occur during the isometric twitch in a half sarcomere ($XBr_{cycles-hs}$) (Eq. 11). The number of cross-bridge cycles per half sarcomere is obtained from the tension-dependent heat per half sarcomere (TDH_{hs}) normalized by the enthalpy per molecule of ATP hydrolysis (56 pico nano Joules) (Eq. 12). The tension-dependent heat per half sarcomere is obtained by normalizing the TDH of the muscle for the number of half sarcomeres in the muscle studied (where L_0 is in mm and a half sarcomere is taken as $1\,\mu m$, with 1000 half sarcomeres per mm; the quantity ($L_0 \times 1000$) defines the number of half sarcomeres in the muscle) (Eq. 13).

$$T_A = I + R \tag{7}$$

$$T_A - R = I \tag{8}$$

$$I = TIH + TDH \tag{9}$$

$$Ca^{2+}\ moles/gm\text{-}beat = \left[K \times (TIH/gm)(Ca^{2+}:CrP\ coupling\ ratio)\right]/(34\ kJ/mole) \tag{10}$$

$$FTI_{XBr} = FTI_{muscle}/(XBr_{cycles-hs}) \tag{11}$$

$$XBr_{cycles-hs} = TDH_{hs}/56\ pnJ \tag{12}$$

$$TDH_{hs} = TDH_{muscle}/(L_o \times 1000) \tag{13}$$

Isometric mechanical and myothermal measurements [7]

The isometric peak force was reduced from $25.9 \pm 3.9\,mN/mm^2$ in the nonfailing strip (NF) to $13.9 \pm 2.0\,mN/mm^2$ in the dilated cardiomyopathic preparations (F) ($p < 0.02$); the rate of tension rise ($+dP/dt$, mN/mm^2-s) is reduced from 193 ± 26 (NF) to 95 ± 11 (F) ($p < 0.003$). Time to peak tension was increased from $189 \pm 9\,ms$ (NF) to $216 \pm 8\,ms$ (F) ($p < 0.03$), while the rate of relaxation ($-dP/dt$, mN/mm^2-s) decreased from 148 ± 23 (NF) to 80 ± 13 ($p < 0.02$). The total activity-related heat (T_A), initial heat (I), tension-dependent heat (TDH), tension-independent heat (TIH), and rate of tension-independent heat ($dTIH/dt$) liberation were significantly reduced in the failing heart strips (table 1). There is no significant difference between NF and F preparations in the ratio of total activity related heat to initial heat (T_A/I). This finding suggests that the mitochondria in the failing preparations are functioning normally. From Eq. 10 we can calculate the amount of calcium cycled per gram-beat and the rate of calcium cycled per gram-beat. In the failing heart preparations, these values are reduced to 31% of those in the nonfailing strips (table 2). From Eqs. 11, 12, and 13, we calculate the average cross-bridge force–time integral (figure 3). In the failing heart, the average cross-bridge force–time integral is increased by 41%. At a molecular level, this increase may result from an increase in the unitary force or the attachment time of the individual cross-bridge during the complete cycle.

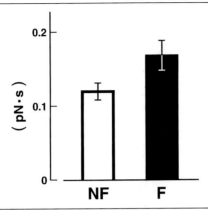

Figure 3. The average cross-bridge force–time integral determined in strips from nonfailing (NF) and failing (F) hearts (Eqs. 11, 12, 13).

Table 1. Myothermal data from nonfailing (NF) and dilated cardiomyopathic failing (F) hearts

Parameter	NF	F	p value
T_A (mJ/g-beat)	7.78 ± 1.32	2.78 ± 0.48	$p < 0.005$
I (mJ/g-beat)	3.89 ± 0.66	1.50 ± 0.26	$p < 0.005$
TDH (mJ/g-beat)	3.39 ± 0.66	1.34 ± 0.22	$p < 0.01$
TIH (mJ/g-beat)	0.51 ± 0.13	0.16 ± 0.05	$p < 0.03$
dTIH/dt (mW/g-beat)	0.82 ± 0.24	0.25 ± 0.09	$p < 0.03$

T_A, total activity-related heat; I, initial heat; TDH, tension-dependent heat; TIH, tension-independent heat; and dTIH/dt, rate of tension-independent heat.

Table 2. The calcium released into the cytosol per gram-beat and the rate of calcium removal from the cytosol per gram-second-beat for nonfailing (NF) and failing (F) hearts

Parameter	NF	F	p value
Ca^{2+} Release (nmoles/g-beat)	22.13 ± 5.61	6.87 ± 2.04	$p < 0.03$
Ca^{2+} Uptake rate (nmoles/g-sec-beat)	35.18 ± 10.28	10.84 ± 3.77	$p < 0.03$

The force–frequency relationship

In the failing preparations, there is clearly a depression in the peak isometric force as well as in the amount of calcium cycled per beat. These alone contribute substantially to the depression in ventricular function. An additional factor that contributes to the profound depression in performance is the altered force–frequency relationship. In nonfailing heart strips, as the frequency of stimulation is increased, there is a substantial increase in the force developed, with the peak force occurring

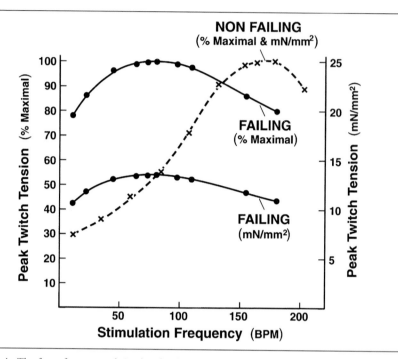

Figure 4. The force–frequency relationship for the nonfailing (NF) and failing (F) preparations.

at a frequency of $177 \pm 4\,\text{min}^{-1}$ (figure 4). In addition to the peak frequency, another index of the contribution of the force–frequency relationship to ventricular perfor-mance is seen in the myocardial reserve, namely, the percent increase in force as the heart rate is increased from 60 to $120\,\text{min}^{-1}$. From the diagram in figure 4 it is clear that the nonfailing preparation has a substantial myocardial reserve. In contrast, the optimum frequency for the failing strips was found to be $81 \pm 22\,\text{min}^{-1}$ with a neg-ative myocardial reserve, i.e., a decrease in force between 60 and $120\,\text{min}^{-1}$. The use of information obtained using strips from nonfailing hearts is supported by com-parable data obtained by others from nonfailing hearts in vivo [12].

DISCUSSION

Peak isometric twitch force and the rate of isometric force development

The depression in isometric force, as well as in the rate of isometric force devel-opment, in strips from the failing hearts is substantial. This depression cannot be attributed to force development of the individual cross-bridge in that the average cross-bridge force–time integral in the failing hearts is increased by 41% (figure 3), so based on the expected interactions at the molecular–motor level, one might antic-ipate a higher force being developed. This is clearly not the case. Because the amount of calcium cycled per beat is so remarkably depressed, it would appear that the most

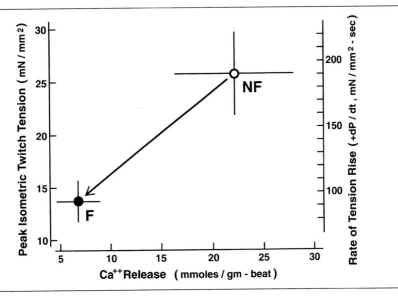

Figure 5. The relationship of peak isometric twitch force and the rate of tension development to the amount of calcium cycled per gram of heart muscle per beat.

likely cause of the depressed peak isometric force and rate of force development might be attributable to the decrease in the amount of calcium cycled per beat. This can be seen in figure 5, where the peak isometric force and the rate of peak isometric force production is plotted against the amount of calcium released into the cytosol per beat. It is also entirely reasonable to attribute the alteration in the force–frequency relationship to the amount of calcium cycled per beat as well as to the rate of calcium uptake, both of which are severely depressed.

The rate of isometric relaxation and time to peak tension

In NYHA Class III and IV heart failure, there is clearly a decrease in the rate of ventricular relaxation and an increase in diastolic pressure. The corollary in the measurement of strip mechanics is found in the rate of isometric relaxation ($-dP/dt$) and in the time to peak tension. The rate of isometric relaxation is decreased while time to peak tension is increased in the failing preparations. These changes are readily attributable to the decrease found in the rate of calcium uptake as measured by and calculated from the rate of tension-independent heat liberation (Eq. 10) (figure 6).

The power output

In the failing heart, one of the key parameters that defines the inadequacy of ventricular performance is the decrease in the rate of work production or power output. At the cross-bridge level, the increase in the average cross-bridge force–time integral (figure 3) ensures an increase in the economy of isometric force production

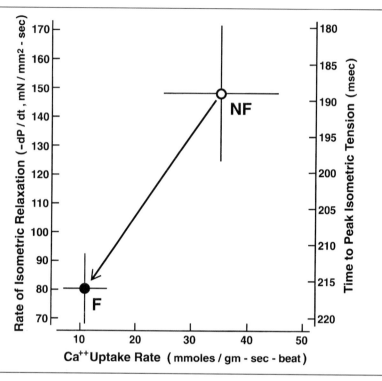

Figure 6. The relationship of the rate of iosometric relaxation $(-dP/dt)$ and time to peak tension to the rate of Ca^{2+} removal from the cytosol.

(force–time integral per ATP hydrolyzed) but has, as a potential consequence, a decrease in the velocity of shortening. From studies on circumferential fiber short-ening in intact hearts, myofibrillar ATPase measurements, and the in vitro motility assay, we know that the velocity of shortening in failing hearts is markedly reduced [3,13–15]. Because the isometric force and the maximum velocity of shortening are reduced in the failing preparations, this means that the force–velocity curve is shifted to the left and down. Power is the product of the force at each velocity, accordingly, with a depressed force–velocity relationship in failing hearts, the power must also be depressed (figure 7).

Calcium cycling

The depression in the amount and rate of calcium cycling calculated from the changes in the tension-independent heat and the rate of tension-independent lib-eration in the strips from the failing ventricles suggests major changes in those strips. If there were a significant replacement of healthy tissue with fibrous tissue, scarring, or substantial apoptosis, this might explain the decrease in the tension-independent heat measurements per gram of tissue. We attempted to reduce this possibility by

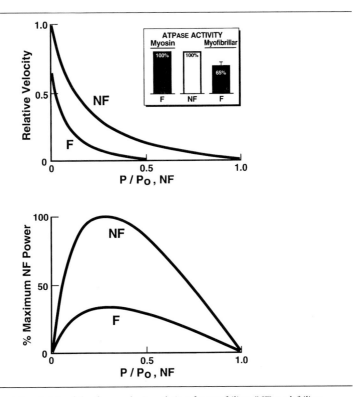

Figure 7. A representative sketch of the force–velocity relation for nonfailing (NF) and failing (F) hearts, with the myofibrillar and myosin ATPase shown in the inset. Power as a percentage of maximum power in the nonfailing (NF) hearts for NF and failing (F) preparations is illustrated in the lower drawing.

preparing strips of failing muscle from the portion of the heart where there was no visible sign of increases in connective tissue or scarring. In support of the improbability that tissue destruction can explain the 70% reduction in tension-independent heat measurements, we never found a reduction in myosin content greater than 20%. A more likely explanation for the reduction in calcium cycling in failing hearts is the observed changes in calcium-cycling proteins, where the sarcolemmal sodium–calcium exchange protein and mRNA are increased, while in the sarcoplasmic reticulum, the SERCA2, phospholamban, and ryanodine receptor are all decreased [16–18].

Cross-bridge cycling

It was unexpected to find that the average cross-bridge force–time integral in the failing hearts was increased by 41%. This finding was especially interesting in that the myofibrillar ATPase was decreased in heart failure, whereas the myosin ATPase was unchanged [14,15]. This finding suggests that the alteration in the failing hearts is not caused by a change in the myosin but rather by a change in the thin fila-ment proteins. One very interesting observation that may offer a mechanism for this change is the finding that the alteration in myofibrillar ATPase activity correlates with a shift in the troponin-T isoforms [19,20]. The shift in the troponin-T isoform may change the movement of tropomyosin following calcium liberation and thus the specific binding sites on the surface of the actin that are available for myosin binding.

CONCLUSIONS

The phenotypic cellular restructuring found in the failing heart has significant effects on the quantity and rate of calcium cycling as well as on the cross-bridge cycle. The increase in sarcolemmal Na–Ca exchange protein and the decrease in the sarcoplasmic reticulum SERCA2 calcium pump, phospholamban, and rynanodine receptor can substantially decrease the amount of calcium available for activation. This may readily explain the results presented here, where the tension-independent heat is reduced 70% and presumably the calcium cycled per beat is accordingly reduced. The alterations in cross-bridge cycling (increase in the average cross-bridge force–time integral, decrease in myofibrillar ATPase activity, and decrease in veloc-ity of shortening) are believed to be associated with the shift in the troponin T isoform from TnT_3 to TnT_4. The change in calcium cycling, resulting in a change in peak force, and the TnT isoform shift, leading to a reduction in shortening velocity, result in a shift in the force–velocity relationship to the left and down (figure 7), with a commensurate reduction in the power output. Future work must be directed at understanding the mechanisms involved in producing the phenotypic changes observed that ultimately involve the progression from compensation to failure.

ACKNOWLEDGMENTS

This work was supported in part by USPHS Grant # USPHS RO1 HL 55641.

NOTES

1. The NYHA category system is based on shortness of breath and fatigue as a function of activity with severe heart failure (NYHA III or IV) involving symptoms with minimal activity or at rest, respectively.

2. For the NF strip preparations, patients gave informed consent. The study was approved by the Committee on Human Research of the University of Vermont. Informed consent was given prior to transplant by patients at the transplant center.

REFERENCES

1. Cowie MR, Mostead A, Wood DA, et al. 1997. The epidemiology of heart failure. Eur Heart J 18:208–225.
2. Califf RM, Adams KF, McKenna WJ, Gheorghiade M, Uretsky BF, McNulty SE, Darius H, Schulman K, Zannad F, Handberg-Thurmond E, Harrell FE Jr, Wheeler W, Soler-Soler J, Swedberg K. 1997. A radomized controlled trial of epoprostenol therapy for severe congestive heart failure: the Flolan Interational Randomizd Survival Trial (FIRST). Am Heart J 134:44–54.

3. The SOLVD Investigators. 1991. Effect of enalapril on survival in patients with reduced left ventricular ejection fractions and congestive heart failure. N Engl J Med 325:293–302.

4. Cohn JN, Ziesche S, Smith R, Anand I, Dunkman WB, Loeb H, Cintron G, Boden W, Baruch L,
Rochin P, Loss L. 1997. Effect of the calcium antagonist felodipine as supplementary vasodilator
therapy in patients with chronic heart failure treated with enalapril: V-HeFT III. Vasodilator-Heart
Failure Trial (V-HeFT) Study Group. Circulation 5;96(3):856–863.

5. Mulieri LA, Hasenfuss G, Ittleman F, Blanchard EM, Alpert NR. 1989. Protection of human left
ventricular myocardium from cutting injury with 2,3-butanedione monoxime. Circ Res
65:1441–1449.

6. Mulieri LA, Luhr G, Treffry J, Alpert NR. 1977. Metal-film thermopiles for use with rabbit right
ventricular papillary muscles. Am J Physiol 233:C146–C156.

7. Hasenfuss G, Mulieri LA, Leavitt JB, Allen PD, Haeberle JR, Alpert NR. 1992. Alterations of
contractile function and excitation–contraction coupling in dilated cardiomyopathy. Circ Res
70:1225–1232.

8. Mulieri LA, Hasenfuss G, Leavit B, Allen PD, Alpert NR. 1992. Altered myocardial force–frequency
relation in human heart failure. Circulation 85:1743–1750.

9. Woledge RC, Reilly PJ. 1988. Molar enthalpy change for the hydrolysis of phosphocreatine under
conditions in muscle cells. Biophys J 54:97–104.

10. Gibbs CL, Chapman JB. 1979. Cardiac heat production. Annu Rev Physiol 41:507–519.

11. Alpert NR, Blanchard EM, Mulieri LA. 1989. Tension-independent heat in rabbit papillary muscle.
J Physiol 414:433–453.

12. Mulieri LA, Alpert NR. 1998. The role of the myocardial force–frequency relation in left ventricular function and progression of human heart failure. In Heart Metabolism in Failure. Ed. R Altschuld
and R Haworth, 47–62. Greenwich, CT: JAI Press.

13. Harris D, Work SS, Wright RK, Alpert NR, Warshaw DM. 1994. Smooth, cardiac and skeletal muscle
myosin force and motion generation by cross-bridge mechanical interactions in vitro. J Mol Res
Cell Motility 15:11–19.

14. Alpert NR, Gordon MS. 1962. Myofibrillar adenosine triphosphatase activity in congestive heart
failure. Am J Physiol 202:940–945.

15. Pagani ED, Alousi AA, Grant AM, Older TM, Dziuban SW Jr, Allen PD. 1988. Changes in myofibrillar content and Mg-ATPase activity in ventricular tissue from patients with heart failure caused
by coronary artery disease, cardiomyopathy or mitral valve insufficiency. Circ Res 63:380–385.

16. Struder R, Reinecke H, Bilger J, Eschenhagen T, Bohm M, Hasenfuss G, Just H, Holtz J, Drexler
H. Gene expression of the cardiac Na^+-Ca^{2+} exchanger in end-stage human heart failure. Circ Res
1994. 75:443–453.

17. Arai M, Alpert NR, MacLennan D, Barton P, Periasamy M. 1993. Alterations in sarcoplasmic reticulum gene expression in human heart failure: a possible mechanism of alterations in systolic and
diastolic properties of the failing myocardium. Circ Res 72:463–469.

18. Mercadier JJ, Lompre AM, Duc P, Boheler KR, Fraysse JB, Wisnewski G, Allen PD, Kokajda M,
Schwartz K. 1990. Altered sarcoplasmic reticulum Ca^{2+}–ATPase gene expression in human ventricle
during end-state failure. J Clin Invest 85:305–309.

19. Anderson PAW, Grieg A, Mark TM, Malouf NN, Oakeley AE, Ungerlieder RM, Allen PD, Kay BK.
1995. Molecular basis for human cardiac troponin T isoform in the developing, adult and failing
heart. Circ Res 76:681–686.

20. Mesnard L, Logeart D, Taviaux S, Diriong S, Mercadier JJ, Samson G. 1995. Human cardiac troponin
T. Cloning and expression of new isoforms in normal and failing heart. Circ Res 76:687–692.

N. Takeda, M. Nagano and N.S. Dhalla
(eds). The Hypertrophied Heart. Copyright
© 2000. pp. 423–439. Kluwer Academic
Publishers. Boston. All rights reserved.

THE STRUCTURAL CORRELATE OF REDUCED CARDIAC FUNCTION IN FAILING HUMAN HEARTS

SAWA KOSTIN

Department of Experimental Cardiology, Max-Planck-Institute, Thoracic and Cardiovascular Surgery, Kerckhoff-Clinic, Benekestr. 2, D-61231 Bad Nauheim, Germany

Summary. The present chapter summarizes and reviews the morphological alterations that are typical of dilated cardiomyopathy (DCM) at the late stage of the disease resulting in heart failure; evidence for the occurrence of myocyte cell loss, chronic cellular degeneration, possible defects in sarcomerogenesis, and disorganization of the cardiomyocyte cytoskeleton and proteins of the cardiac intercalated disk is demonstrated. The data presented show that in DCM many different proteins are subjected to alterations in expression and arrangement, demonstrating a graded sensitivity towards pathological stimuli in that the contractile proteins and sarcomeric skeleton are the most sensitive proteins and the cytoskeleton and its associated proteins show a compensatory increase. From these findings, it is concluded that different reactions of the cardiac protein families to chronic cardiomyopathic processes reflect the survival priorities of the cells. Furthermore, these data show that alterations and extensive but disproportionate reorganization of a whole complex of proteins represent the structural basis for the reduction of contractile function in failing human hearts. In addition, disorganization of gap junctions distribution associated with myocardial scarring and myofiber disarray, and selective disruption of large gap junctions may play an important role in the development of an arrhythmogenic substrate in human DCM.

INTRODUCTION

Heart failure is the final clinical presentation of a variety of cardiovascular diseases, such as coronary artery disease, hypertension, valvular heart disease, myocarditis, and cardiomyopathies. Progressive deterioration of left ventricular function is a characteristic feature of the heart failure state. The mechanisms responsible for this hemodynamic deterioration are not known but have been attributed to a so-called vicious circle of compensatory mechanisms intended to maintain homeostasis, such as ventricular remodeling and enhanced activity of the sympathetic nervous system and renin–angiotensin system, which become factors that accelerate the process of left ventricular dysfunction. Although the etiopathologies of cardiac diseases that progress to heart failure are different, they share almost the same sequence of molecular and biochemical events leading from cardiac hypertrophy to congestive heart failure.

A relevant issue in heart failure concerns the understanding of the structural correlate of depressed left ventricular function. Until recently, a thorough investigation of the morphology of heart failure had been hampered by the insufficient quality of morphological techniques and by the fact that only postmortem tissue or very small catheter biopsies could be studied. Tissue specimens obtained at the time of cardiac transplantation have expanded previous observations on morphological changes associated with cardiac failure. Moreover, the recent availability of human explanted hearts, allowing the optimal tissue preservation by rapid fixation, provides the basis for the use of highly sensitive new methods in morphology, such as electron microscopy, immunoconfocal and molecular biology techniques.

In recent years, we have extensively described the structural changes in the human heart that is failing because of dilated cardiomyopathy (DCM). Specifically, there was a marked heterogeneity in myocyte size as well as in the intracellular alterations, including myocyte cell death, chronic cellular degeneration, cytoskeletal protein abnormalities, myofilament loss, and abnormal sarcomeres [1–6]. Furthermore, the extracellular space was enlarged, and there was an increase in all components of the matrix, including proteins such as fibronectin and laminin, fibrillar collagen, fibroblasts, and macrophages [3,4,7,8]. The changes described are believed to be an important component of the structural correlate of reduced cardiac function in human hearts.

The present chapter will summarize and review the morphological alterations that are typical of DCM at the late stage of the disease. Evidence will be demonstrated for the occurrence of myocyte cell loss, chronic cellular degeneration and proteins involved in this process, possible defects in sarcomerogenesis, and the disorganization of the cardiomyocyte cytoskeleton and proteins forming the cardiac intercalated disc. These will be discussed as potential structural correlates of reduced myocardial function. The data presented here were obtained from patients with severely depressed left ventricular performance (ejection fraction less than 20%) undergoing cardiac transplantation because of intractable heart failure due to DCM. The methods employed are electron microscopy and immunohistochemistry with confocal laser scanning microscopy.

MYOCYTE CELL LOSS IN THE FAILING HUMAN MYOCARDIUM

Recently, data have accumulated to show that progressive deterioration of myocardial function and ventricular remodeling in heart failure is due to ongoing loss of viable cardiomyocytes [9–13]. Numerous morphological studies of human hearts have clearly demonstrated replacement and diffuse interstitial fibrosis, degenerative changes in myocytes, and sequestration of cell fragments—findings that provide some support, albeit indirect, to the concept that ongoing myocyte loss, apoptotic or necrotic in nature, may be taking place in the failing heart [2,14–16]. The electron micrograph in figure 1A shows the disappearance of a single cardiomyocyte with low cellular infiltration, suggestive of apoptosis. Only remnants of the intercalated

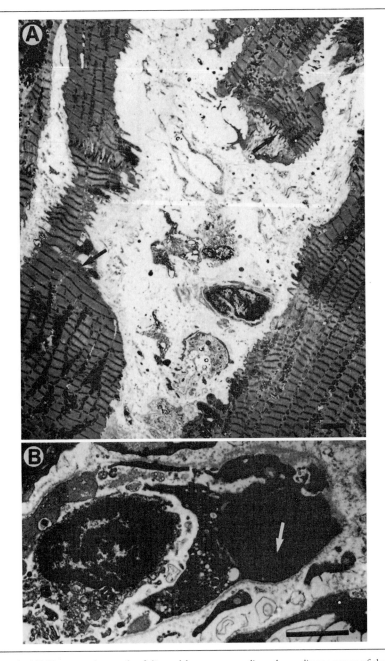

Figure 1. (A) Electron micrograph of diseased human myocardium shows disappearance of the central myocyte. Only remnants of the intercalated disc and preexisting interconnections (arrows) of the former cardiomyocyte can be observed. (B) Simultaneous occurrence of apoptosis and oncosis in ischemic myocardial tissue. At the left side, the nucleus of the endothelial cell shows irregular chromatin clumping typical of oncotic necrosis. On the right side, the pericyte shows dense chromatin condensation typical of apoptosis (arrow). All preparations were doubly stained with uranyl acetate and lead citrate. In all micrographs, bar = 5 µm.

disc and preexisting interconnections and position of the former cardiomyocyte can be observed.

Although myocyte necrosis is an uncommon finding in end-stage heart failure, recent characterizations of apoptosis as the predominant mode of cell death in advanced heart disease has provided further support for the role of cell loss in the progression of cardiac hypertrophy to failure. Apoptosis is a distinct form of cell death that displays characteristic alterations in cell morphology (figures 1B and 2c–e), such as chromatin condensation and margination that result in a "half-moon" or "shoe" appearance of the nucleus. (For comparison with normal nuclear morphology, see figure 2a and 2b). In later stages of apoptosis, nuclear fragmentation becomes evident, the cytoplasm condenses progressively, and one or more apoptotic bodies are formed from each dying cell (figure 2f).

The recognition that myocyte apoptosis is implicated in cardiac diseases and heart failure is important, emphasizing the need for the quantification of this process. The most reliable way to confirm apoptosis, following stringent criteria for definition, remains the identification of characteristic morphological features by transmission electron microscopy (figure 2c–e); however, for routine use, quantitating cells undergoing apoptosis by this method is impractical because of the rather small tissue samples that are investigated. In tissue sections, the TdT-mediated dUTP nick end labeling (TUNEL) or ISEL (in situ end labeling) method for the detection of internucleosomal DNA fragmentation, combined with confocal microscopy, is the only procedure feasible for this purpose until now. DNA laddering as observed in gel electrophoresis, providing biochemical documentation of the pattern of DNA fragmentation, is useful in tissue homogenates. It does not, however, permit the identification of the type of cell in apoptosis, and its sensibility is low. For tissue sections, in own experience, the TUNEL method in combination with electron microscopy has proved to provide reliable, reproducible results.

Only a few studies report the occurrence of apoptosis in human hearts with DCM. In 1996, Mallat et al. [17] and Narula et al. [18] reported the occurrence of apoptotic myocytes in human dilated cardiomyopathy. Their numbers, however, vary greatly and are difficult to compare. Narula et al. found an apoptotic rate ranging from 5% to 35.5% in four patients with DCM, located mostly in the subendocardium. Mallat et al. found 14% of cells to be in apoptosis in right ventricular displasia. The findings of high levels of apoptosis must be interpreted with extreme caution because, assuming that the completion of this process may take 24 hours or even less, these findings would indicate a massive loss of heart tissue over a very short period of time. In our own preliminary study, we found 45 apoptotic myocyte nuclei in more than 1 million myocytes evaluated using the TUNEL method in 20 patients with end-stage heart failure due to DCM [12]. Olivetti et al. [11] studied five patients with DCM and counted 2366 ± 2033 apoptotic nuclei/10^6 nuclei in cardiomyocytes, which amounts to 0.23%. Again, by assuming that apoptosis will take 24 hours to be completed, Olivetti's data would predict a loss of 83% of myocytes by apoptosis per year, and our data per year would result in disappearance of 1.3% of myocytes, indicating that Olivetti's data most probably are too high and ours are too low. Such contradictory results indicate the need for the application of uniform methods for the detection and

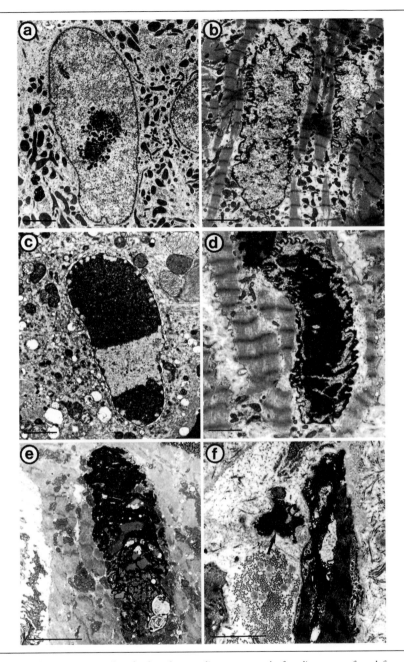

Figure 2. Electron micrographs of cultured rat cardiomyocytes and of cardiomyocyte from left ventricle of normal and diseased human hearts. (**a**) The nucleus from cardiomyocytes in culture or from normal human myocardium (**b**) shows even distribution of chromatin in the nucleoplasm. (**c**) Nuclear condensation in a cardiomyocyte maintained in culture for 10 days undergoing apoptosis. Notice the compaction and segregation of nuclear chromatin into sharply delineated masses, resulting in a typical "shoe-like" appearance of the nucleus. (**d, e**) Ultrastructural evidence of apoptosis in human myocardium: clumping of chromatin in the presence of undamaged mitochondria—a typical ultrastructural sign of apoptosis. (**f**) The formation of an apoptotic body (arrow), containing fragments of condensed nuclear chromatin, is a typical example of an advanced stage of apoptosis. The cytoplasm of the neighboring cardiomyocyte at the right side is electron dense and shows shrinkage, whereas the nucleus is fragmented and shows severe chromatin clumping. All preparations were doubly stained with uranyl acetate and lead citrate. In all micrographs, bar = 5 μm.

quantification of cell death in the myocardium. The possibility exists, however, that apoptosis occurs discontinuously, which renders the interpretation of data on the rate of apoptosis in myocardial tissue even more difficult.

Apart from the unresolved question on how important myocyte apoptosis is in progression of left ventricular dysfunction and the transition to heart failure, we as well as others in recent years have aimed to induce experimentally apoptotic cell death with components typical of heart failure, such as abnormal hemodynamic load or neurohumoral substances. In an experimental model of isometric stretch of papillary muscle, apoptosis of cardiomyocytes could be detected in 0.64% of cardiomyocytes, indicating that elevated end-diastolic pressure may constitute an initiating event for myocyte apoptosis [19]. Interestingly, passive overstretching of isolated papillary muscles produced Fas overexpression; however, myocyte apoptosis seemed to be dependent upon superoxide anion production. In a recent study conducted in isolated adult rat cardiomyocytes in long-term culture, we developed a new model of apoptosis induced by hydrogen peroxide as a challenger, which yielded a 50% incidence of apoptosis, that could be significantly prevented by inhibitors of ICE-like proteases, such as Z-YVAD-fmk (K. Suzuki, unpublished data). This model is relevant, because adult cardiomyocytes in long-term culture show a phenotype closely resembling that of hypertrophic and failing myocardium [20]. Using freshly dissociated adult cardiomyocytes, Kajstura et al. [21] documented an increased incidence of apoptosis in cells exposed to angiotensin II (0.9% apoptotic cardiomyocytes in the angiotensin II-treated group versus 0.2% in the control group), suggesting the possibility that the beneficial effect of angiotensin-converting enzyme inhibitors in heart failure may be in part be attributable to an inhibition of myocyte loss. The observation that tumor necrosis factor-α (TNF-α) is a trigger for apoptosis of a variety of cells in vitro and that serum levels of TNF-α in patients with heart failure are elevated [22] suggests that the cardiotoxicity of this substance may also be complicated by inducing myocyte apoptosis [23].

In summary, our data and published evidence support the contention that cardiac myocyte cell death occurs in different cardiac diseases that progress to heart failure and can be induced experimentally with substances and agents present during the developmental phases of heart failure. However, the determination of apoptosis in cardiac tissue is still hampered by technical difficulties, and the rate of apoptosis reported for DCM and other cardiac diseases therefore varies widely. The duration of the apoptotic process in myocytes is unknown, further complicating our understanding of the role of this form of death in the evolution of the heart failure. Therefore, the importance of apoptosis in the transition from compensated hypertrophy to cardiac failure and in heart failure caused by DCM has still to be established.

CARDIOMYOCYTE PROTEIN COMPOSITION AND CHRONIC CELLULAR DEGENERATION IN FAILING HUMAN HEARTS

The complexity of events involved in the pathogenesis of heart failure cannot be solely attributed to myocyte cell loss. Among other structural correlates of heart failure, chronic myocyte degeneration is the less understood process. In DCM, intracellular degenerative alterations could be observed in about one third of all myocytes and are characterized by loss of the myofilaments, an accumulation of nonspecified cytoplasm, small mitochondria, and myelin figures [2]. In the present study, we have investigated the proteins involved in this process and have compared their distribution and localization with those observed in normal human myocardial tissue or in normal isolated ventricular myocytes.

From the published reports and our own observations, it is evident that the cardiomyocyte contains a multitude of different proteins, which can be categorized into the following families [1]:

1. The contractile proteins
2. The sarcomeric skeleton
3. The cytoskeletal proteins
4. Membrane-associated proteins
5. Focal adhesion molecules
6. Proteins of the intercalated disc

This classification is based on the structural properties of the myocyte, i.e., the contractile and sarcomeric skeleton proteins form the sarcomere; the cytoskeletal proteins are the basis of the cytoskeleton, consisting of microtubules and filamentous structures; the membrane-associated proteins and focal adhesion molecules play a major role in anchoring the entire array of myofibrils and are in close spatial relationship with the cellular membrane and, via the integrins, with the extracellular space; and the proteins of the intercalated disc are involved in the connection of the myocytes in a longitudinal direction and in the conduction of the electrical stimulus for contraction. Following this classification, we tried to investigate the sensitivity and reaction of these proteins families toward the chronic cardiomyopathic process.

Contractile proteins

It was obvious from the electron microscopy studies that the content of myofilaments was significantly reduced in failing human hearts. These ultrastructural findings were confirmed by immunohistochemistry using different monoclonal antibodies against the myosin heavy chain, the α-isoforms of actin, tropomyosin, and troponin T [14]. In control nondiseased myocardium, the contractile proteins were regularly organized in the majority of myocytes, whereas myocardium from human hearts with DCM showed a significant partial or total lack of myosin filaments from many myocytes. This finding was especially evident in hypertrophied or atrophied myocytes. It was concluded that the myofilaments are the proteins that are most sensitive to pathophysiological influences.

The proteins of the sarcomeric skeleton

The contractile proteins are kept in register by different proteins localized in the Z-disc and in the M-band of the sarcomere, as well as by the giant filament-molecule titin, which spans the entire half-sarcomere from the Z-disc to the M-line. The Z-disc is a region of overlapping tails of actin microfilaments, cross-linked by α-actinin. Another component of cardiac Z-disc has been recently identified as a 109 kDa nebulin-related protein, nebulette, which appears to insert only to the periphery of the Z-disc [24]. The M-line is the region where the myosin tails are linked and organized by the M-line proteins—myomesin, M- and C-proteins, and creatine kinase. Titin is anchored with its N-terminus at the Z-disc and reaches the M-line region with its C-terminal head portion where it interacts with M-line protein and with myomesin [25]. Because of the length of the titin molecule, many different epitopes have been isolated and antibodies produced against various regions of the molecule. Depending on the location of the antibody binding, the labeling pattern with monoclonal antibodies will vary. A fine cross-striation is observed by labeling with the T12 antibody against an epitope close to the Z-disc and the T42 antibody against the M-line epitope. Labeling with the T30 antibody results in a rather wide cross-striation at the level of the A-band (figure 3a and c). In cardiac muscle cells, α-actinin shows a clear cross-striation at the level of the Z-disc, while myomesin is localized in the region of the M-band (figure 3b and d).

In failing human myocardium, titin and α-actinin showed disorganization and were partially reduced. In many cells, only remnants of the formerly highly organized support structures of the sarcomeres were found. Typically, these were arranged along the periphery of the myocyte underneath the sarcolemma, whereas in the center only punctate-like structures were observed (figure 3e and f). Since α-actinin and titin bind to each other at the level of the Z-disc, these proteins may interact and jointly disappear in this situation. In the confocal miscrocope after labeling with monoclonal antibodies, remnants of the sarcomeres are still visible, whereas in the electron microscope the sarcomeres will not be detectable anymore. Since titin, myomesin, and α-actinin have been reported to be involved in sarcomerogenesis, we postulated that the defect of these proteins may be more crucial for the structural abnormalities observed in the failing heart than those of the contractile apparatus. Currently in our laboratory, studies are carried out on adult myocytes in culture to test this hypothesis. Involvement of titin in cardiac disease processes has been shown, as reviewed by Labeit et al. [25] and also by Hein et al. [6].

The cytoskeleton

The cardiomyocyte cytoskeleton is composed of a highly organized complex array of specific proteins, arranged to transmit mechanical forces within the cell, to adjacent cells, and to the extracellular matrix, as well as to maintain the internal organization of cellular organelles. A network of intermediate filaments (figure 4A and B) and microtubules (figure 4C) extends throughout the cytoplasm, which therefore plays a central role in maintaining cellular integrity and function of the myocardium.

In failing human hearts, the proteins of the cytoskeleton, namely, desmin and tubulin, show a labeling pattern different from that of the two previous protein groups. Whereas the contractile and sarcomeric skeleton proteins were greatly

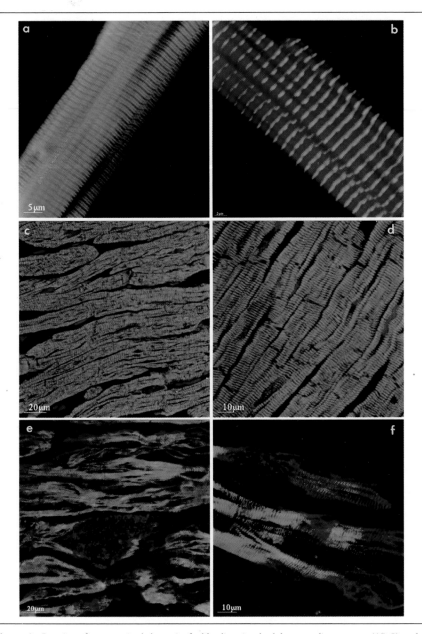

Figure 3. Proteins of sarcomeric skeleton in freshly dissociated adult rat cardiomyocytes (ARC) and in normal or diseased human cardiomyocytes. (**a**) Titin labeling with T30 antibody shows a distinct cross-striation on both sides of the dark M-band. The wider dark line represents the Z-disc, with parts of the I-band of neighboring sarcomeres. (**b**) Myomesin labeling (green) in ARC shows a clear cross-striation at the level of the M-band. Actin filaments are stained with phalloidin conjugated with TRITC (red). Staining of normal human myocardium using monoclonal anti-titin T30 (**c**) and antimyomesin (**d**) showing normal distribution and a clear cross-striation pattern for both proteins. (**e, f**) Double labeling for α-actinin (red) and myomesin (green) shows a few examples of disarrangement and partial lack of both proteins in human DCM.

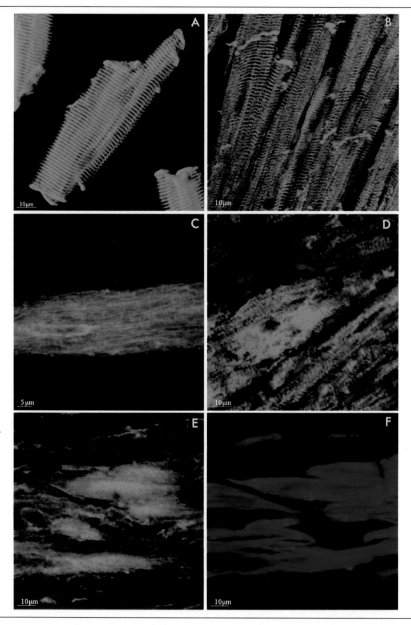

Figure 4. The cytoskeleton in freshly dissociated adult rat cardiomyocytes (ARC) and in normal or diseased human cardiomyocytes. (**A**) Desmin staining in ARC shows a cross-striation pattern at the Z-line level of the sarcomeres. Increased intensity of desmin immunofluorescence at the intercalated disc is evident. (**B**) In normal human myocardium, desmin is regularly distributed in a cross-striated pattern, as well as conspicuously at the intercalated disc regions. (**C**) Staining of tubulin in freshly isolated ARC using monoclonal anti-β-tubulin. Microtubuli surround the nucleus and form a dense network within the myocyte, mostly in the longitudinal direction. (**D**) Different patterns of desmin immunofluorescence intensity and organization in a patient with DCM. Notice the irregular distribution of desmin with loss of cross-striation and marked accumulation in the central cardiomyocyte. (**E**) Densification and disarrangement of microtubuli network is evident in some cardiomyocytes from a patient with DCM. (**F**) The same field as in **E**, showing the overall morphology and organization of the contractile apparatus stained with phalloidin-TRITC.

reduced in amount, the cytoskeletal proteins were partially increased but completely disorganized. This is especially evident for desmin (figure 4D) but applies also to tubulin (figure 4E and F). It was obvious that this increase in cytoskeletal proteins was mainly observed in cells that lacked myofilaments and was interpreted as a compensatory mechanism for the loss of cellular stability due to damage to the contractile apparatus. These data, obtained in human hearts, confirm experimental reports and strongly support the concept of the involvement of cytoskeleton in contractile dysfunction and increased ventricular stiffness in failing hearts, as previously formulated by Cooper and coworkers [26–28]. Furthermore, our data indicate the involvement of desmin intermediate filaments in cardiomyocyte remodeling as well. To date, a progressive increase of desmin protein and filaments was observed during the transition from hypertrophy to heart failure in guinea pig hearts after aortic banding [29]. On the other hand, a desmin null mutation has been reported to give rise to cardiomyopathy, indicating the essential role of desmin for cell survival and sarcomerogenesis [30].

Focal adhesion molecules and membrane-associated proteins

These groups of proteins are referred to cytoskeleton-associated proteins and include the vinculin talin integrin link [31], the dystrophin–glycoprotein–laminin complex [32], and spectrin-based submembranous skeleton [33]. All these proteins have been shown to be present within or in close proximity to the sarcolemma in the cardiac muscle cells of different mammals; however, information regarding the key question—whether these proteins are specifically associated with specialized regions of cardiac sarcolemma (e.g., costamere, T-tubules, etc.)—is still limited, and studies in human myocardium are lacking. In order to resolve these questions, we recently conducted confocal immunocytochemical studies to examine the subcellular localization of cell-matrix focal adhesion molecules (FAM) vinculin, talin, $\beta_1\alpha_5$-integrin, and the membrane-associated proteins (MAP) dystrophin and spectrin in human myocardium. The results are summarized in table 1. The localization

Table 1. Localization of focal adhesion molecules and membrane-associated proteins in cardiomyocytes

Protein	Z-discs	Costameres	T-tubules	"Free" sarcolemma	Intercalated discs
α-Actinin	+	−	−	−	+
Vinculin	−	+	+	−	+
Talin	−	+	+	−	−
α5 Integrin	−	+	+	−	−
Spectrin	−	+	+	+	−
Dystrophin	−	+	+	+	−
Laminin	−	+	+	+	−
Collagen IV	−	+	+	+	−
Fibronectin	−	+	+	+	−

+, present; −, absent.

reported here of FAMs and MAPs in the sarcolemma is in close agreement with published evidence of the costameric localization of vinculin [34,35], talin [36], integrins [37], spectrin [38], and dystrophin [39]. In contrast to the findings of Terracio et al. [40] and Meng et al. [41], we as well as Stevenson et al. [35] find no evidence for the presence of either vinculin or dystrophin within the Z-discs of myofibrils.

In addition to costameric localization of FAMs and MAPs, we found these proteins to be in association with the T-tubules (figure 5A and B). Together with basal lamina proteins (figure 5C and D), they would be predicted to confer integrity to the T-tubular plasma membrane during contraction/relaxation cycles and to maintain a stable position of the T-tubules at the Z-level. This relationship is important for Ca^{2+} exchange and thus for the control of contraction and force generation.

In heart muscle, vinculin has been described as the main protein of the costameres, the circular lattice elements that attach myofibrils to the sarcolemma [34,38]. Talin was found in the skeletal and cardiac costameres as well [36]. Costameres link myofibrils to the extracellular matrix and are sites of force coupling between myofibrils and extracellular matrix [42].

Immunofluorescent staining of normal human cardiac tissue revealed three sites of vinculin reactivity (figure 5E). First, vinculin was organized at the lateral sarcolemma in transverse rib-like bands, the costameres, underlying the central part of the Z-band. Second, vinculin localized also at the lateral sarcolemma in finer strands running parallel to the cellular long axis and interconnecting costameres. Third, vinculin labeling was particularly conspicuous at the transverse plicate regions of the intercalated disks, corresponding to the positions of the fascia adherens junctions. In DCM, vinculin (figure 5F), as well as talin and dystrophin, showed an intense fluorescence at the lateral sarcolemma of cardiac myocytes in failing myocardium. This phenomenon was most pronounced in cells with lack of contractile proteins and of the sarcomeric skeleton and was also interpreted as a mechanism to preserve cellular stability and integrity.

Proteins of the intercalated disc

Cardiac muscle cells are interconnected by three distinct types of intercellular junctions—gap junctions, *fasciae adherentes*, and desmosomes—located in a specialized portion of the plasma membrane, the intercalated disc (ID). Gap junctions form the low-resistance pathway that enables rapid conduction of cardiac action potential throughout the myofibers, thereby synchronizing contractions of the heart. Connexin 43 (Cx43) is the major connexin isoform expressed in the cardiac gap junctions [43,44]. In adult cardiac myocytes, connexin 43 is localized at the ID at the ends of the cell and side branches (figure 6A).

Fasciae adherentes and desmosomes belong to the adhering group of junctions and are responsible for attachment of the contractile filaments and the intermediate filaments to sites of the intercellular adhesion, respectively. These junctions are characterized by the presence of junction-specific sarcoplasmic plaque proteins and transmembrane cadherins.

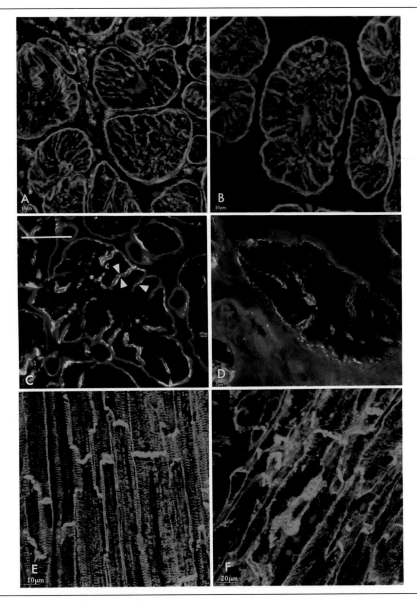

Figure 5. The distribution and localization of membrane-associated proteins (spectrin and dystrophin) and focal adhesion molecules (vinculin and talin) in transverse or longitudinal sections of normal or failing human myocardium. (**A**) Spectrin (green) is present in the interstitial cells as well as in the peripheral and T-tubular sarcolemma of the cardiomyocyte. (**B**) Dystrophin (green) labels the surface sarcolemma as well as the internal T-tubular network as radially oriented finger-like projections. Notice that dystrophin is absent from the membrane of different interstitial cells. (**C**) Double labeling for vinculin (green) with basal lamina protein laminin (red) in normal human myocardium. Laminin is precisely codistributed with vinculin immunofluorescence at the peripheral and T-tubular sarcolemma. (**D**) Double labeling for talin (green) and fibronectin (red). Fibronection colocalizes with talin and is abundantly present in the extracellular space in diseased human myocardium. Notice the dilated appearance of T-tubules in DCM. (**E**) The distribution of vinculin (green) in longitudinal myocardial sections of normal myocardium is visible within the cells (T-tubules), at the intercalated disc, and as fluorescent dots at the peripheral sarcolemma (costameres). (**F**) Vinculin in diseased human myocardium is significantly increased at the lateral sarcolemma and shows severe disorganization. In **A**, **B**, **E**, and **F**, nuclei are stained red with 7-aminoactinomycin. In all figures, bars = 10 μm.

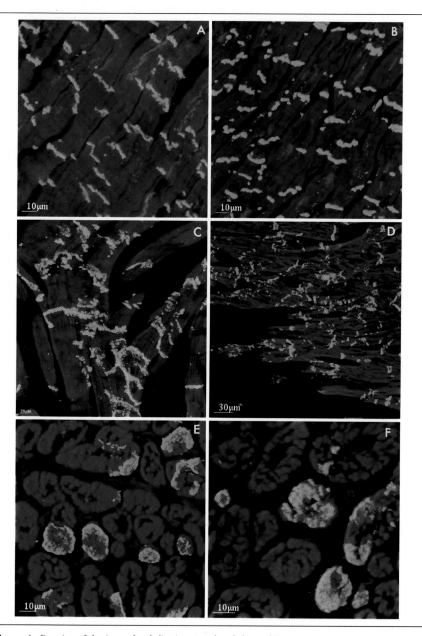

Figure 6. Proteins of the intercalated disc in normal and diseased human myocardium. Immunolabeled gap junctions for connexin 43 (**A**) and fascia adherens for N–cadherin (**B**) in longitudinal cryosections are clearly confined to cell termini at the intercalated disc in normal human myocardium. (**C**) In areas of myofiber disarray of a patient with DCM connexin 43 immunofluorescence shows a random distribution and dispersed gap junctions along the peripheral sarcolemma. (**D**) Myocytes adjacent to the fibrotic tissue (lower left corner, free of label) show a marked disorganization of connexin 43 gap junctions (compare with **A**). (**E**) *En face* view of connexin 43 immunolabeling in normal human myocardium shows that gap junctions appear as ovoid structures with a prominent ring of staining at the edge of disk. (**F**) In transverse sections, some cardiomyocytes from a patient with DCM show loss of large peripheral gap junctions, making disk borders difficult to define. In all figures, the contractile apparatus is labeled with phalloidin-TRITC (red).

The cytoplasmic plaque of the fascia adherens has been shown to be composed of α-, β- and γ-catenin, vinculin, and α-actinin [45]. Immunocytochemical data identified γ-catenin to be identical with plakoglobin, which binds to either desmosomal or classic cadherins [46]. The desmosomal plaque is made up of the cytoplasmic tails of the desmosomal cadherins, plakoglobin and desmoplakins. Desmoplakin I and II are the most abundant proteins of the desmosomal plaque, serving as a cell surface attachment for the intermediate filaments to the cytoplasmic tails of the desmosomal cadherins [47].

Cadherins form a group of cell surface glycoproteins that mediate calcium-dependent homophilic cell-cell adhesion [48]. Different types of cadherin molecules are found in different types of junction forming the cardiac ID: N-cadherin occurs in fascia adherens, whereas desmogleins and desmocollins are found to be present in desmosomes. Immunolabeled fasciae adherentes for N-cadherin in the nondiseased control tissues were uniformly distributed across intercalated discs and clearly demarcate each cardiomyocyte at the cell termini (figure 6B).

In DCM, altered patterns of cardiac intercellular junction distribution were observed in areas featuring myofiber disarray (figure 6C) and at the myocardial interface with areas of replacement fibrosis (figure 6D). In the latter areas, connexin 43 gap junctions, as well as immunolabeled fasciae adherentes for N-cadherin, were arranged in longitudinally orientated arrays along the lateral sarcolemma, forming aberrant side-to-side connections. This abnormality extended in parallel with increasing myocardial scarring. Severe junctional abnormalities were detected in zones of myofiber disarray, including random and dispersed distribution along the cellular membrane of connexin 43 immunolabeling (figure 6C). In areas free from the above mentioned structural changes, many myocytes have a normal disk-like pattern of the distribution of connexin 43; however, in some myocytes, especially those viewed *en face*, there was a striking loss of the larger peripheral gap junctions (figure 6F) as compared with normal tissue (figure 6E). The abnormalities observed in gap junction distribution were interpreted as a potential substrate in the development of a ventricular arrhythmogenic substrate in human DCM.

In conclusion, from the data presented here, it becomes evident that in DCM many different proteins are subjected to alterations in expression and arrangement, demonstrating a graded sensitivity towards pathological stimuli in that the contractile proteins and sarcomeric skeleton are the most sensitive proteins and the cytoskeleton and its associated proteins show a compensatory increase. From these findings, it is concluded that different reactions of the cardiac protein families to chronic cardiomyopathic processes reflect the survival priorities of the cells. Furthermore, these findings show that alterations and extensive but disproportionate reorganization of a whole complex of proteins represent the structural basis for the reduction of contractile function in failing human hearts. The disorganization of connexin 43 distribution associated with myocardial scarring and myofiber disarray and selective disruption of large gap junctions may play an important role in the development of an arrhythmogenic substrate in human DCM.

REFERENCES

1. Kostin S, Heling A, Hein S, Scholz D, Klövekorn WP, Schaper J. 1998. The protein composition of the normal and diseased cardiac myocyte. Heart Fail Rev 2:245–260.
2. Schaper J, Froede R, Hein S, Buck A, Hashizume H, Speiser B, Friedl A, Bleese N. 1991. Impairment of the myocardial ultrastructure and changes of the cytoskeleton in dilated cardiomyopathy. Circulation 83:504–514.
3. Schaper J, Speiser B, Brand T. 1993. The cytoskeleton and extracellular matrix in human hearts with dilated cardiomyopathy. In Idiopathic Dilated Cardiomyopathy. Ed. H Figulla, R Kandolf, and B McManus, 75–80. Berlin, Heidelberg: Springer Verlag.
4. Schaper J, Mollnau H, Hein S, Münkel B. 1995. Interaction between cardiac myocytes and the extracellular matrix in failing human myocardium. In Heart Hypertrophy and Failure. Ed. N Dhalla, G Pierce, R Panagia, and R Beamish, 275–285. Boston, Dordrecht, London: Kluwer Academic Publisher.
5. Scholz D, Diener W, Schaper J. 1994. Altered nucleus/cytoplasm relationship and degenerative structural changes in human dilated cardiomyopathy. Cardioscience 5:127–138.
6. Hein S, Scholz D, Fujitani N, Rennollet H, Brand T, Friedl A, Schaper J. 1994. Altered expression of titin and contractile proteins in failing human myocardium. J Mol Cell Cardiol 26:1291–1306.
7. Speiser B, Riess CF, Schaper J. 1991. The extracellular matrix in human myocardium. Part I: collagens I, II, IV, and VI. Cardioscience 2:225–232.
8. Speiser B, Weihrauch D, Riess CF, Schaper J. 1992. The extracellular matrix in human cardiac tissue. Part II: vimentin, laminin, and fibronectin. Cardioscience 3:41–49.
9. Anversa P, Kajstura J, Olivetti G. 1996. Myocyte death in heart failure. Curr Opin Cardiol 11:245–251.
10. Haunstetter A, Izumo S. 1998. Apoptosis. Basic mechanisms and implications for cardiovascular disease. Circ Res 82:1111–1129.
11. Olivetti G, Abbi R, Quaini F, Kajstura J, Cheng W, Nitahara J, Quaini E, Loreto C, Beltrami C, Krajewski S, Reed J, Anversa P. 1997. Apoptosis in the failing human heart. N Engl J Med 336:1131–1141.
12. Freude B, Masters TN, Kostin S, Robicsek F, Schaper J. 1997. Cardiomyocyte apoptosis in acute and chronic conditions. Bas Res Cardiol 93:85–89.
13. Colucci WS. 1996. Apoptosis in the heart. N Engl J Med 335:1224–1226.
14. Schaper J, Hein S. 1993. The structural correlate of reduced cardiac function in human dilated cardiomyopathy. Heart Failure 9:95–111.
15. Elsässer A, Schlepper M, Klövekorn WP, Cai WJ, Zimmermann R, Müller KD, Strasser R, Kostin S, Gagel C, Münkel B, Schaper W, Schaper J. 1997. Hibernating myocardium—an incomplete adaptation to ischemia. Circulation 96:2920–2931.
16. Schaper J, Hein S, Scholz D, Mollnau H. 1995. Multifaceted morphological alterations are present in the failing human heart. J Mol Cell Cardiol 27:857–861.
17. Mallat Z, Tedgui A, Fontaliran F, Frank R, Durigon M, Fontaine G. 1996. Evidence of apoptosis in arrhythmogenic right ventricular dysplasia. N Engl J Med 335:1190–1196.
18. Narula J, Haider N, Virmani R, DiSalvo TG, Haijjar RJ, Schmidt U, Semigran MJ, Dec GW, Khaw BA. 1996. Apoptosis in myocytes in end stage heart failure. N Engl J Med 335:1182–1189.
19. Cheng W, Li B, Kajstura J, Wolin MS, Sonnenblick EH, Hintze TH, Olivetti G, Anversa P. 1995. Stretch-induced programmed myocyte cell death. J Clin Invest 96:2247–2259.
20. Schaub MC, Hefti MA, Harder BA, Eppenberger HM. 1997. Various hypertrophic stimuli induce distinct phenotypes in cardiomyocytes. J Mol Cell Cardiol 75:901–920.
21. Kajstura J, Cigola E, Malhotra A, Li P, Cheng W, Meggs LG, Anversa A. 1997. Angiotensin II induces apoptosis of adult ventricular myocytes in vitro. J Mol Cell Cardiol 29:859–870.
22. Levine B, Kalman J, Mayer L, Fillit H, Packer M. 1990. Elevated circulating levels of tumor necrosis factor in severe chronic heart failure. N Engl J Med 323:236–241.
23. Krown KA, Page MT, Nguen C, Zechner D, Gutierrez V, Comstock KL, Glembotski G, Quintana PJE, Sabbadini RA. 1996. Tumor necrosis factor alpha-induced apoptosis in cardiac myocytes. J Clin Invest 98:2854–2865.
24. Millevoi S, Trombitas K, Kostin S, Schaper J, Pelin K, Kolmerer B, Granzier H, Labeit S. 1998. Characterization of nebulette and nebulin and emerging concepts of their roles for vertebrate Z-discs. J Mol Biol 282:111–123.
25. Labeit S, Kolmerer B, Linke WA. 1997. The giant protein titin. Emerging roles in physiology and pathophysiology. Circulation Res 80:290–294.

26. Tsutsui H, Ishihara K, Cooper G. 1993. Cytoskeletal role for contractile dysfunction of hypertrophied myocardium. Science 260:682–687.
27. Tsutsui H, Tagawa H, Kent RL, Mc Collam PL, Ishihara K, Nagatsu M, Cooper G 4th. 1994. Role of microtubules in contractile dysfunction of hypertrophied cardiocytes. Circulation 90(1):533–555.
28. Tagawa H, Koide M, Sato I, Cooper G. 1996. Cytoskeletal role in the contractile dysfunction of cardiocytes from hypertrophied and failing right ventricular myocardium. Proc Assoc Am Physicians 108(39):218–229.
29. Wang X, Li F, Campbell SE, Gerdes A. 1999. Chronic pressure overload cardiac hypertrophy and failure in guinea pigs: II. Cytoskeletal remodeling. J Mol Cell Cardiol 31:319–331.
30. Thornell LE, Carlsson L, Li Z, Mericskay M, Paulin D. 1997. Null mutation in the desmin gene gives rise to a cardiomyopathy. J Mol Cell Cardiol 29:2107–2124.
31. Burridge K, Chrzanowska-Wodnicka M. 1996. Focal adhesions, contractility, and signaling. Annu Rev Cell Div 12:463–519.
32. Ohlendieck K. 1996. Towards an understanding of the dystrophin–glycoprotein complex: linkage between the extracellular matrix and the membrane cytoskeleton in muscle fibers. Eur J Cell Biol 69:1–10.
33. Bennett V, Gilligan DM. 1993. The spectrin-based skeleton and micron-scale organization of the plasma membrane. Annu Rev Cell Biol 9:27–66.
34. Pardo JV, Siliciano JD, Craig SW. 1983. Vinculin is a component of an extensive network of myofibril–sarcolemma attachment regions in cardiac muscle fibers. J Cell Biol 97:1081–1088.
35. Stevenson S, Rothery S, Cullen MJ, Severs NJ. 1997. Dystrophin is not a specific component of the cardiac costamere. Circ Res 80:269–280.
36. Belkin AM, Zhidkova NI, Koteliansky VE. 1986. Localization of talin in skeletal and cardiac muscles. FEBS Lett 200:32–36.
37. Carver W, Price RL, Raso DS, Terracio L, Borg TK. 1994. Distribution of β-1 integrin in the developing rat heart. J Histochem Cytochem 42:167–175.
38. Craig SW, Pardo JV. 1983. Gamma actin, spectrin, and intermediate filament proteins colocalize with vinculin at costameres, myofibril-to-sarcolemma attachment sites. Cell Motil 3:449–462.
39. Straub V, Bittner RE, Leger JJ, Voit T. 1992. Direct visualization of the dystrophin network on skeletal muscle fiber membrane. J Cell Biol 119:1183–1191.
40. Terracio L, Simpson DG, Hilenski L, Carver W, Decker RS, Vinson N, Borg TK. 1990. Distribution of vinculin in the Z-disk of striated muscle: analysis by laser scanning confocal microscopy. J Cell Physiol 145:78–87.
41. Meng H, Leddy JJ, Frank J, Holland P, Tuana BS. 1996. The association of cardiac dystrophin with myofibrils/Z-disc regions in cardiac muscle suggests a novel role in the contractile apparatus. J Biol Chem 271:12364–12371.
42. Danowski B, Imanaka-Yoshida K, Sanger JM, Sanger JW. 1992. Costameres are sites of force transmission to the substratum in adult rat cardiomyocytes. J Cell Biol 118:1411–1420.
43. Kanter HL, Laing JG, Beau SL, Beyer EC, Saffitz JE. 1993. Distinct patterns of connexin expression in canine Purkinje fibers and ventricular muscle. Circ Res 72:1124–1131.
44. Severs NJ. 1990. Review. The cardiac gap junction and intercalated disc. Int J Cardiol 26:136–173.
45. Ozawa M, Baribault H, Kemler R. 1989. The cytoplasmic domain of the cell adhesion molecule uvomorulin associates with three independent proteins structurally related in different species. EMBO J 8:1711–1717.
46. Knudsen KA, Wheelock MJ. 1992. Plakoglobin, or an 83 Kd homologue distinct from β-catenin, interacts with E-cadherin and N-cadherin. J Cell Biol 118:671–679.
47. Franke WW, Moll R, Schiller DL, Schmid E, Kartenbeck J, Müller H. 1982. Desmoplakins of epithelial and myocardial desmosomes are immunologically and biochemically related. Differentiation 23:115–127.
48. Takeichi M. 1991. Cadherin cell adhesion receptors as a morphogenetic regulator. Science 251:1451–1455.

N. Takeda, M. Nagano and N.S. Dhalla
(eds). The Hypertrophied Heart. Copyright
© 2000. pp. 441–452. Kluwer Academic
Publishers. Boston. All rights reserved.

DIASTOLIC DYSFUNCTION AND DIASTOLIC HEART FAILURE

KAZUHIRO YAMAMOTO, TOHRU MASUYAMA,
YASUSHI SAKATA, and MASATSUGU HORI

*Department of Internal Medicine and Therapeutics, Osaka University Graduate School of Medicine, 2-2
Yamadaoka, Suita 565-0871, Japan.*

Summary. It has been shown that heart failure frequently occurs in the absence of left
ventricular (LV) systolic dysfunction, and diastolic dysfunction is considered to be the underlying cause for this phenotype of heart failure: *isolated diastolic heart failure*. LV diastolic dysfunction is an important determinant of symptoms and prognosis of heart failure, even in
patients with systolic failure. The development of Doppler echocardiography has provided us
much knowledge about the clinical features of diastolic dysfunction and diastolic failure. In
this chapter, the current concept of diastolic heart failure and diastolic dysfunction will be
discussed.

INTRODUCTION

Left ventricular (LV) diastolic dysfunction precedes systolic dysfunction in cardiovascular diseases, and in the mid-1980s it was reported that some patients develop
heart failure because of diastolic dysfunction in the absence of LV systolic dysfunction [1,2]. In the last decade it has been shown that this phenotype of heart failure,
i.e., *isolated diastolic heart failure*, is observed in 30–50% of patients with heart failure
[3,4]. In addition, even in patients with systolic dysfunction, the symptoms and prognosis of heart failure are determined by the degree of diastolic dysfunction, rather
than systolic dysfunction [5,6]. A recent study in a community population revealed
that prognosis is not different between patients with systolic heart failure and those
with isolated diastolic heart failure [7]. Therefore strategies for the diagnosis and
treatment of diastolic heart failure and/or diastolic dysfunction should be established
so that these can lead to the improvement of morbidity and mortality of patients
with cardiovascular diseases. However, the importance of diastolic dysfunction as the
underlying cause for heart failure is still underestimated, even among cardiologists.

In this chapter, the current concept of diastolic heart failure and/or diastolic dysfunction will be discussed.

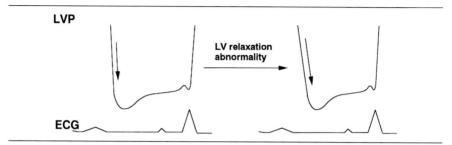

Figure 1. Left ventricular pressure tracing (LVP) and electrocardiogram (ECG). Left ventricular relaxation abnormality is associated with a slow fall of left ventricular pressure as compared with normal left ventricular relaxation.

PATHOPHYSIOLOGY OF DIASTOLIC DYSFUNCTION

LV relaxation and compliance are major determinants of diastolic function. The process of relaxation, an energy-requiring active process, is assessed as the time constant of the drop in isovolumic LV pressure (τ) [8,9]. Impairment of relaxation is associated with a slow rate and prolonged duration of the drop in LV pressure (figure 1). LV compliance is a passive distensibility of the chamber and is primarily determined by loading condition and myocardial characteristics. Ventricular interaction, pericardial restraint, and coronary vascular engorgement also influence LV compliance [10]. Increases in right ventricular diastolic volume augment ventricular interaction, thus shifting the LV diastolic pressure–volume curve upward and elevating LV diastolic pressure at any LV diastolic volume (figure 2). Pericardial restraint also shifts the diastolic pressure–volume curve upward. An increase in coronary vascular engorgement reduces LV compliance. Myocardial characteristics are altered in the presence of myocardial hypertrophy, ischemia, fibrosis, or infiltration. As LV compliance decreases (and LV stiffness increases) with alteration of myocardial characteristics, the slope of the LV diastolic pressure–volume curve steepens, and there is a larger increase in diastolic pressure with any given filling volume (figure 2). Because the LV diastolic pressure–volume relationship shows concave curvilinearity [10], the "operant" compliance can decrease as chamber volume increases, even without changes in myocardial characteristics.

ASSESSMENT OF DIASTOLIC FUNCTION

Diastolic dysfunction augments resistance to LV diastolic filling, resulting in an elevation of LV filling pressures, modulation of LV filling patterns, and progression of clinical signs and symptoms of heart failure. Doppler echocardiography is useful in the noninvasive assessment of LV filling characteristics. Thus, in the last two decades, much knowledge has been gained from the analysis of Doppler transmitral flow velocity curves in clinical practice, leading to the concept of assessment of diastolic function from the viewpoint of LV filling dynamics.

Associated with changes in mechanical interaction of cardiac chambers

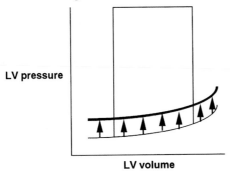

LV pressure

LV volume

Association with alteration of myocardial characteristics

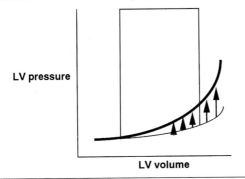

LV pressure

LV volume

Figure 2. Left ventricular diastolic pressure–volume curve in altered left ventricular compliance. (**Upper panel**) Effects of changes in the mechanical interaction of cardiac chambers on the left ventricular diastolic pressure–volume curve. In association with an increase in the interaction, the diastolic pressure–volume curve shifts upward. (**Lower panel**) Effects of changes in myocardial characteristics on the diastolic pressure–volume curve. An alteration of myocardial characteristics steepens the diastolic pressure–volume curve.

The pulsed-wave Doppler transmitral flow velocity curves normally have a biphasic contour consisting of an early diastolic flow velocity (mitral E) and a flow velocity at atrial contraction (mitral A) (figure 3). Following ventricular systole, LV pressure falls rapidly due to relaxation. When LV pressure falls bellow the left atrial pressure, the mitral valve opens and LV pressure continues to fall. This produces a positive left-atrial-to-LV pressure gradient, which causes the mitral E velocity curve. The rate of the LV pressure drop is regulated by the speed and timing of relaxation. As early diastolic filling continues, LV pressure rises, with regulation by multiple factors (viscoelastic forces of the myocardium, pericardial restraint, ventricular interaction), and the transmitral gradient decreases. The rate of reversal of the pres-

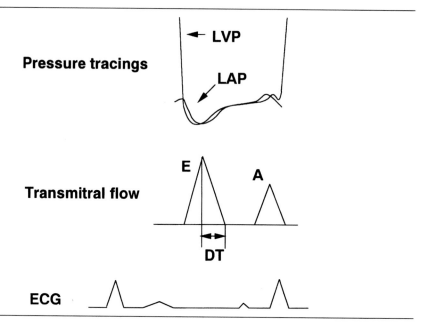

Figure 3. Schema of left atrial and left ventricular pressure tracings (LAP, LVP), transmitral flow velocity curves (Transmitral flow), and electrocardiogram (ECG). See text for discussion. A, mitral A velocity; DT, deceleration time of the mitral E velocity; E, mitral E velocity.

sure gradient, and thus the effective operant compliance of the LV, determines the deceleration rate and deceleration time of mitral E velocity [11]. At the time of atrial contraction, left atrial pressure rises rapidly, followed by a rise of LV pressure from the atrial contribution to ventricular filling. The resultant positive transmitral pressure gradient at atrial contraction produces the mitral A velocity curve. LV compliance regulates the rate of passive LV pressure rise associated with ventricular filling.

LV relaxation abnormality is associated with a slow rate of LV pressure drop. This slow rate will decrease the early diastolic transmitral pressure gradient and the mitral E velocity. Early diastolic filling is decreased, and there is a compensatory increase in filling with atrial contraction to maintain LV diastolic filling. Thus, the mitral flow velocity curve will show a low E, high A, and long deceleration time of mitral E velocity. A decrease in the "operant" LV compliance is associated with a rapid LV pressure rise with any given filling volume, leading to a decrease in transmitral pressure gradient and LV filling volume. To keep the LV filling volume left atrial pressure is elevated and increases the transmitral pressure gradient, resulting in a high mitral E velocity, shortening of the deceleration time, and a low mitral A [12].

It has been hypothesized and subsequently shown in the animal model [12] that there is a progression of the transmitral flow velocity curves associated with the transition from diastolic dysfunction to diastolic heart failure (figure 4). In the early

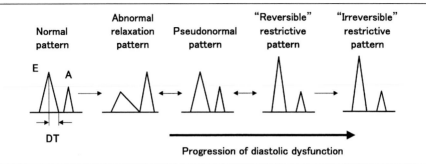

Figure 4. Alteration of transmitral flow velocity curves with the progression of diastolic dysfunction in patients with cardiac disease. The natural progression is from the normal pattern, to the abnormal relaxation pattern, to the pseudonormal pattern, to a reversal restrictive pattern, and finally to an irreversible restriction pattern.

stage of cardiac disease, LV relaxation is impaired, and the transmitral flow velocity curves represent a low mitral E velocity, a long deceleration time of mitral E velocity, and a high mitral A velocity. This is called an *abnormal relaxation pattern*, and patients with this pattern are usually minimally symptomatic at rest. At this stage, LV filling pressures are rarely increased. These patients may complain of dyspnea even at this stage in association with atrial fibrillation due to loss of atrial contraction, shortening of the diastolic filling period (increases in heart rate), and moderate to extreme exertion even in the absence of myocardial ischemia. With progression of the cardiac disease, LV compliance is decreased. To maintain LV filling volume and stroke volume, left atrial pressure must increase. As the left atrial pressure increases, the early diastolic transmitral pressure gradient increases, with a high mitral E velocity [13,14]. The increased early diastolic filling volume and the reduced LV compliance result in a shortened deceleration time and a decrease in the mitral A velocity. Thus, the transmitral flow velocity curves appear normal, and not the abnormal relaxation pattern, in spite of a consistent relaxation abnormality. This phenomenon is referred to as *pseudonormalization*. In this stage, patients usually are more symptomatic, since LV filling pressures increase even at rest. Following progressive alteration in LV compliance and left atrial pressures, the mitral E velocity and E/A ratio increase further, with marked decreases in the deceleration time; this is referred to as *restrictive pattern*. At this stage, patients are most symptomatic.

Several clinical studies have confirmed such a relation between the alteration of transmitral flow velocity curves and severity of heart failure. Klein et al. showed such alteration of the flow velocity curves in the progression of cardiac amyloidosis in individual patients [15]. Pinamonti et al. demonstrated that patients with restrictive pattern have poorer prognosis than other patients. [16]. However, as described above, transmitral flow velocity curves are determined by myocardial characteristics and loading conditions. Since loading conditions are alterable, the restrictive pattern can change into other patterns following preload reduction therapy. Thus, a question may arise as to whether a *reversible restrictive pattern* has similar clinical significance to an *irreversible restrictive pattern*. Recent clinical studies [17,18] have clarified that patients with irreversible restrictive pattern have the poorest prognosis, and that we therefore have to distinguish the reversible restrictive pattern from the irreversible restrictive pattern.

It must be recognized that the flow velocity curves assess only LV filling characteristics and are influenced by multiple parameters such as loading condition, LV systolic function, heart rate, and age [19]. Patients with systolic dysfunction do not have normal diastolic function, and thus, assessment of the severity of diastolic dysfunction with transmitral flow velocity curves alone is not difficult. In patients with normal systolic function in whom isolated diastolic heart failure may occur, it may be difficult to differentiate between a truly normal pattern with normal filling pressures and a pseudonormal pattern with elevated filling pressures through the use of the transmitral flow velocity curves alone [20]. Additional information is required. It has been suggested that a change in preload may be helpful in making this differentiation. A reduction in preload should result in a transition from a pseudonormal to an abnormal relaxation pattern or from a restrictive to a pseudonormal pattern in patients with elevated filling pressures (figure 4). Alternatively, if there is a reduction in preload with a patient who has a truly "normal" pattern, there will be a hypovolemic response, with reduction in both mitral E and A velocities [21]. Another useful method for this differentiation is to detect elevated filling pressures through analysis of flow velocity curves at atrial contraction using pulsed Doppler transmitral and pulmonary venous flow velocity curves. Rossvol and Hatle have reported that the duration of flow with atrial contraction at the pulmonary veins gets longer than that at the mitral valve in patients with elevated filling pressures, and that the difference in these durations correlates with filling pressures [22]. We have confirmed that the correlation between this index and filling pressures exists irrespective of patients' systolic function [20]. Other methods under investigation for detection of abnormal diastolic function include (1) the assessment of the intraventricular flow propagation in early diastolic filling with color M-mode Doppler echocardiography [23], (2) Doppler tissue imaging of mitral annulus motion [24], and (3) the evaluation of τ with continuous-wave Doppler mitral or aortic regurgitant velocity curves [25,26].

TREATMENT OF DIASTOLIC HEART FAILURE

Treatment of diastolic heart failure has not been well established [27]. There have not been large randomized trials examining specific therapy for treatment of diastolic dysfunction. Based upon the increasing knowledge that has been gained over the past few decades, however, some recommendations for therapy can be made.

Patients with an abnormal relaxation pattern of transmitral flow velocity curves are usually asymptomatic at rest; however, they may become symptomatic with exercise because of shortening of the diastolic filling period. A shortening of the diastolic filling period accompanied by an increase in heart rate is associated with an onset of atrial contraction before the cessation of early diastolic filling, resulting in an elevation of LV filling pressures. An optimal therapy for such patients would be a medication that would increase the diastolic filling period. Beta-blockers or calcium channel blockers with negative chronotropic properties are appropriate for this purpose. For patients with a pseudonormal or a restrictive pattern due to decreased effective operant LV compliance, most of the LV filling volume occurs during the early diastolic filling period, and thus a prolongation of the diastolic filling period may not be beneficial. Thus, the treatment strategy for such patients would not be β-blockers or calcium channel blockers.

In patients with an abnormal relaxation pattern, atrial fibrillation disguises signs of heart failure, because atrial contraction largely contributes to the maintenance of LV filling volume. In these patents, aggressive therapy directed at maintaining sinus rhythm should be instituted.

Dual-chamber pacing has been proposed as a therapeutic alternative for severely symptomatic patients with dilated cardiomyopathy, since it provides a mechanical treatment of abnormal diastolic filling [28]. The mechanism behind the beneficial effects of dual-chamber pacing is restoration of proper atrioventricular synchrony in selected patients with first-degree atrioventricular block in whom the occurrence of atrial contraction before the cessation of early diastolic filling leads to an elevation of LV filling pressures.

If patients complain of dyspnea due to diastolic dysfunction and increased LV filling pressure, preload reduction therapy may be useful to relieve symptoms in selected patients depending upon the mechanism of the increased filling pressures. If elevation in filling pressures is due to an augmentation in interventricular interaction and pericardial restriction, shifting the LV diastolic pressure–volume curve upward (figure 2), then preload reduction therapy can decrease right-sided diastolic pressure and pericardial pressure, shifting the diastolic pressure–volume curve downward (figure 5). Therefore, preload reduction therapy can decrease LV filling pressures with little reduction in the LV end-diastolic volume and stroke volume. In contrast, if elevation in filling pressures is due to an alteration in myocardial characteristics, preload reduction will move the LV pressure–volume loop on the same diastolic pressure–volume curve, resulting in a decrease in end-diastolic volume and stroke volume. In some cases with severe alteration in myocardial characteristics, preload reduction induces a large decrease in stroke volume and cardiac shock.

An elevated afterload will increase filling pressures through several mechanisms. An elevation of afterload directly impairs ventricular relaxation. In addition, the high afterload will increase end-systolic volume, especially if there has been an acute increase in blood pressure. This will move the pressure–volume loop rightward on the diastolic pressure–volume curve, further increasing filling pressures (figure 6). Thus, afterload reduction is also effective.

If the underlying cardiovascular process is coronary artery disease and myocardial ischemia, a revascularization procedure may be beneficial. If constrictive pericarditis or the presence of pericardial effusion is a cause of augmented ventricular interaction and pericardial restraint, then pericardiectomy or pericardiocentesis should be performed.

Associated with changes in mechanical interaction of cardiac chambers

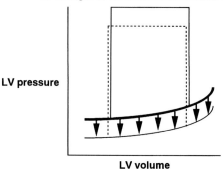

Association with alteration of myocardial characteristics

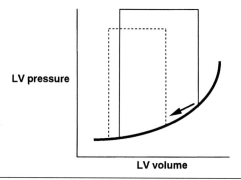

Figure 5. Effects of preload reduction on the left ventricular pressure–volume loop. (**Upper panel**) In a patient in whom an increase in left ventricular end-diastolic pressure is caused by enhanced mechanical interaction of the cardiac chambers, preload reduction decreases right-sided cardiac pressure and induces a downward shift of pressure–volume loop. Thus, left ventricular end-diastolic pressure decreases with little decrease in left ventricular end-diastolic volume and stroke volume. (**Lower panel**) In a patient in whom an increase in left ventricular end-diastolic pressure is caused by changes in myocardial characteristics, preload reduction induces a leftward shift of pressure–volume loop and decreases left ventricular end-diastolic volume and pressure and stroke volume. Pressure–volume loops drawn with solid line and dotted line are before and after preload reduction, respectively.

There have been misconceptions that the calcium channel blockers, specifically verapamil, can directly improve diastolic function by enhancing relaxation. However, this concept was derived from erroneous interpretations of the results of pulsed Doppler transmitral flow velocity curves before and after therapy. Studies showed that verapamil may "normalize" the peak early diastolic filling rate in patients with abnormal relaxation patterns. However, the invasive study that measured filling pressures and τ directly has shown that verapamil-induced "normalization" of early diastolic filling rate is associated with increased filling pressures and prolonged τ, not

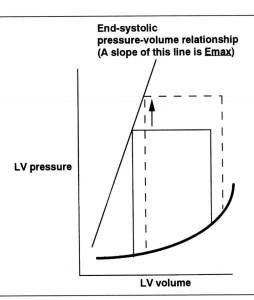

Figure 6. Effects of afterload elevation on left ventricular pressure–volume loop. Following afterload elevation without changes in cardiac contractility (without changes in E_{max}), the pressure–volume loop moves rightward on the same diastolic pressure–volume curve to maintain stroke volume, and thus, left ventricular end-diastolic pressure and volume increase. Pressure–volume loops drawn with solid line and dotted line are before and after afterload elevation, respectively.

with improvement of relaxation (shortening of τ) [29]. Thus, there is no drug at the current time that is known to improve diastolic function.

Future therapy

Recent studies have suggested that there may be other drugs that can directly improve diastolic function. In patients with LV hypertrophy, the intracoronary infusion of angiotensin-converting enzyme inhibitor showed beneficial effects on LV diastolic function, although the beneficial effects were dependent upon the etiology and type of ventricular hypertrophy [30,31]. Brain natriuretic peptide (BNP) also improved LV diastolic function both in animal and in clinical studies [32,33].

In patients with cardiovascular diseases, excessive progression of LV remodeling such as ventricular hypertrophy and myocardial fibrosis contributes to ventricular diastolic dysfunction and heart failure. Thus, drugs to induce regression of ventricular hypertrophy or fibrosis may be beneficial in treating diastolic dysfunction. The angiotensin-converting enzyme inhibitors [34,35], angiotensin II receptor blockers [36], spironolactone [37], and β-blockers [35,38] have been reported to induce regression of ventricular hypertrophy and/or fibrosis. Our recent animal study directly demonstrated that a subdepressor dose of angiotensin II receptor blocker inhibited the transition to isolated diastolic heart failure with the prevention of ventricular hypertrophy and fibrosis in hypertensive heart disease [39]. Endogenous endothelin is considered to play an important role in the progression of ventricular hypertrophy and fibrosis, and endothelin receptor antagonist may be effective in attenuating ventricular hypertrophy and fibrosis [40,41].

CONCLUSIONS

We have summarized the present concept of diastolic dysfunction and diastolic heart failure in this chapter. In spite of the frequent occurrence of isolated diastolic heart failure and the importance of LV diastolic dysfunction as a determinant of morbidity and mortality of patients with heart failure, our tools for the diagnosis and treatment still have many limitations. Further studies are necessary to establish noninvasive assessment of diastolic function and/or to develop new simple markers of diastolic dysfunction. Randomized, controlled clinical trials are mandatory to establish the treatment strategies for patients with diastolic dysfunction.

REFERENCES

1. Soufer R, Wohlgelernter D, Vita NA, Amuchestegui M, Sostman HD, Berger HJ, Zaret BL. 1985. Intact systolic left ventricular function in clinical congestive heart failure. Am J Cardiol 55:1032–1036.
2. Dougherty AH, Naccarelli GV, Gray EL, Hicks CH, Goldstein RA. 1984. Congestive heart failure with normal systolic function. Am J Cardiol 54:778–782.
3. Bonow RO, Udelson JE. 1992. Left ventricular diastolic dysfunction as a cause of congestive heart failure. Am Intern Med 117:502–510.
4. Vasan RS, Benjamin EJ, Levy D. 1995. Prevalence, clinical features and prognosis of diastolic heart failure: an epidemiologic perspective. J Am Coll Cardiol 26:1565–1574.
5. Vanoverschelde JL, Raphael DA, Robert AR, Cosyns JR. 1990. Left ventricular filling in dilated cardiomyopathy: relation to functional class and hemodynamics. J Am Coll Cardiol 15:1288–1295.
6. Rihal CS, Nishimura RA, Hatle LK, Bailey KR, Tajik AJ. 1994. Systolic and diastolic dysfunction in patients with clinical diagnosis of dilated cardiomyopathy. Relation to symptoms and prognosis. Circulation 90:2772–2779.
7. Senni M, Tribouilloy CM, Rodeheffer RJ, Jacobsen SJ, Evans JM, Bailey KR, Redfield MM. 1998. Congestive heart failure in the community: a study of all incident cases in Olmsted County, Minnesota, in 1991. Circulation 98:2282–2289.
8. Raff GL, Glantz SA. 1981. Volume loading slows left ventricular isovolumic relaxation rate: evidence of load-dependent relaxation in the intact dog heart. Circ Res 48:813–824.
9. Weiss JL, Frederiksen JW, Weisfeldt ML. 1976. Hemodynamic determinants of the time-course of fall in canine left ventricular pressure. J Clin Invest 58:751–760.
10. Gilbert JC, Glantz SA. 1989. Determinants of left ventricular filling and of the diastolic pressure–volume relation. Circ Res 64:827–852.
11. Courtois M, Vered Z, Barzilai B, Ricciotti NA, Perez JE, Ludbrook PA. 1988. The transmitral pressure–flow velocity relation: effect of abrupt preload reduction. Circulation 78:1459–1468.
12. Doi R, Masuyama T, Yamaoto K, Doi Y, Mano T, Sakata Y, Ono K, Kuzuya T, Hirota S, Koyama T, Miwa T, Hori M. 2000. Development of different phenotypes of hypertensive heart failure: systolic versus diastolic failure in Dahl salt-sensitive rats. J Hypertens 18:111–120.
13. Yamamoto K, Masuyama T, Tanouchi J, Uematsu M, Doi Y, Naito J, Hori M, Tada M, Kamada T. 1993. Importance of left ventricular minimal pressure as a determinant of transmitral flow velocity pattern in the presence of left ventricular systolic dysfunction. J Am Coll Cardiol 21:662–672.
14. Nishimura RA, Tajik AJ. 1997. Evaluation of diastolic filling of left ventricle in health and disease: Doppler echocardiography is the clinician's Rosetta Stone. J Am Coll Cardiol 30:8–18.
15. Klein AL, Hatle LK, Taliercio CP, Taylor CL, Kyle RA, Bailey KR, Seward JB, Tajik AJ. 1990. Serial Doppler echocardiographic follow-up of left ventricular diastolic function in cardiac amyloidosis. J Am Coll Cardiol 16:1135–1141.
16. Pinamonti B, Lenarda AD, Sinagra G, Camerini F. 1993. Restrictive left ventricular filling pattern in dilated cardiomyopathy assessed by Doppler echocardiography: clinical echocardiographic and hemodynamic correlations and prognostic implications. J Am Coll Cardiol 22:808–815.

17. Pozzoli M, Traversi E, Cioffi G, Stenner R, Sanarico M, Tavazzi L. 1997. Loading manipulations improve the prognostic value of Doppler evaluation of mitral flow in patients with chronic heart failure. Circulation 95:1222–1230.
18. Temporelli PL, Corra U, Imparato A, Bosimini E, Scapellato F, Giannuzzi P. 1998. Reversible restrictive left ventricular diastolic filling with optimized oral therapy predicts a more favorable prognosis in patients with chronic heart failure. J Am Coll Cardiol 31:1591–1597.
19. Yamamoto K, Redfield MM, Nishimura RA. 1996. Analysis of left ventricular diastolic function. Heart 75(Suppl 2):27–35.
20. Yamamoto K, Nishimura RA, Chaliki HP, Appleton CP, Holmes DR Jr, Redfield MM. 1997. Determination of left ventricular filling pressure by Doppler echocardiography in patients with coronary artery disease: critical role of left ventricular systolic function. J Am Coll Cardiol 30:1819–1826.
21. Hurrell DG, Nishimura RA, Ilstrup DM, Appleton CP. 1997. The utility of preload alteration in the assessment of left ventricular filling pressure by Doppler echocardiography: a simultaneous catheterization and Doppler echocardiographic study. J Am Coll Cardiol 30:459–467.
22. Rossvoll O, Hatle LK. 1993. Pulmonary venous flow velocities recorded by transthoracic Doppler ultrasound: relation to left ventricular diastolic pressures. J Am Coll Cardiol 21:1687–1696.
23. Takatsuji H, Mikami T, Urasawa K, Teranishi J, Onozuka H, Takagi C, Makita Y, Matsuo H, Kusuoka H, Kitabatake A. 1996. A new approach for evaluation of left ventricular diastolic function: spatial and temporal analysis of left ventricular filling flow propagation by color M-mode Doppler echocardiography. J Am Coll Cardiol 27:365–371.
24. Nagueh SF, Lakkis NM, Midleton KJ, Spencer WH III, Zoghbi WA, Quinones MA. 1999. Doppler estimation of left ventricular filling pressures in patients with hypertrophic cardiomyopathy. Circulation 99:254–261.
25. Nishimura RA, Schwartz RS, Tajik AJ, Holmes DR Jr. 1993. Noninvasive measurement of rate of left ventricular relaxation by Doppler echocardiography. Validation with simultaneous cardiac catheterization. Circulation 88:146–155.
26. Yamamoto K, Masuyama T, Doi Y, Naito J, Mano T, Kondo H, Nagano R, Tanouchi J, Hori M, Kamada T. 1995. Noninvasive assessment of left ventricular relaxation using continuous-wave Doppler aortic regurgitant velocity curve. Its comparative value to the mitral regurgitation method. Circulation 91:192–200.
27. Williams JF Jr, Bristow MR, Fowler MB, Francis GS, Garson A Jr, Gersh BJ, Hammer DF, Hlatky MA, Leier CV, Packer M, Bertram P, Ullyot DJ, Wexler LF, Winters WL Jr, Ritchie JL, Cheitlin MD, Eagle KA, Gardener TJ, Garson A Jr, Gibbons RJ, Lewis RP, O'Rourke RA, Ryan TJ. 1995. Guidelines for the evaluation and management of heart failure: report of the American College of Cardiology / American Heart Association Task Force on practice guidelines (committee on evaluation and management of heart failure). Circulation 92:2764–2784.
28. Nishimura RA, Hayes DL, Holmes DR Jr, Tajik AJ. 1995. Mechanism of hemodynamic improvement by dual-chamber pacing for severe left ventricular dysfunction: an acute Doppler and catheterization hemodynamic study. J Am Coll Cardiol 25:281–288.
29. Nishimura RA, Schwartz RS, Holmes DR Jr, Tajik AJ. 1993. Failure of calcium channel blockers to improve ventricular relaxation in humans. J Am Coll Cardiol 21:182–188.
30. Friedrich SP, Lorell BH, Rousseau MF, Hayashida W, Hess OM, Douglas PS, Gordon S, Keighley CS, Benedict C, Krayenbuehl HP, Grossman W, Pouleur H. 1994. Intracardiac angiotensin-converting enzyme inhibition improves diastolic function in patients with left ventricular hypertrophy due to aortic stenosis. Circulation 90:2761–2771.
31. Haber HL, Powers ER, Gimple LW, Wu CC, Subbiah K, Johnson WH, Feldman MD. 1994. Intracoronary angiotensin-converting enzyme inhibition improves diastolic function in patients with hypertensive left ventricular hypertrophy. Circulation 89:2616–2625.
32. Clarkson PBM, Wheeldon NM, MacFadyen RJ, Pringle SD, MacDonald TM. 1996. Effects of brain natriuretic peptide on exercise hemodynamics and neurohormones in isolated diastolic heart failure. Circulation 93:2037–2042.
33. Yamamoto K, Burnett JC Jr, Redfield MM. 1997. Effect of endogenous natriuretic peptide system on ventricular and coronary function in failing heart. Am J Physiol 273:H2406–H2414.
34. Lievre M, Gueret P, Gayet C, Roudaut R, Haugh MC, Delair S, Boissel JP, on behalf of the HYCAR Study Group. 1995. Ramipril-induced regression of left ventricular hypertension in treated hypertensive individuals. Hypertension 25:92–97.
35. Gottdiener JS, Reda DJ, Massie BM, Materson BJ, Williams DW, Anderson RJ. 1997. Effect of single-drug therapy on reduction of left ventricular mass in mild to moderate hypertension. Circulation 95:2007–2014.

36. Kojima M, Shiojima I, Yamazaki T, Komuro I, Yunzeng Z, Ying W, Mizuno T, Ueki K, Tobe K, Kadowaki T, Nagai R, Yazaki Y. 1994. Angiotensin II receptor antagonist TCV-116 induces regression of hypertensive left ventricular hypertrophy in vivo and inhibits the intracellular signaling pathway of stretch-mediated cardiomyocyte hypertrophy in vitro. Circulation 89:2204–2211.
37. Weber KT, Sun Y, Guarda E. 1994. Structural remodeling in hypertensive heart disease and the role of hormones. Hypertension 23:869–877.
38. Dahlof B, Pennert K, Hansson L. 1992. Reversal of left ventricular hypertrophy in hypertensive patients. Am J Hypertens 5:95–110.
39. Sakata Y, Masuyama T, Yamamoto K, Doi R, Mano T, Kuzuya T, Miwa T, Takeda H, Hori M. 2000. Renin angiotensin system-dependent hypertrophy as a contributor to heart failure in hypertensive rats: different characteristics from renin angiotensin system-independent hypertrophy. J Am Coll Cardiol (in press).
40. Sakai S, Miyauchi T, Kobayashi M, Yamaguchi I, Goto K, Sugishita Y. 1996. Inhibition of myocardial endothelin pathway improves long-term survival in heart failure. Nature 384:353–355.
41. Mulder P, Richard V, Derumeaux G, Hogie M, Henry JP, Lallemand F, Compagnon P, Mace B, Comoy E, Letac B, Thuillez C. 1997. Role of endogenous endothelin in chronic heart failure: effect of long-term treatment with an endothelin antagonist on survival, hemodynamics, and cardiac remodeling. Circulation 96:1976–1982.

N. Takeda, M. Nagano and N.S. Dhalla
(eds). The Hypertrophied Heart. Copyright
© 2000. pp. 453–461. Kluwer Academic
Publishers. Boston. All rights reserved.

EFFECTS OF MELATONIN ON CARDIAC FUNCTION AND METABOLISM IN THE ISCHEMIC WORKING RAT HEART

KENICHI MASUI, TAKESHI OGUCHI, SATOSHI KASHIMOTO,
TOSHIAKI YAMAGUCHI, and TERUO KUMAZAWA

Department of Anesthesiology, Yamanashi Medical University, Shimokato 1110, Tamaho-cho, Nakakoma-gun,

Yamanashi, 409-3898, Japan

Summary. We investigated the effects of melatonin on function and metabolism in reperfused working rat hearts. Thirty-six hearts were rapidly excised and perfused with modified Krebs–Henseleit biocarbonate buffer. Whole-heart ischemia was induced for 15 minutes followed by reperfusion for 20 minutes. Melatonin in three different concentrations (0.2, 1.0, and 5.0 μg/mL) was administered from the preischemic period until the end of reperfusion. At the end of reperfusion, myocardial metabolites were measured by enzymatic methods. There were no significant differences in cardiac output, left ventricular dP/dt maximum, heart rate, and coronary flow among the groups. In addition, there were also no significant differences in myocardial ATP, lactate, and glycogen. These results suggest that even the highest dose of melatonin has no significant direct effects on function and metabolism in the isolated ischemic heart. If melatonin has the ability to protect myocardium, an indirect process is indicated. Moreover, there is a possibility that the antiarrhythmic actions of melatonin are subject to its antioxidant activity.

INTRODUCTION

Melatonin, N-acetyl-5-methoxytryptamine, is a very old molecule phylogenetically—a hormone metabolite of serotonin derived from the pineal gland. Axelrod [1] showed that melatonin influences the circadian cycle and is secreted throughout the night (its plasma concentration is approximately 50 pg/mL in humans) but not in the daytime [2].

It has been reported that nocturnal secretion of melatonin was impaired in patients with ischemic heart disease [3,4]. However, the effects of melatonin on the ischemic heart have not been well elucidated. Recently, Hardland et al. [5] demonstrated that melatonin had an antioxidant property. Reperfusion injury has been shown to be associated with oxygen free radicals [6]. Therefore, it could be hypothesized that the presence of melatonin brings about a protective property against coronary heart disease. The study described in this chapter was designed to investigate the effects of melatonin on function and metabolism in the reperfused ischemic working rat heart preparation.

MATERIALS AND METHODS

The experiments were approved by the Animal Ethical Committee of the Yamanashi Medical University. Isolation and preparation of hearts as used for this study have been detailed in an earlier study [7]. Thirty-six male Wistar rats weighing 300–330 g were used. In a plastic case, the animals were anesthetized with sevoflurane. The hearts were rapidly excised and perfused according to the Langendorff procedure. Nonrecirculating modified Krebs–Henseleit biocarbonate buffer (KHB) was used as preperfusate. The perfusate was maintained at $37 \pm 0.3°C$ and contained (mM): NaCl 118, KCl 4.7, $CaCl_2$ 2.0, $MgSO_4$ 1.2, KH_2PO_4 1.2, $NaHCO_3$ 25, di-NaEDTA 0.5, and Glucose 11. The solution was equilibrated with a gas mixture of 95% O_2 and 5% CO_2. During the retrograde perfusion, the left atrium was connected via a pulmonary vein to an angled steel cannula. After this preliminary perfusion, the heart was converted to a working heart preparation for a stabilization period. Nonrecirculating KHB was also used in the working heart systems.

Left ventricular pressure was measured with a transducer (P10EZ, Gould, Oxnard, CA, USA) connected to a thin catheter (18G, Argyle Intramedicut Catheter, Sherwood, Tokyo, Japan) inserted into the left ventricle from the angled steel cannula in the left atrium. Rates of tension development (dP/dt) were measured from the derivatives of left ventricular pressure obtained electronically. Aortic outflow was recorded with an electromagnetic blood flow meter (MFV-3200, Nihonkohden, Tokyo, Japan). Coronary flow was measured by timed collection of the pulmonary artery outflow and surface runoff of the heart. Cardiac output was considered as the sum of the aortic and coronary outflows. At no time was the coronary effluent recirculated.

For measurement of oxygen tension of coronary effluent, a catheter was placed in the pulmonary artery. The oxygen tension was measured in an intermittently self-calibrating blood gas analyzer system (Instrumentation Laboratory Model 1306, Lexington, MA, USA). Myocardial oxygen consumption, MVO_2 ($\mu moles \cdot min^{-1} \cdot gram^{-1}$), was calculated as O_2 solubility multiplied by coronary flow per gram of heart tissue multiplied by the difference between inflow O_2 and outflow O_2 tensions. Oxygen delivery (DO_2) was calculated from the inflow O_2 tension multiplied by O_2 solubility multiplied by coronary flow per gram of heart tissue.

Hearts prepared for this study were randomly assigned to one of four groups as follows (each group: $n = 9$): Control (C) group, which received no melatonin during perfusion; Low concentration (L) group, in which melatonin concentration in the perfusate was $0.2 \mu g \cdot mL^{-1}$; Middle concentration (M) group, in which melatonin concentration in perfusate was $1.0 \mu g \cdot mL^{-1}$; and High concentration (H) group, in which melatonin concentration in perfusate was $5.0 \mu g \cdot mL^{-1}$. Melatonin was obtained from Sigma Aldrich Chem. co. (WI, USA). Melatonin was dissolved in methyl alcohol and diluted in KHB (final concentration: methyl alcohol $100 \mu g \cdot mL^{-1}$). After an initial stabilization period (10 minutes), the heart was exposed for 10 minutes to the perfusate with vehicle (C group) or with each concentration of melatonin (L, M, and H groups) under aerobic condition for 10 minutes. Afterward, whole-heart ischemia was induced by clamping the one-way aortic valve bypass for 15 minutes [8]. Only during the ischemic period was the heart paced at 333 beats·min^{-1}. Reperfusion of the heart after this ischemic period of 15 minutes was performed by declamping the one-way aortic valve bypass tube, for 20 minutes. The administration of melatonin lasted until the end of reperfusion.

The heart was quickly frozen in liquid nitrogen at the end of reperfusion and was freeze-dried for 6 days. An aliquot was extracted with perchloric acid and centrifuged at 3000 rpm. Concentrations of adenosine triphosphate (ATP) and lactate were measured spectrophotometrically by enzymatic techniques [9]. We determined the decrease in absorbance at 340 nm that resulted when NADH was oxidized to NAD by ATP and two enzymes (phosphoglycerate phosphokinase and glyceraldehyde phosphate dehydrogenase), and we obtained a measure of the amount of ATP originally presented. To measure lactate, we determined the increase in absorbance at 340 nm due to NADH formation from NAD, lactate, and lactate dehydrogenase. Another piece of freeze-dried sample was placed in 30% potassium hydroxide and digested at 100°C. Tissue glycogen was extracted, hydrolyzed, and assayed as glucose equivalents in neutralized, potassium-hydrated extracts [10]. The values were expressed as μmol per gram dry heart weight.

The data are expressed as means ± SD. Testing for significant differences among the different groups was accomplished by one-way ANOVA, followed by Duncan's multiple range test. Intragroup comparisons were performed by two-way ANOVA for repeated measures, followed by paired t-tests with the Bonferroni correction. The duration of ventricular fibrillation was analyzed by the Kruskal–Wallis test. A probability of $p < 0.05$ was regarded as statistically significant.

RESULTS

During the entire experimental period, there were no significant differences in cardiac output, left ventricular dP/dt maximum, heart rate, and coronary flow among the groups (figures 1–4). Figure 5 shows the relationship between DO_2 and MVO_2. Melatonin did not affect myocardial oxygen balance all the time. There were also no significant differences in myocardial ATP, lactate, glycogen, and pyruvate (table 1). The duration of ventricular fibrillation during reperfusion was 559 seconds, 612 seconds, 449 seconds, and 288 seconds in the C, L, M, and H groups, respectively. Ventricular fibrillation did not last in any heart of the H group until the end of reperfusion (figure 6). However, this reductive effect on the duration of ventricular fibrillation was not statistically significant ($p = 0.08$).

DISCUSSION

Recent investigations [3,4] revealed that nocturnal secretion of melatonin was impaired in patients with coronary heart disease. These facts suggest the possibility that melatonin has some protective properties against the ischemic heart. Therefore,

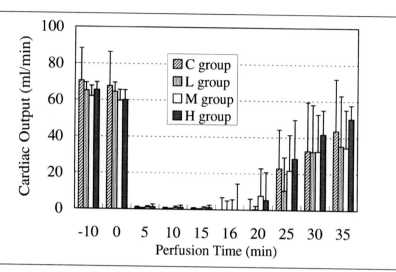

Figure 1. Changes in cardiac output of the C, L, M, and H groups as a function of time. The *x*-axis represents perfusion time in minutes. At zero time, ischemia was induced by the one-way aortic valve procedure. Perfusion as an ischemic heart was continued for 15 minutes followed by reperfusion for 20 minutes. Each point represents mean ± S.D. for the nine hearts.

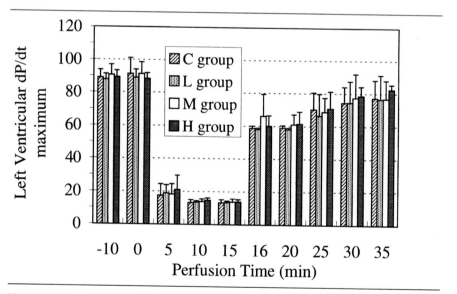

Figure 2. Changes in left ventricular *dP*/*d*t maximum of the C, L, M, and H groups as a function of time. See figure 1 for explanations.

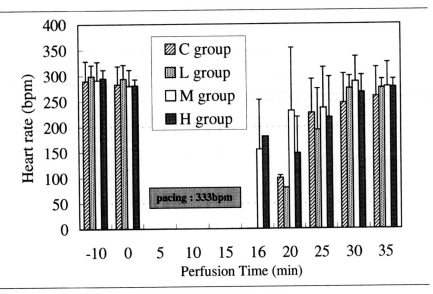

Figure 3. Changes in heart rate of the C, L, M, and H groups as a function of time. See figure 1 for explanations.

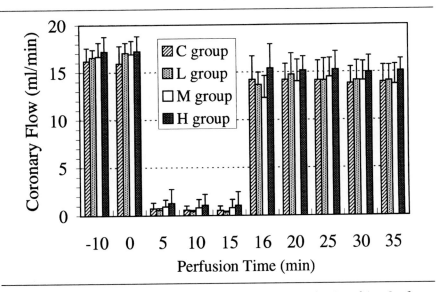

Figure 4. Changes in coronary flow of the C, L, M, and H groups as a function of time. See figure 1 for explanations.

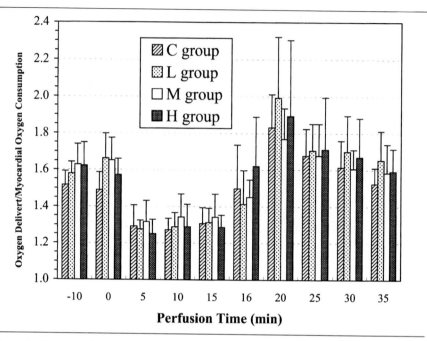

Figure 5. Changes in the oxygen delivery (DO$_2$) to myocardial oxygen consumption (MVO$_2$) ratio of the C, L, M, and H groups as a function of time. See figure 1 for explanations.

Table 1. Myocardial metabolites (μmol/g.d.)

Group	ATP	Lactate	Pyruvate	Glycogen
C	10.3 ± 0.5	33.0 ± 3.4	0.44 ± 0.11	27.5 ± 3.6
L	9.4 ± 1.2	32.1 ± 5.0	0.58 ± 0.29	30.9 ± 7.1
M	9.4 ± 1.5	33.7 ± 2.5	0.43 ± 0.12	32.5 ± 10.5
H	9.6 ± 0.5	33.2 ± 4.1	0.50 ± 0.14	34.0 ± 6.8

we examined the direct effects of melatonin on the ischemic reperfused heart. In the present study, we could not show any beneficial effects on functional and metabolic recovery during reperfusion. However, the duration of ventricular fibrillation during reperfusion tended to decrease in the melatonin-treated groups, though this effect was not statistically significant due to the limited number of hearts in each group. Reperfusion-induced arrhythmia was associated with the high energy demand in the ventricular portion during hypoxemia, while mediated by O$_2$-derived free radicals in the endothelial part [6,11]. Woodward et al. [12] reported that superoxide dismutase, which is a free radical scavenger, reduced reperfusion-induced arrhythmias. Hardeland et al. [5] have shown that melatonin had an antioxidant property. Therefore, the antiarrhythmic actions of melatonin may be related to its

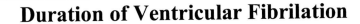

Duration of Ventricular Fibrilation

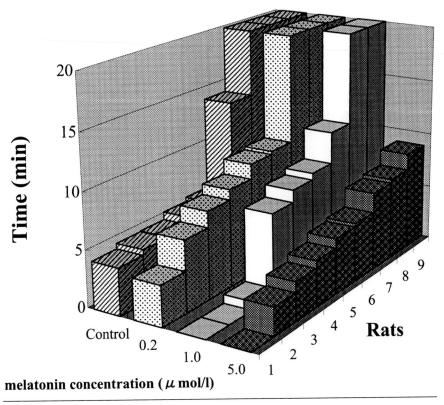

Figure 6. Durations of ventricular fibrillation during reperfusion period of the nine hearts in the C, L, M, and H groups.

antioxidant activity [13–15]. The cellular mechanisms of melatonin remain to be examined to elucidate the antidysrhythmic effect.

Our results show that melatonin had no significant effect on coronary flow during the entire time. Moreover, melatonin also exerted no influence on myocardial oxygen demand relative to oxygen supply during the aerobic, ischemic, and reperfused periods. These observations differ from those of Weekley et al. [16], who reported that melatonin caused a dose-dependent contraction of coronary arteries isolated from normal pigs. They also showed that melatonin had no effect on the contration of the coronary artery in the presence of the α-adrenergic antagonist prazocin, and caused a dose-dependent relaxation in 6-hydroxydopamine-treated vessels (this treatment destroyed sympathetic nerve terminals in the vascular wall [17]). Because we used not isolated coronary vessels but isolated hearts, some chemical mediator around coronary blood vessels might account for the difference between the present study and their studies.

There are still some possibilities that melatonin has protective effects via indirect mechanisms. Melatonin decreases brain serotonin secretion and causes sympathetic inhibition or parasympathetic stimulation, which leads to hypotention and brady-cardia in rats [18]. Moreover, melatonin decreases norepinephrine and epinephrine contents in the adrenal grand of three avian species [19]. Because sympathetic inhibition leads to heart rate decrease or ventricular afterload reduction, melatonin may reduce the occurrence of myocardial ischemia. Our in vitro study did not show any significant beneficial effects on ischemic hearts. Accordingly, further investigations are necessary to reveal the role of melatonin in patients with ischemic heart disease.

In conclusion, melatonin had no beneficial effect on function and metabolism in the reperfused ischemic rat heart. Indirect actions of melatonin on ischemic heart should be investigated in vivo to determine whether melatonin has a protective property against coronary heart disease. Although we employed high doses of melatonin as compared with the physical condition, melatonin had no deleterious effects during ischemia and postischemic reperfusion.

ACKNOWLEDGMENTS

We thank Mr. Koshimizu and Miss Amemiya for their valuable technical assistance.

REFERENCES

1. Axelrod J. 1974. The pineal gland: a neuroendocrine transducer. Science 184:1341–1348.
2. Vaughan GM, Bell R, De La Pana A. 1979. Nocturnal plasma melatonin in humans: episodic pattern and influence of light. Neurosci Lett 14:81–84.
3. Brugger P, Marktl W, Herold M. 1995. Impaired nocturnal secretion of melatonin in coronary heart disease. Lancet 345:1408.
4. Fiorina P, Lattuada G, Ponari O, Silvestrini C, DallAglio P. 1996. Impaired nocturnal melatonin excretion and changes of immunological status in ischaemic stroke patients. Lancet 347:692–693.
5. Hardeland R, Reiter RJ, Poeggeler B, Tan DX. 1993. The significance of the metabolism of the neurohormone melatonin: antioxidative protection and formation of bioactive substances. Neurosci Biobehav Rev 17:347–357.
6. Samaja M, Motterlini R, Santoro F, Dell Antonio G, Corno A. 1994. Oxidative injury in reoxygenated and reperfused hearts. Free Rad Biol Med 16:255–262.
7. Oguchi T, Kashimoto S, Yamaguchi T, Nakamura T, Kumazawa T. 1995. Comparative effects of halothane, enflurane, isoflurane and sevoflurane on function and metabolism in the ischaemic rat heart. Br J Anaesth 74:569–575.
8. Neely JR, Rovetto MJ, Whitner JT, Morgan HE. 1973. Effects of ischemia on function and metabolism of the isolated working rat heart. Am J Physiol 225:651–658.
9. Bergmeyer HU. 1975. Neue Werte Für die molaren Extinktions-Koeffizienten von NADH und NADPH zum Gebrauch im Routine-Laboratorium. Zeit Klin Chemie Klin Biochem 13:507–508.
10. Werner W, Rey HG, Wielinger H. 1970. Über die Eigenschaften eines neuen Chromogens für die Blutzuckerbestimmung nach der GOD/POD-Methode. Zeit Anal Chem 252:224–228.
11. Yamakawa T, Kadowaki Y, Garcia-Alves M, Yokoyama M, Iwashita Y, Nishi K. 1989. Effects of polyoxyethylene-modified superoxide dismutase on reperfusion induced arrhythmias in isolated rat and guinea-pig hearts. J Mol cell Cardiol 21:441–452.
12. Woodward B, Zakaria MNM. 1985. Effects of some free radical scavengers on reperfusion induced arrythmias in the isolated rat heart. J Mol Cell Cardiol 17:485–493.
13. Pieri C, Marra M, Moroni F, Recchioni R, Marcheselli F. 1994. Melatonin: a peroxyl radical scavenger more effective than vitamine E. Life Sci 55:271–276.

14. Reiter RJ, Tan DX, Poeggeler B, Menendez-Pelaez A, Chen LD, Saarela S. 1994. Melatonin as a free radical scavenger: implications for aging and age-related diseases. Ann NY Acad Sci 719:1–12.
15. Pierrefiche G, Topall G, Courboin G, Henriet I, Laborit H. 1993. Antioxidant activity of melatonin in mice. Res Commun Chem Pathol Pharmacol 80:211–223.
16. Weekley LB. 1993. Effects of melatonin on pulmonary and coronary vessels are exerted through perivascular nerves. Clin Autonom Res 3:45–47.
17. Aprigliano O, Hermsmeyer K. 1976. In vitro denervation of the portal vein and caudal artery of the rat. J Pharmacol Exp Ther 198:568–577.
18. Chuang JI, Chen SS, Lin MT. 1993. Melatonin decreases brain serotonin release, arterial pressure and heart heart rate in rats. Pharmacology 47:91–97.
19. Mahata SK, De K. 1991. Effect of melatonin on norepinephrine, epinephrine, and corticosterone contents in the adrenal gland of three avian species. J Comp Physiol B 161:81–84.

INDEX